NUR
POC
DRU
200

C000077723

EDITOR

Judith A. Barberio, PhD, APRN, BC-ANP, GNP, FNP

Assistant Professor
Rutgers, The State University of New Jersey
College of Nursing
Newark, New Jersey

CONSULTING EDITOR

Leonard G. Gomella, MD, FACS

The Bernard W. Godwin, Jr., Professor
Chairman, Department of Urology
Jefferson Medical College
Thomas Jefferson University
Philadelphia, Pennsylvania

McGraw-Hill
MEDICAL PUBLISHING DIVISION

New York Chicago San Francisco Lisbon London Madrid Mexico City Milan
New Delhi San Juan Seoul Singapore Sydney Toronto

Nurse's Pocket Drug Guide 2006

1 2 3 4 5 6 7 8 9 0   WBCWBC   0 9 8 7 6 5 4

ISBN: 0-07-145731-3
ISSN: 1550-2554

Notice

Medicine is an ever-changing science. As new research and clinical experience broaden our knowledge, changes in treatment and drug therapy are required. The authors and the publisher of this work have checked with sources believed to be reliable in their efforts to provide information that is complete and generally in accord with the standards accepted at the time of publication. However, in view of the possibility of human error or changes in medical sciences, neither the authors nor the publisher nor any other party who has been involved in the preparation or publication of this work warrants that the information contained herein is in every respect accurate or complete, and they disclaim all responsibility for any errors or omissions or for the results obtained from use of the information contained in this work. Readers are encouraged to confirm the information contained herein with other sources. For example and in particular, readers are advised to check the product information sheet included in the package of each drug they plan to administer to be certain that the information contained in this work is accurate and that changes have not been made in the recommended dose or in the contraindications for administration. This recommendation is of particular importance in connection with new or infrequently used drugs.

This book was set in Times Roman by Pine Tree Composition, Inc.
The editors were Janet Foltin and Harriet Lebowitz.
The production supervisor was Sherri Souffrance.
Project management was provided by Pine Tree Composition, Inc.
The cover designer was Mary McKeon.
The text designer was Marsha Cohen/Parallelogram Graphics.
The index was prepared by Ann Salinger
Webcom Limited was printer and binder.

This book is printed on acid-free paper.

CONTENTS

ASSOCIATE EDITORS v
PREFACE vii
MEDICATION KEY ix
ABBREVIATIONS xiii
CLASSIFICATION 1
    Allergy 1
    Antidotes 1
    Antimicrobial Agents 1
    Miscellaneous Antibacterial Agents 3
    Antineoplastic Agents 4
    Cardiovascular Agents 6
    Central Nervous System Agents 8
    Dermatologic Agents 9
    Dietary Supplements 10
    Ear (Otic) Agents 11
    Endocrine System Agents 11
    Eye (Ophthalmic) Agents 12
    Gastrointestinal Agents 13
    Hematologic Agents 15
    Immune System Agents 16
    Musculoskeletal Agents 16
    OB/GYN Agents 17
    Pain Medications 18
    Respiratory Agents 19
    Urinary/Genitourinary Agents 21
    Wound Care 21
    Miscellaneous Therapeutic Agents 21
GENERIC DRUG DATA 23
COMMONLY USED MEDICINAL HERBS 255
TABLES 262
INDEX 285

ASSOCIATE EDITORS

PREFACE

On behalf of the entire editorial board, we are pleased to present the second edition of the *Nurse's Pocket Drug Guide*. This book is based on the basic drug presentation style used since 1983 in the *Clinician's Pocket Reference*.

Our goal is to identify the most frequently used and clinically important medications and herbs based on input from our readers and editorial board. The book includes over 1000 generic medications and herbs and is designed to represent a cross section of those used in health care practices across the country.

The style of drug presentation includes key "must know" facts of commonly used medications and herbs, which represents the essential information for both the student and practicing nurse, and health care provider. A unique feature is the inclusion of common uses of medications and herbs rather than just the official labeled indications. These recommendations are based on the actual uses of the medication and herbs supported by publications and community standards of care. All uses have been reviewed by our editorial board. New in this edition is the inclusion of antimicrobial spectrum for the majority of antibiotics, useful for accurate prescribing practices.

It is essential that students, registered nurses, and advanced-practice nurses learn more than the name and dose of the medications they prescribe and administer. Certain common side effects and significant contraindications are associated with most prescription medications. Although nurses and other health care practitioners should ideally be completely familiar with the entire package insert of any medication prescribed, such a requirement is unreasonable. References such as the *Physician's Desk Reference* and in many cases the drug manufacturer's Web site make package inserts readily available for many medications, but may not provide key data for generic drugs and those available over the counter. The limitations of difficult-to-read package inserts were acknowledged by the Food and Drug Administration in early 2001, when it noted that health care providers do not have time to read the many pages of small print in the typical package insert. In the future, package inserts will likely be redesigned to ensure that important drug interactions, contraindications, and common side effects are highlighted for easier practitioner reference. We have made this key prescribing information available to you now in this pocket-sized book. Information in this book is meant for use by health care professionals who are familiar with these commonly prescribed medications.

We are pleased about the popularity of the first edition. The previous edition has been completely reviewed and updated by our editorial board. Over three dozen key new medications and thirty herbs have been added, with changes in indications and available forms of other drugs updated based on new FDA approvals.

We express special thanks to our families for their support of this book and the entire project. The contributions of the members of the editorial board are deeply appreciated. Janet Foltin, Linda Davoli, and the team at McGraw-Hill have been supportive in our goal of creating a pocket reference for nursing professionals.

Your comments and suggestions are always welcome and encouraged because improvements to this book would be impossible without the interest and feedback of our readers. We hope this book will help you learn some of the key elements in prescribing medications and allow you to care for your patients in the best way possible.

Judith A. Barberio, PhD, APRN, BC-ANP, GNP, FNP

Newark, NJ

JABPHD83@aol.com

Leonard G. Gomella, MD, FACS

Philadelphia, PA

Leonard.Gomella@jefferson.edu

MEDICATION KEY

Medications are listed by prescribing class, and the individual medications are then listed in alphabetical order by generic name. Some of the more commonly recognized trade names are listed for each medication (in parentheses after the generic name).

Generic Drug Name (Selected Common Brand Names [Controlled Substance]) WARNING: Summary of the "Black Box" precautions that are deemed necessary by the FDA. These are significant precautions and contraindications concerning the individual medication. **Uses:** This includes both FDA labeled indications bracketed by * and other "off label" uses of the medication. Because many medications are used to treat various conditions based on the medical literature and not listed in their package insert, we list common uses of the medication rather than the official "labeled indications" (FDA approved) based on input from our editorial board **Action:** How the drug works. This information is helpful in comparing classes of drugs and understanding side effects and contraindications. *Spectrum:* Included for most antibiotics **Dose:** *Adults.* Where no specific pediatric dose is given, the implication is that this drug is not commonly used or indicated in that age group. At the end of the dosing line, important dosing modifications may be noted (ie, take with food, avoid antacids, etc) **Caution:** [pregnancy/fetal risk categories, breast-feeding] cautions concerning the use of the drug in specific settings **Contra:** Contraindications **Supplied:** Common dosing forms **SE:** Common or significant side effects **Notes:** Other key information about the drug. **Interactions:** Common drug—drug, drug—herb, and drug—food interactions that may change the drug response **Labs:** Common laboratory test results that are changed by the drug or significant lab monitoring requirements **NIPE:** Nursing Indications and/or Patient Education) Significant information that the nurse must be aware of with administration of the drug or information that should be given to any patient taking the drug.

CONTROLLED SUBSTANCE CLASSIFICATION

Medications under the control of the US Drug Enforcement Agency (Schedule I–V controlled substances) are indicated by the symbol [C]. Most medications are "uncontrolled" and do not require a DEA prescriber number on the prescription. The following is a general description for the schedules of DEA controlled substances:

Schedule (C-I) I: All nonresearch use forbidden (eg, heroin, LSD, mescaline, etc).

Schedule (C-II) II: High addictive potential; medical use accepted. No telephone call-in prescriptions; no refills. Some states require special prescription form (eg, cocaine, morphine, methadone).

Schedule (C-III) III: Low to moderate risk of physical dependence, high risk of psychologic dependence; prescription must be rewritten after 6 months or five refills (eg, acetaminophen plus codeine).

Schedule (C-IV) IV: Limited potential for dependence; prescription rules same as for schedule III (eg, benzodiazepines, propoxyphene).

Schedule (C-V) V: Very limited abuse potential; prescribing regulations often same as for uncontrolled medications; some states have additional restrictions.

FDA FETAL RISK CATEGORIES

Category A: Adequate studies in pregnant women have not demonstrated a risk to the fetus in the first trimester of pregnancy; there is no evidence of risk in the last two trimesters.

Category B: Animal studies have not demonstrated a risk to the fetus, but no adequate studies have been done in pregnant women.

or

Animal studies have shown an adverse effect, but adequate studies in pregnant women have not demonstrated a risk to the fetus during the first trimester of pregnancy and there is no evidence of risk in the last two trimesters.

Category C: Animal studies have shown an adverse effect on the fetus, but no adequate studies have been done in humans. The benefits from the use of the drug in pregnant women may be acceptable despite its potential risks.

or

No animal reproduction studies and no adequate studies in humans have been done.

Category D: There is evidence of human fetal risk, but the potential benefits from the use of the drug in pregnant women may be acceptable despite its potential risks.

Category X: Studies in animals or humans or adverse reaction reports, or both, have demonstrated fetal abnormalities. The risk of use in pregnant women clearly outweighs any possible benefit.

Category ?: No data available (not a formal FDA classification; included to provide complete data set).

BREAST-FEEDING

No formally recognized classification exists for drugs and breast-feeding. This shorthand was developed for the *Clinician's Pocket Drug Reference*.

+	Compatible with breast-feeding
M	Monitor patient or use with caution
+/–	Excreted, or likely excreted, with unknown effects or at unknown concentrations
?/–	Unknown excretion, but effects likely to be of concern
–	Contraindicated in breast-feeding
?	No data available

ABBREVIATIONS

ac: before meals (*ante cibum*)
ABMT: autologous bone marrow transplantation
ACE: angiotensin-converting enzyme
ACEI: angiotensin-converting enzyme inhibitor
ACLS: advanced cardiac life support
ACS: acute coronary syndrome
ADH: antidiuretic hormone
ADHD: attention-deficit hyperactivity disorder
AF: atrial fibrillation
Al: aluminum
ALL: acute lymphocytic leukemia
ALT: alanine aminotransferase
AMI: acute myocardial infarction
AML: acute myelogenous leukemia
amp: ampule
ANC: absolute neutrophil count
aPTT: activated partial thromboplastin time
APAP: acetaminophen [*N*-acetyl-*p*-aminophenol]
ARB: angiotensin II receptor blocker
ARDS: adult respiratory distress syndrome
ASA: aspirin (acetylsalicylic acid)
AUC: area under the curve
AV: atrioventricular
AVM: arteriovenous malformation
BB: beta-blocker
BCL: B-cell lymphoma

BMT: bone marrow transplantation
BSA: body surface area
BUN: blood urea nitrogen
Ca: calcium
CA: cancer
CAD: coronary artery disease
cap: capsule
CAP: cancer of prostate
CBC: complete blood count
CCB: calcium channel blocker
CF: cystic fibrosis
CHF: congestive heart failure
CLL: chronic lymphocytic leukemia
CML: chronic myelogenous leukemia
CMV: cytomegalovirus
CNS: central nervous system
Contra: contraindicated
COPD: chronic obstructive pulmonary disease
CP: chest pain
CPP: central precocious puberty
CR: controlled release
CrCl: creatinine clearance
CRF: chronic renal failure
CV: cardiovascular
CVA: cerebrovascular accident
CVH: common variable hypergammaglobulinemia
D_5LR: 5% dextrose in lactated Ringer's solution
D_5NS: 5% dextrose in normal saline
D_5W: 5% dextrose in water

xiii

DC: discontinue
DI: diabetes insipidus
DKA: diabetic ketoacidosis
dL: deciliter
DN: diabetic nephropathy
DVT: deep venous thrombosis
Dz: disease
EC: enteric-coated
ECC: emergency cardiac care
ECG: electrocardiogram
ELISA: enzyme-linked immunosor-
bent assay
EPS: extrapyramidal symptoms
ESRD: end-stage renal disease
ET: endotracheal
EtOH: ethanol
ext: extract
Fe: iron
FSH: follicle-stimulating hormone
5-FU: fluorouracil
Fxn: function
g: gram
GABA: gamma-aminobutyric acid
G-CSF: granulocyte colony-stimulat-
ing factor
GERD: gastroesophageal reflux dis-
ease
GFR: glomerular filtration rate
GH: growth hormone
GI: gastrointestinal
GIST: gastrointestinal stromal tumor
GM-CSF: granulocyte-macrophage
colony-stimulating factor
GnRH: gonadotropin-releasing hor-
mone
gt, gtt: drop, drops (*gutta*)
HA: headache
HCL: hairy cell leukemia
Hct: hematocrit
HCTZ: hydrochlorothiazide
HF: heart failure
Hgb: hemoglobin

HIT: heparin-induced thrombocy-
topenia
HIV: human immunodeficiency virus
HMG-CoA: hydroxymethylglutaryl
coenzyme A
hs: at bedtime (*hora somni*)
HSV: herpes simplex virus
5-HT: 5-hydroxytryptamine
HTN: hypertension
Hx: history
I: iodine
IBD: irritable bowel disease
IBS: irritable bowel syndrome
ICP: intracranial pressure
Ig: immunoglobulin
IM: intramuscular
inf: infusion
INH: isoniazid
inj: injection
INR: international normalized ratio
I&O: intake and output
ISA: intrinsic sympathomimetic ac-
tivity
IT: intrathecal
ITP: idiopathic thrombocytopenic
purpura
IV: intravenous
K: potassium
L/d: liters per day
LDL: low-density lipoprotein
LFT: liver function test
LH: luteinizing hormone
LHRH: luteinizing hormone-releas-
ing hormone
Li: lithium
liq: liquid
LMW: low molecular weight
LVD: left ventricular dysfunction
LVEF: left ventricular ejection frac-
tion
MAC: *Mycobacterium avium* com-
plex

MAO/MAOI: monoamine oxidase/inhibitor

mEq: milliequivalent

Mg: magnesium

MI: myocardial infarction, mitral insufficiency

mL: milliliter

MRSA: methicillin-resistant *Staphylococcus aureus*

MS: multiple sclerosis

MSSA: methicillin-sensitive *Staphylococcus aureus*

MTT: monotetrazolium

MTX: methotrexate

MyG: myasthenia gravis

Na: sodium

ng: nanogram

NG: nasogastric

NHL: non-Hodgkin's lymphoma

NIDDM: non-insulin-dependent diabetes mellitus

NPO: nothing by mouth (*nil per os*)

NS: normal saline

NSAID: nonsteroidal antiinflammatory drug

N/V: nausea and vomiting

N/V/D: nausea, vomiting, diarrhea

OCP: oral contraceptive pill

OD: overdose

OTC: over the counter

P: phosphorus

PAT: paroxysmal atrial tachycardia

pc: after eating (*post cibum*)

PCP: *Pneumocystis jiroveci* pneumonia

PCWP: pulmonary capillary wedge pressure

PDGF: platelet-derived growth factor

PE: pulmonary embolus, physical examination, pleural effusion

PFT: pulmonary function test

pg: picogram

PID: pelvic inflammatory disease

plt: platelet

PMDD: premenstrual dysphoric disorder

PO: by mouth (*per os*)

PPD: purified protein derivative

PR: by rectum

prep: preparation

PRG: pregnancy

PRN: as often as needed (*pro re nata*)

PSA: prostate-specific antigen

PSVT: paroxysmal supraventricular tachycardia

Pt: patient

PT: prothrombin time

PTCA: percutaneous transluminal coronary angioplasty

PTH: parathyroid hormone

PTT: partial thromboplastin time

PUD: peptic ulcer disease

PVC: premature ventricular contraction

PVD: peripheral vascular disease

PWP: pulmonary wedge pressure

q: every (*quaque*)

q_h: every _ hours

qd: every day

qh: every hour

qhs: every hour of sleep (before bedtime)

qid: four times a day (*quater in die*)

qod: every other day

RA: rheumatoid arthritis

RCC: renal cell carcinoma

RDA: recommended dietary allowance

RDS: respiratory distress syndrome

RSV: respiratory syncytial virus

RT: reverse transcriptase

RTA: renal tubular acidosis

Rx: treatment

Rxn: reaction

SCr: serum creatinine
SIADH: syndrome of inappropriate
  antidiuretic hormone
SL: sublingual
SLE: systemic lupus erythematosus
SPAG: small particle aerosol genera-
  tor
SQ: subcutaneous
SSRI: selective serotonin reuptake in-
  hibitor
SSS: sick sinus syndrome
S/Sxs: signs and symptoms
stat: immediately (*statim*)
suppl: supplement
supp: suppository
SVT: supraventricular tachycardia
Sx: symptom
Sz: seizure
tab/tabs: tablet/tablets
TB: tuberculosis
TCA: tricyclic antidepressant
TFT: thyroid function test
TIA: transient ischemic attack
tid: three times a day (*ter in die*)
tinc: tincture
TMP: trimethoprim

TMP–SMX: trimethoprim–sul-
  famethoxazole
TPA: tissue plasminogen activator
tri: trimester
tsp: teaspoon
TTP: thrombotic thrombocytopenic
  purpura
ULN: upper limits of normal
URI: upper respiratory infection
UTI: urinary tract infection
VF: ventricular fibrillation
VT: ventricular tachycardia
w/: with
WHI: Women's Health Initiative
w/in: within
wk: week
WNL: within normal limits
w/o: without
WPW: Wolff–Parkinson–White syndrome
wt: weight
ZE: Zollinger–Ellison (syndrome)
<: less than, younger than
>: greater than, older than
↑: increase
↓: decrease
⊘: not recommended, do not take

CLASSIFICATION (Generic and common brand names)

ALLERGY

Antihistamines

Azelastine (Astelin, Optivar)
Cetirizine (Zyrtec)
Chlorpheniramine (Chlor-Trimeton)
Clemastine Fumarate (Tavist)

Cyproheptadine (Periactin)
Desloratadine (Clarinex)
Diphenhydramine (Benadryl)

Fexofenadine (Allegra)
Hydroxyzine (Atarax, Vistaril)
Loratadine (Claritin, Alavert)

Miscellaneous Antiallergenic Agents

Budesonide (Rhinocort, Pulmicort)

Cromolyn Sodium (Intal, NasalCrom, Opticrom)

Montelukast (Singulair)

ANTIDOTES

Acetylcysteine (Mucomyst)
Amifostine (Ethyol)
Charcoal (Superc
Actidose, Liqui-Char
Activated)

Dexrazoxane (Zinecard)
Digoxin Immune Fab (Digibind)
Flumazenil (Romazicon)
Ipecac Syrup (OTC Syrup)

Mesna (Mesnex)
Naloxone (Narcan)
Physostigmine (Antilirium)
Succimer (Chemet)

ANTIMICROBIAL AGENTS

Antibiotics

AMINOGLYCOSIDES
Amikacin (Amikin)
Gentamicin (Garamycin, G-Mycitin)

Neomycin
Streptomycin

Tobramycin (Nebcin)

CARBAPENEMS
Ertapenem (Invanz)

Imipenem–Cilastatin (Primaxin)

Meropenem (Merrem)

CEPHALOSPORINS, FIRST GENERATION

Cefadroxil (Duricef, Ultracef)

Cefazolin (Ancef, Kefzol)

Cephalexin (Keflex, Keftab)

Cephradine (Velosef)

CEPHALOSPORINS, SECOND GENERATION

Cefaclor (Ceclor)

Cefmetazole (Zefazone)

Cefonicid (Monocid)

Cefotetan (Cefotan)

Cefoxitin (Mefoxin)

Cefprozil (Cefzil)

Cefuroxime (Ceftin [oral], Zinacef [parenteral])

Loracarbef (Lorabid)

CEPHALOSPORINS, THIRD GENERATION

Cefdinir (Omnicef)

Cefditoren (Spectracef)

Cefixime (Suprax)

Cefoperazone (Cefobid)

Cefotaxime (Claforan)

Cefpodoxime (Vantin)

Ceftazidime (Fortaz, Cep-taz, Tazidime, Tazicef)

Ceftibuten (Cedax)

Ceftizoxime (Cefizox)

Ceftriaxone (Rocephin)

CEPHALOSPORINS, FOURTH GENERATION

Cefepime (Maxipime)

FLUOROQUINOLONES

Ciprofloxacin (Cipro)

Gatifloxacin (Tequin)

Levofloxacin (Levaquin, Quixin Ophthalmic)

Lomefloxacin (Maxaquin)

Moxifloxacin (Avelox)

Norfloxacin (Noroxin)

Ofloxacin (Floxin, Ocuflox Ophthalmic)

Sparfloxacin (Zagam)

Trovafloxacin (Trovan)

MACROLIDES

Azithromycin (Zithromax)

Clarithromycin (Biaxin)

Dirithromycin (Dynabac)

Erythromycin (E-Mycin, E.E.S., Ery-Tab)

Erythromycin and Sulfisoxazole (Eryzole, Pediazole)

KETOLIDE

Telithromycin (Ketek)

PENICILLINS

Amoxicillin (Amoxil, Polymox)

Amoxicillin and Clavu-lanic Acid (Augmentin)

Ampicillin (Amcill, Omnipen)

Ampicillin–Sulbactam (Unasyn)

Dicloxacillin (Dynapen, Dycill)

Mezlocillin (Mezlin)

Nafcillin (Nallpen)

Oxacillin (Bactocill, Prostaphlin)

Penicillin G, Aqueous (Potassium or Sodium) (Pfizerpen, Pentids)

Penicillin G Benzathine
(Bicillin)
Penicillin G Procaine
(Wycillin)

Penicillin V (Pen-Vee K,
Veetids)
Piperacillin (Pipracil)
Piperacillin–Tazobactam
(Zosyn)

Ticarcillin (Ticar)
Ticarcillin/Potassium
Clavulanate
(Timentin)

TETRACYCLINES

Doxycycline
(Vibramycin)

Tetracycline
(Achromycin V,
Sumycin)

MISCELLANEOUS ANTIBACTERIAL AGENTS

Aztreonam (Azactam)
Clindamycin (Cleocin,
Cleocin-T)
Fosfomycin (Monurol)
Linezolid (Zyvox)
Metronidazole (Flagyl,
MetroGel)

Quinupristin–Dalfo-
pristin (Synercid)
Trimethoprim–
Sulfamethoxazole
[Co-Trimoxazole]
(Bactrim, Septra)

Vancomycin (Vancocin,
Vancoled)

Antifungals

Amphotericin B
(Fungizone)
Amphotericin B Choles-
teryl (Amphotec)
Amphotericin B Lipid
Complex (Abelcet)
Amphotericin B Liposo-
mal (AmBisome)
Caspofungin (Cancidas)

Clotrimazole (Lotrimin,
Mycelex)
Clotrimazole and
Betamethasone
(Lotrisone)
Econazole (Spectazole)
Fluconazole (Diflucan)
Itraconazole (Sporanox)
Ketoconazole (Nizoral)

Miconazole (Monistat)
Nystatin (Mycostatin)
Oxiconazole (Oxistat)
Sertaconazole (Ertaczo)
Terbinafine (Lamisil)
Triamcinolone and
Nystatin (Mycolog-II)
Voriconazole (VFEND)

Antimycobacterials

Clofazimine (Lamprene)
Dapsone (Avlosulfon)
Ethambutol (Myambutol)

Isoniazid (INH)
Pyrazinamide
Rifabutin (Mycobutin)

Rifampin (Rifadin)
Rifapentine (Priftin)
Streptomycin

Antiprotozoals

Nitazoxanide (Alinia)

Antiretrovirals

Abacavir (Ziagen)
Amprenavir (Agenerase)

Delavirdine (Rescriptor)
Didanosine [ddI] (Videx)

Efavirenz (Sustiva)
Fosamprenavir (Lexiva)

Indinavir (Crixivan)
Lamivudine (Epivir, Epivir-HBV)
Lopinavir/Ritonavir (Kaletra)

Nelfinavir (Viracept)
Nevirapine (Viramune)
Ritonavir (Norvir)
Saquinavir (Fortovase)
Stavudine (Zerit)

Tenofovir (Viread)
Zalcitabine (Hivid)
Zidovudine (Retrovir)
Zidovudine and Lamivudine (Combivir)

Antivirals

Acyclovir (Zovirax)
Adefovir (Hepsera)
Amantadine (Symmetrel)
Atazanavir (Reyataz)
Cidofovir (Vistide)
Emtricitabine (Emtriva)
Enfuvirtide (Fuzeon)
Famciclovir (Famvir)

Foscarnet (Foscavir)
Ganciclovir (Cytovene, Vitrasert)
Interferon Alfa-2b and Ribavirin Combination (Rebetron)
Oseltamivir (Tamiflu)
Palivizumab (Synagis)

Peg Interferon Alfa 2a (Pegasys)
Penciclovir (Denavir)
Ribavirin (Virazole)
Rimantadine (Flumadine)
Valacyclovir (Valtrex)
Valganciclovir (Valcyte)
Zanamivir (Relenza)

Miscellaneous Antimicrobial Agents

Atovaquone (Mepron)
Atovaquone/Proguanil (Malarone)

Pentamidine (Pentam 300, NebuPent)

Trimetrexate (Neutrexin)

ANTINEOPLASTIC AGENTS

Alkylating Agents

Altretamine (Hexalen)
Busulfan (Myleran, Busulfex)

Carboplatin (Paraplatin)
Cisplatin (Platinol)
Procarbazine (Matulane)

Triethylenetriphosphamide (Thio-Tepa, Tespa, TSPA)

NITROGEN MUSTARDS

Chlorambucil (Leukeran)
Cyclophosphamide (Cytoxan, Neosar)

Ifosfamide (Ifex, Holoxan)
Mechlorethamine (Mustargen)

Melphalan [L-PAM] (Alkeran)

NITROSOUREAS

Carmustine [BCNU] (BiCNU, Gliadel)

Streptozocin (Zanosar)

Antibiotics

Bleomycin Sulfate (Blenoxane)

Dactinomycin (Cosmegen)

Daunorubicin (Daunomycin, Cerubidine)

Doxorubicin (Adriamycin, Rubex)

Epirubicin (Ellence)
Idarubicin (Idamycin)

Mitomycin (Mutamycin)

Antimetabolites

Cytarabine [ARA-C] (Cytosar-U)
Cytarabine Liposome (DepoCyt)
Floxuridine (FUDR)
Fludarabine Phosphate (Flamp, Fludara)

Fluorouracil [5-FU] (Adrucil)
Gemcitabine (Gemzar)
Mercaptopurine [6-MP] (Purinethol)
Methotrexate (MRX, Folex, Rheumatrex)

6-Thioguanine [6-TG] (Tabloid)

Hormones

Abarelix (Plenaxis)
Anastrozole (Arimidex)
Bicalutamide (Casodex)
Estramustine Phosphate (Estracyt, Emcyt)
Exemestane (Aromasin)

Fluoxymesterone (Halotestin)
Flutamide (Eulexin)
Fulvestrant (Faslodex)
Goserelin (Zoladex)
Leuprolide (Lupron, Viadur, Eligard)

Levamisole (Ergamisol)
Megestrol Acetate (Megace)
Nilutamide (Nilandron)
Tamoxifen (Nolvadex)
Triptorelin (Trelstar Depot, Trelstar LA)

Mitotic Inhibitors

Etoposide [VP-16] (VePesid)
Vinblastine (Velban, Velbe)

Vincristine (Oncovin, Vincasar PFS)

Vinorelbine (Navelbine)

Miscellaneous Antineoplastic Agents

Aldesleukin [Interleukin-2, IL-2] (Proleukin)
Aminoglutethimide (Cytadren)
L-Asparaginase (Elspar, Oncaspar)
BCG [Bacillus Calmette-Guérin] (TheraCys, Tice BCG)
Bevacizumab (Avastin)
Bortezomib (Velcade)
Cladribine (Leustatin)

Dacarbazine (DTIC)
Docetaxel (Taxotere)
Gefitinib (Iressa)
Gemtuzumab Ozogamicin (Mylotarg)
Hydroxyurea (Hydrea, Droxia)
Imatinib (Gleevec)
Irinotecan (Camptosar)
Letrozole (Femara)
Leucovorin (Wellcovorin)
Mitotane (Lysodren)

Mitoxantrone (Novantrone)
Paclitaxel (Taxol)
Pemetrexed (Alimta)
Rasburicase (Elitek)
Thalidomide (Thalomid)
Topotecan (Hycamtin)
Trastuzumab (Herceptin)
Tretinoin, Topical [Retinoic Acid] (Retin-A, Avita, Renova)

CARDIOVASCULAR AGENTS

Aldosterone Antagonist

Eplerenone (Inspra)

Alpha$_1$-Adrenergic Blockers

Doxazosin (Cardura)   Prazosin (Minipress)   Terazosin (Hytrin)

Angiotensin-Converting Enzyme Inhibitors

Benazepril (Lotensin)   Lisinopril (Prinivil,   Quinapril (Accupril)
Captopril (Capoten)   Zestril)   Ramipril (Altace)
Enalapril (Vasotec)   Moexipril (Univasc)   Trandolapril (Mavik)
Fosinopril (Monopril)   Perindopril Erbumine
                               (Aceon)

Angiotensin II Receptor Antagonists

Candesartan (Atacand)   Irbesartan (Avapro)   Telmisartan (Micardis)
Eprosartan (Teveten)   Losartan (Cozaar)   Valsartan (Diovan)

Antiarrhythmic Agents

Adenosine (Adenocard)   Dofetilide (Tikosyn)   Procainamide (Pronestyl,
Amiodarone (Cordarone,   Esmolol (Brevibloc)   Procan)
  Pacerone)   Flecainide (Tambocor)   Propafenone (Rythmol)
Atropine   Ibutilide (Corvert)   Quinidine (Quinidex,
Digoxin (Lanoxin,   Lidocaine (Anestacon   Quinaglute)
  Lanoxicaps)   Topical, Xylocaine)   Sotalol (Betapace,
Disopyramide (Norpace,   Mexiletine (Mexitil)   Betapace AF)
  NAPamide)

Beta-Adrenergic Blockers

Acebutolol (Sectral)   Carvedilol (Coreg)   Pindolol (Visken)
Atenolol (Tenormin)   Labetalol (Trandate,   Propranolol (Inderal)
Atenolol and Chlorthali-   Normodyne)   Timolol (Blocadren)
  done (Tenoretic)   Metoprolol (Lopressor,
Betaxolol (Kerlone)   Toprol XL)
Bisoprolol (Zebeta)   Nadolol (Corgard)
Carteolol (Cartrol,   Penbutolol (Levatol)
  Ocupress Ophthalmic)

Calcium Channel Antagonists

Amlodipine (Norvasc)
Bepridil (Vascor)
Diltiazem (Cardizem,
    Cartia XT, Dilacor,
    Diltia XT, Tiamate,
    Tiazac)

Felodipine (Plendil)
Isradipine (DynaCirc)
Nicardipine (Cardene)
Nifedipine (Procardia,
    Procardia XL, Adalat,
    Adalat CC)

Nimodipine (Nimotop)
Nisoldipine (Sular)
Verapamil (Calan,
    Isoptin)

Centrally Acting Antihypertensive Agents

Clonidine (Catapres)

Methyldopa (Aldomet)

Diuretics

Acetazolamide (Diamox)
Amiloride (Midamor)
Bumetanide (Bumex)
Chlorothiazide (Diuril)
Chlorthalidone
    (Hygroton)
Furosemide (Lasix)
Hydrochlorothiazide (Hy-
    droDIURIL, Esidrix)

Hydrochlorothiazide and
    Amiloride
    (Moduretic)
Hydrochlorothiazide and
    Spironolactone
    (Aldactazide)
Hydrochlorothiazide and
    Triamterene (Dyazide,
    Maxzide)

Indapamide (Lozol)
Mannitol
Metolazone (Mykrox,
    Zaroxolyn)
Spironolactone
    (Aldactone)
Torsemide (Demadex)
Triamterene (Dyrenium)

Inotropic/Pressor Agents

Digoxin (Lanoxin,
    Lanoxicaps)
Dobutamine (Dobutrex)
Dopamine (Intropin)
Epinephrine (Adrenalin,
    Sus-Phrine, EpiPen)

Inamrinone (Inocor)
Isoproterenol (Isuprel)
Milrinone (Primacor)
Nesiritide (Natrecor)
Norepinephrine
    (Levophed)

Phenylephrine
    (Neo-Synephrine)

Lipid-Lowering Agents

Atorvastatin (Lipitor)
Cholestyramine
    (Questran,
    LoCHOLEST)
Colesevelam (Welchol)
Colestipol (Colestid)

Ezetimibe (Zetia)
Fenofibrate (Tricor)
Fluvastatin (Lescol)
Gemfibrozil (Lopid)
Lovastatin (Mevacor,
    Altocor)

Niacin (Niaspan)
Pravastatin (Pravachol)
Rosuvastatin (Crestor)
Simvastatin (Zocor)

Lipid-Lowering/Antihypertensive Combinations

Amlodipine/Atorvastatin
  (Caduet)

Vasodilators

Alprostadil
  [Prostaglandin E₁]
  (Prostin VR)
Epoprostenol (Flolan)
Fenoldopam (Corlopam)
Hydralazine (Apresoline)
Isosorbide Dinitrate
  (Isordil, Sorbitrate,
  Dilatrate-SR)

Isosorbide Mononitrate
  (Ismo, Imdur)
Minoxidil (Loniten,
  Rogaine)
Nitroglycerin (Nitrostat,
  Nitrolingual, Nitro-
  Bid Ointment, Nitro-
  Bid IV, Nitrodisc,
  Transderm-Nitro)

Nitroprusside (Nipride,
  Nitropress)
Tolazoline (Priscoline)
Treprostinil Sodium
  (Remodulin)

CENTRAL NERVOUS SYSTEM AGENTS

Antianxiety Agents

Alprazolam (Xanax)
Buspirone (BuSpar)
Chlordiazepoxide (Lib-
  rium, Mitran, Libritabs)
Clorazepate (Tranxene)

Diazepam (Valium)
Doxepin (Sinequan,
  Adapin)
Hydroxyzine (Atarax,
  Vistaril)

Lorazepam (Ativan)
Meprobamate (Equanil,
  Miltown)
Oxazepam (Serax)

Anticonvulsants

Carbamazepine (Tegretol)
Clonazepam (Klonopin)
Diazepam (Valium)
Ethosuximide (Zarontin)
Fosphenytoin (Cerebyx)
Gabapentin (Neurontin)

Lamotrigine (Lamictal)
Levetiracetam (Keppra)
Lorazepam (Ativan)
Oxcarbazepine (Trileptal)
Pentobarbital (Nembutal)
Phenobarbital

Phenytoin (Dilantin)
Tiagabine (Gabitril)
Topiramate (Topamax)
Valproic Acid (Depak-
  ene, Depakote)
Zonisamide (Zonegran)

Antidepressants

Amitriptyline (Elavil)
Bupropion (Wellbutrin,
  Zyban)
Citalopram (Celexa)
Desipramine (Norpramin)
Doxepin (Sinequan,
  Adapin)

Escitalopram (Lexapro)
Fluoxetine (Prozac,
  Sarafem)
Fluvoxamine (Luvox)
Imipramine (Tofranil)
Mirtazapine (Remeron)
Nefazodone (Serzone)

Nortriptyline (Aventyl,
  Pamelor)
Paroxetine (Paxil)
Phenelzine (Nardil)
Sertraline (Zoloft)
Trazodone (Desyrel)
Venlafaxine (Effexor)

Antiparkinson Agents

Amantadine (Symmetrel)
Apomorphine (Apokyn)
Benztropine (Cogentin)
Bromocriptine (Parlodel)

Carbidopa/Levodopa (Sinemet)
Entacapone (Comtan)
Pergolide (Permax)
Pramipexole (Mirapex)

Ropinirole (Requip)
Selegiline (Eldepryl)
Tolcapone (Tasmar)
Trihexyphenidyl (Artane)

Antipsychotics

Aripiprazole (Abilify)
Chlorpromazine (Thorazine)
Clozapine (Clozaril)
Fluphenazine (Prolixin, Permitil)
Haloperidol (Haldol)
Lithium Carbonate (Eskalith, Lithobid)

Mesoridazine (Serentil)
Molindone (Moban)
Olanzapine (Zyprexa)
Perphenazine (Trilafon)
Prochlorperazine (Compazine)
Quetiapine (Seroquel)
Risperidone (Risperdal)

Thioridazine (Mellaril)
Thiothixene (Navane)
Trifluoperazine (Stelazine)
Ziprasidone (Geodon)

Sedative Hypnotics

Chloral Hydrate (Aquachloral, Supprettes)
Diphenhydramine (Benadryl)
Estazolam (ProSom)
Flurazepam (Dalmane)

Hydroxyzine (Atarax, Vistaril)
Midazolam (Versed)
Pentobarbital (Nembutal)
Phenobarbital
Propofol (Diprivan)

Quazepam (Doral)
Secobarbital (Seconal)
Temazepam (Restoril)
Triazolam (Halcion)
Zaleplon (Sonata)
Zolpidem (Ambien)

Miscellaneous CNS Agents

Atomoxetine (Strattera)
Galantamine (Reminyl)
Memantine (Namenda)

Nimodipine (Nimotop)
Rivastigmine (Exelon)

Sodium Oxybate (Xyrem)
Tacrine (Cognex)

DERMATOLOGIC AGENTS

Acitretin (Soriatane)
Acyclovir (Zovirax)
Alefacept (Amevive)
Anthralin (Anthra-Derm)
Amphotericin B (Fungizone)

Bacitracin, Topical (Baciguent)
Bacitracin and Polymyxin B, Topical (Polysporin)
Bacitracin, Neomycin, and Polymyxin B,

Topical (Neosporin Ointment)
Bacitracin, Neomycin, Polymyxin B, and Hydrocortisone, Topical (Cortisporin)

Bacitracin, Neomycin, Polymyxin B, and Lidocaine, Topical (Clomycin)
Calcipotriene (Dovonex)
Capsaicin (Capsin, Zostrix)
Ciclopirox (Loprox)
Ciprofloxacin (Cipro)
Clindamycin (Cleocin)
Clotrimazole and Betamethasone (Lotrisone)
Dibucaine (Nupercainal)
Doxepin, Topical (Zonalon)
Econazole (Spectazole)
Efalizumab (Raptiva)
Erythromycin, Topical (A/T/S, Eryderm, Erycette, T-Stat)
Finasteride (Proscar, Propecia)
Gentamicin, Topical (Garamycin, G-Mycitin)
Haloprogin (Halotex)

Imiquimod Cream, 5% (Aldara)
Isotretinoin [13-*cis* Retinoic acid] (Accutane, Amnesteem, Claravis, Sotret)
Ketoconazole (Nizoral)
Lactic Acid and Ammonium Hydroxide [Ammonium Lactate] (Lac-Hydrin)
Lindane (Kwell)
Metronidazole (Flagy, MetroGel)
Miconazole (Monistat)
Minoxidil (Loniten, Rogaine)
Mupirocin (Bactroban)
Naftifine (Naftin)
Neomycin Sulfate (Myciguent)
Nystatin (Mycostatin)
Oxiconazole (Oxistat)
Penciclovir (Denavir)
Permethrin (Nix, Elimite)
Pimecrolimus (Elidel)

Podophyllin (Podocon-25, Condylox Gel 0.5%, Condylox)
Pramoxine (Anusol Ointment, Proctofoam-NS)
Pramoxine and Hydrocortisone (Enzone, Proctofoam-HC)
Selenium Sulfide (Exsel Shampoo, Selsun Blue Shampoo, Selsun Shampoo)
Silver Sulfadiazine (Silvadene)
Steroids, Topical (Table 5, page 272)
Tacrolimus (Prograf, Protopic)
Tazarotene (Tazorac)
Terbinafine (Lamisil)
Tolnaftate (Tinactin)
Tretinoin, Topical [Retinoic Acid] (Retin-A, Avita, Renova)

DIETARY SUPPLEMENTS

Calcium Acetate (Calphron, Phos-Ex, PhosLo)
Calcium Glubionate (Neo-Calglucon)
Calcium Salts [Chloride, Gluconate, Glucepate]
Cholecalciferol [Vitamin D_3] (Delta D)
Cyanocobalamin [Vitamin B_{12}]

Ferric Gluconate Complex (Ferrlecit)
Ferrous Gluconate (Fergon)
Ferrous Sulfate
Folic Acid
Iron Dextran (DexFerrum, InFeD)
Iron Sucrose (Venofer)
Magnesium Oxide (Mag-Ox 400)
Magnesium Sulfate

Phytonadione [Vitamin K] (AquaMEPHYTON)
Potassium Supplements (Kaon, Kaochlor, K-Lor, Slow-K, Micro-K, Klorvess)
Pyridoxine [Vitamin B_6]
Sodium Bicarbonate [$NaHCO_3$]
Thiamine [Vitamin B_1]

EAR (OTIC) AGENTS

Acetic Acid and
  Aluminum Acetate
  (Otic Domeboro)
Benzocaine and
  Antipyrine (Auralgan)
Ciprofloxacin, Otic
  (Cipro HC Otic)
Neomycin, Colistin, and
  Hydrocortisone
  (Cortisporin-TC Otic
  Drops)

Neomycin, Colistin,
  Hydrocortisone, and
  Thonzonium
  (Cortisporin-TC Otic
  Suspension)
Neomycin, Polymyxin,
  and Hydrocortisone
  (Cortisporin
  Ophthalmic and Otic)

Polymyxin B and
  Hydrocortisone
  (Otobiotic Otic)
Sulfacetamide and Pred-
  nisolone (Blephamide)
Triethanolamine
  (Cerumenex)

ENDOCRINE SYSTEM AGENTS

Antidiabetic Agents

Acarbose (Precose)
Chlorpropamide
  (Diabinese)
Glimepiride (Amaryl)
Glipizide (Glucotrol)
Glyburide (DiaBeta,
  Micronase, Glynase)

Glyburide/Metformin
  (Glucovance)
Insulins (Table 6, page
  275)
Metformin (Glucophage)
Miglitol (Glyset)
Nateglinide (Starlix)

Pioglitazone (Actos)
Repaglinide (Prandin)
Rosiglitazone (Avandia)
Tolazamide (Tolinase)
Tolbutamide (Orinase)

Hormone and Synthetic Substitutes

Calcitonin (Cibacalcin,
  Miacalcin)
Calcitriol (Rocaltrol)
Cortisone Systemic,
  Topical
Desmopressin (DDAVP,
  Stimate)
Dexamethasone
  (Decadron)

Fludrocortisone Acetate
  (Florinef)
Glucagon
Hydrocortisone Topical
  & Systemic (Cortef,
  Solu-Cortef)
Methylprednisolone
  (Solu-Medrol)
Prednisolone

Prednisone
Testosterone (AndroGel,
  Androderm, Striant,
  Testim, Testoderm)
Vasopressin [Antidi-
  uretic Hormone,
  ADH] (Pitressin)

Hypercalcemia Agents

Etidronate Disodium
  (Didronel)

Gallium Nitrate (Ganite)
Pamidronate (Aredia)

Zoledronic acid
  (Zometa)

Obesity

Sibutramine (Meridia)

Osteoporosis Agents

Alendronate (Fosamax)   Risedronate (Actonel)   Zoledronic Acid
Raloxifene (Evista)   Teriparatide (Forteo)   (Zometa)

Thyroid/Antithyroid

Levothyroxine   Potassium iodide   Propylthiouracil [PTU]
   (Synthroid, Levoxyl)   [Lugol's solution]
Liothyronine (Cytomel)   (SSKI, Thyro-Block)
Methimazole (Tapazole)

Miscellaneous Endocrine Agents

Cinacalcet (Sensipar)   Demeclocycline   Diazoxide (Hyperstat,
                                  (Declomycin)   Proglycem)

EYE (OPHTHALMIC) AGENTS

Glaucoma Agents

Acetazolamide (Diamox)   Dipivefrin (Propine)   Levobunolol (A-K Beta,
Apraclonidine (Iopidine)   Dorzolamide (Trusopt)   Betagan)
Betaxolol, Ophthalmic   Dorzolamide and   Levocabastine (Livostin)
   (Betoptic)   Timolol (Cosopt)   Lodoxamide (Alomide)
Brimonidine (Alphagan)   Echothiophate Iodine   Rimexolone (Vexol
Brinzolamide (Azopt)   (Phospholine   Ophthalmic)
Carteolol (Cartrol,   Ophthalmic)   Timolol, Ophthalmic
   Ocupress Ophthalmic)   Latanoprost (Xalatan)   (Timoptic)

Ophthalmic Antibiotics

Bacitracin, Ophthalmic   Bacitracin, Neomycin,   Neomycin and Dexa-
   (AK-Tracin   Polymyxin B, and   methasone (AK-Neo-
   Ophthalmic)   Hydrocortisone, Oph-   Dex Ophthalmic,
Bacitracin and   thalmic (AK Spore HC   NeoDecadron Oph-
   Polymyxin B,   Ophthalmic, Cor-   thalmic)
   Ophthalmic (AK Poly   tisporin Ophthalmic)   Neomycin, Polymyxin
   Bac Ophthalmic,   Ciprofloxacin,   B, and Dexametha-
   Polysporin   Ophthalmic (Ciloxan)   sone (Maxitrol)
   Ophthalmic)   Erythromycin,   Neomycin, Polymyxin
Bacitracin, Neomycin,   Ophthalmic (Ilotycin   B, and Prednisolone
   and Polymyxin B (AK   Ophthalmic)   (Poly-Pred
   Spore Ophthalmic,   Gentamicin, Ophthalmic   Ophthalmic)
   Neosporin   (Garamycin, Genoptic,   Ofloxacin (Floxin,
   Ophthalmic)   Gentacidin, Gentak)   Ocuflox Ophthalmic)

Silver Nitrate (Dey-Drop)
Sulfacetamide (Bleph-10, Cetamide, Sodium Sulamyd)

Sulfacetamide and Prednisolone (Blephamide)
Tobramycin, Ophthalmic (AKTob, Tobrex)

Tobramycin and Dexamethasone (TobraDex)
Trifluridine (Viroptic)

Other Ophthalmic Agents

Artificial Tears (Tears Naturale)
Cromolyn Sodium (Opticrom)
Cyclopentolate (Cyclogyl)
Dexamethasone, Ophthalmic (AK-Dex Ophthalmic, Decadron Ophthalmic)

Emedastine (Emadine)
Ketorolac, Ophthalmic (Acular)
Ketotifen (Zaditor)
Lodoxamide (Alomide)
Naphazoline and Antazoline (Albalon-A Ophthalmic)

Naphazoline and Pheniramine Acetate (Naphcon A)
Olopatadine (Patanol)
Pemirolast (Alamast)
Rimexolone (Vexol Ophthalmic)

GASTROINTESTINAL AGENTS

Antacids

Alginic Acid (Gaviscon)
Aluminum Hydroxide (Amphojel, AlternaGEL)
Aluminum Hydroxide with Magnesium Carbonate (Gaviscon)
Aluminum Hydroxide with Magnesium Hydroxide (Maalox)

Aluminum Hydroxide with Magnesium Hydroxide and Simethicone (Mylanta, Mylanta II, Maalox Plus)
Aluminum Hydroxide with Magnesium Trisilicate (Gaviscon, Gaviscon-2)

Calcium Carbonate (Tums, Alka-Mints)
Magaldrate (Riopan, Lowsium)
Simethicone (Mylicon)

Antidiarrheals

Bismuth Subsalicylate (Pepto-Bismol)
Diphenoxylate with Atropine (Lomotil)

Kaolin-Pectin (Kaodene, Kao-Spen, Kapectolin, Parepectolin)
Lactobacillus (Lactinex Granules)

Loperamide (Imodium)
Octreotide (Sandostatin, Sandostatin LAR)
Paregoric [Camphorated Tincture of Opium]

Antiemetics

Aprepitant (Emend)
Chlorpromazine (Thorazine)

Dimenhydrinate (Dramamine)
Dolasetron (Anzemet)

Dronabinol (Marinol)
Droperidol (Inapsine)
Granisetron (Kytril)

Meclizine (Antivert)
Metoclopramide
  (Reglan, Clopra,
  Octamide)
Ondansetron (Zofran)

Palonosetron (Aloxi)
Prochlorperazine
  (Compazine)
Promethazine
  (Phenergan)

Scopolamine (Scopace)
Thiethylperazine
  (Torecan)
Trimethobenzamide
  (Tigan)

Antiulcer Agents

Cimetidine (Tagamet)
Esomeprazole (Nexium)
Famotidine (Pepcid)
Lansoprazole (Prevacid)

Nizatidine (Axid)
Omeprazole (Prilosec)
Pantoprazole (Protonix)
Rabeprazole (Aciphex)

Ranitidine Hydrochlo-
  ride (Zantac)
Sucralfate (Carafate)

Cathartics/Laxatives

Bisacodyl (Dulcolax)
Docusate Calcium
  (Surfak)
Docusate Potassium
  (Dialose)
Docusate Sodium (DOS,
  Colace)
Glycerin Suppository
Lactulose (Chronulac,
  Cephulac, Enulose)

Magnesium Citrate
Magnesium Hydroxide
  (Milk of Magnesia)
Mineral Oil
Polyethylene Glycol-
  Electrolyte Solution
  (GoLYTELY, CoLyte)

Psyllium (Metamucil,
  Serutan, Effer-
  Syllium)
Sodium Phosphate
  (Visicol)
Sorbitol

Enzymes

Pancreatin (Pancrease,
  Cotazym, Creon,
  Ultrase)

Miscellaneous GI Agents

Alosetron (Lotronex)
Balsalazide (Colazal)
Dexpanthenol (Ilopan-
  Choline Oral, Ilopan)
Dibucaine (Nupercainal)
Dicyclomine (Bentyl)
Hydrocortisone, Rectal
  (Anusol-HC Supposi-
  tory, Cortifoam
  Rectal, Proctocort)

Hyoscyamine
  (Anaspaz, Cystospaz,
  Levsin)
Hyoscyamine, Atropine,
  Scopolamine, and
  Phenobarbital
  (Donnatal)
Infliximab (Remicade)
Mesalamine (Rowasa,
  Asacol, Pentasa)

Metoclopramide (Reglan,
  Clopra, Octamide)
Misoprostol (Cytotec)
Olsalazine (Dipentum)
Pramoxine (Anusol
  Ointment, Procto-
  foam-NS)
Pramoxine with Hydro-
  cortisone (Enzone,
  Proctofoam-HC)

Propantheline (Pro-Banthine)
Sulfasalazine (Azulfidine)

Tegaserod Maleate (Zelnorm)

Vasopressin (Pitressin)

HEMATOLOGIC AGENTS

Anticoagulants

Ardeparin (Normiflo)
Argatroban (Acova)
Bivalirudin (Angiomax)
Dalteparin (Fragmin)

Enoxaparin (Lovenox)
Fondaparinux (Arixtra)
Heparin
Lepirudin (Refludan)

Protamine
Tinzaparin (Innohep)
Warfarin (Coumadin)

Antiplatelet Agents

Abciximab (ReoPro)
Aspirin (Bayer, Ecotrin, St. Joseph's)
Clopidogrel (Plavix)

Dipyridamole (Persantine)
Dipyridamole and Aspirin (Aggrenox)

Eptifibatide (Integrilin)
Reteplase (Retavase)
Ticlopidine (Ticlid)
Tirofiban (Aggrastat)

Antithrombotic Agents

Alteplase, Recombinant [tPA] (Activase)
Aminocaproic Acid (Amicar)
Anistreplase (Eminase)

Aprotinin (Trasylol)
Danaparoid (Orgaron)
Dextran 40 (Rheomacrodex)
Reteplase (Retavase)

Streptokinase (Streptase, Kabikinase)
Tenecteplase (TNKase)
Urokinase (Abbokinase)

Hematopoietic Stimulants

Darbepoetin Alfa (Aranesp)
Epoetin Alfa [Erythropoietin, EPO] (Epogen, Procrit)

Filgrastim [G-CSF] (Neupogen)
Oprelvekin (Neumega)
Pegfilgrastim (Neulasta)

Sargramostim [GM-CSF] (Prokine, Leukine)

Volume Expanders

Albumin (Albuminar, Buminate, Albutein)

Dextran 40 (Rheomacrodex)
Hetastarch (Hespan)

Plasma Protein Fraction (Plasmanate)

Miscellaneous Hematologic Agents

Antihemophilic Factor VIII (Monoclate)

Desmopressin (DDAVP, Stimate)

Pentoxifylline (Trental)

IMMUNE SYSTEM AGENTS

Immunomodulators

Adalimumab (Humira)
Anakinra (Kineret)
Etanercept (Enbrel)
Interferon Alfa (Roferon-A, Intron A)

Interferon Alfacon-1 (Infergen)
Interferon Beta-1b (Betaseron)

Interferon Gamma-1b (Actimmune)
Peg Interferon Alfa-2b (PEG-Intron)

Immunosuppressive Agents

Azathioprine (Imuran)
Basiliximab (Simulect)
Cyclosporine (Sandimmune, NePO)
Daclizumab (Zenapax)

Lymphocyte Immune Globulin [Antithymocyte Globulin, ATG] (Atgam)
Muromonab-CD3 (Orthoclone OKT3)

Mycophenolate Mofetil (CellCept)
Sirolimus (Rapamune)
Steroids, Systemic (Table 4, page 271)
Tacrolimus (Prograf, Protopic)

Vaccines/Serums/Toxoids

Cytomegalovirus Immune Globulin [CMV-IG IV] (CytoGam)
Diphtheria, Tetanus Toxoids, and Acellular Pertussis Adsorbed, Hepatitis B (recombinant), and Inactivated Poliovirus Vaccine (IPV) Combined (Pediarix)
Haemophilus B Conjugate Vaccine (ActHIB, HibTITER, Pedvax-HIB, Prohibit)
Hepatitis A Vaccine (Havrix, Vaqta)

Hepatitis A (Inactivated) and Hepatitis B Recombinant Vaccine (Twinrix)
Hepatitis B Immune Globulin (HyperHep, H-BIG)
Hepatitis B Vaccine (Engerix-B, Recombivax HB)
Immune Globulin, IV (Gamimune N, Sandoglobulin, Gammar IV)
Influenza Vaccine (Fluzone, FluShield, Fluvirin)

Influenza Virus Vaccine Live, Intranasal (FluMist)
Meningococcal Polysaccharide Vaccine (Menomune)
Pneumococcal 7-Valent Conjugate Vaccine (Prevnar)
Pneumococcal Vaccine, Polyvalent (Pneumovax-23)
Tetanus Immune Globulin
Tetanus Toxoid
Varicella Virus Vaccine (Varivax)

MUSCULOSKELETAL AGENTS

Antigout Agents

Allopurinol (Zyloprim, Lopurin, Alloprim)

Colchicine
Probenecid (Benemid)

Sulfinpyrazone (Anturane)

Muscle Relaxants

Baclofen (Lioresal)
Carisoprodol (Soma)
Chlorzoxazone
  (Paraflex, Parafon
  Forte DSC)

Cyclobenzaprine
  (Flexeril)
Dantrolene (Dantrium)
Diazepam (Valium)
Metaxalone (Skelaxin)

Methocarbamol
  (Robaxin)
Orphenadrine (Norflex)

Neuromuscular Blockers

Atracurium (Tracrium)
Pancuronium (Pavulon)
Rocuronium (Zemuron)

Succinylcholine
  (Anectine, Quelicin,
  Sucostrin)

Vecuronium (Norcuron)

Miscellaneous Musculoskeletal Agents

Edrophonium (Tensilon)
Leflunomide (Arava)

Methotrexate (Folex,
  Rheumatrex)

OB/GYN AGENTS

Contraceptives

Estradiol Cypionate and
  Medroxyprogesterone
  Acetate (Lunelle)
Etonogestrel/Ethinyl
  Estradiol (NuvaRing)
Levonorgestrel Implant
  (Norplant)

Medroxyprogesterone
  (Provera, Depo-
  Provera)
Norgestrel (Ovrette)
Oral Contraceptives,
  Monophasic (Table 7,
  page 276)

Oral Contraceptives,
  Multiphasic (Table 7,
  page 276)
Oral Contraceptives,
  Progestin Only (Table
  7, page 276)

Emergency Contraceptives

Ethinyl Estradiol, and
  Levonorgestrel
  (Preven)

Levonorgestrel (Plan B)

Estrogen Supplementation Agents

Esterified Estrogens
  (Estratab,
  Menest)
Esterified Estrogens with
  Methyltestosterone
  (Estratest)

Estradiol (Estrace)
Estradiol, Transdermal
  (Estraderm, Climara,
  Vivelle)
Estrogen, Conjugated
  (Premarin)

Estrogen, Conjugated-
  Synthetic (Cenestin)
Estrogen, Conjugated
  with Medroxyproges-
  terone (Prempro,
  Premphase)

Estrogen, Conjugated with Methylprogesterone (Premarin with Methylprogesterone)

Estrogen, Conjugated with Methyltestosterone (Premarin with Methyltestosterone)

Ethinyl Estradiol (Estinyl, Feminone) Norethindrone Acetate/Ethinyl Estradiol (FemHRT)

Vaginal Preparations

Amino-Cerv pH 5.5 Cream
Miconazole (Monistat)

Nystatin (Mycostatin)
Terconazole (Terazol 7)

Tioconazole (Vagistat)

Miscellaneous Ob/Gyn Agents

Dinoprostone (Cervidil Vaginal Insert, Pre-pidil Vaginal Gel)
Gonadorelin (Lutrepulse)
Leuprolide (Lupron, Viadur, Eligard)

Magnesium Sulfate
Medroxyprogesterone (Provera, Depo-Provera)
Methylergonovine (Methergine)

Mifepristone [RU 486] (Mifeprex)
Oxytocin (Pitocin)
Terbutaline (Brethine, Bricanyl)

PAIN MEDICATIONS

Local Anesthetics

Benzocaine and An-tipyrine (Auralgan)
Bupivacaine (Marcaine)
Capsaicin (Capsin, Zostrix)

Cocaine
Dibucaine (Nupercainal)
Lidocaine (Anestacon Topical, Xylocaine)

Lidocaine and Prilocaine (EMLA, LMX)
Pramoxine (Anusol Ointment, Procto-foam-NS)

Migraine Headache Medications

Acetaminophen with Bu-talbital w/wo Caffeine (Fioricet, Medigesic, Repan, Sedapap-10 Two-Dyne, Triapin, Axocet, Phrenilin Forte)

Almotriptan (Axert)
Aspirin and Butalbital Compound (Fiorinal)
Aspirin with Butalbital, Caffeine, and Codeine (Fiorinal with Codeine)

Frovatriptan (Frova)
Naratriptan (Amerge)
Serotonin Receptor Agonists (See Table 11, page 283)
Sumatriptan (Imitrex)
Zolmitriptan (Zomig)

Narcotics

Acetaminophen with Codeine (Tylenol No. 1, 2, 3, 4)

Alfentanil (Alfenta)
Aspirin with Codeine (Empirin No. 2, 3, 4)

Buprenorphine (Buprenex)
Butorphanol (Stadol)

Codeine
Dezocine (Dalgan)
Fentanyl (Sublimaze)
Fentanyl, Transdermal
  (Duragesic)
Fentanyl, Transmucosal
  (Actiq System)
Hydrocodone and Aceta-
  minophen (Lorcet,
  Vicodin)
Hydrocodone and
  Aspirin (Lortab ASA)
Hydrocodone and Ibupro-
  fen (Vicoprofen)
Hydromorphone
  (Dilaudid)

Levorphanol (Levo-
  Dromoran)
Meperidine (Demerol)
Methadone (Dolophine)
Morphine (Avinza XR,
  Duramorph, MS
  Contin, Kadian SR,
  Oramorph SR,
  Roxanol)
Nalbuphine (Nubain)
Oxycodone (OxyContin,
  OxyIR, Roxicodone)
Oxycodone and Aceta-
  minophen (Percocet,
  Tylox)

Oxycodone and Aspirin
  (Percodan, Percodan-
  Demi)
Oxymorphone (Numor-
  phan)
Pentazocine (Talwin)
Propoxyphene (Darvon)
Propoxyphene and
  Acetaminophen
  (Darvocet)
Propoxyphene and
  Aspirin (Darvon
  Compound-65,
  Darvon-N with
  Aspirin)

Nonnarcotic Agents

Acetaminophen [APAP]
  (Tylenol)
Aspirin (Bayer, Ecotrin,
  St. Joseph's)

Tramadol (Ultram)
Tramadol/Aceta-
  minophen (Ultracet)

Nonsteroidal Antiinflammatory Agents

Celecoxib (Celebrex)
Diclofenac (Cataflam,
  Voltaren)
Diflunisal (Dolobid)
Etodolac (Lodine)
Fenoprofen (Nalfon)
Flurbiprofen
  (Ansaid)

Ibuprofen (Motrin,
  Rufen, Advil)
Indomethacin (Indocin)
Ketoprofen (Orudis,
  Oruvail)
Ketorolac (Toradol)
Meloxicam (Mobic)
Nabumetone (Relafen)

Naproxen (Aleve,
  Naprosyn, Anaprox)
Oxaprozin (Daypro)
Piroxicam (Feldene)
Rofecoxib (Vioxx)
Sulindac (Clinoril)
Tolmetin (Tolectin)
Valdecoxib (Bextra)

Miscellaneous Pain Medications

Amitriptyline (Elavil)

Imipramine (Tofranil)

Tramadol (Ultram)

RESPIRATORY AGENTS

Antitussives, Decongestants, and Expectorants

Acetylcysteine
  (Mucomyst)

Benzonatate (Tessalon
  Perles)

Codeine

Dextromethorphan (Mediquell, Benylin DM, PediaCare 1)
Guaifenesin (Robitussin)
Guaifenesin and Codeine (Robitussin AC, Brontex)
Guaifenesin and Dextromethorphan
Hydrocodone and Guaifenesin (Hycotuss Expectorant)
Hydrocodone and Homatropine (Hycodan, Hydromet)
Hydrocodone and Pseudoephedrine (Detussin, Histussin-D)
Hydrocodone, Chlorpheniramine, Phenylephrine, Acetaminophen, and Caffeine (Hycomine)
Potassium Iodide (SSKI, Thyro-Block)
Pseudoephedrine (Sudafed, Novafed, Afrinol)

Bronchodilators

Albuterol (Proventil, Ventolin, Volmax)
Albuterol and Ipratropium (Combivent)
Aminophylline
Bitolterol (Tornalate)
Ephedrine
Epinephrine (Adrenalin, Sus-Phrine, EpiPen)
Formoterol (Foradil Aerolizer)
Isoproterenol (Isuprel)
Levalbuterol (Xopenex)
Metaproterenol (Alupent, Metaprel)
Pirbuterol (Maxair)
Salmeterol (Serevent)
Terbutaline (Brethine, Bricanyl)
Theophylline (Theolair, Somophyllin)

Respiratory Inhalants

Acetylcysteine (Mucomyst)
Beclomethasone (Beconase, Vancenase Nasal Inhaler)
Beclomethasone (QVAR)
Beractant (Survanta)
Budesonide (Rhinocort, Pulmicort)
Calfactant (Infasurf)
Colfosceril Palmitate (Exosurf Neonatal)
Cromolyn Sodium (Intal, NasalCrom, Opticrom)
Dexamethasone, Nasal (Dexacort Phosphate Turbinaire)
Flunisolide (AeroBid, Nasalide)
Fluticasone, Oral, Nasal (Flonase, Flovent)
Fluticasone Propionate and Salmeterol Xinafoate (Advair Diskus)
Ipratropium (Atrovent)
Nedocromil (Tilade)
Tiotropium (Spiriva)
Triamcinolone (Azmacort)

Miscellaneous Respiratory Agents

Alpha$_1$-Protease Inhibitor (Prolastin)
Dornase Alfa (Pulmozyme)
Montelukast (Singulair)
Omalizumab (Xolair)
Zafirlukast (Accolate)
Zileuton (Zyflo)

URINARY/GENITOURINARY AGENTS

Alprostadil, Intracavernosal (Caverject, Edex)
Alprostadil, Urethral Suppository (Muse)
Ammonium Aluminum Sulfate [Alum]
Belladonna and Opium Suppositories (B & O Supprettes)
Bethanechol (Urecholine, Duvoid)
Dimethyl Sulfoxide [DMSO] (Rimso 50)
Flavoxate (Urispas)
Hyoscyamine (Anaspaz, Cystospaz, Levsin)

Methenamine (Hiprex, Urex)
Neomycin-Polymyxin Bladder Irrigant [Neosporin GU Irrigant]
Nitrofurantoin (Macrodantin, Furadantin, Macrobid)
Oxybutynin (Ditropan, Ditropan XL)
Oxybutynin Transdermal System (Oxytrol)
Pentosan Polysulfate (Elmiron)
Phenazopyridine (Pyridium)

Potassium Citrate (Urocit-K)
Potassium Citrate and Citric Acid (Polycitra-K)
Sildenafil (Viagra)
Sodium Citrate (Bicitra)
Tadalafil (Cialis)
Tolterodine (Detrol, Detrol LA)
Trimethoprim (Trimpex, Proloprim)
Trospium Chloride (Sanctura)
Vardenafil (Levitra)

Benign Prostatic Hyperplasia Medications

Alfuzosin (Uroxatral)
Doxazosin (Cardura)
Dutasteride (Avodart)

Finasteride (Proscar, Propecia)

Tamsulosin (Flomax)
Terazosin (Hytrin)

WOUND CARE

Becaplermin (Regranex Gel)

Silver Nitrate (Dey-Drop)

MISCELLANEOUS THERAPEUTIC AGENTS

Cilostazol (Pletal)
Drotrecogin Alfa (Xigris)
Megestrol Acetate (Megace)
Naltrexone (ReVia)
Nicotine Gum (Nicorette)

Nicotine Nasal Spray (Nicotrol NS)
Nicotine Transdermal (Habitrol, Nicoderm, Nicotrol)
Orlistat (Xenical)

Potassium Iodide [Lugol's Solution] (SSKI, Thyro-Block)
Sevelamer (Renagel)
Sodium Polystyrene Sulfonate (Kayexalate)
Talc (Sterile Talc Powder)

Commonly Used Medicinal Herbs

Arnica (*Arnica montana*)
Astragalus (*Astragalus membranaceus*)

Butcher's Broom (*Ruscus aculeatus*)

Black Cohosh (*Cimicifuga racemosa*)

Chamomile (*Matricaria recutita*)

Chondroitin Sulfate

Dong Quai (*Angelica polymorpha, sinensis*)

Echinacea (*Echinacea purpurea*)

Ephedra/Ma Huang

Feverfew (*Tanacetum parthenium*)

Garlic (*Allium sativum*)

Ginger (*Zingiber officinale*)

Ginkgo biloba

Ginseng (*Panax quinquefolius*)

Glucosamine Sulfate (chitosamine)

Hawthorn (*Crataegus laevigata*)

Kava Kava (*Piper methysticum*)

Licorice (*Glycyrrhiza glabra*)

Melatonin, (MEL)

Milk thistle (*Silybum marianum*)

Saw Palmetto (*Serenoa repens*)

Spirulina (*Spirulina* spp)

St. John's Wort (*Hypericum perforatum*)

Tea Tree (*Melaleuca alternifolia*)

Valerian (*Valeriana officinalis*)

Yohimbine (*Pausinystalia yohimbe*)

GENERIC DRUG DATA

Abacavir (Ziagen) WARNING: Hypersensitivity (fever, rash, fatigue, GI, esp) reported; lactic acidosis & hepatomegaly/steatosis reported Uses: *HIV infection* Action: Nucleoside RT inhibitor Dose: *Adults.* 300 mg PO bid *Peds.* 8 mg/kg bid Caution: [C, –] CDC recommends HIV-infected mothers not breastfeed due to risk of infant HIV transmission Supplied: Tabs 300 mg; soln 20 mg/mL SE: See Warning, ↑d LFTs, fat redistribution Notes: Numerous drug interactions Interactions: EtOH ↓ drug elimination and ↑ drug exposure Labs: Monitor LFTs, FBS, CBC & differential, BUN & creatinine, triglycerides NIPE: ⊘ EtOH; monitor & teach Pt about hypersensitivity Rxns; DC drug immediately if hypersensitivity Rxn occurs and ⊘ rechallenge; take w/ or w/o food

Abarelix (Plenaxis) WARNING: Immediate-onset systemic allergic Rxns (eg, hypotension & syncope), w/ initial & ↑d risk w/ subsequent doses possible. Following dose, observe for at least 30 min; allergic Rxns should be managed appropriately. Only physicians enrolled in the Plenaxis PLUS Program (Plenaxis User Safety Program) may prescribe (www.plenaxis.com). Effectiveness beyond 12 mo not established. Follow serum testosterone to document effectiveness. Uses: *Palliation of advanced symptomatic CAP where LHRH agonists are not appropriate* Action: GnRH antagonist; does not cause flare seen w/ agonists Dose: 100 mg IM (buttock) day 1, 15, 29 & q4wk. Check testosterone before day 29 dose & q8wk to confirm suppression Caution: [X, N/A] Body weight >225 lb, prolonged QT interval or liver dysfunction, w/ class IA or III antiarrhythmics Contra: Women or children Supplied: 100 mg inj vial SE: Immediate allergic Rxns (urticaria, pruritus, hypotension, syncope), gynecomastia, hot flashes, sleep disturbances, nipple tenderness Interactions: None known with drugs, herbs, or food Labs: ↑ hgb NIPE: Use within 1 h of reconstitution, baseline EKG to measure QT interval

Abciximab (ReoPro) Uses: *Prevent acute ischemic complications in PTCA,* MI Action: Inhibits plt aggregation (glycoprotein IIb/IIIa inhibitor) Dose: 0.25 mg/kg bolus 10–60 min pre PTCA, then 0.125 µg/kg/min (max = 10 µg/min) cont inf × 12 h Caution: [C, ?/–] Contra: Active or recent (w/in 6 wk) internal hemorrhage, CVA w/in 2 y or CVA w/ significant neurologic deficit, bleeding diathesis or PO anticoagulants use w/in 7 d (unless PT ≥ 2× control), thrombocytopenia (<100,000 cells/µL), recent trauma or major surgery (w/in 6 wk), CNS tumor, AVM, aneurysm, severe uncontrolled HTN, vasculitis, use of dextran prior to or during PTCA, hypersensitivity to murine proteins Supplied: Inj 2 mg/mL SE: Allergic Rxns, bleeding, thrombocytopenia possible **Notes:** Use w/ heparin **Interactions:** May ↑ bleeding w/ anticoagulants, antiplts, NSAIDs, thrombolytics **Labs:** Monitor CBC, PT, PTT, INR, guaiac stools, urine for blood **NIPE:** Monitor for ↑ bleeding & bruising; ⊘ shake vial or mix w/ another drug, contact sports ⊘

Acarbose (Precose) **Uses:** *Type 2 DM* **Action:** α-Glucosidase inhibitor; delays digestion of carbohydrates, to ↓ glucose **Dose:** 25–100 mg PO tid (w/ 1st bite each meal) **Caution:** [B, ?] ⊘ if CrCl <25 mL/min **Contra:** IBD, cirrhosis **Supplied:** Tabs 25, 50, 100 mg **SE:** Abdominal pain, diarrhea, flatulence, ↑ LFTs **Notes:** OK w/ sulfonylureas; can affect digoxin levels; check LFTs q3mo for 1st yr **Interactions:** ↑ Hypoglycemic effect w/ sulfonylureas, juniper berries, ginseng, garlic, coriander, celery; ↓ effects w/ intestinal absorbents, digestive enzyme preps, diuretics, corticosteroids, phenothiazines, estrogens, phenytoin, INH, sympathomimetics, CCBs, thyroid hormones; ↓ conc of digoxin **Labs:** LFTs, FBS, HbA1c, LFTs, Hgb & Hct **NIPE:** Take drug tid w/ first bite of food, ↓ GI side effects by ↓ dietary starch, treat hypoglycemia w/ dextrose instead of sucrose, continue diet & exercise program

Acebutolol (Sectral) **Uses:** *HTN, arrhythmias* **Action:** Competitively blocks β-adrenergic receptors, β₁, & ISA **Dose:** 200–800 mg/d, ↓ if CrCl <50 mL/min **Caution:** [B, D in 2nd & 3rd tri, +] Can exacerbate ischemic heart Dz, ⊘ DC abruptly **Contra:** 2nd-, 3rd-degree heart block **Supplied:** Caps 200, 400 mg **SE:** Fatigue, HA, dizziness, bradycardia **Interactions:** ↓ Antihypertensive effect w/ NSAIDs, salicylates, thyroid preps, anesthetics, antacids, α-adrenergic stimulants, ma-huang, ephedra, licorice; ↓ hypoglycemic effect of glyburide; ↑ hypotensive response w/ other antihypertensives, nitrates, EtOH, diuretics, black cohash, hawthorn, goldenseal, parsley; ↑ bradycardia w/ digoxin, amiodarone; ↑ hypoglycemic effect of insulin **Labs:** Monitor lipids, uric acid, K⁺, FBS, LFTs, thyroxin, ECG **NIPE:** Teach Pt to monitor BP, pulse, S/Sxs CHF

Acetaminophen [APAP, N-acetyl-p-aminophenol] (Tylenol, other generic) [OTC] **Uses:** *Mild to moderate pain, HA, & fever* **Action:** Nonnarcotic analgesic; inhibits CNS synthesis of prostaglandins & hypothalamic heat-regulating center **Dose:** *Adults.* 650 mg PO or PR q4–6h or 1000 mg PO q6h; max 4 g/24 h. *Peds <12 y.* 10–15 mg/kg/dose PO or PR q4–6h; max 2.6 g/24 h. See quick dosing Table 1, page 263. Administer q6h if CrCl 10–50 mL/min & q8h if CrCl <10 mL/min **Caution:** [B, +] Hepatotoxicity in elderly & w/ EtOH use w/ >4 g/day; alcoholic liver Dz **Contra:** G6PD deficiency **Supplied:** Tabs 160, 325, 500, 650 mg; chew tabs 80, 160 mg; liq 100 mg/mL, 120 mg/2.5 mL, 120 mg/5 mL, 160 mg/5 mL, 167 mg/5 mL, 325 mg/5 mL, 500 mg/15 mL; gtt 48 mg/mL, 60 mg/0.6 mL; supp 80, 120, 125, 300, 325, 650 mg **SE:** OD causes hepatotoxicity, Rx w/ N-acetylcysteine **Notes:** No antiinflammatory or plt-inhibiting action; ⊘ ETOH **Interactions:** ↑ Hepatotoxicity w/ ETOH, barbiturates, carbamazepine, INH, rifampin, phenytoin; ↑ risk of bleeding w/ NSAIDs, salicylates, warfarin, feverfew, ginkgo biloba, red clover; ↓ absorption w/ antacids, cholestyramine, colestipol **Labs:** Monitor LFTs, CBC, BUN, creatinine, PT, INR; ↓lse ↑ urine 5-HIAA, urine glucose, serum uric acid; false ↓ serum glucose, amy- ase **NIPE:** Delayed absorption if given w/ food, ⊘ EtOH, teach S/Sxs hepatotoxi-city, consult health provider if temp ↑103° F/>3 d

Acetaminophen + Butalbital ± Caffeine (Fioricet, Medigesic, Repan, Sedapap-10, Two-Dyne, Triapin, Axocet, Phrenilin Forte) [C-III] Uses: *Tension HA,* mild pain **Action:** Nonnarcotic analgesic w/ barbiturate **Dose:** 1–2 tabs or caps PO q4/6h PRN; ↓ dose in renal/hepatic impairment; 4 g/24 h APAP max **Caution:** [D, +] Alcoholic liver Dz **Contra:** G6PD deficiency **Supplied:** Caps Medigesic, Repan, Two-Dyne: butalbital 50 mg, caf-feine 40 mg, + APAP 325 mg. Caps Axocet, Phrenilin Forte: butalbital 50 mg + APAP 650 mg; Triapin: butalbital 50 mg + APAP 325 mg. Tabs Medigesic, Fioricet, Repan: butalbital 50 mg, caffeine 40 mg, + APAP 325 mg; Phrenilin: bu-talbital 50 mg + APAP 325 mg; Sedapap-10: butalbital 50 mg + APAP 650 mg **SE:** Drowsiness, dizziness, "hangover" effect **Notes:** Butalbital is habit-forming; ⊘ ETOH intake **Interactions:** ↑ Effects of benzodiazepines, opioid analgesics, seda-ives/hypnotics, ETOH, methylphenidate hydrochloride; ↓ effects of MAOIs, TCAs, corticosteroids, theophylline, oral contraceptives, BBs, doxycycline **NIPE:** ⊘ EtOH & CNS depressants, may impair coordination, monitor for depression, use barrier protection contraception

Acetaminophen + Codeine (Tylenol No. 1, No. 2, No. 3, No. 4) [C-III, C-V] Uses: *Mild–moderate pain (No. 1, 2, 3); moderate–se-vere pain (No. 4)* **Action:** Combined APAP & a narcotic analgesic **Dose:** Adults. 1–2 tabs q3–4h PRN (max dose APAP = 4 g/d). Peds. APAP 10–15 mg/kg/dose; codeine 0.5–1 mg/kg dose q4–6h (dosing guide: 3–6 y, 5 mL/dose; 7–12 y, 10 mL/dose); ↓ in renal/hepatic impairment **Caution:** [C, +] Alcoholic liver Dz **Con-tra:** G6PD deficiency **Supplied:** Tabs 300 mg of APAP + codeine; caps 325 mg of APAP + codeine; helix, susp (C-V) APAP 120 mg + codeine 12 mg/5 mL **SE:** Drowsiness, dizziness, N/V **Notes:** Codeine in No. 1 = 7.5 mg, No. 2 = 15 mg, No. 3 = 30 mg, No. 4 = 60 mg **Interactions:** ↑ Effects of benzodiazepines, opioid anal-gesics, sedatives/hypnotics, EtOH, methylphenidate hydrochloride; ↓ effects of MAOIs, TCAs, corticosteroids, theophylline, oral contraceptives, BBs, doxycy-cline **NIPE:** ⊘ EtOH & CNS depressants, may impair coordination, monitor for depression, use barrier protection contraception

Acetazolamide (Diamox) Uses: *Diuresis, glaucoma, prevent high alti-tude sickness, & refractory epilepsy* **Action:** Carbonic anhydrase inhibitor; ↓ renal excretion of hydrogen & ↑ renal excretion of Na^+, K^+, HCO_3^-, & H_2O **Dose:** Adults. Diuretic: 250–375 mg IV or PO q24h. Glaucoma: 250–1000 mg PO q24h in ÷ doses. Epilepsy: 8–30 mg/kg/d PO in ÷ doses. Altitude sickness: 250 mg PO q8–12h or SR 500 mg PO q12–24h start 24–48 h before ascent & 48 h after highest ascent. Peds. Epilepsy: 8–30 mg/kg/24 h PO in ÷ doses; max 1 g/d. Diuretic: 5 mg/kg/24 h PO or IV. Alkalinization of urine: 5 mg/kg/dose PO bid–tid. Glau-

coma: 5–15 mg/kg/24 h PO in ÷ doses; max 1 g/d; adjust in renal impairment; ⊘ CrCl <10 mL/min **Caution:** [C, +] **Contra:** Renal/hepatic failure, sulfa hypersensitivity **Supplied:** Tabs 125, 250 mg; SR caps 500 mg; inj 500 mg/vial **SE** Malaise, metallic taste, drowsiness, photosensitivity, hyperglycemia **Notes:** Follow Na⁺ & K⁺; SR forms ⊘ in epilepsy **Interactions:** Causes ↑ effects of amphetamines, quinidine, procainamide, TCAs, ephedrine; ↓ effects of Li, phenobarbital salicylates, barbiturates; ↑ K⁺ loss w/ corticosteroids and amphotericin B **Labs** Monitor serum electrolytes, FBS, CBC, creatinine, intraocular pressure; false + fo urinary protein, urinary urobilinogen; ↓ I uptake; ↑ serum and urine glucose, uri acid, Ca²⁺, serum ammonia **NIPE:** ↓ GI distress w/ food, monitor for S/Sxs metabolic acidosis, ↑ fluid to ↓ risk of kidney stones

Acetic Acid & Aluminum Acetate (Otic Domeboro) Uses: *Oti tis externa* Action: Antiinfective Dose: 4–6 gtt in ear(s) q2–3h Caution: [C, ?] Contra: Perforated tympanic membranes Supplied: 2% otic soln NIPE: Burnin w/ instillation or irrigation

Acetylcysteine (Mucomyst) Uses: *Mucolytic* agent as adjuvant R for chronic bronchopulmonary Dzs & CF; *antidote to APAP hepatotoxicity* Action: Splits disulfide linkages between mucoprotein molecular complexes; protect liver by restoring glutathione in APAP OD Dose: *Adults & Peds.* Nebulizer: 3–! mL of 20% soln diluted w/ equal vol of water or NS tid–qid. *Antidote:* PO or NG 140 mg/kg load, then 70 mg/kg q4h for 17 doses. (Dilute 1:3 in carbonated bever age or orange juice; best if used w/in 24 h) Caution: [C, ?] Supplied: Soln 10% 20% SE: Bronchospasm (inhalation), N/V, drowsiness Notes: Activated charcoa adsorbs acetylcysteine when given PO for acute APAP ingestion Interactions Discolors rubber, Fe, Cu, Ag; incompatible w/ multiple antibiotics—administe drugs separately Labs: Monitor ABGs & pulse oximetry w/ bronchospasm NIPE Inform Pt of ↑ productive cough, clear airway before aerosol administration, ↑ flu ids to liquefy secretions, unpleasant odor will disappear & may cause N/V

Acitretin (Soriatane) WARNING: Must not be used by females who are PRG or intend to become PRG during therapy or for up to 3 y following discontin uation of therapy; ⊘ EtOH during therapy or for 2 mo following cessation of ther apy; ⊘ donate blood during or up to 3 y following cessation of therapy Uses *Severe psoriasis*; other keratinization disorders (lichen planus, etc) Action Retinoid-like activity Dose: 25–50 mg/d PO, w/ main meal; ↑ if no response by < wk to 75 mg/d Caution: [X, –] Renal/hepatic impairment; in women of reproductive potential Contra: See Warning Supplied: Caps 10, 25 mg SE: Cheilitis, skin peeling, alopecia, pruritus, rash, arthralgia, GI upset, photosensitivity, thrombocytosis, hypertriglyceridemia Notes: Follow LFTs; response often takes 2–3 mo must sign a Pt agreement/informed consent prior to use Interactions: ↑ ½ life w EtOH use, ↑ hepatotoxicity w/ MRX, ↓ effects of progestin-only contraceptives Labs: Monitor LFTs, lipids, FBS, HbA1c NIPE: Use effective contraception; ⊘ donate blood for 3 y after Rx, teach Pt S/Sxs pancreatitis

Acyclovir (Zovirax) Uses: *Herpes simplex & zoster infections* Action: Interferes w/ viral DNA synthesis Dose: *Adults. PO: Initial genital herpes:* 200 mg PO q4h while awake, 5 caps/d × 10 d or 400 mg PO tid × 7–10 d. *Chronic suppression:* 400 mg PO bid. *Intermittent Rx:* As for initial Rx, except treat for 5 d, or 800 mg PO bid, at earliest prodrome. *Herpes zoster:* 800 mg PO 5×/d for 7–10 d. *IV:* 5–10 mg/kg/dose IV q8h. *Topical: Initial herpes genitalis:* Apply q3h (6×/d) for 7 d. *Peds.* 5–10 mg/kg/dose IV or PO q8h or 750 mg/m²/24 h ÷ q8h. *Chickenpox:* 20 mg/kg/dose PO qid; ↓ for CrCl <50 mL/min Caution: [C, +] Supplied: Caps 200 mg; tabs 400, 800 mg; susp 200 mg/5 mL; inj 500 mg/vial; oint 5% SE: Dizziness, lethargy, confusion, rash, inflammation at IV site Notes: PO better than topical for herpes genitalis Interactions: ↑ CNS SE w/ MRX & zidovudine, ↑ blood levels w/ probenecid Labs: Monitor BUN, SCr, LFTs, CBC NIPE: Start immediately w/ Sxs, ↑ hydration w/ IV dose, ↑ risk cervical cancer w/ genital herpes, ↑ length of Rx in immunocompromised Pts

Adalimumab (Humira) WARNING: Cases of TB have been observed; check tuberculin skin test prior to use Uses: *Moderate–severe RA w/ an inadequate response to one or more DMARDs* Action: TNF-α inhibitor Dose: 40 mg SQ every other week; may ↑ 40 mg qwk if not on MTX Caution: [B, ?/–] Serious infections & sepsis reported Supplied: Prefilled 1 mL (40 mg) syringe SE: Inj site Rxns, serious infections, neurologic events, malignancies Notes: Refrigerate prefilled syringe, rotate inj sites, OK w/ other DMARDs Interactions: ↑ Effects w/ MRX Labs: May ↑ lipids, alkaline phosphatase NIPE: ⊘ exposure to infection; ⊘ admin live-virus vaccines

Adefovir (Hepsera) WARNING: Acute exacerbations of hepatitis may occur on discontinuation of therapy (monitor LFTs); chronic administration may lead to nephrotoxicity especially in Pts w/ underlying renal dysfunction (monitor renal Fxn); HIV resistance may emerge; lactic acidosis & severe hepatomegaly w/ steatosis have been reported when used alone or in combination w/ other antiretrovirals Uses: *Chronic active hepatitis B virus* Action: Nucleotide analog Dose: CrCl > 50 mL/min: 10 mg PO qd; CrCl 20–49 mL/min: 10 mg PO q48h; CrCl 10–19 mL/min: 10 mg PO q72h; hemodialysis: 10 mg PO q7d post dialysis; adjust w/ CrCl < 50 mL/min Caution: [C, –] Supplied: Tabs 10 mg SE: Asthenia, HA, abdominal pain; see Warning Interactions: See Warning Labs: LFTs, BUN, creatinine, creatine kinase, amylase NIPE: Effects on fetus & baby not known—⊘ breast-feed; use barrier contraception

Adenosine (Adenocard) Uses: *PSVT;* including associated w/ WPW Action: Class IV antiarrhythmic; slows AV node conduction Dose: *Adults.* 6 mg IV bolus; may repeat in 1–2 min; max 12 mg IV. *Peds.* 0.05 mg/kg IV bolus; may repeat q1⁄2 min to 0.25 mg/kg max Caution: [C, ?] Contra: 2nd- or 3rd-degree AV block or SSS (w/o pacemaker); recent MI or cerebral hemorrhage Supplied: Inj 6 mg/2 mL SE: Facial flushing, HA, dyspnea, chest pressure, hypotension Notes: Doses >12 mg ⊘; can cause momentary asystole when administered. Inter-

actions: ↓ Effects w/ theophylline, caffeine, guarana; ↑ effects w/ dipyridamole; ↑ risk of hypotension & chest pain w/ nicotine; ↑ risk of bradycardia w/ BBs; ↑ risk of heart block w/ carbamazepine; ↑ risk of ventricular fibrillation w/ digitalis glycosides. **Labs:** Monitor ECG during administration. **NIPE:** Monitor BP & pulse during therapy, monitor resp status—↑ risk of bronchospasm in asthmatics, discard unused or unclear soln

Albumin (Albuminar, Buminate, Albutein) **Uses:** *Plasma volume expansion for shock* (eg, burns, hemorrhage) **Action:** Maint of plasma colloid oncotic pressure **Dose:** *Adults.* Initially, 25 g IV; subsequent dose based on response 250 g/48h max. *Peds.* 0.5–1 g/kg/dose; inf at 0.05–0.1 g/min **Caution:** [C, ?] Severe anemia; cardiac; renal, or hepatic insufficiency due to added protein load & possible hypervolemia **Contra:** Cardiac failure **Supplied:** Soln 5%, 25% **SE:** Chills, fever, CHF, tachycardia, hypotension, hypervolemia **Notes:** Contain 130–160 mEq Na/L; may precipitate pulmonary edema **Interactions:** Atypica Rxns w/ ACEI—withhold 24 h prior to plasma administration **Labs:** ↑ Alkaline phosphatase; monitor Hmg, Hct, electrolytes, serum protein **NIPE:** Monitor BP & DC if hypotensive, monitor intake & output, admin to all blood types

Albuterol (Proventil, Ventolin, Volmax) **Uses:** *Asthma; prevent exercise-induced bronchospasm* **Action:** β-Adrenergic sympathomimetic bronchodilator; relaxes bronchial smooth muscle **Dose:** *Adults.* Inhaler: 2 inhal q4–6h PRN; 1 Rotacap inhaled q4–6h. *PO:* 2–4 mg PO tidóqid. *Neb:* 1.25–5 mg (0.25–1 mL of 0.5% soln in 2–3 mL of NS) tid-qid. *Peds.* Inhaler: 2 inhal q4–6h. *PO.* 0.1–0.2 mg/kg/dose PO; max 2–4 mg PO tid; *Neb:* 0.05 mg/kg (max 2.5 mg) in 2–3 mL of NS tid–qid **Caution:** [C, +] **Supplied:** Tabs 2, 4 mg; XR tabs 4, 8 mg syrup 2 mg/5 mL; 90 (18 µg)/dose met-dose inhaler; Rotacaps 200 µg; soln for neb 0.083, 0.5% **SE:** Palpitations, tachycardia, nervousness, GI upset **Interactions:** ↑ Effects w/ other sympathomimetics; ↑ CV effects w/ MAOI, TCA, inhaled anesthetics; ↓ effects w/ BBs; ↑ effectiveness of insulin, oral hypoglycemics, digoxin **Labs:** Transient ↑ in serum glucose after inhalation; transient ↓ K+ after inhalation **NIPE:** Monitor HR, BP, ABGs, s&s bronchospasm & CNS stimulation; instruct on use of inhaler, must use as 1st inhaler, & rinse mouth after use

Albuterol & Ipratropium (Combivent) **Uses:** *COPD* **Action:** Combination of β-adrenergic bronchodilator & quaternary anticholinergic compound **Dose:** 2 inhal qid **Caution:** [C, +] **Contra:** Allergy to peanut/soybean **Supplied:** Met-dose inhaler, 18 µg ipratropium/103 µg albuterol/puff **SE:** Palpitations, tachycardia, nervousness, GI upset, dizziness, blurred vision **Interactions:** ↑ Effects w/ anticholinergics, including ophthalmic meds; ↓ effects w/ herb jaborand tree, pill-bearing spurge **NIPE:** See Albuterol; may cause transient blurre vision/irritation or urinary changes

Aldesleukin [IL-2] (Proleukin) **WARNING:** Use restricted to Pts w normal pulmonary & cardiac Fxn **Uses:** *Metastatic RCC, melanoma* **Action:**

cts via IL-2 receptor; numerous immunomodulatory effects **Dose:** 600,000 IU/kg ˙h × 14 doses (FDA-approved dose/schedule for RCC). Multiple cont inf & alter˙te schedules (including "high dose" using 24 × 10⁶ IU/m² IV q8h on days 1–5 & ˙–16) **Caution:** [C, ?/–] **Contra:** Organ allografts **Supplied:** Inj 1.1 mg/mL (22 × ˙⁶ IU) **SE:** Flu-like syndrome (malaise, fever, chills), N/V/D, ↑ bilirubin; capil˙ry leak syndrome w/ ↓ BP, pulmonary edema, fluid retention, & weight gain; ˙nal toxicity & mild hematologic toxicity (anemia, thrombocytopenia, leukope˙a) & secondary eosinophilia; cardiac toxicity (myocardial ischemia, atrial ar˙ythmias); neurologic toxicity (CNS depression, somnolence, rarely coma, ˙lirium). Pruritic rashes, urticaria, & erythroderma common. **Notes:** Cont inf Rx ˙ss likely to cause severe hypotension & fluid retention **Interactions:** May ↑ toxi˙y of cardiotoxic, hepatotoxic, myelotoxic, & nephrotoxic drugs; ↑ hypotension ˙ antihypertensive drugs; ↓ effects w/ corticosteroids; acute Rxn w/ iodinated ˙ntrast media up to several months after inf; CNS effects w/ psychotropics **Labs:** ˙ay cause ↑ alkaline phosphatase, bilirubin, BUN, SCr, LFTs. **NIPE:** Thoroughly ˙plain serious SE of drug & that some SE are expected; ⊘ NSAIDs, ASA

┃efacept (Amevive) **WARNING:** Must monitor CD4 before each dose; ˙hold if <250; DC if <250 × 1 month **Uses:** *Moderate/severe chronic plaque ˙oriasis* **Action:** Fusion protein inhibitor **Dose:** 7.5 mg IV or 15 mg IM once ˙eekly × 12 wk **Caution:** [B, ?/–] PRG registry; associated w/ serious infections ˙ontra:** Lymphopenia **Supplied:** 7.5-, 15-mg vials **SE:** Pharyngitis, myalgia, inj ˙e Rxn, malignancy **Notes:** IV or IM different formulations; may repeat course 12 ˙k later if CD4 acceptable **Interactions:** No studies performed **Labs:** Monitor ˙BCs, CD4+ T lymphocyte counts **NIPE:** ↑ Risk of infection; ⊘ exposure to in˙ctions; inj site inflammation; rotate sites

┃lendronate (Fosamax) **Uses:** *Rx & prevention of osteoporosis, Rx of ˙eroid-induced osteoporosis & Paget's Dz* **Action:** ↓ Normal & abnormal bone ˙sorption **Dose:** *Osteoporosis: Rx:* 10 mg/d PO or 70 mg qwk. *Steroid-induced os˙oporosis: Rx:* 5 mg/d PO. *Prevention:* 5 mg/d PO or 35 mg qwk. *Paget's Dz:* 40 ˙g/d PO **Caution:** [C, ?] ⊘ if CrCl <35 mL/min; w/ NSAID use **Contra:** Abnor˙alities of the esophagus, inability to sit or stand upright for 30 min, hypocalcemia ˙upplied:** Tabs 5, 10, 35, 40, 70 mg **SE:** GI disturbances, HA, pain **Notes:** Take ˙st thing in AM w/ water (8 oz) > 30 min before 1st food/beverage of the day. ⊘ Lie ˙own for 30 min after. Adequate Ca²⁺ & vitamin D suppl necessary **Interactions:** ↓ Absorption w/ antacids, Ca suppls, Fe, food; ↑ risk of upper GI bleed w/ ASA & ˙SAIDs **Labs:** May cause transient ↑ serum Ca & phosphate **NIPE:** Adequate Ca ˙ vitamin D suppl needed, ↑ weight-bearing activity, ↓ smoking, EtOH use

┃lfentanil (Alfenta) [C-II] **Uses:** *Adjunct in the maint of anesthesia; ˙nalgesia* **Action:** Short-acting narcotic analgesic **Dose:** *Adults & Peds >12 y.* ˙–75 μg/kg IV inf; total depends on duration of procedure **Caution:** [C, +/–] ↑ ˙CP, resp depression **Supplied:** Inj 500 μg/mL **SE:** Bradycardia, hypotension, cardiac arrhythmias, peripheral vasodilation, ↑ ICP, drowsiness, resp depression **Interactions:** ↓ Effect w/ phenothiazines; ↑ effects w/ BBs, CNS depressants, erythromycin **NIPE:** Monitor HR, BP, resp rate

Alfuzosin (Uroxatral) **WARNING:** May prolong QTc interval **Uses:** *Benign prostatic hypertrophy* **Action:** α-Blocker **Dose:** 10 mg PO daily immediately after the same meal **Caution:** [B, –] **Contra:** Concomitant CYP3A4 inhibitors; moderate/severe hepatic impairment **Supplied:** Tabs 10 mg **SE:** Postural hypotension, dizziness, HA, fatigue **Notes:** XR tablet–⊘ cut or crush; fewest reports of ejaculatory disorders compared w/ other drugs in class **Interactions:** ↑ Effects w/ atenolol, azole antifungals, cimetidine, ritonavir; ↑ effects of antihypertensives **NIPE:** Not indicated for use in women or children; take w/ food; ↑ risk of postural hypotension; ⊘ take other meds that prolong QT interval

Alginic Acid + Aluminum Hydroxide & Magnesium Trisilicate (Gaviscon) [OTC] **Uses:** *Heartburn*; pain from hiatal hernia **Action:** Forms protective layer to block gastric acid **Dose:** 2–4 tabs or 15–30 mL PO qid followed by water; caution in renal impairment or w/ Na-restricted diet **Supplied:** Tabs, susp **SE:** Diarrhea, constipation **Interactions:** ↓ Absorption of tetracyclines

Allopurinol (Zyloprim, Lopurin, Alloprim) **Uses:** *Gout, hyperuricemia of malignancy, & uric acid urolithiasis* **Action:** Xanthine oxidase inhibitor; ↓ uric acid production **Dose:** *Adults. PO:* Initial 100 mg/d; usual 300 mg/d; max 800 mg/d. *IV:* 200–400 mg/m²/d (max 600 mg/24 h) (take after meal w/ plenty of fluid). *Peds.* Use only for treating hyperuricemia of malignancy in <10 y 10 mg/kg/24 h PO or 200 mg/m²/d IV ÷ q6–8h (max 600 mg/24 h); ↓ in renal impairment **Caution:** [C, M] **Supplied:** Tabs 100, 300 mg; inj 500 mg/30 mL (Alloprim) **SE:** Skin rash, N/V, renal impairment, angioedema **Notes:** Aggravates acute gout; begin after acute resolves; IV dose of 6 mg/mL final conc as single daily inf or ÷ 6-, 8-, or 12-h intervals **Interactions:** ↑ Effect of theophylline, oral anticoagulants; ↑ hypersensitivity Rxns w/ ACEIs, thiazide diuretics; ↑ risk of rash w/ ampicillin/amoxicillin; ↑ bone marrow depression w/ cyclophosphamide, azathioprine, mercaptopurine; ↓ effects w/ EtOH **Labs:** ↑ Alkaline phosphatase, bilirubin, LFTs **NIPE:** ↑ fluids to 2–3 L/day, take pc, may ↑ drowsiness

Almotriptan (Axert) See Table 11, page 283

Alosetron (Lotronex) **WARNING:** Serious GI side effects, some fatal, including ischemic colitis, have been reported. May be prescribed only through participation in the prescribing program for Lotronex **Uses:** *Severe diarrhea-predominant IBS in women who have failed conventional therapy* **Action:** Selective 5-HT₃ receptor antagonist **Dose:** *Adults.* 1 mg PO qd × 4 wk; titrate to max of 1 mg bid; DC after 4 wk at max dose if IBS Sxs not controlled **Caution:** [B, ?/–] **Contra:** Hx chronic or severe constipation, GI obstruction, strictures, toxic megacolon, GI perforation, adhesions, ischemic colitis, Crohn's Dz, ulcerative colitis, diverticulitis, thrombophlebitis, or hypercoagulable state. **Supplied:** Tabs 1 m

Alprostadil, Intracavernosal

31

SE: Constipation, abdominal pain, nausea **Notes:** DC immediately if constipation or Sxs of ischemic colitis develop; must sign a Pt agreement/informed consent prior to use. **Interactions:** ↑ Risk constipation w/ other drugs that ↓ GI motility, inhibits *N*-acetyltransferase & may influence metabolism of INH, procainamide, hydralazine **NIPE:** Administer w/o regard to food, eval effectiveness >4 w

Alpha₁-Protease Inhibitor (Prolastin) **Uses:** *α₁-Antitrypsin deficiency*; panacinar emphysema **Action:** Replace human α₁-protease inhibitor **Dose:** 60 mg/kg IV once/wk **Caution:** [C, ?] **Contra:** Selective IgA deficiencies w/ known IgA antibodies **Supplied:** Inj 500 mg/20 mL, 1000 mg/40 mL **SE:** Fever, dizziness, flu-like Sxs, allergic Rxns **NIPE:** Infuse over 30 min, ⊘ mix w/ other drugs, use w/in 3 h of reconstitution

Alprazolam (Xanax) [C-IV] **Uses:** *Anxiety & panic disorders,* anxiety w/ depression **Action:** Benzodiazepine; antianxiety agent **Dose:** *Anxiety:* Initially, 0.25–0.5 mg tid; ↑ to a max of 4 mg/d in ÷ doses. *Panic:* Initially, 0.5 mg tid; may gradually ↑ to desired response; ↓ dose in elderly, debilitated, & hepatic impairment **Caution:** [D, –] **Contra:** Narrow-angle glaucoma, concomitant itra-/ketoconazole **Supplied:** Tabs 0.25, 0.5, 1, 2 mg; soln 1 mg/1 mL **SE:** Drowsiness, fatigue, irritability, memory impairment, sexual dysfunction **Notes:** ⊘ abrupt discontinuation after prolonged use **Interactions:** ↑ CNS depression w/ EtOH, other CNS depressants, narcotics, MAOIs, anesthetics, antihistamines, theophylline, & herbs: kava kava, valerian; ↑ effect w/ oral contraceptives, cimetidine, INH, disulfiram, omeprazole, valproic acid, ciprofloxacin, erythromycin, clarithromycin, phenytoin, verapamil, grapefruit juice; ↑ risk of ketoconazole, itraconazole, & digitalis toxicity, ↓ effectiveness of levodopa; ↓ effect w/ carbamazepine, rifampin, rifabutin, barbiturates, cigarette smoking **Labs:** ↑ Alkaline phosphatase, may cause ↓ Hct & neutropenia **NIPE:** Monitor for resp depression

Alprostadil [Prostaglandin E₁] (Prostin VR) **Uses:** *Any state in which blood flow must be maintained through the ductus arteriosus* to sustain either pulmonary or systemic circulation until surgery can be performed (eg, pulmonary atresia, pulmonary stenosis, tricuspid atresia, transposition, severe tetralogy of Fallot) **Action:** Vasodilator, plt aggregation inhibitor; smooth muscle of the ductus arteriosus is especially sensitive **Dose:** 0.05 µg/kg/min IV; ↓ dose to lowest that maintains response **Caution:** [X, –] **Contra:** Neonatal resp distress syndrome **Supplied:** Injectable forms **SE:** Cutaneous vasodilation, Sz-like activity, jitteriness, ↑ temp, hypocalcemia, apnea, thrombocytopenia, ↓ BP; may cause apnea **Notes:** Keep intubation kit at bedside if Pt is not intubated **Interactions:** ↑ effects of anticoagulants & antihypertensives, ↓ effects of cyclosporine **Labs:** ↓ fibrinogen **NIPE:** Dilute drug before administration, refrigerate & discard >24 h, apnea & bradycardia indicates drug overdose, central line preferred, flushing indicates catheter malposition

Alprostadil, Intracavernosal (Caverject, Edex) **Uses:** *Erectile dysfunction* **Action:** Relaxes smooth muscles, dilates cavernosal arteries, ↑s lacu-

nar spaces & entrapment of blood by compressing venules against tunica albuginea
Dose: 2.5–60 μg intracavernosal; adjusted to individual **Caution:** [X, –] **Contra:**
Conditions predisposing to priapism; anatomic deformities of the penis; penile implants; men in whom sexual activity is inadvisable **Supplied:** *Caverject:* 6–10 or
6–20 μg vials w/wo diluent syringes. *Caverject Impulse:* Self-contained syringe
(29 gauge) 10 & 20 μg. *Edex:* 5, 10, 20, 40 μg vials w/ syringes **SE:** Local pain w/
inj **Notes:** Counsel Pts about possible priapism, penile fibrosis, & hematoma;
titrate dose at health care provider's office **Interactions:** ↑ Effects of anticoagulants & antihypertensives, ↓ effects of cyclosporine **Labs:** ↓ Fibrinogen **NIPE:**
Vaginal itching and burning in female partners, ⊘ inj >3×/wk or closer than 24
h/dose

Alprostadil, Urethral Suppository (Muse) Uses: *Erectile dysfunction* **Action:** Alprostadil (PGE₁) absorbed through urethral mucosa; vasodilator & smooth muscle relaxant of corpus cavernosa **Dose:** 125–1000 μg system
5–10 min prior to sexual activity **Caution:** [X, –] **Contra:** Conditions predisposing
to priapism; anatomic deformities of the penis; penile implants; men in whom sexual activity is inadvisable **Supplied:** 125, 250, 500, 1000 μg w/ a transurethral delivery system **SE:** ↓ BP, dizziness, syncope, penile pain, testicular pain, urethral
burning/bleeding, priapism **Notes:** Dose titration under health care provider's supervision **Interactions:** ↑ effects of anticoagulants & antihypertensives, ↓ effects
of cyclosporine **Labs:** ↓ Fibrinogen; **NIPE:** No more than 2 supp/24 h, urinate
prior to use

Alteplase, Recombinant [tPA] (Activase) Uses: *AMI, PE, acute
ischemic stroke, & CV cath occlusion* **Action:** Thrombolytic; initiates local fibrinolysis by binding to fibrin in the thrombus **Dose:** *AMI & PE:* 100 mg IV over 3
(10 mg over 2 min, then 50 mg over 1 h, then 40 mg over 2 h). *Stroke:* 0.9 mg/kg
(max 90 mg) inf over 60 min. *Cath occlusion:* 10–29 kg 1 mg/mL, ≥30 kg 2
mg/mL **Caution:** [C, ?] **Contra:** Active internal bleeding; uncontrolled HTN (systolic BP = 185 mm Hg/diastolic = 110 mm Hg); recent (w/in 3 mo) CVA, GI bleed,
trauma, surgery, prolonged internal cardiac massage; intracranial neoplasm, suspected aortic dissection, AVM/aneurysm, bleeding diathesis, hemostatic defects, S
at the time of stroke, suspicion of subarachnoid hemorrhage **Supplied:** Powder fo
inj 50, 100 mg **SE:** Bleeding, bruising (especially from venipuncture sites), hypotension **Notes:** Give heparin to prevent reocclusion; in AMI doses of >150 mg
associated w/ intracranial bleeding **Interactions:** ↑ Risk of bleeding w/ heparin,
ASA, NSAIDs, abciximab, dipyridamole, eptifibatide, tirofiban; ↓ effects w/ nitroglycerine **Labs:** ↓ Fibrinogen **NIPE:** Compress venipuncture site at least 30 min,
monitor PT/PTT, bed rest during inf

Altretamine (Hexalen) Uses: *Epithelial ovarian CA* **Action:** Unknown; cytotoxic agent, possibly alkylating agent; inhibits nucleotide incorporation into DNA/RNA **Dose:** 260 mg/m²/d in 4 ÷ doses for 14–21 d of a 28-d R
cycle; dose ↑ to 150 mg/m²/d for 14 d in multiagent regimens (see specific proto

ls) Caution: [D, ?/–]. Contra: Preexisting BM depression or neurologic toxicity upplied: Caps 50, 100 mg SE: Vomiting, diarrhea, & cramps; neurologic (periph- al neuropathy, CNS depression); minimally myelosuppressive Interactions: ↓ ffect w/ phenobarbital, ↓ antibody response w/ live virus vaccines, ↑ risk of toxi- ty w/ cimetidine & hypotension w/ MAOIs, ↑ bone marrow depression w/ radia- on Labs: ↑ Alkaline phosphatase, BUN, & SCr NIPE: Use barrier contraception, ke w/ food, monitor CBC

Aluminum Hydroxide (Amphojel, AlternaGEL) [OTC] Uses:
Relief of heartburn, upset or sour stomach, or acid indigestion*; suppl to Rx of yperphosphatemia Action: Neutralizes gastric acid; binds phosphate Dose: dults. 10–30 mL or 2 tabs PO q4–6h. Peds. 5–15 mL PO q4–6h or 50–150 g/kg/24 h PO q4–6h (hyperphosphatemia) Caution: [C, ?] Supplied: Tabs 300, 00 mg; chew tabs 500 mg; susp 320, 600 mg/5 mL SE: constipation Notes: OK in enal failure Interactions: ↓ Absorption & effects of allopurinol, benzodiazepines, orticosteroids, chloroquine, cimetidine, digoxin, INH, phenytoin, quinolones, ran- idine, tetracycline Labs: ↑ Serum gastrin, ↓ serum phosphate NIPE: Separate ther drug administration by 2 h, ↑ effectiveness of liquid form

Aluminum Hydroxide + Magnesium Carbonate (Gaviscon) [OTC] Uses: *Relief of heartburn, acid indigestion* Action: Neutralizes gastric cid Dose: Adults. 15–30 mL PO pc & hs. Peds. 5–15 mL PO qid or PRN; ⊘ in enal impairment Caution: [C, ?] Supplied: Liq w/ Al hydroxide 95 mg + Mg car- onate 358 mg/15 mL SE: May cause ↑ Mg²⁺ (w/ renal insufficiency), constipa- ion, diarrhea Notes: Doses qid are best given pc & hs; may affect absorption of ome drugs Interactions: In addition to Al hydroxide ↓ effects of histamine block- rs, hydantoins, nitrofurantoin, phenothiazines, ticlopidine, ↑ effects of quinidine, ulfonylureas NIPE: ⊘ Concurrent drug use & separate by 2 h, ↑ fiber

Aluminum Hydroxide + Magnesium Hydroxide (Maalox) [OTC] Uses: *Hyperacidity* (peptic ulcer, hiatal hernia, etc) Action: Neutral- zes gastric acid Dose: Adults. 10–60 mL or 2–4 tabs PO qid or PRN. Peds. 5–15 mL PO qid or PRN Caution: [C, ?] Supplied: Tabs, susp SE: May cause ↑ Mg²⁺ n renal insufficiency, constipation, diarrhea Notes: Doses best given pc & hs Interactions: In addition to Al hydroxide, ↓ effects of digoxin, quinolines, pheny- oin, Fe suppl, and ketoconazole NIPE: ⊘ Concurrent drug use; separate by 2 h

Aluminum Hydroxide + Magnesium Hydroxide + Sime- thicone (Mylanta, Mylanta II, Maalox Plus) [OTC] Uses: *Hy- peracidity w/ bloating* Action: Neutralizes gastric acid & defoaming Dose: Adults. 10–60 mL or 2–4 tabs PO qid or PRN. Peds. 5–15 mL PO qid or PRN; ⊘ n renal impairment Caution: [C, ?] Supplied: Tabs, susp SE: Hypermagnesemia n renal insufficiency, diarrhea, constipation Notes: Mylanta II contains twice the Al & Mg hydroxide of Mylanta; may affect absorption of some drugs Interac- tions: In addition to Al hydroxide, ↓ effects of digoxin, quinolones, phenytoin, Fe suppl, and ketoconazole NIPE: ⊘ Concurrent drug use; separate by 2 h

Aluminum Hydroxide + Magnesium Trisilicate (Gaviscon Gaviscon-2) [OTC] Uses: *Relief of heartburn, upset or sour stomach, o acid indigestion* Action: Neutralizes gastric acid Dose: Chew 2–4 tabs qid; ⊘ i renal impairment Caution: [C, ?] Contra: Mg sensitivity Supplied: *Gaviscon:* A hydroxide 80 mg & Mg trisilicate 20 mg; *Gaviscon-2:* Al hydroxide 160 mg & M trisilicate 40 mg SE: Hypermagnesemia in renal insufficiency, constipation, diar rhea Notes: Concomitant administration may affect absorption of some drugs In teractions: In addition to Al hydroxide, ↓ effects of digoxin, quinolones phenytoin, Fe suppl, and ketoconazole NIPE: ⊘ Concurrent drug use; separate b 2 h

Amantadine (Symmetrel) Uses: *Rx or prophylaxis for influenza A viral infections, parkinsonism, & drug-induced EPS* Action: Prevents release o infectious viral nucleic acid into the host cell; releases dopamine from intac dopaminergic terminals Dose: *Adults. Influenza A:* 200 mg/d PO or 100 mg PC bid. *Parkinsonism:* 100 mg PO daily or bid. *Peds.1–9 y:* 4.4–8.8 mg/kg/24 h to 150 mg/24 h max ÷ doses qd–bid. *10–12 y:* 100–200 mg/d in 1–2 ÷ doses; reduce dose in renal impairment Caution: [C, M] Supplied: Caps 100 mg; tabs 100 mg; soln 50 mg/5 mL SE: Orthostatic hypotension, edema, insomnia, depression, irritabil ity, hallucinations, dream abnormalities Interactions: ↑ Effects w/ HCTZ, tri amterene, amiloride, pheasant's eye herb, scopolia root, benztropine Labs: ↑ BUN, SCr, CPK, alkaline phosphatase, bilirubin, LDH, AST, ALT NIPE: ⊘ Dis continue abruptly, take at least 4 h before sleep if insomnia occurs, eval for menta status changes, take w/ meals, ⊘ EtOH

Amifostine (Ethyol) Uses: *Xerostomia prophylaxis during RT (head & neck, ovarian, or non-small-cell lung CA). Reduces renal toxicity associated w/ re peated administration of cisplatin* Action: Prodrug, dephosphorylated by alkaline phosphatase to the pharmacologically active thiol metabolite Dose: 910 mg/m²/d as a 15-min IV inf 30 min prior to chemotherapy Caution: [C, +/–] Supplied: 500-mg vials of lyophilized drug w/ 500 mg of mannitol, reconstituted in sterile NS SE: Transient hypotension in >60%, N/V, flushing w/ hot or cold chills, dizzi ness, hypocalcemia, somnolence, & sneezing. Notes: Does not reduce the effec tiveness of cyclophosphamide plus cisplatin chemotherapy Interactions: ↑ Effects w/ antihypertensives Labs: ↓ Calcium levels NIPE: Monitor BP, ensure adequate hydration, infuse over 15 min w/Pt supine

Amikacin (Amikin) Uses: *Serious infections caused by gram(–) bacteria & mycobacteria* Action: Aminoglycoside antibiotic; inhibits protein synthesis *Spectrum:* Good gram(–) bacterial coverage including *Pseudomonas* sp; *Mycobac terium* sp Dose: *Adults & Peds.* 5–7.5 mg/kg/dose ÷ q8–24h based on renal Fxn *Neonates <1200 g, 0–4 wk:* 7.5 mg/kg/dose q12h–18h. *Postnatal age <7 d, 1200–2000 g:* 7.5 mg/kg/dose q12h; *>2000 g:* 10 mg/kg/dose q12h. *Postnatal age >7 d, 1200–2000 g:* 7 mg/kg/dose q8h; *>2000 g:* 7.5–10 mg/kg/dose q8h Cau tion: [C, +/–] Supplied: Inj 100, 500 mg/2 mL SE: Nephrotoxicity, ototoxicity eurotoxicity; ⊘ use w/ potent diuretics **Notes:** May be effective against gram(−) acteria resistant to gentamicin & tobramycin; monitor renal Fxn carefully for osage adjustments; monitor serum levels (see Table 2, page 265) **Interactions:** ↑ isk of ototoxicity and nephrotoxicity w/ acyclovir, amphotericin B, ephalosporins, cisplatin, loop diuretics, methoxyflurane, polymyxin B, van-omycin; ↑ neuromuscular blocking effect w/ muscle relaxants & anesthetics **abs:** ↑ BUN, SCr, AST, ALT, serum alkaline phosphatase, bilirubin, LDH **NIPE:** Fluid consumption

Amiloride (Midamor) Uses: *HTN, CHF, & thiazide-induced hy-okalemia* **Action:** K-sparing diuretic; interferes w/ K⁺/Na⁺ exchange in distal ubules **Dose:** *Adults.* 5–10 mg PO qd. *Peds.* 0.625 mg/kg/d; ↓ dose in renal im-airment **Caution:** [B, ?] **Contra:** Hyperkalemia, SCr > 1.5, BUN > 30 **Supplied:** abs 5 mg **SE:** Hyperkalemia possible; monitor serum K⁺ levels; HA, dizziness, ehydration, impotence **Interactions:** ↑ Risk of hyperkalemia w/ ACE-I, K-spar-ng diuretics, NSAIDs, & K salt substitutes; ↑ effects of Li, digoxin, antihypertens-ives, amantadine; ↑ risk of hypokalemia w/ licorice **NIPE:** Take w/ food, I&O, aily weights, ⊘ salt substitutes, bananas, & oranges

Aminocaproic Acid (Amicar) Uses: *Excessive bleeding from systemic yperfibrinolysis & urinary fibrinolysis* **Action:** Inhibits fibrinolysis via inhibition f tPA substances **Dose:** *Adults.* 5 g IV or PO (1st h) followed by 1–1.25 g/h IV or O. *Peds.* 100 mg/kg IV (1st h) (max dose/d: 30 g), then 1 g/m²/h; max 18 g/m²/d; in renal failure **Caution:** [C, ?] Hematuria of upper urinary tract **Contra:** Dis-eminated intravascular coagulation **Supplied:** Tabs 500 mg; syrup 250 mg/mL; nj 250 mg/mL **SE:** ↓ BP, bradycardia, dizziness, HA, fatigue, rash, GI distur-ance, ↓ plt Fxn **Notes:** Administer for 8 h or until bleeding is controlled; not for pper urinary tract bleeding **Interactions:** ↑ Coagulation w/ estrogens & oral con-raceptives **Labs:** ↑ K⁺ levels, false ↑ urine amino acids **NIPE:** Creatine kinase nonitoring w/ long-term use, eval for thrombophlebitis & difficulty urinating

Amino-Cerv pH 5.5 Cream Uses: *Mild cervicitis,* postpartum cer-vicitis/cervical tears, postcauterization, postcryosurgery, & postconization **Action:** Hydrating agent; removes excess keratin in hyperkeratotic conditions **Dose:** 1 Ap-olicatorful intravaginally hs for 2–4 wk **Caution:** [C, ?] Use in viral skin infection **Supplied:** Vaginal cream **SE:** Transient stinging, local irritation **Notes:** AKA car-oamide or urea; contains 8.34% urea, 0.5% sodium propionate, 0.83% methionine, 0.35% cystine, 0.83% inositol, & benzalkonium chloride

Aminoglutethimide (Cytadren) Uses: Adrenocortical carcinoma, *Cushing's syndrome,* breast CA & CAP **Action:** Inhibits adrenal steroidogenesis & conversion of androgens to estrogens **Dose:** 750–1500 mg/d in ÷ doses plus hy-drocortisone 20–40 mg/d; ↓ dose in renal insufficiency **Caution:** [D, ?] **Supplied:** Tabs 250 mg **SE:** Adrenal insufficiency ("medical adrenalectomy"), hypothy-roidism, masculinization, hypotension, vomiting, rare hepatotoxicity, rash, myal-gia, fever **Interactions:** ↓ Effects w/ dexamethasone & hydrocortisone, ↓ effects of warfarin, theophylline, medroxyprogesterone **NIPE:** Masculinization reversible after DC drug, ⊘ PRG

Aminophylline
Uses: *Asthma, COPD* & bronchospasm **Action:** Relaxes smooth muscle of the bronchi, pulmonary blood vessels; stimulates diaphragm **Dose:** *Adults. Acute asthma:* Load 6 mg/kg IV, then 0.4–0.9 mg/kg/h IV cont inf. *Chronic asthma:* 24 mg/kg/24 h PO or PR ÷ q6h. *Peds.* Load 6 mg/kg IV, then 1 mg/kg/h IV cont inf; ↓ in hepatic insufficiency & w/ certain drugs (macrolide & quinolone antibiotics, cimetidine, & propranolol) **Caution:** [C, +] Uncontrolled arrhythmias, hyperthyroidism, peptic ulcers, uncontrolled Sz disorder **Supplied:** Tabs 100, 200 mg; soln 105 mg/5 mL; supp 250, 500 mg; inj 25 mg/mL **SE:** N/V, irritability, tachycardia, ventricular arrhythmias, & Szs **Notes:** Individualize dosage; follow serum levels (as theophylline, Table 2, page 265; aminophylline is about 85% theophylline; erratic absorption w/ rectal doses **Interactions:** ↓ Effects of Li, phenytoin, adenosine; ↓ effects w/ phenobarbital, aminoglutethamide, barbiturates, rifampin, ritonavir, thyroid meds; ↑ effects w/ cimetidine, ciprofloxacin, erythromycin, INH, oral contraceptives, verapamil, tobacco, charcoal-broiled foods, St. John's wort **Labs:** ↑ Uric acid levels, falsely ↑ levels w/ furosemide, probenecid, acetaminophen, coffee, tea, cola, chocolate **NIPE:** ⊘ Chew or crush time-released capsules & take on empty stomach, immediate release can be taken w/ food, ↑ fluids 2 L/d, tobacco ↑ drug elimination

Amiodarone (Cordarone, Pacerone)
Uses: *Recurrent VF or hemodynamically unstable VT,* supraventricular arrhythmias, AF **Action:** Class III antiarrhythmic **Dose:** *Adults. Ventricular arrhythmias: IV:* 15 mg/min for 10 min, then 1 mg/min for 6 h, then maint 0.5 mg/min cont. inf or *PO:* Load: 800–1600 mg/d PO for 1–3 wk. Maint: 600–800 mg/d PO for 1 mo, then 200–400 mg/d. *Supraventricular arrhythmias: IV:* 300 mg IV over 1 h, then 20 mg/kg for 24 h, then 600 mg PO qd for 1 wk, then maint 100–400 mg qd or *PO:* Load: 600–800 mg/d PO for 1–4 wk. Maint: Gradually ↓ to 100–400 mg q day. *Peds.* 10–15 mg/kg/24 h ÷ q12h PO for 7–10 d, then 5 mg/kg/24 h ÷ q12h or qd (infants/neonates require a higher loading dose); ↓ in severe liver insufficiency **Caution:** [D, –] **Contra:** Sinus node dysfunction, 2nd- or 3rd-degree AV block, sinus bradycardia (w/o pacemaker) **Supplied:** Tabs 200 mg; inj 50 mg/mL **SE:** Pulmonary fibrosis, exacerbation of arrhythmias, prolongs QT interval; CHF, arrhythmias, hypo-/hyperthyroidism, ↑ LFTs, liver failure, corneal microdeposits, optic neuropathy/neuritis, peripheral neuropathy, photosensitivity **Notes:** Half-life is 53 d; IV conc of >0.2 mg/mL administered via a central catheter; alters digoxin levels, may require reduced digoxin dose **Interactions:** ↑ Serum levels of digoxin, quinidine, procainamide, flecainide, phenytoin, warfarin, theophylline, cyclosporine; ↑ levels w/ cimetidine, indinavir, ritonavir; ↓ levels w/ cholestyramine, rifampin, St. John's wort; ↑ cardiac effects w/ BBs, CCB **Labs:** ↑ T_4 & RT_3, ANA titer, ↓ T_3 **NIPE:** Monitor cardiac rhythm, BP, LFTs, thyroid Fxn, ophthalmologic exam; ↑ photosensitivity—use sunscreen; take w/ food

Amitriptyline (Elavil) Uses: *Depression,* peripheral neuropathy, chronic pain, & tension HAs Action: TCA; inhibits reuptake of serotonin & norepinephrine by the presynaptic neurons Dose: *Adults.* Initially, 30–50 mg PO hs; may ↑ to 300 mg hs. *Peds.* ⊘ if <12 y unless for chronic pain; initially 0.1 mg/kg PO hs, advance over 2–3 wk to 0.5–2 mg/kg PO hs; caution in hepatic impairment; taper when discontinuing Caution: [D, +/–] Narrow-angle glaucoma Contra: W/ MAOIs, during acute recovery following MI Supplied: Tabs 10, 25, 50, 75, 100, 150 mg; inj 10 mg/mL SE: Strong anticholinergic SEs; OD may be fatal; urine retention & sedation, ECG changes, photosensitivity Interactions: ↓ Dffects w/ carbamazepine, phenobarbital, rifampin, cholestyramine, colestipol, tobacco; ↑ effects w/ cimetidine, quinidine, indinavir, ritonavir, CNS depressants, SSRIs, haloperidol, oral contraceptives, BBs, phenothiazines, EtOH, evening primrose oil; ↑ effects of amphetamines, anticholinergics, epinephrine, hypoglycemics, phenylephrine Labs: ↑ Glucose, false ↑ carbamazepine levels NIPE: ↑ photosensitivity—use sunscreen, appetite, & craving for sweets, ⊘ DC abruptly, may turn urine blue-green

Amlodipine (Norvasc) Uses: *HTN & stable or unstable angina* Action: CCB; relaxes coronary vascular smooth muscle Dose: 2.5–10 mg/d PO Caution: [C, ?] Supplied: Tabs 2.5, 5, 10 mg SE: Peripheral edema, HA, palpitations, flushing Notes: May be taken w/out regard to meals

Amlodipine/Atorvastatin (Caduet) Uses: * HTN, chronic stable angina, vasospastic angina, control ↑d cholesterol & triglycerides* Action: CCB & HMG-CoA reductase inhibitor Dose: Amlodipine 5–10 mg PO daily/ Atorvastatin 10–80 mg PO daily Caution: [X, –] Contra: Active liver Dz, unexplained elevation of serum transaminases Supplied: Tabs amlodipine/atorvastatin: 5/10, 5/20, 5/40, 5/80, 10/10, 10/20, 10/40, 10/80 mg SE: Peripheral edema, HA, palpitations, flushing, myopathy, arthralgia, myalgia, GI upset Interactions: ↑ Hypotension w/ fentanyl, nitrates, EtOH, quinidine, other antihypertensives, grapefruit juice; ↑ effects w/ diltiazem, erythromycin, H₂ blockers, proton pump inhibitors, quinidine; ↓ effects w/ NSAIDs, barbiturates, rifampin Labs: Monitor LFTs NIPE: ⊘ DC abruptly, ↑ photosensitivity—use sunscreen

Ammonium Aluminum Sulfate [Alum] [OTC] Uses: *Hemorrhagic cystitis when bladder irrigation fails* Action: Astringent Dose: 1–2% soln used w/ constant bladder irrigation w/ NS Caution: [+/–] Supplied: Powder for reconstitution SE: Encephalopathy possible; obtain Al levels, especially in renal insufficiency; can precipitate & occlude catheters Notes: Safe to use w/out anesthesia & w/ vesicoureteral reflux

Amoxicillin (Amoxil, Polymox) Uses: *Ear, nose, & throat, lower resp, skin, urinary tract infections resulting from susceptible gram(+) bacteria (streptococci) & gram(–) bacteria (H. influenzae, E. coli, P. mirabilis), H. pylori,* endocarditis prophylaxis Action: β-Lactam antibiotic; inhibits cell wall synthesis from Spectrum: Gram(+) including Streptococcus sp, Enterococcus sp; some gram(−) including *H. influenzae, E. coli, N. gonorrhoeae,* & *P. mirabilis* **Dose: Adults.** 250–500 mg PO tid or 500–875 mg bid. **Peds.** 25–100 mg/kg/24 h PO ÷ q8h. 200–400 mg PO bid (equivalent to 125–250 mg tid); ↓ dose in renal impairment **Caution:** [B, +] **Supplied:** Caps 250, 500 mg; chew tabs 125, 200, 250, 400 mg; susp 50 mg/mL, 125, 250 mg/5 mL; tabs 500, 875 mg **SE:** Diarrhea; skin rash common **Notes:** Cross-hypersensitivity w/ penicillin; many hospital strains of *E. coli*-resistant **Interactions:** ↑ Effects of warfarin, ↑ effects w/ probenecid, disulfiram, ↑ risk of rash w/ allopurinol, ↓ effects of oral contraceptives, ↓ effects w/ tetracyclines, chloramphenicol **Labs:** ↑ Serum alkaline phosphatase, LDH, LFTs, false + direct Coombs test **NIPE:** Space meds over 24/h, eval for superinfection, use barrier contraception

Amoxicillin & Clavulanic Acid (Augmentin, Augmentin 600 ES, Augmentin XR)

Uses: *Ear, lower resp, sinus, urinary tract, skin infections caused by β-lactamase-producing *H. influenzae, S. aureus,* & *E. coli** **Action:** Combination of a β-lactam antibiotic & a β-lactamase inhibitor. *Spectrum:* Gram(+) coverage same as amoxicillin alone, MSSA; gram(−) coverage as w/ amoxicillin alone, β-lactamase-producing *H. influenzae, Klebsiella* sp, *M. catarrhalis* **Dose: Adults.** 250–500 mg PO q8h or 875 mg q12h; XR 2000 mg PO q12h. **Peds.** 20–40 mg/kg/d as amoxicillin PO ÷ q8h or 45 mg/kg/d ÷ q12h; ↓ in renal impairment (take w/ food) **Caution:** [B, ?] **Supplied** (expressed as amoxicillin/clavulanic acid): Tabs 250/125, 500/125, 875/125 mg; chew tabs 125/31.25, 200/28.5, 250/62.5, 400/57 mg; susp 125/31.25, 250/62.5, 200/28.5, 400/57 mg/5 mL; 600-ES 600/42.9 mg tab; XR tab 1000/62.5 mg **SE:** Abdominal discomfort, N/V/D, allergic Rxn, vaginitis **Notes:** ⊘ Substitute two 250-mg tabs for one 500-mg tab or an OD of clavulanic acid will occur **Interactions:** ↑ Effects of warfarin, ↑ effects w/ probenecid, disulfiram, ↑ risk of rash w/ allopurinol, ↓ effects of oral contraceptives, ↓ effects w/ tetracyclines, chloramphenicol **Labs:** ↑ Serum alkaline phosphatase, LDH, LFTs, false + direct Coombs' test **NIPE:** Space meds over 24/h, eval for superinfection, use barrier contraception

Amphotericin B (Fungizone)

Uses: *Severe, systemic fungal infections; oral & cutaneous candidiasis* **Action:** Binds ergosterol in the fungal membrane, altering membrane permeability **Dose: Adults & Peds.** 1 mg adults or 0.1 mg/kg to 1 mg in children, then 0.25–1.5 mg/kg/24 h IV over 2–6 h (range 25–50 mg/d or qod). Total dose varies w/ indication. *PO:* 1 mL qid. *Topical:* Apply bid–qid for 1–4 wk depending on infection; ↓ dose in renal impairment **Caution:** [B, ?] **Supplied:** Powder for inj 50 mg/vial; PO susp 100 mg/mL; cream, lotion, oint 3% **SE:** Reduced K+/Mg2+ from renal wasting; anaphylaxis reported **Notes:** Monitor renal Fxn/LFTs; pretreatment w/ APAP & antihistamines (Benadryl) minimizes adverse effects w/ IV inf (eg, fever, chills, HA, nephrotoxicity, hypotension anemia) **Interactions:** ↑ Nephrotoxic effects w/ antineoplastics, cyclosporine furosemide, vancomycin, aminoglycosides, ↑ hypokalemia w/ corticosteroids skeletal muscle relaxants **Labs:** ↑ Serum bilirubin, serum cholesterol **NIPE:** Monitor CNS effects & ⊘ take hs; topical cream discolors skin

Amphotericin B Cholesteryl (Amphotec)
Uses: *Aspergillosis in Pts intolerant or refractory to conventional amphotericin B,* systemic candidiasis **Action:** Binds sterols in the cell membrane, alters membrane permeability **Dose: Adults & Peds.** Test dose 1.6–8.3 mg, over 15–20 min, then 3–4 mg/kg/d; 1 mg/kg/h inf; ↓ in renal insufficiency **Caution:** [B, ?] **Supplied:** Powder for inj 50 mg, 100 mg/vial (final conc 0.6 mg/mL) **SE:** Anaphylaxis reported; fever, chills, HA, ↓ K⁺, ↓ Mg²⁺, nephrotoxicity, ↓ BP, anemia **Notes:** ⊘ Use in-line filter; monitor LFT & electrolytes **Interactions:** See Amphotericin B

Amphotericin B Lipid Complex (Abelcet)
Uses: *Refractory invasive fungal infection in Pts intolerant to conventional amphotericin B* **Action:** Binds sterols in cell membrane, alters membrane permeability **Dose: Adults & Peds.** 5 mg/kg/d IV as a single daily dose; 2.5 mg/kg/h inf **Caution:** [B, ?] **Supplied:** Inj 5 mg/mL **SE:** Anaphylaxis reported; fever, chills, HA, ↓ K⁺, ↓ Mg²⁺, nephrotoxicity, hypotension, anemia **Notes:** Filter soln w/ a 5-mm filter needle; ⊘ mix in electrolyte-containing solns; if inf >2 h, manually mix bag **Interactions:** See Amphotericin B

Amphotericin B Liposomal (AmBisome)
Uses: *Refractory invasive fungal infection in Pts intolerant to conventional amphotericin B, cryptococcal meningitis in HIV, empiric Rx for febrile neutropenia, visceral leishmaniasis* **Action:** Binds to sterols in the cell membrane, results in changes in membrane permeability **Dose: Adults & Peds.** 3–5 mg/kg/d, inf 60–120 min; ↓ in renal insufficiency **Caution:** [B, ?] **Supplied:** Powder for inj 50 mg **SE:** Anaphylaxis reported; fever, chills, HA, ↓ K⁺, ↓ Mg²⁺ nephrotoxicity, hypotension, anemia **Notes:** Filter w/no less than 1-μm filter **Interactions:** See Amphotericin B

Ampicillin (Amcill, Omnipen)
Uses: *Resp tract, GU tract, GI tract infections & meningitis due to susceptible gram(−) & gram(+) bacteria; endocarditis prophylaxis* **Action:** β-Lactam antibiotic; inhibits cell wall synthesis. *Spectrum:* Gram(+) coverage, including *Streptococcus* sp, *Staphylococcus* sp, *Listeria;* gram(−) coverage, including *Klebsiella* sp, *E. coli, H. influenzae, P. mirabilis, Shigella* sp, *Salmonella* sp **Dose: Adults.** 500 mg–2 g IM or IV q6h or 250–500 mg PO q6h. **Peds.** *Neonates <7 d:* 50–100 mg/kg/24 h IV ÷ q8h. *Term infants:* 75–150 mg/kg/24 h ÷ q6–8h IV or PO. *Children >1 mo:* 100–200 mg/kg/24 h ÷ q4–6h IM or IV; 50–100 mg/kg/24 h ÷ q6h PO up to 250 mg/dose. *Meningitis:* 200–400 mg/kg/24 h ÷ q4–6h IV; ↓ in renal impairment (take on an empty stomach) **Caution:** [B, M] Cross-hypersensitivity w/ penicillin **Supplied:** Caps 250, 500 mg; susp 100 mg/mL (reconstituted as drops), 125 mg/5 mL, 250 mg/5 mL, 500 mg/5 mL; powder for inj 125 mg, 250 mg, 500 mg, 1 g, 2 g, 10 g/vial **SE:** Diarrhea, skin rash, allergic Rxn **Notes:** Many strains of *E. coli* now resistant **Interactions:** ↓ Effects of oral contraceptives & atenolol, ↓ effects w/ chloramphenicol,

erythromycin, tetracycline, & food; ↑ effects of anticoagulants & MRX; ↑ risk of rash w/ allopurinol; ↑ effects w/ probenecid & disulfiram **Labs:** ↑ LFTs, serum protein, serum theophylline, serum uric acid; ↓ serum estrogen, serum cholesterol, serum folate; false + direct Coombs' test, urine glucose, & urine amino acids **NIPE:** Take on empty stomach & around the clock; may cause candidal vaginitis; use barrier contraception

Ampicillin–Sulbactam (Unasyn) Uses: *Gynecologic, intraabdominal, skin infections caused by β-lactamase-producing strains of *S. aureus, Enterococcus, H. influenzae, P. mirabilis,* & *Bacteroides* sp* **Action:** Combination of a β-lactam antibiotic & a β-lactamase inhibitor. *Spectrum:* Gram(+) coverage as ampicillin alone, gram(–) coverage as ampicillin alone; also *Enterobacter, Acinetobacter, Bacteroides* **Dose:** *Adults.* 1.5–3 g IM or IV q6h. *Peds.* 100–200 mg ampicillin/kg/d (150–300 mg Unasyn) q6h; ↓ in renal failure **Caution:** [B, M] **Supplied:** Powder for inj 1.5, 3.0 g/vial **SE:** Hypersensitivity Rxns, rash, diarrhea, pain at inj site **Notes:** A 2:1 ratio of ampicillin:sulbactam **Interactions:** See Ampicillin

Amprenavir (Agenerase) WARNING: PO soln contra in children <4 y due to potential toxicity from large volume of excipient polypropylene glycol in the formulation Uses: *HIV infection* **Action:** Protease inhibitor; prevents the maturation of the virion to mature viral particle **Dose:** *Adults.* 1200 mg bid. *Peds.* 20 mg/kg bid or 15 mg/kg tid up to 2400 mg/d **Caution:** [C, ?] CDC recommends HIV-infected mothers not breast-feed due to risk of transmission of HIV to infant; previous allergic Rxn to sulfonamides **Contra:** CYP450 3A4 substrates (ergot derivatives, midazolam, triazolam, etc); soln < 4 y, PRG, hepatic or renal failure, disulfram, or metronidazole **Supplied:** Caps 50, 150 mg; soln 15 mg/mL **SE:** Life-threatening rash, hyperglycemia, hypertriglyceridemia, fat redistribution, N/V/D, depression **Notes:** Caps & soln contain vitamin E exceeding RDA intake amounts; ⊘ high-fat meals w/ administration; many drug interactions **Interactions:** ↑ Effects w/ abacavir, cimetidine, delavirdine, indinavir, itraconazole, ketoconazole, macrolides, ritonavir, zidovudine, grapefruit juice; ↑ effects of cisapride, clozapine, ergotamine, loratadine, nelfinavir, dapsone, pimozide, rifabutin, saquinavir, sildenafil, terfenadine, triazolam, warfarin, zidovudine, HMG-CoA reductase inhibitors; ↓ effects w/ antacids, barbiturates, carbamazepine, nevirapine, phenytoin, rifampin, St. John's wort, high-fat food; ↓ effects of oral contraceptives **Labs:** ↑ Serum glucose, cholesterol, & triglyceride levels **NIPE:** Use barrier contraception, may take w/ food other than high-fat food, ⊘ take vitamin E

Anakinra (Kineret) WARNING: Associated w/ ↑ incidence of serious infections; DC w/ serious infection Uses: *Reduce signs & Sxs of moderately to severely active RA, failed 1 or more Dz-modifying antirheumatic drugs* **Action:** Human IL-1 receptor antagonist **Dose:** 100 mg SQ qd **Caution:** [B, ?] **Contra:** Hypersensitivity to *E. coli*-derived proteins, active infection, <18 y **Supplied:** 100-mg prefilled syringes **SE:** Neutropenia especially when used w/ TNF-blocking gents, inj site Rxns, infections **Interactions:** ↓ Effects of immunizations; ↑ risk of infections if combined w/ TNF-blocking drugs **Labs:** ↓ WBCs, plts, absolute neutrophil count **NIPE:** Store drug in refrigerator, ⊘ light exposure, & discard any unused portion; ⊘ use soln if discolored or has particulate matter

Anastrozole (Arimidex) **Uses:** *Breast CA: postmenopausal women w/ metastatic breast CA, adjuvant Rx of postmenopausal women w/ early hormone-receptor-+ breast CA* **Action:** Selective nonsteroidal aromatase inhibitor; ↓ circulating estradiol **Dose:** 1 mg/d **Caution:** [C, ?] **Contra:** PRG **Supplied:** Tabs 1 mg **SE:** May ↑ cholesterol; diarrhea, hypertension, flushing, ↑d bone & tumor pain, HA, somnolence **Notes:** No effect on adrenal corticosteroids or aldosterone **Interactions:** None noted **Labs:** ↑ GTT, LFTs, alkaline phosphatase, total & LDL cholesterol **NIPE:** May ↓ fertility & cause fetal damage, eval for pain & administer adequate analgesia, may cause vaginal bleeding first few weeks

Anistreplase (Eminase) **Uses:** *AMI* **Action:** Thrombolytic; activates conversion of plasminogen to plasmin, promoting thrombolysis **Dose:** 30 units IV over 2–5 min **Caution:** [C, ?] **Contra:** Active internal bleeding, Hx CVA, recent (<2 mo) intracranial or intraspinal surgery or trauma, intracranial neoplasm, AVM, aneurysm, bleeding diathesis, severe uncontrolled HTN **Supplied:** Vials w/30 units **SE:** Bleeding, hypotension, hematoma **Notes:** May not be effective if readministered >5 d after the previous dose of anistreplase or streptokinase, or streptococcal infection, because of the production of antistreptokinase antibody **Interactions:** ↑ Risk of hemorrhage w/ warfarin, oral anticoagulants, ASA, NSAIDs, dipyridamole; ↓ effectiveness w/ aminocaproic acid **Labs:** ↓ Plasminogen & fibrinogen, ↑ transaminase level, thrombin time, APTT & PT **NIPE:** Store powder in refrigerator & use w/in 30 min of reconstitution, initiate therapy ASAP after MI, monitor S/Sxs internal bleeding

Anthralin (Anthra-Derm) **Uses:** *Psoriasis* **Action:** Keratolytic **Dose:** Apply qd **Caution:** [C, ?] **Contra:** Acutely inflamed psoriatic eruptions, erythroderma **Supplied:** Cream, oint 0.1, 0.2, 0.25, 0.4, 0.5, 1% **SE:** Irritation; discoloration of hair, fingernails, skin **Interactions:** ↑ Toxicity if used immediately after long-term topical corticosteroid therapy **NIPE:** May stain fabric; external use only; ⊘ sunlight-medicated areas

Antihemophilic Factor [AHF, Factor VIII] (Monoclate) **Uses:** *Classic hemophilia A, von Willebrand's Dz* **Action:** Provides factor VIII needed to convert prothrombin to thrombin **Dose:** *Adults & Peds.* 1 AHF unit/kg ↑ factor VIII level ≈2%. Units required = (kg) (desired factor VIII ↑ as % normal) × (0.5). Prophylaxis of spontaneous hemorrhage = 5% normal. Hemostasis after trauma/surgery = 30% normal. Head injuries, major surgery, or bleeding = 80–100% normal. Determine Pt's % of normal factor VIII before dosing **Caution:** [C, ?] **Supplied:** Check each vial for units contained **SE:** Rash, fever, HA, chills, N/V **Interactions:** None **Labs:** Monitor CBC & direct Coombs' test **NIPE:** ⊘ ASA, immunize against Hep B, DC if tachycardic

Antithymocyte Globulin [ATG] (ATGAM) Uses: *RX allograft rejection in transplant Pts* **Action:** Reduces the number of circulating, thymus-dependent lymphocytes **Dose:** 10–15 mg/kg/d **Caution:** [C, ?/–] **Contra:** ⊘ Use w/ a Hx of severe systemic Rxn to other equine gamma globulin prep **Supplied:** Inj 50 mg/mL **SE:** Thrombocytopenia, leukopenia **Notes:** DC if severe thrombocytopenia/leucopenia **Interactions:** ↑ Risk of infection with antineoplastics, corticosteroids, cyclosporines **Labs:** Baseline hematopoietic function & periodically during drug therapy **NIPE:** Refrigerate & keep out of light, reconstitute at room temperature, soln stable for 4 h after reconstitution, 1st dose infused over 6 h

Apomorphine (Apokyn) WARNING: ⊘ Administer IV **Uses:** *Acute, intermittent hypomobility ("off") episodes of Parkinson's Dz* **Action:** Dopamine agonist **Dose:** *Adults.* 0.2-mL SQ test dose under medical supervision; if BP OK, initial 0.2 mL SQ during "off" periods; only 1 dose per "off" period; requires careful titration; 0.6 mL max single doses; requires concomitant antiemetic; ↓ in renal impairment **Caution:** [C, +/–] ⊘ EtOH; antihypertensives, vasodilators, cardio or cerebrovascular Dz, hepatic impairment **Contra:** 5HT₃ antagonists, sulfite hypersensitivity **Supplied:** Inj 10 mg/mL, 3-mL prefilled pen cartridges; 2-mL amp **SE:** Emesis, syncope, QT interval prolongation, orthostatic hypotension, somnolence, ischemia, inj site Rxn, abuse potential, dyskinesia, fibrotic conditions, priapism **Notes:** Potential for daytime somnolence may limit Pts activities; trimethobenzamide 300 mg tid PO or other non-5HT₃ antagonist antiemetic given 3 d prior to & up to 2 mo following initiation **Interactions:** ↑ Risk of hypotension with alosetron, dolasetron, granisetron, ondansetron, palonosetron **Labs:** ECG–monitor for prolongation of QT interval **NIPE:** Start antiemetic 3 d before therapy and for 2 mo after therapy ends

Apraclonidine (Iopidine) Uses: *Glaucoma, postop intraocular HTN* **Action:** α₂-Adrenergic agonist **Dose:** 1–2 gtt of 0.5% tid **Caution:** [C, ?] **Contra:** MAOI use **Supplied:** 0.5, 1% soln **SE:** Ocular irritation, lethargy, xerostomia **Interactions:** ↓ Intraocular pressure w/ pilocarpine or topical BBs **NIPE:** Monitor CV status of Pts w/ CAD, potential for dizziness

Aprepitant (Emend) Uses: *Prevents N/V assoc w/ highly emetogenic CA chemotherapy (eg, cisplatin) (used in combination w/ other antiemetic agents)* **Action:** Substance P/neurokinin 1(NK₁) receptor antagonist **Dose:** 125 mg PO day 1, 1 h before chemo, then 80 mg PO q AM on days 2 & 3 **Caution:** [B, ?/–]; substrate & moderate inhibitor of CYP3A4; inducer of CYP2C9 **Contra:** Use w/ pimozide **Supplied:** Caps 80, 125 mg **SE:** Fatigue, asthenia, hiccups **Notes:** ↓ Effectiveness of PO contraceptives; ↓ anticoagulant effect of warfarin **Interactions:** ↑ Effects w/ clarithromycin, diltiazem, itraconazole, ketoconazole, nefazodone, nelfinavir, ritonavir, troleandomycin; ↑ effects of alprazolam, astemizole, cisapride, dexamethasone, methylprednisolone, midazolam, pimozide, terfenadine, triazolam and chemotherapeutic agents eg docetaxel, etoposide, ifosfamide, imatinib, irinotecan, paclitaxel, vinblastine, vincristine, vinorelbine; ↓ effects w/

paroxetine, rifampin; ↓ effects of oral contraceptives, paroxetine, phenytoin, tolbu-
amide, warfarin **Labs:** ↑ ALT, AST, BUN, alkaline phosphatase, leukocytes
NIPE: Use barrier contraception, take w/o regard to food

Aprotinin (Trasylol) **Uses:** *↓/Prevents blood loss in Pts undergoing
CABG* **Action:** Protease inhibitor, antifibrinolytic **Dose:** 1-mL IV test dose. *High
dose:* 2 million KIU load, 2 million KIU to prime pump, then 500,000 KIU/h until
surgery ends. *Low dose:* 1 million KIU load, 1 million KIU to prime pump, then
250,000 KIU/h until surgery ends; 7 million KIU max total **Caution:** [B, ?]
Thromboembolic Dz requiring anticoagulants or blood factor administration **Supplied:** Inj 1.4 mg/mL (10,000 KIU/mL) **SE:** AF, MI, HF, dyspnea, postop renal
dysfunction **Notes:** 1000/KIU = 0.14 mg of aprotinin **Interactions:** ↑ Clotting
time w/ heparin, ↓ effects of fibrinolytics, captopril **Labs:** Monitor aPTT, ACT,
CBC, BUN, creatinine **NIPE:** Monitor cardiac and pulmonary status during inf

Ardeparin (Normiflo) **Uses:** *Prevents DVT/PE following knee replacement* **Action:** LMW heparin **Dose:** 35–50 units/kg SQ q12h. Begin day of
surgery, continue up to 14 d; caution in ↓ renal Fxn **Caution:** [C, ?] **Contra:** Active hemorrhage; hypersensitivity to pork products **Supplied:** Inj 5000, 10,000
IU/0.5 mL **SE:** Bleeding, bruising, thrombocytopenia, pain at inj site, ↑ serum
transaminases **Notes:** Lab monitoring usually not necessary

Argatroban (Acova) **Uses:** *Prophylaxis or Rx of thrombosis in HIT, PCI
in Pts w/ risk of HIT* **Action:** Anticoagulant, direct thrombin inhibitor **Dose:** 2
μg/kg/min IV; adjust until aPTT 1.5–3× baseline not to exceed 100 s; 10 μg/kg/min
max; ↓ dose in hepatic impairment. **Caution:** [B, ?] ⊘ PO anticoagulants, ↑ bleeding risk; ⊘ concomitant use of thrombolytics **Contra:** Overt major bleed **Supplied:** Inj 100 mg/mL **SE:** AF, cardiac arrest, cerebrovascular disorder,
hypotension, VT, N/V/D, sepsis, cough, renal toxicity, ↓ Hgb **Interactions:** ↑ Risk
of bleeding w/ anticoagulants, feverfew, garlic, ginger, ginkgo, ↑ risk of intracranial bleed w/ thrombolytics **Labs:** ↑ aPTT, PT, INR, ACT, thrombin time **NIPE:**
Report ↑ bruising & bleeding, ⊘ breast-feed

Aripiprazole (Abilify) **Uses:** *Schizophrenia* **Action:** Dopamine & serotonin antagonist **Dose:** *Adults.* 10–15 mg PO qd; ↓ when used w/ potent CYP3A4
or CYP2D6 inhibitors; ↑ when used in combination w/ inducer of CYP3A4 **Caution:** [C, –] **Supplied:** Tabs 10, 15, 20, 30 mg **SE:** Neuroleptic malignant syndrome, tardive dyskinesia, orthostatic hypotension, cognitive & motor impairment
Interactions: ↑ Effects w/ ketoconazole, quinidine, fluoxetine, paroxetine, ↓ effects w/ carbamazepine **NIPE:** ⊘ Breast-feed, consume EtOH, or use during PRG;
use barrier contraception; ↑ fluid intake

Artificial Tears (Tears Naturale) [OTC] **Uses:** *Dry eyes* **Action:**
Ocular lubricant **Dose:** 1–2 gtt tid–qid **Caution:** N/A **Supplied:** OTC soln **SE:**
N/A

ʟ-Asparaginase (Elspar, Oncaspar) **Uses:** *ALL* (in combination
w/ other agents) **Action:** Protein synthesis inhibitor **Dose:** 500–20,000 IU/m²/d for

1–14 d (see specific protocols) **Caution:** [C, ?] **Contra:** Active/Hx pancreatitis **Supplied:** Inj 10,000 IU **SE:** Hypersensitivity Rxn in 20–35% (spectrum of urticaria to anaphylaxis); test dose recommended; rare GI toxicity (mild nausea/anorexia, pancreatitis) **Interactions:** ↑ Effects w/ prednisone, vincristine; ↓ effects of MRX, sulfonylureas, insulin **Labs:** ↓ T_4 & T_4-binding globulin, serum albumin, total cholesterol, plasma fibrinogen; ↑ BUN, glucose, uric acid, LFTs, alkaline phosphatase **NIPE:** ↑ Fluid intake, monitor for bleeding, monitor I&O and weight, ⊘ EtOH or ASA

Aspirin (Bayer, Ecotrin, St. Joseph's) [OTC]

Uses: *Angina, CABG, PTCA, carotid endarterectomy, ischemic stroke, TIA, MI, arthritis, pain,* HA, *fever,* * inflammation, Kawasaki Dz **Action:** Prostaglandin inhibitor **Dose:** *Adults. Pain, fever:* 325–650 mg q4–6h PO or PR. *RA:* 3–6 g/d PO in ÷ doses. *Plt inhibitor:* 81–325 mg PO qd. *Prevent MI:* 81–325 mg PO qd. **Peds.** Antipyretic: 10–15 mg/kg/dose PO or PR q4h up to 80 mg/kg/24 h. *RA:* 60–100 mg/kg/24 h PO ÷ q4–6h (keep levels between 15 & 30 mg/dL); ⊘ w/ CrCl <10 mL/min, in severe liver Dz **Caution:** [C, M] Use linked to Reye's syndrome; ⊘ use w/ viral illness in children **Contra:** Allergy to ASA, chickenpox or flu Sxs, syndrome of nasal polyps, asthma, rhinitis **Supplied:** Tabs 325, 500 mg; chew tabs 81 mg; EC tabs 165, 325, 500, 650, 975 mg; SR tabs 650, 800 mg; effervescent tabs 325, 500 mg; supp 120, 200, 300, 600 mg **SE:** GI upset & erosion **Notes:** DC 1 wk prior to surgery to ⊘ postoperative bleeding; ⊘ or limit EtOH use **Interactions:** ↑ effects w/ anticoagulants, ammonium chloride, antibiotics, ascorbic acid, furosemide, methionine, nizatidine, NSAIDs, verapamil, EtOH, feverfew, garlic, ginkgo biloba, horse chestnut, kelpware (black-tang), prickly ash, red clover; ↓ effects w/ antacids, activated charcoal, corticosteroids, griseofulvin, $NaHCO_3$, ginseng, food; ↑ effects of ACEI, hypoglycemics, insulin, Li, MRX, phenytoin, sulfonamides, valproic acid; ↓ effects of BBs, probenecid, spironolactone, sulfinpyrazone **Labs:** False − results of urinary glucose & urinary ketone tests, serum albumin, total serum phenytoin, T_3 & T_4 **NIPE:** Chronic ASA use may result in ↓ folic acid, Fe-deficiency anemia, & hypernatremia; ⊘ foods ↑ salicylate, eg curry powder, paprika, licorice, prunes, raisins, tea; take ASA w/ food or milk; report S/Sxs bleeding/GI pain/ringing in ears

Aspirin & Butalbital Compound (Fiorinal) [C-III]

Uses: *Tension HA,* * pain **Action:** Combination barbiturate & analgesic **Dose:** 1–2 PO q4h PRN, max 6 tabs/d; ⊘ use w/ CrCl <10 mL/min & in severe liver Dz **Caution:** [C (D if used for prolonged periods or high doses at term), ?] **Contra:** Allergy to ASA, GI ulceration, bleeding disorder, porphyria, syndrome of nasal polyps, angioedema, & bronchospasm to NSAIDs **Supplied:** Caps Fiorgen PF, Fiorinal. Tabs Fiorinal, Lanorinal: ASA 325 mg/butalbital 50 mg/caffeine 40 mg **SE:** Drowsiness, dizziness, GI upset, ulceration, bleeding **Notes:** Butalbital habit-forming; ⊘ or limit EtOH intake See Aspirin. **Additional Interactions:** ↑ Effect of benzodiazepines,

CNS depressants, chloramphenicol, methylphenidate, propoxyphene, valproic acid; ↓ effects of BBs, corticosteroids, chloramphenicol, cyclosporines, doxycycline, griseofulvin, haloperidol, oral contraceptives, phenothiazines, quinidine, TCAs, theophylline, warfarin **NIPE:** Use barrier contraception; ⊘ EtOH

Aspirin + Butalbital, Caffeine, & Codeine (Fiorinal + Codeine) [C-III] Uses: Mild *pain*, HA, especially when associated w/ stress **Action:** Sedative analgesic, narcotic analgesic **Dose:** 1–2 tabs (caps) PO q4–6h PRN **Caution:** [D, ?] **Contra:** Allergy to ASA **Supplied:** Cap/tab contains 325 mg ASA, 40 mg caffeine, 50 mg of butalbital, 30 mg of codeine **SE:** Drowsiness, dizziness, GI upset, ulceration, bleeding See Aspirin + Butalbital **Additional Interactions:** ↑ Effects w/ narcotic analgesics, MAOIs, neuromuscular blockers, ↓ effects w/ tobacco smoking; ↑ effects of digitoxin, phenytoin, rifampin; ↑ resp & CNS depression w/ cimetidine **Labs:** ↑ Plasma amylase & lipase **NIPE:** May cause constipation, ↑ fluids & fiber, take w/ milk to ↓ GI distress

Aspirin + Codeine (Empirin No. 2, No. 3, No. 4) [C-III] Uses: Mild to *moderate pain* **Action:** Combined effects of ASA & codeine **Dose:** **Adults.** 1–2 tabs PO q4–6h PRN. **Peds.** ASA 10 mg/kg/dose; codeine 0.5–1.0 mg/kg/dose q4h **Caution:** [D, M] **Contra:** Allergy to ASA/codeine, PUD, bleeding, anticoagulant Rx, children w/ chickenpox or flu Sxs **Supplied:** Tabs 325 mg of ASA & codeine (Codeine in No. 2 = 15 mg, No. 3 = 30 mg, No. 4 = 60 mg) **SE:** Drowsiness, dizziness, GI upset, ulceration, bleeding See Aspirin. **Additional Interactions** ↑ Effects w/ narcotic analgesics, MAOIs, neuromuscular blockers, ∅ effects w/ tobacco smoking; ↑ effects of digitoxin, phenytoin, rifampin; ↑ resp & CNS depression w/ cimetidine **Labs:** ↑ Plasma amylase & lipase **NIPE:** May cause constipation, ↑ fluids & fiber, take w/ milk to ↓ GI distress

Atazanavir (Reyataz) WARNING: Hyperbilirubinemia may require drug discontinuation **Uses:** *HIV-1 infection* **Action:** Protease inhibitor **Dose:** 400 mg PO daily w/ food; when given w/ efavirenz 600 mg, administer atazanavir 300 mg + ritonavir 100 mg once/d; separate doses from buffered didanosine administration; ↓ in hepatic impairment **Caution:** [B, –]; ↑ levels of statins, sildenafil, antiarrhythmics, warfarin, cyclosporine, tricyclics; atazanavir conc ↓ by St. John's wort **Contra:** Concomitant use of midazolam, triazolam, ergots, cisapride, pimozide **Supplied:** 100-mg, 150-mg, 200-mg caps **SE:** Headache, N/V/D, rash, abdominal pain, DM, photosensitivity; ↑ PR interval **Notes:** May have ↓ effects on cholesterol profile **Interactions:** ↑ Effects w/ amprenavir, clarithromycin, indinavir, lamivudine, lopinavir, ritonavir, saquinavir, stavudine, tenofovir, zalcitabine, zidovudine; ↑ effects of amiodarone, atorvastatin, CCBs, clarithromycin, cyclosporine, diltiazem, irinotecan, lidocaine, lovastatin, oral contraceptives, rifabutin, quinidine, saquinavir, sildenafil, simvastatin, sirolimus, tacrolimus, TCAs, warfarin; ↓ effects w/ antacids, antimycobacterials, efavirenz, esomeprazole, H2 receptor antagonists, lansoprazole, omeprazole, rifampin, St. John's wort **Labs:** ↑

ALT, AST, total bilirubin, amylase, lipase, serum glucose, ↓ Hgb, neutrophils **NIPE:** Take w/ food; will not cure HIV or ↓ risk of transmission; use barrier contraception; ↑ risk of skin and/or scleral yellowing

Atenolol (Tenormin) **Uses:** *HTN, angina, MI* **Action:** Competitively blocks β-adrenergic receptors, β₁ **Dose:** *HTN & angina:* 50–100 mg/d PO. *AMI:* 5 mg IV ×2 over 10 min, then 50 mg PO bid if tolerated; ↓ in renal impairment **Caution:** [D, M] DM, bronchospasm; abrupt DC can exacerbate angina & MI risk **Contra:** Bradycardia, cardiogenic shock, cardiac failure, 2nd- or 3rd- degree AV block **Supplied:** Tabs 25, 50, 100 mg; inj 5 mg/10 mL **SE:** Bradycardia, ↓ BP, 2nd- or 3rd-degree AV block, dizziness, fatigue **Interactions:** ↑ Effects w/ other antihypertensives especially diltiazem & verapamil, nitrates, EtOH; ↑ bradycardia w/ adenosine, digitalis glycosides, dipyridamole, physostigmine, tacrine; ↓ effects w/ ampicillin, antacids, NSAIDs, salicylates; ↑ effects of lidocaine; ↓ effects of dopamine, glucagons, insulin, sulfonylureas **Labs:** ↑ ANA titers, BUN, glucose, serum lipoprotein, K⁺, triglyceride, uric acid levels; ↓ HDL **NIPE:** May mask S/Sxs hypoglycemia, may ↑ sensitivity to cold, may ↑ depression, wheezing, orthostatic hypotension

Atenolol & Chlorthalidone (Tenoretic) **Uses:** *HTN* **Action:** β-Adrenergic blockade w/ diuretic **Dose:** 50–100 mg/d PO; ↓ in renal impairment **Caution:** [D, M] DM, bronchospasm **Contra:** See atenolol; anuria **Supplied:** *Tenoretic 50:* Atenolol 50 mg/chlorthalidone 25 mg; *Tenoretic 100:* Atenolol 100 mg/chlorthalidone 25 mg **SE:** Bradycardia, ↓ BP, 2nd- or 3rd-degree AV block, dizziness, fatigue, ↓ K⁺, photosensitivity See Atenolol. **Additional Interactions:** ↑ Effects w/ other antihypertensives; ↓ effects w/ cholestyramine, NSAIDs; ↑ effects of Li, digoxin, ↓ effects of sulfonylureas **Labs:** False ↓ urine esriol; ↑ CPK, serum ammonia, amylase, Ca²⁺, Cl⁻, cholesterol, glucose; ↓ serum Cl⁻, Mg²⁺, K⁺, Na⁻ **NIPE:** Take in AM to prevent nocturia, use sunblock >SPF 15, monitor S/Sxs gout

Atomoxetine (Strattera) **Uses:** *ADHD* **Action:** Selective norepinephrine reuptake inhibitor **Dose:** *Adults & children >70kg.* 40 mg × 3 days, titrate ↑ to 80–100 mg + qd–bid. *Peds < 70 kg:* 0.5 mg/kg × 3 d, then titrate to max of 1.2 mg/kg given qd or bid **Caution:** [C, ? /–] **Contra:** Narrow-angle glaucoma, use w/ or w/in 2 wk of DC an MAOI **Supplied:** Caps 10, 18, 25, 40, 60 mg **SE:** ↑ BP, tachycardia, weight loss, sexual dysfunction **Notes:** ↓ Dose w/ hepatic insufficiency, ↓ dose in combination w/ inhibitors of CYP2D6

Atorvastatin (Lipitor) **Uses:** *↑ Cholesterol & triglycerides* **Action:** HMG-CoA reductase inhibitor **Dose:** Initial dose 10 mg/d, may be ↑ to 80 mg/d **Caution:** [X, –] **Contra:** Active liver Dz, unexplained ↑ of serum transaminases **Supplied:** Tabs 10, 20, 40, 80 mg **SE:** May cause myopathy, HA, arthralgia, myalgia, GI upset **Notes:** monitor LFTs regularly **Interactions:** ↑ Effects w/ azole antifungals, erythromycin, nefazodone, protease inhibitors, grapefruit juice; ↓ effects w/ antacids, bile acid sequestrants; ↑ effects of digoxin, levothyroxine, oral contraceptives **Labs:** ↑ LFTs, CPK, ↓ lipid levels **NIPE:** ⊘ EtOH, breast-feeding, or while PRG

Atovaquone (Mepron)
Uses: *Rx & prevention PCP* **Action:** ↓ Nucleic acid & ATP synthesis **Dose:** *Rx:* 750 mg PO bid for 21 d. *Prevention:* 1500 mg PO once/d (w/ meals) **Caution:** [C, ?] **Supplied:** Suspension 750 mg/5 mL **SE:** Fever, HA, anxiety, insomnia, rash, N/V **Interactions:** ↓ Effects w/ metoclopramide, rifabutin, rifampin, tetracycline **NIPE:** ↑ Absorption w/ meal esp ↑ fat, monitor LFTs w/ long-term use

Atovaquone/Proguanil (Malarone)
Uses: *Prevention or Rx Pseudomonas falciparum malaria* **Action:** Antimalarial **Dose:** *Adults: Prevention:* 1 tab PO 2 d before, during, & 7 d after leaving endemic region; *Rx:* 4 tabs PO single dose qd ×3 d. *Peds.* See insert **Caution:** [C, ?] **Contra:** CrCl < 30 mL/min **Supplied:** Tab atovaquone 250 mg/proguanil 100 mg; pediatric 62.5/25 mg **SE:** HA, fever, myalgia. See Atovaquone

Atracurium (Tracrium)
Uses: *Adjunct to anesthesia to facilitate ET intubation* **Action:** Nondepolarizing neuromuscular blocker **Dose:** *Adults & Peds.* 0.4–0.5 mg/kg IV bolus, then 0.08–0.1 mg/kg q20–45 min PRN **Caution:** [C, ?] **Supplied:** Inj 10 mg/mL **SE:** Flushing **Notes:** Pt must be intubated & on controlled ventilation; use adequate amounts of sedation & analgesia **Interactions:** ↑ Effects w/ general anesthetics, aminoglycosides, bacitracin, BBs, β agonists, clindamycin, CCBs, diuretics, lidocaine, Li, Mg sulfate, narcotic analgesics, procainamide, quinidine, succinylcholine, trimethaphan, verapamil; ↓ effects w/ Ca, carbamazepine, phenytoin, theophylline, caffeine **Labs:** Monitor BUN, creatinine, LFTs **NIPE:** Drug does not effect consciousness or pain, inability to speak until drug wears off

Atropine
Uses: *Preanesthetic; symptomatic bradycardia & asystole* **Action:** Antimuscarinic agent; blocks acetylcholine at parasympathetic sites **Dose:** *Adults. ECC:* 0.5–1 mg IV q3–5min. *Preanesthetic:* 0.3–0.6 mg IM. *Peds. ECC:* 0.01–0.03 mg/kg IV q2–5min, max 1 mg, min dose 0.1 mg. *Preanesthetic:* 0.01 mg/kg/dose SC/IV (max 0.4 mg) **Caution:** [C, +] **Contra:** Glaucoma **Supplied:** Tabs 0.3, 0.4, 0.6 mg; inj 0.05, 0.1, 0.3, 0.4, 0.5, 0.8, 1 mg/mL; ophthalmic 0.5, 1, 2% **SE:** Blurred vision, urinary retention, constipation, dried mucous membranes **Interactions:** ↑ Effects w/ amantadine, antihistamines, disopyramide, procainamide, quinidine, TCA, thiazides, betel palm, squaw vine; ↓ effects w/ antacids, levodopa; ↓ effects of phenothiazines **Labs:** ↓ Gastric motility & emptying may effect results of upper GI series **NIPE:** Monitor I&O, ↑ fluids & oral hygiene, wear dark glasses to ↓ photophobia

Azathioprine (Imuran)
Uses: *Adjunct to prevent rejection following kidney transplantation, RA,* SLE **Action:** Immunosuppressive; antagonizes purine metabolism **Dose:** *Adults & Peds.* 1–3 mg/kg/d IV or PO (↓ in renal failure) **Caution:** [D, ?] **Contra:** PRG **Supplied:** Tabs 50 mg; inj 100 mg/20 mL **SE:** GI intol-

erance, fever, chills, leukopenia, thrombocytopenia; chronic use may ↑ neoplasia **Notes:** Handle inj w/ cytotoxic precautions; interaction w/ allopurinol; ⊘ administer live vaccines to a Pt taking azathioprine **Interactions:** ↑ Effects w/ allopurinol; ↑ effects of antineoplastic drugs, cyclosporine, myelosuppressive drugs, MRX; ↑ risk of severe leucopenia w/ ACEI; ↓ effects of nondepolarizing neuromuscular blocking drugs, warfarin **Labs:** Monitor BUN, creatinine, CBC, LFTs during therapy **NIPE:** ⊘ PRG, breast-feeding, immunizations, take w/ or pc

Azelastine (Astelin, Optivar) **Uses:** *Allergic rhinitis (rhinorrhea, sneezing, nasal pruritus); allergic conjunctivitis* **Action:** Histamine H₁-receptor antagonist **Dose:** *Nasal:* 2 sprays/nostril bid. *Ophthalmic:* 1 gt into each affected eye bid **Caution:** [C, ?/–] **Contra:** Component sensitivity **Supplied:** Nasal spray 137 μg/spray; ophthalmic soln 0.05% **SE:** Somnolence, bitter taste **Interactions:** ↑ Effects with cimetidine; ↑ effects of EtOH, CNS depressants **Labs:** ↑ AST, ↓ skin reactions to antigen skin tests **NIPE:** Systemically absorbed; clear nares before admin; prime pump before use

Azithromycin (Zithromax) **Uses:** *Community-acquired pneumonia, pharyngitis, otitis media, skin infections, nongonococcal urethritis, & PID; Rx & prevention of MAC in HIV* **Action:** Macrolide antibiotic; inhibits protein synthesis. *Spectrum: Chlamydia, Haemophilus ducreyi, H. influenzae, Legionella, Moraxella catarrhalis, Mycoplasma pneumoniae, M. hominis, Neisseria gonorrhoeae, Staphylococcus aureus, Streptococcus agalactiae, S. pneumoniae, S. pyogenes* **Dose:** *Adults. PO: Resp tract infections:* 500 mg day 1, then 250 mg/d PO ×4 d or 500 mg/d PO × 3 days. *Nongonococcal urethritis:* 1 g PO single dose. *Prevention of MAC:* 1200 mg PO once/wk. *IV:* 500 mg ×2 d, then 500 mg PO ×7–10 d. *Peds. Otitis media:* 10 mg/kg PO day 1, then 5 mg/kg/d days 2–5. *Pharyngitis:* 12 mg/kg/d PO ×5 d (take susp on an empty stomach; tabs may be taken w/o food) **Caution:** [B, +] **Supplied:** Tabs 250, 600 mg; Z-Pack (5-day regimen); Tri-Pak (500-mg tabs × 3); susp 1-g single-dose packet; susp 100, 200 mg/5 mL; inj 500 mg **SE:** GI upset **Interactions:** ↓ Effects w/ Al- & Mg-containing antacids, atovaquone, food (suspension); ↑ effects of alfentanil, barbiturates, bromocriptine, carbamazepine, cyclosporine, digoxin, disopyramide, ergot alkaloids, phenytoin, pimozide, terfenadine, theophylline, triazolam, warfarin; ↓ effects of penicillins **Labs:** May ↑ serum bilirubin, alkaline phosphatase, BUN, creatinine, CPK, glucose, K+, LFTs, LDH, PT; may ↓ WBC, plt count, serum folate **NIPE:** Monitor S/Sxs superinfection, use sunscreen & protective clothing

Aztreonam (Azactam) **Uses:** *Aerobic gram(–) UTIs, lower resp, intraabdominal, skin, gynecologic infections & septicemia* **Action:** Monobactam antibiotic; inhibits cell wall synthesis. *Spectrum:* Gram(–) coverage including *Pseudomonas, E. coli, Klebsiella, H. influenzae, Serratia, Proteus, Enterobacter, Citrobacter* **Dose:** *Adults.* 1–2 g IV/IM q6–12h. *Peds. Premature:* 30 mg/kg/dose IV q12h. *Term, children:* 30 mg/kg/dose q6–8h; ↓ in renal impairment **Caution:** [B, +] **Supplied:** Inj 500 mg, 1 g, 2 g **SE:** N/V/D, rash, pain at inj site **Notes:** No gram(+) or anaerobic activity; OK in penicillin-allergic Pts **Interactions:** ↑ Effects w/ probenecid, aminoglycosides, β-lactam antibiotics; ↓ effects w/ cefoxitin, chloramphenicol, imipenem **Labs:** ↑ LFTs, alkaline phosphatase, SCr, PT, PTT, & Coombs' test **NIPE:** Monitor S/Sxs superinfection, taste changes w/ IV administration

Bacitracin, Ophthalmic (AK-Tracin Ophthalmic); Bacitracin & Polymyxin B, Ophthalmic (AK Poly Bac Ophthalmic, Polysporin Ophthalmic); Bacitracin, Neomycin, & Polymixin B, Ophthalmic (AK Spore Ophthalmic, Neosporin Ophthalmic); Bacitracin, Neomycin, Polymyxin B, & Hydrocortisone, Ophthalmic (AK Spore HC Ophthalmic, Cortisporin Ophthalmic) Uses: *Steroid-responsive inflammatory ocular conditions* **Action:** Topical antibiotic plus antiinflammatory components **Dose:** Apply q3–4h into conjunctival sac **Caution:** [C, ?] **Contra:** Viral, mycobacterial, or fungal eye infection **Supplied:** See Bacitracin, Topical equivalents, below **Interactions:** ↑ Effects w/ neuromuscular blocking agents, anesthetics, nephrotoxic drugs **NIPE:** May cause blurred vision

Bacitracin, Topical (Baciguent); Bacitracin & Polymyxin B, Topical (Polysporin); Bacitracin, Neomycin, & Polymyxin B, Topical (Neosporin Ointment); Bacitracin, Neomycin, Polymyxin B, & Hydrocortisone, Topical (Cortisporin); Bacitracin, Neomycin, Polymyxin B, & Lidocaine, Topical (Clomycin) Uses: Prevent/Rx of *minor skin infections* **Action:** Topical antibiotic w/ added effects based on components (antiinflammatory & analgesic) **Dose:** Apply sparingly bid–qid **Caution:** [C, ?] **Supplied:** Bacitracin 500 U/g oint; Bacitracin 500 U/polymyxin B sulfate 10,000 U/g oint & powder; Bacitracin 400 U/neomycin 3.5 mg/polymyxin B 5000 U/g oint (for Neosporin Cream, see page 178); Bacitracin 400 U/neomycin 3.5 mg/polymyxin B/10,000 U/hydrocortisone 10 mg/g oint; Bacitracin 500 U/neomycin 3.5 g/ polymyxin B 5000 U/lidocaine 40 mg/g oint **SE:** N/A **Notes:** Systemic & irrigation forms of bacitracin available but not generally used due to potential toxicity

Baclofen (Lioresal) Uses: *Spasticity secondary to severe chronic disorders such as MS, ALS, or spinal cord lesions,* trigeminal neuralgia, hiccups **Action:** Centrally acting skeletal muscle relaxant; inhibits transmission of both monosynaptic & polysynaptic spinal cord reflexes **Dose:** *Adults.* Initial, 5 mg PO tid; ↑ q3d to effect; max 80 mg/d. *Intrathecal:* Through implantable pump *Peds* 2–7 y: 10–15 mg/d ÷ q8h; titrate, max of 40 mg/d. >8 y: Max of 60 mg/d. *IT:* Through implantable pump; ↓ in renal impairment; ↓ abrupt withdrawal; take w/ food or milk **Caution:** [C, +] Epilepsy & neuropsychiatric disturbances; withdrawal may occur w/ abrupt discontinuation **Supplied:** Tabs 10, 20 mg; IT inj 10 mg/20 mL, 10 mg/5 mL **SE:** Dizziness, drowsiness, insomnia, ataxia, weakness, hypotension **Interactions:** ↑ CNS depression w/ CNS depressants, MAOIs, EtOH, antihistamines, opioid analgesics, sedatives, hypnotics; ↑ effects of antihypertensives, clindamycin, guanabenz; ↑ risk of resp paralysis & renal failure w/ aminoglycosides **Labs:** ↑ Serum glucose, AST, ammonia, alkaline phosphatase; ↓ bilirubin **NIPE:** Take oral meds w/ food

Balsalazide (Colazal) **Uses:** *Ulcerative colitis* **Action:** 5-Aminosalicylic acid derivative, antiinflammatory, ↓ leukotriene synthesis **Dose:** 2.25 g (3 caps) tid ×8–12 wk **Caution:** [B, ?] Severe renal/hepatic failure **Contra:** Hypersensitivity to mesalamine or salicylates **Supplied:** Caps 750 mg **SE:** Dizziness, HA, nausea, agranulocytosis, pancytopenia, renal impairment, allergic Rxns **Notes:** Each daily dose of 6.75 g is equivalent to 2.4 g of mesalamine **Interactions:** Oral antibiotics may interfere w/ mesalamine release in the colon **Labs:** ↑ Bilirubin, CPK, LFTs, LDH, plasma fibrinogen; ↓ Ca^{2+}, K^+, protein **NIPE:** ⊘ if ASA allergy, take w/ food & swallow capsule whole

Basiliximab (Simulect) **Uses:** *Prevention of acute organ transplant rejections* **Action:** IL-2 receptor antagonists **Dose:** *Adults.* 20 mg IV 2 h before transplant, then 20 mg IV 4 d posttransplant. *Peds.* 12 mg/m² ↑ to max of 20 mg 2 h prior to transplant; the same dose IV 4 d posttransplant **Caution:** [B, ?/–] **Contra:** Known hypersensitivity to murine proteins **Supplied:** Inj 20 mg **SE:** Edema, HTN, HA, dizziness, fever, pain, infection, GI effects, electrolyte disturbances **Notes:** Murine/human monoclonal antibody **Interactions:** May ↑ immunosuppression w/ other immunosuppressive drugs **Labs:** ↑ Serum cholesterol, BUN, creatinine, uric acid; ↓ serum Mg phosphate, plts; ↑ or ↓ in Hgb, Hct, serum glucose, K^+, Ca^{2+} **NIPE:** Monitor for infection, hypersensitivity Rxns, IV dose over 20–30 min

BCG [Bacillus Calmette-Guérin] (TheraCys, Tice BCG) **Uses:** *Bladder carcinoma (superficial),* TB prophylaxis **Action:** Immunomodulator **Dose:** Bladder CA, 1 vial prepared & instilled in bladder for 2 h. Repeat once/wk for 6 wk; then maint 3/wk at 3, 6, 12, 18, & 24 mo after initial therapy **Caution:** [C, ?] Asthma, ⊘ administer w/ traumatic catheterization or UTI **Contra:** Immunosuppression, UTI steroid use, acute illness, fever of unknown origin **Supplied:** Inj 81 mg (10.5 ± 8.7 × 10⁸ CFU vial) (TheraCys), 1–8 × 10⁸ CFU/vial (Tice BCG) **SE:** *Intravesical:* Hematuria, urinary frequency, dysuria, bacterial UTI, rare BCG sepsis **Notes:** Routine US adult BCG immunization ⊘; occasionally used in high-risk children who are PPD– & cannot take INH **Interactions:** ↓ Effects w/ antimicrobials, immunosuppressives, radiation **Labs:** Prior BCG may cause false + PPD **NIPE:** Monitor for S/Sxs systemic infection, report persistent pain on urination or blood in urine

Becaplermin (Regranex Gel) **Uses:** Adjunct to local wound care in *diabetic foot ulcers* **Action:** Recombinant PDGF, enhances formation of granulation tissue **Dose:** Based on lesion; 1⅓-in. ribbon from 2-g tube, ⅔-in. ribbon from 7.5- or 15-g tube/in.² of ulcer; apply & cover w/moist gauze; rinse after 12h; ⊘ reapply; repeat in 12 h **Caution:** [C, ?] **Contra:** Neoplasm or active infection at site **Supplied:** 0.01% gel in 2-, 7.5-, 15-g tubes **SE:** Erythema, local pain **Notes:** Use along w/ good wound care; wound must be vascularized **Interactions:** None known **NIPE:** Dosage recalculated q1–2wk

Beclomethasone (Beconase, Vancenase Nasal Inhaler) **Uses:** Allergic *rhinitis* refractory to antihistamines & decongestants; *nasal polyps* **Action:** Inhaled steroid **Dose: Adults.** 1 spray intranasally bid–qid. *Aqueous inhal:* 1–2 sprays/nostril daily–bid. *Peds 6–12 y:* 1 spray intranasally tid **[C, ?] Supplied:** Nasal met-dose inhaler **SE:** Local irritation, burning, epistaxis **Notes:** Nasal spray delivers 42 μg/dose & 84 μg/dose **Interactions:** None noted **NIPE:** Prior use of decongestant nasal gtt if edema or secretions, may take several days for full steroid effect

Beclomethasone (QVAR) **Uses:** Chronic *asthma* **Action:** Inhaled corticosteroid **Dose:** *Adults & Peds.* 1–4 inhal bid (Rinse mouth/throat after use) **Caution:** [C, ?] **Contra:** Acute asthma **Supplied:** PO met-dose inhaler; 40, 80 μg/inhal **SE:** HA, cough, hoarseness, oral candidiasis **Notes:** Not effective for acute asthmatic **Interactions:** None noted **NIPE:** Use inhaled bronchodilator prior to inhaled steroid, rinse mouth after inhaled steroid

Belladonna & Opium Suppositories (B & O Supprettes) [C-II] **Uses:** *Bladder spasms; moderate/severe pain* **Action:** Antispasmodic, analgesic **Dose:** 1 supp PR q6h PRN; 15A = 30 mg powdered opium/16.2 mg belladonna extract; 16A = 60 mg powdered opium/16.2 mg belladonna extract **Caution:** [C, ?] **Supplied:** Supp 15A, 16A **SE:** Anticholinergic side effects (sedation, urinary retention, & constipation) **Interactions:** ↑ Effects w/ CNS depressants, TCAs; ↓ effects w/ phenothiazines **Labs:** ↑ LFTs **NIPE:** ⊘ Refrigerate, moisten finger & supp before insertion, may cause blurred vision

Benazepril (Lotensin) **Uses:** *HTN,* DN, CHF **Action:** ACEI **Dose:** 10–40 mg/d PO **Caution:** [C (1st tri), D (2nd & 3rd tri), +] **Contra:** Angioedema, Hx edema **Supplied:** Tabs 5, 10, 20, 40 mg **SE:** Symptomatic ↓ BP w/ diuretics; dizziness, HA, ↓ K⁺, nonproductive cough **Interactions:** ↑ Effects w/ α-blockers, diuretics, capsaicin; ↓ effects w/ NSAIDs, ASA; ↑ effects of insulin, Li; ↑ risk of hyperkalemia w/ trimethoprim & K-sparing diuretics **Labs:** ↑ BUN, SCr, K⁺; ↓ hemoglobin; ECG changes **NIPE:** Persistent cough and/or taste changes may develop, ⊘ PRG, DC if angioedema

Benzocaine & Antipyrine (Auralgan) **Uses:** *Analgesia in severe otitis media* **Action:** Antipyretic w/local decongestant **Dose:** Fill the ear & insert a moist cotton plug; repeat 1–2 h PRN **Caution:** [C, ?] **Contra:** ⊘ Use w/ perforated eardrum **Supplied:** Soln **SE:** Local irritation **Interactions:** May ↓ effects of sulfonamides

Benzonatate (Tessalon Perles) **Uses:** Symptomatic relief of *cough* **Action:** Anesthetizes the stretch receptors in the resp passages **Dose:** *Adults & Peds >10 y.* 100 mg PO tid **Caution:** [C, ?] **Supplied:** Caps 100 mg **SE:** Sedation, dizziness, GI upset **Notes:** ⊘ Chew or puncture the caps **Interactions:** ↑ CNS depression w/ antihistamines, EtOH, hypnotics, opioids, sedatives **NIPE:** ↑ Fluid intake to liquefy secretions

Benztropine (Cogentin) **Uses:** *Parkinsonism & drug-induced extrapyramidal disorders* **Action:** Partially blocks striatal cholinergic receptors **Dose:** ***Adults.*** 0.5–6 mg PO, IM, or IV in ÷ doses/d. ***Peds >3 y.*** 0.02–0.05 mg/kg/dose 1–2/d **Caution:** [C, ?] **Contra:** < 3 y **Supplied:** Tabs 0.5, 1, 2 mg; inj 1 mg/mL **SE:** Anticholinergic side effects **Notes:** Physostigmine 1–2 mg SC/IV to reverse severe Sxs **Interactions:** ↑ Sedation and depressant effects w/ EtOH & CNS depressants; ↑ anticholinergic effects w/ antihistamines, phenothiazines, quinidine, disopyramide, TCAs, MAOIs; ↑ effect of digoxin; ↓ effect of levodopa; ↓ effects w/ antacids and antidiarrheal drugs **NIPE:** May ↑ susceptibility to heat stroke, take w/ meals to avoid GI upset

Bepridil (Vascor) **Uses:** Chronic stable angina **Action:** CCB agent **Dose:** 200–400 mg/d PO **Caution:** [C, ?] **Contra:** QT interval prolongation, Hx ventricular arrhythmias, sick sinus syndrome, hypotension (DBP <90 mm Hg) **Supplied:** Tabs 200, 300, 400 mg **Notes/SE:** Dizziness, nausea, agranulocytosis, bradycardia, and serious ventricular arrhythmias, including torsades de pointes **Interactions:** ↑ Effects w/ amprenavir, ritonavir, moxifloxacin, gatifloxacin, sparfloxacin; ↑ effects of digitalis glycoside, cyclosporine, BBs; ↑ QT prolongation w/ procainamide, quinidine, TCAs **Labs:** ↑ LFTs, CPK, LDH **NIPE:** Take w/ food if GI upset, monitor K+ & ECG

Beractant (Survanta) **Uses:** *Prevention & Rx of RDS in premature infants* **Action:** Replaces pulmonary surfactant **Dose:** 100 mg/kg via ET tube; may repeat 3× q6h; max 4 doses/48 h **Caution:** [N/A, N/A] **Supplied:** Suspension 25 mg of phospholipid/mL **SE:** Transient bradycardia, oxygen desaturation, apnea **Notes:** Administer via 4-quadrant method **Interactions:** None noted **NIPE:** ↑ Risk of nosocomial sepsis after Rx w/ this drug

Betaxolol (Kerlone) **Uses:** *HTN* **Action:** Competitively blocks β-adrenergic receptors, β$_1$ **Caution:** [C (1st tri), D (2nd or 3rd tri), +/–] **Contra:** Sinus bradycardia, AV conduction abnormalities, cardiac failure **Dose:** 10–20 mg/d **Supplied:** Tabs 10, 20 mg **SE:** Dizziness, HA, bradycardia, edema, CHF **Interactions:** ↑ Effects w/ anticholinergics, verapamil, general anesthetics; ↓ effects w/ thyroid drugs, amphetamine, cocaine, ephedrine, epinephrine, norepinephrine, phenylephrine, pseudoephedrine, NSAIDs; ↑ effects of insulin, digitalis glycosides; ↓ effects of theophylline, dopamine, glucagon **Labs:** ↑ BUN, serum lipoprotein, glucose, K+, triglyceride, uric acid, ANA titers **NIPE:** May ↑ sensitivity to cold, ⊘ DC abruptly

Betaxolol, Ophthalmic (Betoptic) **Uses:** Glaucoma **Action:** Competitively blocks β-adrenergic receptors, β$_1$ **Dose:** 1 gt bid **Caution:** [C (1st tri), D (2nd or 3rd tri), ?/–] **Supplied:** Soln 0.5%; susp 0.25% **SE:** Local irritation. See Betaxolol + **NIPE:** Use sunglasses to ⊘ exposure, may cause photophobia, review installation procedures

Bethanechol (Urecholine, Duvoid, others) Uses: *Neurogenic bladder atony w/ retention,* acute *postoperative* & postpartum functional *(nonobstructive) urinary retention* **Action:** Stimulates cholinergic smooth muscle receptors in bladder & GI tract **Dose:** *Adults.* 10–50 mg PO tid–qid or 2.5–5 mg SQ tid–qid & PRN. *Peds.* 0.6 mg/kg/24 h PO ÷ tid–qid or 0.15–2 mg/kg/d SQ ÷ 3–4× (take on empty stomach) **Caution:** [C, ?/–] **Contra:** Bladder outlet obstruction, PUD, epilepsy, hyperthyroidism, bradycardia, COPD, AV conduction defects, parkinsonism, hypotension, vasomotor instability **Supplied:** Tabs 5, 10, 25, 50 mg; inj 5 mg/mL **SE:** Abdominal cramps, diarrhea, salivation, hypotension **Notes:** ⊘ use IM/IV **Interactions:** ↑ Effects w/ BBs, tacrine, cholinesterase inhibitors; ↓ effects w/ atropine, anticholinergic drugs, procainamide, quinidine, epinephrine **Labs:** ↑ In serum AST, ALT, amylase, lipase, bilirubin **NIPE:** May cause blurred vision, monitor I&O, take on an empty stomach

Bevacizumab (Avastin) WARNING: Associated w/ GI perforation, wound dehiscence, & fatal hemoptysis Uses: *Colorectal metastatic carcinoma, w/ 5-FU* **Action:** Vascular endothelial growth factor inhibitor **Dose:** *Adults.* 5 mg/kg IV q14d; 1st dose over 90 min; 2nd over 60 min, 3rd over 30 min if tolerated **Caution:** [C, –] **Contra:** ⊘ Use w/in 28 d of surgery if time for separation of drug & anticipated surgical procedures is unknown; DC w/ serious adverse events **Supplied:** 100 mg/4 mL, 400 mg/16 mL vials **SE:** Wound dehiscence, GI perforation, hemoptysis, hemorrhage, hypertension, proteinuria, CHF, inf Rxns, diarrhea, leucopenia, thromboembolism **Labs:** Monitor for ↑ BP & proteinuria

Bicalutamide (Casodex) Uses: *Advanced CAP* (w/ GnRH agonists [eg, leuprolide, goserelin]) **Action:** Nonsteroidal antiandrogen **Dose:** 50 mg/d **Caution:** [X, ?] **Contra:** Women **Supplied:** Caps 50 mg **SE:** Hot flashes, loss of libido, impotence, diarrhea, N/V, gynecomastia, & LFT elevation **Interactions:** ↑ Effects of anticoagulants, TCAs, phenothiazines; ↓ effects of antipsychotic drugs **Labs:** ↑ LFTs, alkaline phosphatase, bilirubin, BUN, creatinine; ↓ Hgb, WBCs **NIPE:** Monitor PSA, may experience hair loss

Bicarbonate (See Sodium Bicarbonate, page 219)

Bisacodyl (Dulcolax) [OTC] Uses: *Constipation; preop bowel prep* **Action:** Stimulates peristalsis **Dose:** *Adults.* 5–15 mg PO or 10 mg PR PRN. *Peds* <2 y: 5 mg PR PRN. >2 y: 5 mg PO or 10 mg PR PRN (⊘ chew tabs; ⊘ give w/in 1 h of antacids or milk) **Caution:** [B, ?] **Contra:** Acute abdomen or bowel obstruction, appendicitis, gastroenteritis **Supplied:** EC tabs 5 mg; supp 10 mg **SE:** Abdominal cramps, proctitis, & inflammation w/ suppositories **Interactions:** Antacids & milk ↑ dissolution of enteric coating causing abdominal irritation **Labs:** False ↓ urine glucose **NIPE:** ↑ Fluid intake & high-fiber foods, ⊘ take w/ milk or antacids

Bismuth Subsalicylate (Pepto-Bismol) [OTC] Uses: Indigestion, nausea, & *diarrhea;* combination for Rx of *H. pylori infection* **Action:** Antisecretory & antiinflammatory effects **Dose:** *Adults.* 2 tabs or 30 mL PO PRN (max 8

doses/24 h). **Peds.** *3–6 y:* ⅛ tab or 5 mL PO PRN (max 8 doses/24 h). *6–9 y:* ⅔ tab or 10 mL PO PRN (max 8 doses/24 h). *9–12 y:* 1 tab or 15 mL PO PRN (max 8 doses/24 h) **Caution:** [C, D (3rd tri), –] ⊘ in renal failure **Contra:** Influenza or chickenpox (↑ risk of Reye's syndrome), ASA allergy **Supplied:** Chew tabs 262 mg; liq 262, 524 mg/15 mL **Interactions:** ↑ Effects of ASA, MRX, valproic acid; ↓ effects of tetracyclines, quinolones, probenecid; ↓ effects w/ corticosteroids **Labs:** False ↑ uric acid, AST; may interfere w/ GI tract x-rays; ↓ K⁺, T₃, & T₄ **NIPE:** May darken tongue & stool, chew tab, ⊘ swallow whole

Bisoprolol (Zebeta)
Uses: *HTN* **Action:** Competitively blocks β₁-adrenergic receptors **Dose:** 5–10 mg/d (max dose 20 mg/d); ↓ in renal impairment **Caution:** [C (D 2nd & 3rd tri), +/–] **Contra:** Sinus bradycardia, AV conduction abnormalities, cardiac failure **Supplied:** Tabs 5, 10 mg **SE:** Fatigue, lethargy, HA, bradycardia, edema, CHF **Notes:** Not dialyzed **Interactions:** ↑ Bradycardia w/ adenosine, amiodarone, digoxin, dipyridamole, neostigmine, physostigmine, tacrine; ↑ effects w/ cimetidine, fluoxetine, prazosin; ↓ effects w/ NSAIDs, rifampin; ↓ effects of theophylline, glucagon **Labs:** ↑ T₄, cholesterol, glucose, triglycerides, uric acid; ↓ HDL **NIPE:** ⊘ DC abruptly, may mask S/Sxs hypoglycemia, take w/o regard to food

Bitolterol (Tornalate)
Uses: Prophylaxis & Rx of *asthma* & reversible bronchospasm **Action:** Sympathomimetic bronchodilator; stimulates β₂-adrenergic receptors in the lungs **Dose:** *Adults & Peds >12 y.* 2 inhal q8h **Caution:** [C, ?] **Supplied:** Aerosol 0.8% **SE:** Dizziness, nervousness, trembling, HTN, palpitations **Interactions:** ↑ Cardiac effects of theophylline; ↑ hypokalemia w/ furosemide; ↑ effects w/ other β-adrenergic bronchodilators, MAOIs, TCAs, inhaled anesthetics; ↓ effects w/ β-adrenergic blockers; **Labs:** ↑ AST, ↓ plts, WBCs, proteinuria **NIPE:** Wait 15 min after use of this drug before using an adrenocorticoid inhaler. Shake inhaler well before use

Bivalirudin (Angiomax)
Uses: *Anticoagulant w/ASA in unstable angina undergoing PTCA* **Action:** Anticoagulant, thrombin inhibitor **Dose:** 1 mg/kg IV bolus, then 2.5 mg/kg/h over 4 h; PRN, use 0.2 mg/kg/h for up to 20 h (give w/ ASA 300–325 mg/d; start pre-PTCA) **Caution:** [B, ?] **Contra:** Major bleeding **Supplied:** Powder for inj **SE:** Bleeding, back pain, nausea, HA **Interactions:** ↑ Cardiac effects of theophylline; ↑ hypokalemia w/ furosemide; ↑ effects w/ other β-adrenergic bronchodilators, MAOIs, TCAs, inhaled anesthetics; ↓ effects w/ β-adrenergic blockers; **Labs:** ↑ AST, ↓ plts, WBCs, proteinuria **NIPE:** Wait 15 min after use of this drug before using an adrenocorticoid inhaler. Shake inhaler well before use

Bleomycin Sulfate (Blenoxane)
Uses: *Testis CA; Hodgkin's & NHLs; cutaneous lymphomas; & squamous cell CA (head & neck, larynx, cervix, skin, penis); sclerosing agent for malignant pleural effusion* **Action:** Induces breakage (scission) of single-/double-stranded DNA **Dose:** 10–20 mg (U)/m² 1–2/wk (refer to specific protocols); ↓ in renal impairment **Caution:** [D, ?] Severe

pulmonary Dz **Supplied:** Inj 15 mg (15 U) **SE:** Hyperpigmentation (skin staining) & hypersensitivity (rash to anaphylaxis); fever in 50%; lung toxicity (idiosyncratic & dose-related); pneumonitis may progress to fibrosis; Raynaud's phenomenon, N/V **Notes:** Test dose 1 mg (U) recommended, especially in lymphoma Pts; lung toxicity w/total dose >400 mg (U) **Interactions:** ↑ Effects w/ cisplatin & other antineoplastic drugs; ↓ effects of digoxin & phenytoin **Labs:** Monitor CBC, LFTs, BUN, creatinine; pulmonary Fxn tests **NIPE:** ⊘ Immunizations, breast-feeding; use contraception method

Bortezomib (Velcade) **WARNING:** May worsen preexisting neuropathy
Uses: *Progression of multiple myeloma despite two previous Rxs* **Action:** Proteasome inhibitor **Dose:** 1.3 mg/m² bolus IV 2×/wk × 2 wk, w/ 10-day rest period (= 1 cycle); ↓ dose for hematologic toxicity, neuropathy **Caution:** [D, ?/–] **Supplied:** 3.5-mg vial **SE:** Asthenia, GI upset, anorexia, dyspnea, headache, orthostatic hypotension, edema, insomnia, dizziness, rash, pyrexia, arthralgia, neuropathy **Notes:** May interact w/ drugs metabolized via CYP450 system **Interactions:** ↑ Risk of peripheral neuropathy and/or hypotension w/ amiodarone, antivirals, INH, nitrofurantoin, statins **Labs:** Monitor for ↑ uric acid, ↓ K⁺, Ca²⁺, neutrophils, plts **NIPE:** ⊘ PRG or breast-feeding; use contraception; caution w/ driving due to fatigue/dizziness; ↑ fluids if C/O N/V

Brimonidine (Alphagan)
Uses: *Open-angle glaucoma, ocular HTN* **Action:** α₂-Adrenergic agonist **Dose:** 1 gt in eye(s) tid (wait 15 min to insert contacts) **Caution:** [B, ?] **Contra:** MAOI therapy **Supplied:** 0.2% soln **SE:** Local irritation, HA, fatigue **Interactions:** ↑ Effects of antihypertensives, BBs, cardiac glycosides, CNS depressants; ↓ effects w/ TCAs **NIPE:** ⊘ EtOH, insert soft contact lenses 15 + min after drug use

Brinzolamide (Azopt)
Uses: *Open-angle glaucoma, ocular HTN* **Action:** Carbonic anhydrase inhibitor **Dose:** 1 gt in eye(s) tid **Caution:** [C, ?] **Supplied:** 1% susp **SE:** Blurred vision, dry eye, blepharitis, taste disturbance **Interactions:** ↑ Effects w/ oral carbonic anhydrase inhibitors **Labs:** Check LFTs, BUN, creatinine **NIPE:** ⊘ Use drug if ↑ renal & hepatic studies or allergies to sulfonamides; shake well before use; insert soft contact lenses 15 + min after drug use; wait 10 min before use of other topical ophthalmic drugs

Bromocriptine (Parlodel)
Uses: *Parkinson's Dz, hyperprolactinemia, acromegaly, pituitary tumors* **Action:** Direct-acting on the striatal dopamine receptors; inhibits prolactin secretion **Dose:** Initial, 1.25 mg PO bid; titrate to effect **Caution:** [C, ?] **Contra:** Severe ischemic heart Dz or PVD **Supplied:** Tabs 2.5 mg; caps 5 mg **SE:** ↓ BP, Raynaud's phenomenon, dizziness, nausea, hallucinations **Interactions:** ↑ Effects w/ erythromycin, fluvoxamine, nefazodone, sympathomimetics; ↓ effects w/ phenothiazines, antipsychotics; **Labs:** ↑ BUN, AST, ALT, CPK, alkaline phosphatase, uric acid **NIPE:** ⊘ Breast-feeding, PRG, oral contraceptives; drug may cause intolerance to EtOH, return of menses & suppression of galactorrhea may take 6–8 wk

Budesonide (Rhinocort, Pulmicort) Uses: *Allergic & nonallergic rhinitis, asthma* Action: Steroid Dose: *Intranasal:* 2 sprays/nostril bid or 4 sprays/nostril/d. *Aqueous:* 1 spray/nostril/d. *PO inhaled:* 1–4 inhal bid. Peds. 1–2 inhal bid (Rinse mouth after PO use) Caution: [C, ?/–] Supplied: Met-dose Turbuhaler, nasal inhaler, & aqueous spray SE: HA, cough, hoarseness, *Candida* infection, epistaxis Interactions: ↑ Effects w/ ketoconazole, itraconazole, ritonavir, indinavir, saquinavir, erythromycin, and grapefruit juice NIPE: Shake inhaler well before use, rinse mouth & wash inhaler after use, swallow capsules whole, ⊘ exposure chickenpox or measles.

Bumetanide (Bumex) Uses: *Edema from CHF, hepatic cirrhosis, & renal Dz* Action: Loop diuretic; inhibits reabsorption of Na & Cl in the ascending loop of Henle & the distal renal tubule Dose: *Adults.* 0.5–2 mg/d PO; 0.5–1 mg IV q8–24h (max 10 mg/d). *Peds.* 0.015–0.1 mg/kg/d PO, IV, or IM ÷ q6–24h Caution: [D, ?] Contra: Anuria, hepatic coma, severe electrolyte depletion Supplied: Tabs 0.5, 1, 2 mg; inj 0.25 mg/mL SE: ↓ K+, ↓ Na+, ↑ creatinine, ↑ uric acid, dizziness, ototoxicity Notes: Monitor fluid & electrolytes Interactions: ↑ Effects w/ antihypertensives, thiazides, nitrates, EtOH, clofibrate; ↑ effects of Li, warfarin, thrombolytic drugs, anticoagulants; ↑ K+ loss w/ carbenoxolone, corticosteroids, terbutaline; ↑ ototoxicity w/ aminoglycosides, cisplatin; ↓ effects w/ cholestyramine, colestipol, NSAIDs, probenecid, barbiturates, phenytoin Labs: ↑ T_4, T_3, BUN, serum glucose, creatinine uric acid; ↓ serum K+, Ca²⁺, Mg²⁺ NIPE: Take drug w/ food, take early to prevent nocturia, daily weights

Bupivacaine (Marcaine) Uses: *Local, regional, & spinal anesthesia, local & regional analgesia* Action: Local anesthetic Dose: *Adults & Peds.* Dose-dependent on procedure (ie, tissue vascularity, depth of anesthesia, etc) Caution: [C, ?] Contra: Severe bleeding, severe hypotension, shock & arrhythmias, local infections at anesthesia site, septicemia Supplied: Inj 0.25, 0.5, 0.75% SE: ↓ BP, bradycardia, dizziness, anxiety Interactions: ↑ Effects w/ BBs, hyaluronidase, ergot-type oxytocics, MAOI, TCAs, phenothiazines, vasopressors, CNS depressants; ↓ effects w/ chloroprocaine NIPE: Anesthetized area has temporary loss of sensation & Fxn

Buprenorphine (Buprenex) [C-V] Uses: *Moderate/severe pain* Action: Opiate agonist–antagonist Dose: 0.3–0.6 mg IM or slow IV push q6h PRN Caution: [C, ?/–] Supplied: Inj 0.324 mg/mL (= 0.3 mg of buprenorphine) SE: Sedation, ↓ BP, resp depression Notes: May induce withdrawal syndrome in opioid-dependent Pts Interactions: ↑ Effects of resp & CNS depression w/ EtOH, opiates, benzodiazepines, TCAs, MAOIs, other CNS depressants Labs: ↑ Eerum amylase and lipase NIPE: ⊘ EtOH & other CNS depressants

Bupropion (Wellbutrin, Wellbutrin SR, Wellbutrin XL, Zyban) Uses: *Depression, adjunct to smoking cessation* Action: Weak inhibitor of neuronal uptake of serotonin & norepinephrine; inhibits the neuronal reuptake of dopamine Dose: *Depression:* 100–450 mg/d ÷ bid–tid; SR 100–200 mg bid; XL 150–300 mg daily. *Smoking cessation:* 150 mg/d × 3 d, then 150 mg bid ×8–12 wk; ↓ in renal/hepatic impairment **Caution:** [B, ?/–] **Contra:** Sz disorder, prior diagnosis of anorexia nervosa or bulimia, MAOI, abrupt discontinuation of EtOH or sedatives **Supplied:** Tabs 75, 100 mg; SR tabs 100, 150, 200 mg; XL tabs 150, 300 mg **SE:** Associated w/ Szs; agitation, insomnia, HA, tachycardia **Notes:** ⊘ Use of EtOH & other CNS depressants **Interactions:** ↑ Effects w/ cimetidine, levodopa, MAOIs; ↑ risk of Szs w/ EtOH, phenothiazines, antidepressants, theophylline, TCAs, or abrupt withdrawal of corticosteroids, benzodiazepines **Labs:** ↓ Prolactin level **NIPE:** Drug may cause Szs, take 3–4 wk for full effect, ⊘ EtOH or abrupt DC

Buspirone (BuSpar)   **WARNING:** Closely monitor for worsening depression or emergence of suicidality **Uses:** Short-term relief of *anxiety* **Action:** Antianxiety; selectively antagonizes CNS serotonin receptors **Dose:** 5–10 mg PO tid; ↑ to desired response; usual 20–30 mg/d; max 60 mg/d; ↓ in severe hepatic/renal insufficiency **Caution:** [B, ?/–] **Supplied:** Tabs 5, 10, 15, 30 mg ÷ dose **SE:** Drowsiness, dizziness; HA, nausea **Notes:** No abuse potential or physical or psychologic dependence **Interactions:** ↑ Effects w/ erythromycin, clarithromycin, itraconazole, ketoconazole, diltiazem, verapamil, grapefruit juice; ↓ effects w/ carbamazepine, rifampin, phenytoin, dexamethasone, phenobarbital, fluoxetine **Labs:** ↑ AST, ALT, growth hormone, prolactin **NIPE:** ↑ Sedation w/ EtOH, therapeutic effects may take up to 4 wk

Busulfan (Myleran, Busulfex)   **Uses:** *CML,* preparative regimens for allogeneic & ABMT in high doses **Action:** Alkylating agent **Dose:** 4–12 mg/d for several wks; 16 mg/kg once or 4 mg/kg/d for 4 d w/ another agent in transplant regimens. Refer to specific protocol **Caution:** [D, ?] **Supplied:** Tabs 2 mg, inj 60 mg/10 mL **SE:** Myelosuppression, pulmonary fibrosis, nausea (high-dose therapy), gynecomastia, adrenal insufficiency, & skin hyperpigmentation **Interactions:** ↑ Effects w/ acetaminophen; ↑ bone-marrow suppression w/ antineoplastic drugs & radiation therapy; ↑ uric acid levels w/ probenecid & sulfinpyrazone; ↓ effects w/ itraconazole, phenytoin **Labs:** ↑ Uric acid; monitor CBC, LFTs **NIPE:** ⊘ Immunizations, PRG, breast-feeding; ↑ fluids; use barrier contraception; ↑ risk of hair loss, rash, darkened skin pigment; ↑ susceptibility to infection

Butorphanol (Stadol) [C-IV]   **Uses:** *Anesthesia adjunct, pain* & migraine HA **Action:** Opiate agonist–antagonist w/ central analgesic actions **Dose:** 1–4 mg IM or IV q3–4h PRN. *HA:* 1 spray in 1 nostril; may repeat ×1 if pain not relieved in 60–90 min; ↓ dose in renal impairment **Caution:** [C (D if high doses or prolonged periods at term), +] **Supplied:** Inj 1, 2 mg/mL; nasal spray 10 mg/mL **SE:** Drowsiness, dizziness, nasal congestion **Notes:** May induce withdrawal in opioid dependence **Interactions:** ↑ Effects w/ EtOH, antihistamines, cimetidine, CNS depressants, phenothiazines, barbiturates, skeletal-muscle relaxants, MAOIs; ↓ effects of opioids **Labs:** ↑ Serum amylase & lipase **NIPE:** ⊘ EtOH or other CNS depressants

Calcipotriene (Dovonex) Uses: *Plaque psoriasis* Action: Keratolytic Dose: Apply bid Caution: [C, ?] Contra: ↑ Ca²⁺; vitamin D toxicity; ⊘ apply to face Supplied: Cream; oint; soln 0.005% SE: Skin irritation, dermatitis Interactions: None noted Labs: Monitor serum Ca NIPE: Wash hands after application or wear gloves to apply, DC drug if ↑ Ca

Calcitonin (Cibacalcin, Miacalcin) Uses: *Paget's Dz of bone, hypercalcemia,* osteogenesis imperfecta, *postmenopausal osteoporosis* Action: Polypeptide hormone Dose: *Paget's salmon form:* 100 units/d IM/SC initially, 50 units/d or 50–100 units q1–3d maint. *Paget's human form:* 0.5 mg/d initially; maint 0.5 mg 2–3 ×/wk or 0.25 mg/d, max 0.5 mg bid. *Hypercalcemia salmon calcitonin:* 4 units/kg IM/SC q12h; ↑ to 8 units/kg q12h, max q6h. *Osteoporosis salmon calcitonin:* 100 units/d IM/SQ; intranasal 200 units = 1 nasal spray/d Caution: [C, ?] Supplied: Spray, nasal 200 units/activation; inj, human (Cibacalcin) 0.5 mg/vial, salmon 200 units/mL (2 mL) SE: Facial flushing, nausea, edema at inj site, nasal irritation, polyuria Notes: Human (Cibacalcin) & salmon forms; human only approved for Paget's bone Dz Interactions: None noted Labs: ↓ Serum Li NIPE: Allergy skin test prior to use

Calcitriol (Rocaltrol) Uses: *Reduction of ↑ PTH levels, ↓ Ca²⁺ on dialysis* Action: 1,25-Dihydroxycholecalciferol (vitamin D analogue) Dose: *Adults. Renal failure:* 0.25 µg/d PO, ↑ 0.25 µg/d q4–6wk PRN; 0.5 µg 3×/wk IV, ↑ PRN. *Hyperparathyroidism:* 0.5–2 µg/d. *Renal failure:* 15 ng/kg/d, ↑ PRN; maint 30–60 ng/kg/d. *Peds. Hyperparathyroidism:* <5 y, 0.25–0.75 µg/d >6 y, 0.5–2 µg/d Caution: [C, ?] Contra: ↑ Ca²⁺; vitamin D toxicity Supplied: Inj 1, 2 µg/mL (in 1-mL); caps 0.25, 0.5 µg SE: ↑ Ca²⁺ possible Notes: Monitor dose to keep Ca²⁺ WNL Interactions: ↑ Effect w/ thiazide diuretics; ↓ effect w/ cholestyramine, colestipol Labs: ↑ Ca²⁺, cholesterol, Mg²⁺, BUN, AST, ALT; ↑ alkaline phosphatase; NIPE: ⊘ Mg-containing antacids or suppls

Calcium Acetate (Calphron, Phos-Ex, PhosLo) Uses: *ESRD-associated hyperphosphatemia* Action: Ca suppl to treat hyperphosphatemia w/o Al Dose: 2–4 tabs PO w/ meals Caution: [C, ?] Contra: ↑ Ca²⁺ Supplied: Caps Phos-Ex 500 mg (125 mg Ca); tabs Calphron & PhosLo 667 mg (169 mg Ca) SE: Can cause ↑ Ca²⁺, hypophosphatemia, constipation Notes: Monitor Ca²⁺ Interactions: ↑ Effects of quinidine; ↓ effects w/ large intake of dietary fiber, spinach, rhubarb; ↓ effects of atenolol, CCB, etidronate, tetracyclines, fluoroquinolones, phenytoin, Fe salts Labs: ↑ Ca²⁺, ↓ Mg²⁺ NIPE: ⊘ EtOH, caffeine, tobacco; separate Ca suppls and other meds by 1–2 h

Calcium Carbonate (Tums, Alka-Mints) [OTC] Uses: *Hyperacidity associated w/ peptic ulcer Dz, hiatal hernia,* etc Action: Neutralizes gastric acid Dose: 500 mg–2 g PO PRN; ↓ in renal impairment Caution: [C, ?] Supplied: Chew tabs 350, 420, 500, 550, 750, 850 mg; susp SE: ↑ Ca²⁺, hypophosphatemia, constipation Interactions: ↓ Effect of tetracyclines, fluoroquinolones, Fe salts, and ASA; ↓ Ca absorption w/ high intake of dietary fiber Labs: ↑ Ca²⁺, ↓ Mg²⁺ NIPE:

↑ Fluids, may cause constipation, ⊘ EtOH, caffeine, tobacco; separate Ca suppls and other meds by 1–2 h, chew tablet well

Calcium Glubionate (Neo-Calglucon) [OTC]
Uses: *Rx & prevent Ca deficiency* Action: Ca suppl Dose: Adults. 6–18 g/d ÷ doses. Peds. 600–2000 mg/kg/d ÷ qid (9 g/d max); ↓ in renal impairment Caution: [C, ?] Contra: ↑ Ca²⁺ Supplied: Ca syrup 1.8 g/5 mL = Ca 115 mg/5 mL SE: Hypercalcemia, hypophosphatemia, constipation Interactions: ↑ Effects of quinidine; ↓ effect of tetracyclines; ↓ Ca absorption w/ high intake of dietary fiber; Labs: ↑ Ca²⁺, ↓ Mg²⁺ NIPE: ⊘ EtOH, caffeine, tobacco, separate Ca suppls and other meds by 1–2 h, chew tablet well

Calcium Salts (Chloride, Gluconate, Gluceptate)
Uses: *Ca replacement,* VF, Ca blocker toxicity, Mg intoxication, tetany, *hyperphosphatemia in ESRD* Action: Ca suppl/replacement Dose: Adults. Replacement: 1–2 g/d PO. Cardiac emergencies: CaCl 0.5–1 g IV q 10 min or Ca gluconate 1–2 g IV q 10 min. Tetany: 1 g CaCl over 10–30 min; repeat in 6 h PRN. Peds. Replacement: 200–500 mg/kg/24 h PO or IV ÷ qid. Cardiac emergency: 100 mg/kg/dose IV of gluconate salt q 10 min. Tetany: 10 mg/kg CaCl over 5–10 min; repeat in 6 h or use inf (200 mg/kg/d max). Adult & Peds. Hypocalcemia due to citrated blood inf: 0.45 mEq Ca/100 mL citrated blood inf (↓ in renal impairment) Caution: [C, ?] Contra: Hypercalcemia Supplied: CaCl inj 10% = 100 mg/mL = Ca 27.2 mg/mL = 10-mL amp; Ca gluconate inj 10% = 100 mg/mL = Ca 9 mg/mL; tabs 500 mg = 45 mg Ca, 650 mg = 58.5 mg Ca, 975 mg = 87.75 mg Ca, 1 g = 90 mg Ca; Ca gluceptate inj 220 mg/mL = 18 mg/mL Ca SE: Bradycardia, cardiac arrhythmias, ↑ Ca²⁺ Notes: CaCl 270 mg (13.6 mEq) elemental Ca/g, & Ca gluconate 90 mg (4.5 mEq) Ca/g. RDA for Ca: Adults = 800 mg/d; Peds = <6 mo 360 mg/d, 6 mo–1 y 540 mg/d, 1–10 y 800 mg/d, 10–18 y 1200 mg/d Interactions: ↑ Effects of quinidine and digitalis; ↓ effects of tetracyclines, quinolones, verapamil, CCBs, Fe salts, ASA, atenolol; ↓ Ca absorption w/ high intake of dietary fiber Labs: ↑ Ca²⁺, ↓ Mg²⁺ NIPE: ⊘ EtOH, caffeine, tobacco; separate Ca suppls and other meds by 1–2 h, chew tablet well

Calfactant (Infasurf)
Uses: *Prevention & Rx of RSD in infants* Action: Exogenous pulmonary surfactant Dose: 3 mL/kg instilled into lungs. Can retreat for a total of 3 doses given 12 h apart Caution: [?, ?] Supplied: Intratracheal susp 35 mg/mL SE: Monitor for cyanosis, airway obstruction, bradycardia during administration Interactions: None noted NIPE: ⊘ Reconstitute, dilute, or shake vial; refrigerate & keep away from light; no need to warm soln prior to use

Candesartan (Atacand)
Uses: *HTN,* DN, CHF Action: Angiotensin II receptor antagonists Dose: 2–32 mg/d (usual 16 mg) Caution: [X, –] Contra: Primary hyperaldosteronism; bilateral renal artery stenosis Supplied: Tabs 4, 8, 16, 32 mg SE: Dizziness, HA, flushing, angioedema Interactions: ↑ Effects w/ cimetidine; ↑ risk of hyperkalemia w/ amiloride, spironolactone, triamterene, K suppls, trimethoprim; ↑ effects of Li; ↓ effects w/ phenobarbital, rifampin Labs: ↑

Creatine phosphatase; monitor for albuminuria, hyperglycemia, triglyceridemia, uricemia. **NIPE:** ⊘ Breast-feeding or PRG, use barrier contraception, may take 4–6 wk for full effect, adequate fluid intake, take w/o regard to food

Capsaicin (Capsin, Zostrix, others) [OTC]
Uses: Pain due to *postherpetic neuralgia,* chronic neuralgia, *arthritis,* diabetic neuropathy,* postoperative pain, psoriasis, intractable pruritus **Action:** Topical analgesic **Dose:** Apply tid–qid **Caution:** [?, ?] **Supplied:** OTC creams; gel; lotions; roll-ons **SE:** Local irritation, neurotoxicity, cough **Interactions:** May ↑ cough w/ ACEIs **NIPE:** External use only, ⊘ contact w/ eyes or broken/irritated skin, apply w/ gloves, transient stinging/burning

Captopril (Capoten, others)
Uses: *HTN, CHF, MI,* LVD, DN **Action:** ACEI **Dose:** *Adults. HTN:* Initially, 25 mg PO bid–tid; ↑ to maint q1–2wk by 25-mg increments/dose (max 450 mg/d) to effect. *CHF:* Initially, 6.25–12.5 mg PO tid; titrate PRN *LVD:* 50 mg PO tid. *DN:* 25 mg PO tid. *Peds. Infants <2 mo:* 0.05–0.5 mg/kg/dose PO q8–24h. *Children:* Initially, 0.3–0.5 mg/kg/dose PO; ↑ to 6 mg/kg/d max (Take 1 h ac) **Caution:** [C (1st tri); D (2nd & 3rd tri); ? in renal impairment +] **Contra:** Hx angioedema **Supplied:** Tabs 12.5, 25, 50, 100 mg **SE:** Rash, proteinuria, cough, ↑ K⁺ **Interactions:** ↑ Effects w/ antihypertensives, diuretics, nitrates, probenecid, black catechu; ↓ effects w/ antacids, ASA, NSAIDs, food; ↑ effects of digoxin, insulin, oral hypoglycemics, Li **Labs:** False + urine acetone; may ↑ urine protein, serum BUN, creatinine, K⁺, prolactin, LFTs; may ↓ FBS **NIPE:** ⊘ PRG, breast-feeding, K-sparing diuretics; take w/o food, may take 2 wk for full therapeutic effect

Carbamazepine (Tegretol)
WARNING: Aplastic anemia & agranulosytosis have been reported w/ carbamazepine **Uses:** *Epilepsy, trigeminal neuralgia,* EtOH withdrawal **Action:** Anticonvulsant **Dose:** *Adults.* Initially, 200 mg PO bid; ↑ by 200 mg/d; usual 800–1200 mg/d ÷ doses. *Peds. <6 y:* 5 mg/kg/d, ↑ to 10–20 mg/kg/d ÷ in 2–4 doses. *6–12 y:* Initial, 100 mg PO bid or 10 mg/kg/24 h PO ÷ qd–bid; ↑ to maint 20–30 mg/kg/24 h ÷ tid–qid; ↓ dose in renal impairment (take w/ food) **Caution:** [D, +] **Contra:** MAOI use, Hx bone marrow depression **Supplied:** Tabs 200 mg; chew tabs 100 mg; XR tabs 100, 200, 400 mg; susp 100 mg/5 mL **SE:** Drowsiness, dizziness, blurred vision, N/V, rash, ↓ Na⁺, leukopenia, agranulocytosis **Notes:** Monitor CBC & serum levels (see Table 2, page 265); generic products not interchangeable **Interactions:** ↑ Effects w/ cimetidine, clarithromycin, danazol, diltiazem, felbamate, fluconazole, fluoxetine, fluvoxamine, INH, itraconazole, ketoconazole, macrolides, metronidazole, propoxyphene, protease inhibitors, valproic acid, verapamil, grapefruit juice; ↑ effects of Li, MAOIs; ↓ effects w/ phenobarbital, phenytoin, primidone, plantain; ↓ effects of benzodiazepines, corticosteroids, cyclosporine, doxycycline, felbamate, haloperidol, oral contraceptives, phenytoin, theophylline, thyroid hormones, TCAs, warfarin **Labs:** ↑ BUN, LFTs, bilirubin, alkaline phosphatase; ↓ Ca²⁺, T₃, T₄, Na; false − PRG test & uric acid **NIPE:** Take w/ food, may cause photosensitivity—use sunscreen, use barrier contraception, abrupt withdrawal may cause Szs, ⊘ breast-feeding or PRG

Carbidopa/Levodopa (Sinemet) Uses: *Parkinson's Dz* Action: ↑ CNS levels of dopamine Dose: 25/100 mg bid–qid; ↑ as needed (max 200/2000 mg/d) Caution: [C, ?] Contra: Narrow-angle glaucoma, suspicious skin lesion (may activate melanoma), melanoma, MAOI use Supplied: Tabs (mg carbidopa/mg levodopa) 10/100, 25/100, 25/250; tabs SR (mg carbidopa/mg levodopa) 25/100, 50/200 SE: Psychiatric disturbances, orthostatic hypotension, dyskinesias, & cardiac arrhythmias Interactions: ↑ Effects w/ antacids; ↓ effects w/ anticonvulsants, benzodiazepines, haloperidol, Fe, methionine, papaverine, phenothiazines, phenytoin, pyridoxine, spiramycin, tacrine, thioxanthenes, high protein food Labs: ↑ Urine amino acids, serum acid phosphatase, aspartate aminotransferase; ↓ serum bilirubin, BUN, creatinine, glucose, uric acid NIPE: Darkened urine & sweat may result, ⊘ crush or chew sustained release tabs, take w/o food

Carboplatin (Paraplatin) Uses: *Ovarian, lung, head & neck, testicular, urothelial,* & brain *CA, NHL* & allogeneic & ABMT in high doses Action: DNA cross-linker; forms DNA-platinum adducts Dose: 360 mg/m^2 (ovarian carcinoma); AUC dosing 4–7 mg/mL (using Culvert's formula: mg = AUC × [25 + calculated GFR]); adjusted based on pretreatment plt count, CrCl, & BSA (Egorin's formula); up to 1500 mg/m^2 used in ABMT setting (refer to specific protocols) Caution: [D, ?] Contra: Severe bone marrow suppression, excessive bleeding Supplied: Inj 50, 150, 450 mg SE: Myelosuppression, N/V/D, nephrotoxicity, hematuria, neurotoxicity, ↑ LFTs Notes: Physiologic dosing based on either Culvert's or Egorin's formula allows ↑ doses to reduce toxicity Interactions: ↑ Myelosuppression w/ myelosuppressive drugs; ↑ hemotologic effects w/ bonemarrow suppressants; ↑ bleeding w/ ASA; ↑ nephrotoxicity w/ nephrotoxic drugs; ↓ effects of phenytoin; ↓ effects w/ food and w/ Al Labs: ↓ Mg^{2+}, K$^+$, Na$^+$, Ca^{2+}; ↑ LFTs NIPE: ⊘ Use w/ Al needles or IV administration sets, PRG, breast-feeding; antiemetics prior to admin may prevent N/V, maintain adequate food & fluid intake

Carisoprodol (Soma) Uses: *Adjunct to sleep & physical therapy for the relief of painful musculoskeletal conditions* Action: Centrally acting muscle relaxant Dose: 350 mg PO tid–qid Caution: [C, M] Tolerance may result; caution in renal/hepatic impairment Contra: Hypersensitivity to meprobamate; acute intermittent porphyria Supplied: Tabs 350 mg SE: CNS depression, drowsiness, dizziness, tachycardia Notes: ⊘ EtOH & other CNS depressants; available in combination w/ ASA or codeine. Interactions: ↑ Effects w/ CNS depressants, phenothiazines, EtOH NIPE: ⊘ Breast-feeding, take w/ food if GI upset

Carmustine [BCNU] (BiCNU, Gliadel) Uses: *Primary brain tumors, melanoma, Hodgkin's lymphoma & NHLs, multiple myeloma, & induction for allogeneic & ABMT in high doses; adjunct to surgery in Pts w/ recurrent glioblastoma multiforme* Action: Alkylating agent; nitrosourea forms DNA cross-links; inhibits DNA Dose: 150–200 mg/m^2 q6–8wk single or ÷ dose daily inj over 2d; 20–65 mg/m^2 q4–6wk; 300–900 mg/m^2 in BMT (see specific protocols); ↓ dose in hepatic impairment **Caution:** [D, ?] In ↓ WBC, RBC, plt counts, renal or hepatic impairment **Contra:** Myelosuppression, PRG **Supplied:** Inj 100 mg/vial; wafer: 7.7 mg/vial **SE:** Hypotension, N/V, myelosuppression (WBC & plt), phlebitis, facial flushing, hepatic & renal dysfunction, pulmonary fibrosis, & optic neuroretinitis; hematologic toxicity may persist up to 4–6 wk after dose **Notes:** ⊘ give course more frequently than q6wk (cumulative toxicity); baseline PFTs recommended **Interactions:** ↑ Bleeding w/ ASA, anticoagulants; ↑ hepatic dysfunction w/ etoposide; ↑ myelosuppression w/ cimetidine; ↑ suppression of bone marrow w/ radiation or additional antineoplastics; ↓ effects of phenytoin, digoxin; ↓ pulmonary Fxn **Labs:** ↑ AST, alkaline phosphatase, bilirubin; monitor CBC, plts, LFTs, PFTs **NIPE:** ⊘ PRG, breast-feeding, exposure to infections, ASA products

Carteolol (Cartrol, Ocupress Ophthalmic) **Uses:** *HTN, ↑ intraocular pressure, chronic open-angle glaucoma* **Action:** Blocks β-adrenergic receptors (β_1, β_2), mild ISA **Dose:** PO 2.5–5 mg/d; ophth 1 gt in eye(s) bid; ↓ in renal impairment **Caution:** [C (1st tri); D (2nd & 3rd tri), ?/–] Cardiac failure, asthma **Contra:** Sinus bradycardia; heart block >1st degree; bronchospasm **Supplied:** Tabs 2.5, 5 mg; ophth soln 1% **SE:** Drowsiness, sexual dysfunction, bradycardia, edema, CHF; *ocular:* conjunctival hyperemia, anisocoria, keratitis, eye pain **Notes:** Not shown to be of value in CHF **Interactions:** ↑ Effects w/ amiodarone, adenosine, barbiturates, CCBs, digoxin, dipyridamole, fluoxetine, rifampin, tacrine, nitrates, EtOH; ↑ α-adrenergic effects w/ amphetamines, cocaine, ephedrine, epinephrine, phenylephrine; ↑ effects of theophylline; ↓ effects w/ antacids, NSAIDs, thyroid drugs, clonidine; ↓ effects of hypoglycemics, theophylline, dopamine **Labs:** ↑ BUN, uric acid, K^+, serum lipoprotein, triglycerides, glucose, ANA titers **NIPE:** Ophthalmic drug may cause photophobia & risk of burning; may ↑ cold sensitivity, mental confusion

Carvedilol (Coreg) **Uses:** *HTN, CHF, MI* **Action:** Blocks adrenergic receptors, β_1, β_2, α **Dose:** *HTN:* 6.25–12.5 mg bid. *CHF:* 3.125–25 mg bid; take w/ food to minimize hypotension **Caution:** [C (1st tri); D (2nd & 3rd tri), ?/–] Bradycardia, asthma, diabetes **Contra:** Decompensated cardiac failure, 2nd-/3rd-degree heart block, SSS, severe hepatic impairment **Supplied:** Tabs 3.125, 6.25, 12.5, 25 mg **SE:** Dizziness, fatigue, hyperglycemia, bradycardia, edema, hypercholesterolemia **Notes:** ⊘ DC abruptly; **Interactions:** ↑ Effects w/ cimetidine, clonidine, MAOIs, reserpine, verapamil, fluoxetine, paroxetine; ↑ effects of digoxin, hypoglycemics, cyclosporine, CCBs; ↓ effects w/ rifampin, NSAIDs; **Labs:** ↑ LFTs, K^+, triglycerides, uric acid, BUN, creatinine, alkaline phosphatase; ↓ HDL **NIPE:** Food slows absorption, may cause dry eyes w/ contact lenses

Caspofungin (Cancidas) **Uses:** *Invasive aspergillosis refractory/intolerant to standard therapy, esophageal candidiasis* **Action:** An echinocandin; inhibits fungal cell wall synthesis; highest activity in regions of active cell growth **Dose:** 70 mg IV load day 1, 50 mg/d IV; slow inf; ↓ dose in hepatic impairment **Caution:** [C, ?/–] ⊘ use w/ cyclosporine; not studied as initial therapy **Contra:** Hypersensitivity to any component **Supplied:** IV inf **SE:** Fever, HA, N/V, thrombophlebitis at site, ↑ LFTs **Notes:** Monitor during inf; limited experience beyond 2 wk of therapy **Interactions:** ↑ Effects w/ cyclosporine; ↓ effects w/ carbamazepine, dexamethasone, efavirenz, nelfinavir, nevirapine, phenytoin, rifampin; ↓ effect of tacrolimus **Labs:** ↑ LFTs, serum alkaline phosphatase, eosinophils, PT, urine protein & RBCs; ↓ K⁺, albumin, WBCs, Hgb, Hct, plts, neutrophils; **NIPE:** Infuse slowly over 1 h & ⊘ mix w/ other drugs

Cefaclor (Ceclor) **Uses:** *Rx bacterial infections of the upper & lower resp tract, skin, bone, urinary tract, abdomen, & gynecologic system* **Action:** 2nd-gen cephalosporin; inhibits cell wall synthesis. *Spectrum:* More gram(+) activity than 1st-gen cephalosporins; effective against gram(+) including *S. aureus*; good gram(−) coverage against *H. influenzae* **Dose:** *Adults.* 250–500 mg PO tid; XR 375–500 mg bid. *Peds.* 20–40 mg/kg/d PO ÷ 8–12h; ↓ renal impairment **Caution:** [B, +] **Contra:** Allergy to cephalosporins **Supplied:** Caps 250, 500 mg; XR tabs 375, 500 mg; susp 125, 187, 250, 375 mg/5 mL **SE:** Diarrhea, rash, eosinophilia, ↑ transaminases **Interactions:** ↑ Bleeding w/ anticoagulants; ↑ nephrotoxicity w/ aminoglycosides, loop diuretics; ↑ effects w/ probenecid; ↓ effects w/ antacids, chloramphenicol **Labs:** + Direct Coombs' test; ↑ LFTs, alkaline phosphatase, bilirubin, LDH, BUN, creatinine; false + of serum or UCr, false + urine glucose **NIPE:** Food w/ ER tabs ↑ absorption, monitor for superinfection, ⊘ breast-feeding

Cefadroxil (Duricef, Ultracef) **Uses:** *Rx infections involving skin, bone, upper & lower resp tract, & urinary tract* **Action:** 1st-gen cephalosporin; inhibits cell wall synthesis. *Spectrum:* Good gram(+) coverage, including group A β-hemolytic *Streptococcus*; gram(−) coverage against *E. coli, Proteus, Klebsiella* **Dose:** *Adults.* 1–2 g/d PO, 2 ÷ doses *Peds.* 30 mg/kg/d ÷ bid; ↓ dose in renal impairment **Caution:** [B, +] **Contra:** Hypersensitivity to cephalosporins **Supplied:** Caps 500 mg; tabs 1 g; susp 125, 250, 500 mg/5 mL **SE:** Diarrhea, N/V, rash, eosinophilia, ↑ transaminases **Interactions:** ↑ Bleeding w/ anticoagulants; ↑ nephrotoxicity w/ aminoglycosides, loop diuretics; ↑ effects w/ probenecid; ↓ effects w/ antacids, chloramphenicol **Labs:** + Direct Coombs' test; ↑ LFTs, alkaline phosphatase, bilirubin, LDH, BUN, creatinine; false + of serum or UCr, false + urine glucose **NIPE:** Food w/ ER tabs ↑ absorption, monitor for superinfection, ⊘ breast-feeding; give w/o regard to food

Cefazolin (Ancef, Kefzol) **Uses:** *Rx infections of skin, bone, upper & lower resp tract, & urinary tract* **Action:** 1st-gen cephalosporin; inhibits cell wall synthesis. *Spectrum:* Good coverage against gram(+) bacilli & cocci, *Streptococcus, Staphylococcus* (except *Enterococcus*); some gram(−) coverage (*E. coli, Proteus, Klebsiella*) **Dose:** *Adults.* 1–2 g IV q8h *Peds.* 25–100 mg/kg/d IV ÷ q6–8h; ↓ in renal impairment **Caution:**[B, +] **Contra:** Hypersensitivity to cephalosporins **Supplied:** Inj **SE:** Diarrhea, rash, eosinophilia, elevated transaminases, pain at inj site **Notes:** Widely used for surgical prophylaxis **Interactions:** ↑ Bleeding w/ anticoagulants; ↑ nephrotoxicity w/ aminoglycosides, loop diuretics; ↑ effects w/

probenecid; ↓ effects w/ antacids, chloramphenicol **Labs:** + Direct Coombs' test; ↑ LFTs, alkaline phosphatase, bilirubin, LDH, BUN, creatinine; false + of serum or UCr, false + urine glucose **NIPE:** Food W/ ER tabs ↑ absorption, monitor for superinfection, ⊘ breast-feeding; monitor renal Fxn, I&O

Cefdinir (Omnicef) **Uses:** *Rx infections of the resp tract, skin, bone, & urinary tract* **Action:** 3rd-gen cephalosporin; inhibits cell wall synthesis *Spectrum:* Active in vitro against a wide range of gram(+) & gram(−) organisms; more active than cefaclor & cephalexin against *Streptococcus, Staphylococcus*; active against some anaerobes **Dose:** *Adults.* 300 mg PO bid or 600 mg/d PO. *Peds.* 7 mg/kg PO bid or 14 mg/kg/d PO; ↓ in renal impairment **Caution:** [B, +] In penicillin-sensitive Pts; serum sickness-like Rxns have been reported **Contra:** Hypersentivity to cephalosporins **Supplied:** Caps 300 mg; susp 125 mg/5 mL **SE:** Anaphylaxis, diarrhea, rare pseudomembranous colitis **Interactions:** ↑ Bleeding w/ anticoagulants; ↑ nephrotoxicity w/ aminoglycosides, loop diuretics; ↑ effects w/ probenecid; ↓ effects w/ antacids, chloramphenicol; ↓ effects w/ Fe suppls **Labs:** + Direct Coombs' test; ↑ LFTs, alkaline phosphatase, bilirubin, LDH, BUN, creatinine; false + of serum or UCr, false + urine glucose **NIPE:** Food w/ ER tabs ↑ absorption, monitor for superinfection, ⊘ breast-feeding; stools may initially turn red in color, sucrose in suspension

Cefditoren (Spectracef) **Uses:** *Acute exacerbations of chronic bronchitis, pharyngitis, tonsillitis; skin infections* **Action:** 3rd-gen cephalosporin; inhibits cell wall synthesis. *Spectrum:* Good gram(+) activity against *Streptococcus* & *Staphylococcus* infections; gram(−) *H. influenzae* & *M. catarrhalis* **Dose:** *Adults & Peds >12 y.* Skin: 200 mg PO bid × 10 days. *Chronic bronchitis, pharyngitis, tonsillitis:* 400 mg PO bid × 10 days; ⊘ antacids w/in 2 h; take w/ meals; adjust dose in renal impairment **Caution:** [B, ?] Renal or hepatic impairment **Contra:** Hypersensitivity to cephalosporins/penicillins, milk protein, or carnitine deficiency **Supplied:** 200-mg tabs **SE:** HA, N/V/D, colitis, nephrotoxicity, hepatic dysfunction, Stevens–Johnson syndrome, toxic epidermal necrolysis, hypersensitivity Rxns **Notes:** Causes renal excretion of carnitine **Interactions:** ↑ Bleeding w/ anticoagulants; ↑ nephrotoxicity w/ aminoglycosides, loop diuretics; ↑ effects w/ probenecid; ↓ effects w/ antacids, chloramphenicol **Labs:** + Direct Coombs' test; ↑ LFTs, alkaline phosphatase, bilirubin, LDH, BUN, creatinine; false + of serum or UCr, false + urine glucose **NIPE:** Food w/ ER tabs ↑ absorption, monitor for superinfection, ⊘ breast-feeding, sensitive to milk protein; monitor for Sz activity

Cefepime (Maxipime) **Uses:** *UTI, pneumonia, febrile neutropenia, skin/soft tissue infections* **Action:** 4th-gen cephalosporin; inhibits cell wall synthesis. *Spectrum:* S. pneumoniae, S. aureus, K. pneumoniae, E. coli, P. aeruginosa, & Enterobacter sp **Dose:** *Adults.* 1–2 g IV q12h. *Peds.* 50 mg/kg q8h for febrile neutropenia; 50 mg/kg bid for skin/soft tissue infections; ↓ dose in renal impairment **Caution:** [B, +] **Contra:** Hypersensitivity to cephalosporins **Supplied:** Inj

500 mg, 1, 2 g **SE:** Rash, pruritus, N/V/D, fever, HA, + direct Coombs' test w/out hemolysis **Notes:** Administered as IM or IV **Interactions:** ↑ Bleeding w/ anticoagulants; ↑ nephrotoxicity w/ aminoglycosides, loop diuretics; ↑ effects w/ probenecid; ↓ effects w/ antacids, chloramphenicol; ↓ effects of oral contraceptives **Labs:** + Direct Coombs' test; ↑ LFTs, alkaline phosphatase, bilirubin, LDH, BUN, creatinine; false + of serum or UCr, false + urine glucose **NIPE:** Food w/ ER tabs ↑ absorption, monitor for superinfection, ⊘ breast-feeding or use EtOH w/ drug or w/in 3 d of taking drug

Cefixime (Suprax) Uses: *Rx infections of the resp tract, skin, bone, & urinary tract* **Action:** 3rd-gen cephalosporin; inhibits cell wall synthesis. *Spectrum: S. pneumoniae, S. pyogenes, H. influenzae, & enterobacteria.* **Dose: Adults.** 400 mg PO qd–bid. **Peds.** 8 mg/kg/d PO ÷ daily–bid; ↓ dose in renal impairment **Caution:** [B, +] **Contra:** Hypersensitivity to cephalosporins **Supplied:** Tabs 200, 400 mg; susp 100 mg/5 mL **SE:** N/V/D, flatulence, & abdominal pain **Notes:** Monitor renal & hepatic Fxn; use susp for otitis media **Interactions:** ↑ Bleeding w/ anticoagulants; ↑ nephrotoxicity w/ aminoglycosides, loop diuretics; ↑ effects w/ probenecid; ↓ effects w/ antacids, chloramphenicol; ↓ effects of oral contraceptives **Labs:** + Direct Coombs' test; ↑ LFTs, alkaline phosphatase, bilirubin, LDH, BUN, creatinine; false + of serum or UCr, false + urine glucose **NIPE:** Food w/ ER tabs ↑ absorption, monitor for superinfection, ⊘ breast-feeding

Cefmetazole (Zefazone) Uses: *Rx infections of the upper & lower resp tract, skin, bone, urinary tract, abdomen, & gynecologic system* **Action:** 2nd-gen cephalosporin; inhibits cell wall synthesis. *Spectrum:* Gram(+) against *S. aureus;* gram(−) activity & some anaerobic activity; use in mixed aerobic–anaerobic infections where *Bacteroides fragilis* likely **Dose: Adults.** 2 g IV q6–12h; ↓ in renal impairment **Caution:** [B, +] **Contra:** Hypersensitivity to cephalosporins **Supplied:** Inj 1, 2 g **SE:** Eosinophilia, leukopenia, N/V/D, ↑ LFTs, bleeding risk, rash, pseudomembranous colitis, disulfram Rxn **Notes:** Safety not established in children **Interactions:** ↑ Bleeding w/ anticoagulants; ↑ nephrotoxicity w/ aminoglycosides, loop diuretics; ↑ effects w/ probenecid; ↓ effects w/ antacids, chloramphenicol **Labs:** + Direct Coombs' test; ↑ LFTs, alkaline phosphatase, bilirubin, LDH, BUN, creatinine; false + of serum or UCr, false + urine glucose **NIPE:** Food w/ ER tabs ↑ absorption, monitor for superinfection, ⊘ breast-feeding or use EtOH w/ drug or w/in 3 d of taking drug

Cefonicid (Monocid) Uses: *Rx bacterial infections (resp tract, skin, bone & joint, urinary tract, gynecologic, sepsis)* **Action:** 2nd-gen cephalosporin; inhibits bacterial cell wall synthesis. *Spectrum:* Gram(+) including MSSA & many streptococci; gram(−) bacilli including *E. coli, Klebsiella, P. mirabilis, H. influenzae, & Moraxella* **Dose:** 0.5–2 g/24 h IM/IV; ↓ in renal impairment **Caution:** [B, +] **Contra:** Hypersensitivity to cephalosporins **Supplied:** Powder for inj 500 mg, 1 g, 10 g **SE:** Diarrhea, rash, ↑ plts, eosinophilia, ↑ transaminases **Interactions:** ↑

Bleeding w/ anticoagulants; ↑ nephrotoxicity w/ aminoglycosides, loop diuretics; ↑ effects w/ probenecid; ↓ effects w/ antacids, chloramphenicol **Labs:** + Direct Coombs' test; ↑ LFTs, alkaline phosphatase, LDH, BUN, creatinine; false + of serum or UCr, false + urine glucose **NIPE:** Food w/ ER tabs ↑ absorption, monitor for superinfection, ⊘ breast-feeding

Cefoperazone (Cefobid)

Uses: *Rx infections of the resp, skin, urinary tract, sepsis* **Action:** 3rd-gen cephalosporin; inhibits bacterial cell wall synthesis. *Spectrum:* Gram(−) (eg, *E. coli, Klebsiella*); variable against *Streptococcus* & *Staphylococcus* sp; active *P. aeruginosa* but < ceftazidime **Dose:** *Adults.* 2–4 g/d IM/IV ÷ q 8–12h (12 g/d max). *Peds.* (not approved) 100–150 mg/kg/d IM/IV ÷ bid–tid (12 g/d max); ↓ in renal/hepatic impairment **Caution:** [B, +] May ↑ risk of bleeding **Contra:** Hypersensitivity to cephalosporins **Supplied:** Powder for inj 1, 2 g **SE:** Diarrhea, rash, eosinophilia, ↑ LFTs, hypoprothrombinemia, & bleeding (due to MTT side chain) **Notes:** May interfere w/ warfarin **Interactions:** ↑ Bleeding w/ anticoagulants; ↑ nephrotoxicity w/ aminoglycosides, loop diuretics; ↑ effects w/ probenecid; ↓ effects w/ antacids, chloramphenicol **Labs:** + Direct Coombs' test; ↑ LFTs, alkaline phosphatase, bilirubin, LDH, BUN, creatinine; false + of serum or UCr, false + urine glucose **NIPE:** Food w/ ER tabs ↑ absorption, monitor for superinfection, ⊘ breast-feeding or use EtOH w/ drug or w/in 3 d of taking drug

Cefotaxime (Claforan)

Uses: *Rx infections of resp tract, skin, bone, urinary tract, meningitis, sepsis* **Action:** 3rd-gen cephalosporin; inhibits cell wall synthesis. *Spectrum:* Most gram(−) (not *Pseudomonas*), some gram(+) cocci (not *Enterococcus*); many penicillin-resistant pneumococci **Dose:** *Adults.* 1–2 g IV q4–12h. *Peds.* 50–200 mg/kg/d IV ÷ q 4–12h; ↓ dose renal/hepatic impairment **Caution:** [B, +] Arrhythmia associated w/ rapid inj; caution in colitis **Contra:** Hypersensitivity to cephalosporins **Supplied:** Powder for inj 500 mg, 1, 2, 10 g **SE:** Diarrhea, rash, pruritus, colitis, eosinophilia, ↑ transaminases **Interactions:** ↑ Bleeding w/ anticoagulants; ↑ nephrotoxicity w/ aminoglycosides, loop diuretics; ↑ effects w/ probenecid; ↓ effects w/ antacids, chloramphenicol **Labs:** + Direct Coombs' test; ↑ LFTs, alkaline phosphatase, bilirubin, LDH, BUN, creatinine; false + of serum or UCr, false + urine glucose **NIPE:** Food w/ ER tabs ↑ absorption, monitor for superinfection, ⊘ breast-feeding or use EtOH w/ drug or wi/n 3 d of taking drug

Cefotetan (Cefotan)

Uses: *Rx infections of the upper & lower resp tract, skin, bone, urinary tract, abdomen, & gynecologic system* **Action:** 2nd-gen cephalosporin; inhibits cell wall synthesis. *Spectrum:* Less active against gram(+); anaerobes including *B. fragilis*; gram(−), including *E. coli, Klebsiella,* & *Proteus* **Dose:** *Adults.* 1–2 g IV q12h. *Peds.* 20–40 mg/kg/d IV ÷ q12h; ↓ in renal impairment **Caution:** [B, +] May ↑ bleeding risk; in those Hx of penicillin allergies **Contra:** Hypersensitivity to cephalosporins **Supplied:** Powder for inj 1, 2, 10 g **SE:** Diarrhea, rash, eosinophilia, ↑ transaminases, hypoprothrombinemia, & bleeding (due to MTT side chain) **Notes:** Caution w/ other nephrotoxic drugs; may interfere w/ warfarin **Interactions:** ↑ Bleeding w/ anticoagulants; ↑ nephrotoxicity w/ aminoglycosides, loop diuretics; ↑ effects w/ probenecid; ↓ effects w/ antacids, chloramphenicol **Labs:** + Direct Coombs' test; ↑ LFTs, alkaline phosphatase, bilirubin, LDH, BUN, creatinine; false + of serum or UCr, false + urine glucose **NIPE:** Food w/ ER tabs ↑ absorption, monitor for superinfection, ⊘ breast-feeding or use EtOH w/ drug or w/in 3 d of taking drug

Cefoxitin (Mefoxin) Uses: *Rx infections of the upper & lower resp tract, skin, bone, urinary tract, abdomen, & gynecologic system* **Action:** 2nd-gen cephalosporin; inhibits cell wall synthesis. *Spectrum:* Good gram(−) against enteric bacilli (ie, *E. coli, Klebsiella, & Proteus*); anaerobic activity against *B. fragilis* **Dose:** *Adults.* 1–2 mg IV q6–8h. *Peds.* 80–160 mg/kg/d ÷ q4–6h; ↓ in renal impairment **Caution:** [B, +] **Contra:** Hypersensitivity to cephalosporins **Supplied:** Powder for inj 1, 2, 10 g **SE:** Diarrhea, rash, eosinophilia, ↑ transaminases **Interactions:** ↑ Bleeding w/ anticoagulants; ↑ nephrotoxicity w/ aminoglycosides, loop diuretics; ↑ effects w/ probenecid; ↓ effects w/ antacids, chloramphenicol **Labs:** + Direct Coombs' test; ↑ LFTs, alkaline phosphatase, bilirubin, LDH, BUN, creatinine; false + of serum or UCr, false + urine glucose **NIPE:** Food w/ ER tabs ↑ absorption, monitor for superinfection, ⊘ breast-feeding

Cefpodoxime (Vantin) Uses: *Rx resp, skin, & urinary tract infections* **Action:** 3rd-gen cephalosporin; inhibits cell wall synthesis. *Spectrum: S. pneumoniae* or non-β-lactamase-producing *H. influenzae*; acute uncomplicated *N. gonorrhoeae*; some uncomplicated gram(−)(*E. coli, Klebsiella, Proteus*) **Dose:** *Adults.* 200–400 mg PO q12h. *Peds.* 10 mg/kg/d PO ÷ bid; ↓ dose in renal impairment, take w/ food **Caution:** [B, +] **Contra:** Hypersensitivity to cephalosporins **Supplied:** Tabs 100, 200 mg; susp 50, 100 mg/5 mL **SE:** Diarrhea, rash, HA, eosinophilia, elevated transaminases **Notes:** Drug interactions w/ agents that ↑ gastric pH **Interactions:** ↑ Bleeding w/ anticoagulants; ↑ nephrotoxicity w/ aminoglycosides, loop diuretics; ↑ effects w/ probenecid; ↓ effects w/ antacids, chloramphenicol **Labs:** + Direct Coombs' test; ↑ LFTs, alkaline phosphatase, bilirubin, LDH, BUN, creatinine; false + of serum or UCr, false + urine glucose **NIPE:** Food w/ ER tabs ↑ absorption, monitor for superinfection, ⊘ breast-feeding. See Cefaclor. **Additional Interactions:** ↑ Effects if taken w/ food

Cefprozil (Cefzil) Uses: *Rx resp tract, skin, & urinary tract infections* **Action:** 2nd-gen cephalosporin; inhibits cell wall synthesis. *Spectrum:* Active against MSSA, strep, & gram(−) bacilli (*E. coli, Klebsiella, P. mirabilis, H. influenzae, Moraxella*) **Dose:** *Adults.* 250–500 mg PO daily–bid. *Peds.* 7.5–15 mg/kg/d PO ÷ bid; ↓ dose in renal impairment **Caution:** [B, +] **Contra:** Hypersensitivity to cephalosporins **Supplied:** Tabs 250, 500 mg; susp 125, 250 mg/5 mL **SE:** Diarrhea, dizziness, rash, eosinophilia, ↑ transaminases **Notes:** Use higher doses for otitis & pneumonia **Interactions:** ↑ Bleeding w/ anticoagulants; ↑ nephrotoxicity w/ aminoglycosides, loop diuretics; ↑ effects w/ probenecid; ↓ effects w/ antacids, chloramphenicol **Labs:** + Direct Coombs' test; ↑ LFTs, alkaline phosphatase, bilirubin, LDH, BUN, creatinine; false + of serum or UCr, false + urine glucose **NIPE:** Food w/ ER tabs ↑ absorption, monitor for superinfection, ⊘ breast-feeding

Ceftazidime (Fortaz, Ceptaz, Tazidime, Tazicef) ☉ Uses: *Rx resp tract, skin, bone, urinary tract infections, meningitis, & septicemia* **Action:** 3rd-gen cephalosporin; inhibits cell wall synthesis. *Spectrum: P. aeruginosa* sp, good gram(–)activity **Dose: Adults.** 500–2 g IV q8–12h. **Peds.** 30–50 mg/kg/dose IV q8h; ↓ dose in renal impairment **Caution:** [B, +] **Contra:** Hypersensitivity to cephalosporins **Supplied:** Powder for inj 1, 2, 10 g **SE:** Diarrhea, rash, eosinophilia, ↑ transaminases **Interactions:** ↑ Bleeding w/ anticoagulants; ↑ nephrotoxicity w/ aminoglycosides, loop diuretics; ↑ effects w/ probenecid; ↓ effects w/ antacids, chloramphenicol **Labs:** + Direct Coombs' test; ↑ LFTs, alkaline phosphatase, bilirubin, LDH, BUN, creatinine; false + of serum or UCr, false + urine glucose **NIPE:** Food w/ ER tabs ↑ absorption, monitor for superinfection, ⊘ breast-feeding or use EtOH w/in 3 d of taking drug

Ceftibuten (Cedax) Uses: *Rx resp tract, skin, urinary tract infections & otitis media* **Action:** 3rd-gen cephalosporin; inhibits cell wall synthesis. *Spectrum: H. influenzae* & *M. catarrhalis*; weak against *S. pneumoniae* **Dose: Adults.** 400 mg/d PO. **Peds.** 9 mg/kg/d PO; ↓ dose in renal impairment; take on an empty stomach **Caution:** [B, +] **Contra:** Hypersensitivity to cephalosporins **Supplied:** Caps 400 mg; susp 90, 180 mg/5 mL **SE:** Diarrhea, rash, eosinophilia, ↑ transaminases **Interactions:** ↑ Bleeding w/ anticoagulants; ↑ nephrotoxicity w/ aminoglycosides, loop diuretics; ↑ effects w/ probenecid; ↓ effects w/ antacids, chloramphenicol **Labs:** + Direct Coombs' test; ↑ LFTs, alkaline phosphatase, bilirubin, LDH, BUN, creatinine; false + of serum or UCr, false + urine glucose **NIPE:** Food w/ ER tabs ↑ absorption, monitor for superinfection, ⊘ breast-feeding or use EtOH w/in 3 d of taking drug

Ceftizoxime (Cefizox) Uses: *Rx resp tract, skin, bone, & urinary tract infections, meningitis, & septicemia* **Action:** 3rd-gen cephalosporin; inhibits cell wall synthesis. *Spectrum:* Good against gram(–) bacilli (not *Pseudomonas*), some gram(+) cocci (not *Enterococcus*), & some anaerobes **Dose: Adults.** 1–2 g IV q8–12h. **Peds.** 150–200 mg/kg/d IV ÷ q6–8h; ↓ dose in renal impairment **Caution:** [B, +] **Contra:** Hypersensitivity to cephalosporins **Supplied:** Inj 500 mg, 1, 2, 10 g **SE:** Diarrhea, fever, rash, eosinophilia, thrombocytosis, ↑ transaminases **Interactions:** ↑ Bleeding w/ anticoagulants; ↑ nephrotoxicity w/ aminoglycosides, loop diuretics; ↑ effects w/ probenecid; ↓ effects w/ antacids, chloramphenicol **Labs:** + Direct Coombs' test; ↑ LFTs, alkaline phosphatase, bilirubin, LDH, BUN, creatinine; false + of serum or UCr, false + urine glucose **NIPE:** Food w/ ER tabs ↑ absorption, monitor for superinfection, ⊘ breast-feeding

Ceftriaxone (Rocephin) Uses: *Resp tract, skin, bone, & urinary tract infections, meningitis, & septicemia; pneumonia* **Action:** 3rd-gen cephalosporin; inhibits cell wall synthesis. *Spectrum:* Moderate against gram(+); excellent against

β-lactamase producers **Dose:** *Adults.* 1–2 g IV q12–24h. *Peds.* 50–100 mg/kg/d IV ÷ q12–24h; ↓ dose in renal impairment **Caution:** [B, +] **Contra:** Hypersensitivity to cephalosporins; hyperbilirubinemic neonates (displaces bilirubin from binding sites) **Supplied:** Powder for inj 250 mg, 500 mg, 1, 2 g **SE:** Diarrhea, rash, leukopenia, thrombocytosis, eosinophilia, ↑ transaminases **Interactions:** ↑ Bleeding w/ anticoagulants; ↑ nephrotoxicity w/ aminoglycosides, loop diuretics; ↑ effects w/ probenecid; ↓ effects w/ antacids, chloramphenicol **Labs:** + Direct Coombs' test; ↑ LFTs, alkaline phosphatase, bilirubin, LDH, BUN, creatinine; false + of serum or UCr, false + urine glucose **NIPE:** Food w/ ER tabs ↑ absorption, monitor for superinfection, Ⓢ breast-feeding or use EtOH w/in 3 d of taking drug (NR) mix w/ other antimicrobials

Cefuroxime (Ceftin [PO], Zinacef [parenteral]) Uses: *Upper & lower resp tract, skin, bone, urinary tract, abdomen, & gynecologic infections* **Action:** 2nd-gen cephalosporin; inhibits cell wall synthesis *Spectrum:* Staphylococci, group B streptococci, *H. influenzae, E. coli, Enterobacter, Salmonella,* & *Klebsiella* **Dose:** *Adults.* 750 mg–1.5 g IV q8h or 250–500 mg PO bid. *Peds.* 100–150 mg/kg/d IV ÷ q8h or 20–30 mg/kg/d PO ÷ bid; ↓ dose in renal impairment; take w/ food **Caution:** [B, +] **Contra:** Hypersensitivity to cephalosporins **Supplied:** Tabs 125, 250, 500 mg; susp 125, 250 mg/5 mL; powder for inj 750 mg, 1.5, 7.5 g **SE:** Diarrhea, rash, eosinophilia, ↑ LFTs **Notes:** Cefuroxime axetil film-coated tablets & PO susp not bioequivalent; Ⓢ substitute on a mg/mg basis; IV crosses blood–brain barrier **Interactions:** ↑ Bleeding w/ anticoagulants; ↑ nephrotoxicity w/ aminoglycosides, loop diuretics; ↑ effects w/ probenecid; ↓ effects w/ antacids, chloramphenicol **Labs:** + Direct Coombs' test; ↑ LFTs, alkaline phosphatase, bilirubin, LDH, BUN, creatinine; false + of serum or UCr, false + urine glucose **NIPE:** Food w/ ER tabs ↑ absorption, monitor for superinfection, Ⓢ breast-feeding or use EtOH w/ drug or w/in 3 d of taking drug, food will ↓ GI distress & ↑ absorption, swallow tabs whole

Celecoxib (Celebrex) Uses: *Osteoarthritis & RA*; acute pain, primary dysmenorrhea; preventive in familial adenomatous polyposis **Action:** NSAID; inhibits the COX-2 pathway **Dose:** 100–200 mg/d or bid; ↓ in hepatic impairment; take w/ food/milk to lessen GI SE **Caution:** [C/D (3rd tri), ?] Caution in renal impairment **Contra:** Allergy to sulfonamides **Supplied:** Caps 100, 200 mg **SE:** GI upset, HTN, edema, renal failure, HA **Notes:** Watch for Sxs of GI bleeding; no effect on plt/bleeding time; can affect drugs metabolized by P-450 pathway **Interactions:** ↑ Effects w/ fluconazole; ↑ effects of Li; ↑ risks of GI upset &/or bleeding w/ ASA, NSAIDs, warfarin, EtOH; ↓ effects w/ Al- & Mg-containing antacids, ↓ effects of thiazide diuretics, loop diuretics, ACEIs **Labs:** ↑ LFTs, BUN, creatinine, CPK, alkaline phosphatase; monitor for hypercholesterolemia, hyperglycemia, hypokalemia, hypophosphatemia, albuminuria, hematuria **NIPE:** Take w/ food if GI distress

Cephalexin (Keflex, Keftab) Uses: *Skin, bone, upper/lower resp tract, & urinary tract infections* **Action:** 1st-gen cephalosporin; inhibits cell wall synthesis. *Spectrum: Streptococcus, Staphylococcus, E. coli, Proteus, Klebsiella* **Dose: Adults.** 250–500 mg PO qid. *Peds.* 25–100 mg/kg/d PO ÷ qid; ↓ dose in renal impairment; take on an empty stomach **Caution:** [B, +] **Contra:** Hypersensitivity to cephalosporins **Supplied:** Caps 250, 500 mg; tabs 250, 500, 1000 mg; susp 125, 250 mg/5 mL **SE:** Diarrhea, rash, eosinophilia, ↑ LFTs **Interactions:** ↑ Bleeding w/ anticoagulants; ↑ nephrotoxicity w/ aminoglycosides, loop diuretics; ↑ effects w/ probenecid; ↓ effects w/ antacids, chloramphenicol **Labs:** + Direct Coombs' test; ↑ LFTs, alkaline phosphatase, bilirubin, LDH, BUN, creatinine; false + of serum or UCr, false + urine glucose **NIPE:** Food w/ ER tabs ↑ absorption, monitor for superinfection, ⊘ breast-feeding

Cephradine (Velosef) **Uses:** *Rx resp, genitourinary, GI, skin, soft tissue, bone, & joint infections* **Action:** 1st-gen cephalosporin; inhibits cell wall synthesis. *Spectrum:* Gram(+) bacilli & cocci (not *Enterococcus*); some gram(−) bacilli (*E. coli, Proteus, & Klebsiella*) **Dose: Adults.** 250–500 mg q6–12h (8 g/d max). *Peds >9 mo.* 25–100 mg/kg/d ÷ bid–qid (4 g/d max); ↓ dose in renal impairment **Caution:** [B, +] **Contra:** Hypersensitivity to cephalosporins **Supplied:** Caps 250, 500 mg; powder for susp 125, 250 mg/5 mL, injectable **SE:** Diarrhea, rash, eosinophilia, ↑ LFTs, N/V **Interactions:** ↑ Bleeding w/ anticoagulants; ↑ nephrotoxicity w/ aminoglycosides, loop diuretics; ↑ effects w/ probenecid; ↓ effects w/ antacids, chloramphenicol **Labs:** + Direct Coombs' test; ↑ LFTs, alkaline phosphatase, bilirubin, LDH, BUN, creatinine; false + of serum or UCr, false + urine glucose **NIPE:** Food w/ ER tabs ↑ absorption, monitor for superinfection, ⊘ breast-feeding or use EtOH w/ drug or w/in 3 d of taking drug, ⊘ take w/ any other antibiotic, take w/ food

Cetirizine (Zyrtec) **Uses:** *Allergic rhinitis & other allergic Sxs including urticaria* **Action:** Nonsedating antihistamine **Dose: Adults & Children >6 y.** 5–10 mg/d. *Peds.* 6–11 mo: 2.5 mg qd. 12–23 mo: 2.5 mg qd–bid; ↓ dosage in renal/hepatic impairment **Caution:** [B, ?/–] Elderly & nursing mothers; doses >10 mg/d may cause drowsiness **Contra:** Hypersensitivity to cetirizine, hydroxyzine **Supplied:** Tabs 5, 10 mg; syrup 5 mg/5 mL **SE:** HA, drowsiness, xerostomia **Notes:** Can cause sedation **Interactions:** ↑ Effects w/ anticholinergics, CNS depressants, theophylline, EtOH **Labs:** May cause false − w/ allergy skin tests **NIPE:** ⊘ take w/ EtOH or CNS depressants

Charcoal, Activated (Supterchar, Actidose, Liqui-Char) **Uses:** *Emergency Rx in poisoning by most drugs & chemicals* **Action:** Adsorbent detoxicant **Dose:** Give w/70% sorbitol (2 mL/kg); repeated dose of sorbitol ⊘ **Adults. Acute intoxication:** 30–100 g/dose. *GI dialysis:* 20–50 g q6h for 1–2 d. *Peds 1–12 y.* **Acute intoxication:** 1–2 g/kg/dose. *GI dialysis:* 5–10 g/dose q4–8h **Caution:** [C, ?] May cause vomiting (hazardous in petroleum distillate & caustic ingestions); ⊘ mix w/ milk, ice cream, or sherbet **Contra:** Not effective for cyanide, mineral acids, caustic alkalis, organic solvents, Fe, EtOH, methanol poisoning, Li; ⊘ use sorbitol in Pts w/ fructose intolerance **Supplied:** Powder, liq, aps **SE:** Some liq dosage forms in sorbitol base (a cathartic); vomiting, diarrhea, black stools, constipation **Notes:** Charcoal w/ sorbitol is ⊘ in children < 1 y; monitor for hypokalemia & hypomagnesemia; protect the airway in lethargic or comatose Pts **Interactions:** ↓ Effects if taken w/ ice cream, milk, or sherbet; ↓ effects of digoxin & absorption of other oral meds, ↓ effects of syrup of ipecac **NIPE:** Most effective if given w/in 30 min of acute poisoning, only give to conscious patients

Chloral Hydrate (Aquachloral, Suprettes) [C-IV] Uses: *Short-term nocturnal & preoperative sedation* **Action:** Sedative hypnotic; active metabolite trichloroethanol **Dose:** *Adults. Hypnotic:* 500 mg–1 g PO or PR 30 min as or before procedure. *Sedative:* 250 mg PO or PR tid. *Peds. Hypnotic:* 20–50 mg/kg/24 h PO or PR 30 min hs or before procedure. *Sedative:* 5–15 mg/kg/dose q8h; ⊘ w/ CrCl <50 mL/min or severe hepatic impairment **Caution:** [C, +] Porphyria & neonates **Contra:** Hypersensitivity to components; severe renal, hepatic or cardiac Dz **Supplied:** Caps 500 mg; syrup 250, 500 mg/5 mL; supp 324, 500, 648 mg **SE:** GI irritation, drowsiness, ataxia, dizziness, nightmares, rash **Notes:** May accumulate; tolerance may develop >2 wk; taper dose; mix syrup in water or fruit juice; ⊘ EtOH & CNS depressants **Interactions:** ↑ Effects w/ antihistamines, barbiturates, paraldehyde, CNS depressants, opioid analgesics, EtOH; ↑ effects of anticoagulants **Labs:** False + of urine glucose; may interfere w/ tests for catecholamines and urinary 17-hydroxycorticosteroids **NIPE:** ⊘ Take w/ EtOH, CNS depressants; ⊘ chew or crush capsules

Chlorambucil (Leukeran) Uses: *CLL, Hodgkin's Dz, Waldenström's macroglobulinemia* **Action:** Alkylating agent **Dose:** 0.1–0.2 mg/kg/d for 3–6 wk or 0.4 mg/kg/dose q2wk (refer to specific protocol) **Caution:** [D, ?] Sz disorder & bone marrow suppression; affects human fertility **Contra:** Previous resistance; hypersensitivity to alkylating agents **Supplied:** Tabs 2 mg **SE:** Myelosuppression, CNS stimulation, N/V, drug fever, skin rash, chromosomal damage that can result in secondary leukemias, alveolar dysplasia, pulmonary fibrosis, hepatotoxicity **Notes:** Monitor LFTs, CBC, leukocyte counts, plts, serum uric acid; reduce initial dosage if Pt has received radiation therapy **Interactions:** ↑ Bone marrow suppression w/ antineoplastic drugs and immunosuppressants; ↑ risk of bleeding w/ ASA, anticoagulants **Labs:** ↑ Urine and serum uric acid, ALT, alkaline phosphatase **NIPE:** ⊘ PRG, breast-feeding, infection; ↑ fluids to 2–3 L/d; monitor lab work periodically & CBC w/ differential weekly during drug use, may cause hair loss

Chlordiazepoxide (Librium, Mitran, Libritabs) [C-IV] Uses: *Anxiety, tension, EtOH withdrawal,* & *preoperative apprehension* **Action:** Benzodiazepine; antianxiety agent **Dose:** *Adults. Mild anxiety:* 5–10 mg PO tid–qid or PRN. *Severe anxiety:* 25–50 mg IM, IV, or PO q6–8h or PRN. *EtOH withdrawal:* 50–100 mg IM or IV; repeat in 2–4 h if needed, up to 300 mg in 24 h; gradually taper daily dose. *Peds >6 y.* 0.5 mg/kg/24 h PO or IM ÷ q6–8h; ↓ dose in renal impairment, elderly **Caution:** [D, ?] Resp depression, CNS impairment, or a Hx of drug dependence; ⊘ in hepatic impairment **Contra:** Preexisting CNS depression **Supplied:** Caps 5, 10, 25 mg; tabs 10, 25 mg; inj 100 mg **SE:** Drowsiness, CP, rash, fatigue, memory impairment, xerostomia, weight gain **Notes:** Erratic IM absorption **Interactions:** ↑ Effects w/ antidepressants, antihistamines, anticonvulsants, barbiturates, general anesthetics, MAOIs, narcotics, phenothiazines cimetidine, disulfiram, fluconazole, itraconazole, ketoconazole, oral contraceptives, INH, metoprolol, propoxyphene, propranolol, valproic acid, EtOH, grapefruit juice, kava kava, valerian; ↑ effects of digoxin, phenytoin; ↓ effects w/ aminophylline, antacids, carbamazepine, theophylline, rifampin, rifabutin, tobacco; ↓ effects of levodopa **Labs:** ↑ LFTs, alkaline phosphatase, bilirubin, triglycerides; false ↑ urine 5-HIAA, urine 17-ketosteroids; false + urine PRG test; false ↓ urine 17 ketogenic steroids; ↓ HDL **NIPE:** ⊘ EtOH, PRG, breast-feeding; risk of photosensitivity—use sunscreen, orthostatic hypotension, tachycardia

Chlorothiazide (Diuril) Uses: *HTN, edema* Action: Thiazide diuretic
Dose: *Adults.* 500 mg–1 g PO qd–bid; 100–500 mg/d IV (for edema only). *Peds >6 mo.* 20–30 mg/kg/24 h PO ÷ bid; 4 mg/kg/d IV **Caution:** [D, +] ⊘ administer inj IM or SQ **Contra:** Cross-sensitivity to thiazides/sulfonamides, anuria **Supplied:** Tabs 250, 500 mg; susp 250 mg/5 mL; inj 500 mg/vial **SE:** ↓ K⁺, ↓ Na⁺, dizziness, hyperglycemia, hyperuricemia, hyperlipidemia, photosensitivity **Notes:** May be taken w/ food/milk; take early in the day to ⊘ nocturia; use sunblock; monitor electrolytes **Interactions:** ↑ Effects w/ ACEI, amphotericin B, corticosteroids; ↑ effects of diazoxide, Li, MRX; ↓ effects w/ colestipol, cholestyramine, NSAIDs; ↓ effects of hypoglycemics **Labs:** ↑ CPK, ammonia, amylase, Ca²⁺, Cl⁻, cholesterol, glucose, Mg²⁺, K⁺, Na⁺, uric acid **NIPE:** Monitor for gout, hyperglycemia, photosensitivity—use sunscreen, I&O, weight

Chlorpheniramine (Chlor-Trimeton, others [OTC]) Uses: *Allergic Rxns; common cold* Action: Antihistamine Dose: *Adults.* 4 mg PO q4–6h or 8–12 mg PO bid of SR *Peds.* 0.35 mg/kg/24 h PO ÷ q4–6h or 0.2 mg/kg/24 h SR **Caution:** [C, ?/–] bladder obstruction; narrow-angle glaucoma; hepatic insufficiency **Contra:** Hypersensitivity **Supplied:** Tabs 4 mg; chew tabs 2 mg; SR tabs 8, 12 mg; syrup 2 mg/5 mL; inj 10, 100 mg/mL **SE:** Anticholinergic SE & sedation common, postural hypotension, QT changes, extrapyramidal Rxns, photosensitivity **Interactions:** ↑ Effects w/ other CNS depressants, EtOH, opioids, sedatives, MAOIs, atropine, haloperidol, phenothiazines, quinidine, disopyramide; ↑ effects of epinephrine; ↓ effects of heparin, sulfonylureas **Labs:** False – w/ allergy testing **NIPE:** Stop drug 4 d prior to allergy testing, take w/ food if GI distress

Chlorpromazine (Thorazine) Uses: *Psychotic disorders, N/V,* apprehension, intractable hiccups Action: Phenothiazine antipsychotic; antiemetic **Dose:** *Adults. Psychosis:* 10–25 mg PO or PR bid–tid (usual 30–800 mg/d in ÷ doses). *Severe Sxs:* 25 mg IM/IV initial; may repeat in 1–4 h; then 25–50 mg PO or PR tid. *Hiccups:* 25–50 mg PO bid–tid. *Children >6 mo. Psychosis & N/V:* 0.5–1 mg/kg/dose PO q4–6h or IM/IV q6–8h; ⊘ in severe hepatic impairment **Caution:**

[C, ?/–] Safety in children <6 mo not established; caution in known Szs, BM suppression **Contra:** Cross-sensitivity w/ other phenothiazines; ⊘ in narrow-angle glaucoma **Supplied:** Tabs 10, 25, 50, 100, 200 mg; SR caps 30, 75, 150 mg; syrup 10 mg/5 mL; conc 30, 100 mg/mL; supp 25, 100 mg; inj 25 mg/mL **SE:** Extrapyramidal SE & sedation; α-adrenergic blocking properties; ↓ BP; prolongs QT interval **Notes:** ⊘ Stop abruptly; dilute PO concentrate in 2–4 oz of liquid **Interactions:** ↑ Effects w/ amodiaquine, chloroquine, sulfadoxine–pyrimethamine, antidepressants, narcotic analgesics, propranolol, quinidine, BBs, MAOIs, TCAs, EtOH, kava kava; ↑ effects of anticholinergics, centrally acting antihypertensives, propranolol, valproic acid; ↓ effects w/ antacids, antidiarrheals, barbiturates, Li, tobacco; ↓ effects of anticonvulsants, guanethidine, levodopa, Li, warfarin **Labs:** False ↑ for amylase, phenylketonuria, urine bilirubin, urine protein, uroporphyrins, urobilinogen, PRG test; ↑ plasma cholesterol **NIPE:** Risk of photosensitivity—use sunscreen & tardive dyskinesia, take w/ food if GI upset, may darken urine

Chlorpropamide (Diabinese)
Uses: *Type 2 DM* **Action:** Sulfonylurea; ↑ release of insulin from pancreas; ↑ peripheral insulin sensitivity; ↓ hepatic glucose output **Dose:** 100–500 mg/d; take w/ food **Caution:** [C, ?/–] ⊘ use in CrCl < 50 mL/min; ↓ in hepatic impairment **Contra:** Cross-sensitivity w/ sulfonamides **Supplied:** Tabs 100, 250 mg **SE:** HA, dizziness, rash, photosensitivity, hypoglycemia, SIADH **Notes:** ⊘ EtOH (disulfiram-like Rxn) **Interactions:** ↑ Effects w/ ASA, NSAIDs, anticoagulants, BBs, chloramphenicol, guanethidine, insulin, MAOIs, phenytoin, probenecid, rifampin, sulfonamides, EtOH, juniper berries, ginseng, garlic, fenugreek, coriander, dandelion root, celery, bitter melon, ginkgo biloba; ↑ effects of anticoagulants, phenytoin, ASA, NSAIDs; ↓ effects w/ diazoxide, thiazide diuretics **Labs:** False ↑ serum Ca

Chlorthalidone (Hygroton, others)
Uses: *HTN* **Action:** Thiazide diuretic **Dose:** *Adults.* 50–100 mg PO daily. *Peds.* (not approved) 2 mg/kg/dose PO 3×/wk or 1–2 mg/kg/d PO; ↓ in renal impairment **Caution:** [D, +] **Contra:** Cross-sensitivity w/ thiazides or sulfonamides; anuria **Supplied:** Tabs 15, 25, 50, 100 mg **SE:** ↑ K⁺, dizziness, photosensitivity, hyperglycemia, hyperuricemia, sexual dysfunction **Interactions:** ↑ Effects w/ ACEIs, diazoxide; ↑ effects of digoxin, Li, MRX; ↓ effects w/ cholestyramine, colestipol, NSAIDs; ↓ effects of hypoglycemics; ↓ K⁺ w/ amphotericin B, carbenoxolone, corticosteroids **Labs:** ↑ CPK, amylase, Ca²⁺, Cl⁻, cholesterol, glucose, uric acid; ↓ Cl⁻, Mg²⁺, K⁺, Na⁺ **NIPE:** May take w/ food, and milk, take early in day, use sunscreen

Chlorzoxazone (Paraflex, Parafon Forte DSC, others)
Uses: *Adjunct to rest & physical therapy for the relief of discomfort associated w/ acute, painful musculoskeletal conditions* **Action:** Centrally acting skeletal muscle relaxant **Dose:** *Adults.* 250–500 mg PO tid–qid. *Peds.* 20 mg/kg/d in 3–4 ÷ doses **Caution:** [C, ?] ⊘ EtOH & CNS depressants **Contra:** Severe liver Dz **Supplied:** Tabs 250; caps 250, 500 mg **SE:** Drowsiness, tachycardia, dizziness, hepatotoxicity, angioedema **Interactions:** ↑ Effects w/ antihistamines, CNS depressants,

MAOIs, TCAs, opioids, EtOH, watercress **Labs:** Monitor LFTs **NIPE:** Urine ma turn reddish purple or orange

Cholecalciferol [Vitamin D₃] (Delta D) **Uses:** Dietary suppl to Rx vi tamin D deficiency **Action:** Increases intestinal Ca absorption **Dose:** 400–100 IU/d PO **Caution:** [A (D doses above the RDA), +] **Contra:** Hypercalcemia, hy pervitaminosis, hypersensitivity **Supplied:** Tabs 400, 1000 IU **SE:** Vitamin D toxi city (renal failure, HTN, psychosis) **Notes:** 1 mg of cholecalciferol = 40,000 IU o vitamin D activity

Cholestyramine (Questran, LoCHOLEST) **Uses:** *Hyperchole: terolemia; Rx pruritus associated w/ partial biliary obstruction; diarrhea associate w/ excess fecal bile acids* **Action:** Binds intestinal bile acids to form insolubl complexes **Dose:** *Adults.* Individualize: 4 g/d–bid (↑ to max 24 g/d & 6 doses/d) *Peds.* 240 mg/kg/d in 3 ÷ doses **Caution:** [C, ?] Constipation & phenylketonuri **Contra:** Complete biliary obstruction; hypolipoproteinemia types III, IV, V **Sup plied:** 4 g of cholestyramine resin/9 g of powder; w/ aspartame: 4 g resin/5 g o powder **SE:** Constipation, abdominal pain, bloating, HA, rash **Notes:** OD may re sult in GI obstruction; mix 4 g of cholestyramine in 2–6 oz of noncarbonated bev erage **Interactions:** ↓ Effects of acetaminophen, amiodarone, anticoagulants ASA, cardiac glycosides, clindamycin, corticosteroids, diclofenac, fat-soluble vita mins, gemfibrozil, glipizide, Fe salts, MRX, methyldopa, nicotinic acid, peni cillins, phenobarbital, phenytoin, propranolol, thiazide diuretics, tetracyclines thyroid drugs, troglitazone, warfarin **Labs:** ↑ LFTs, PT, P, Cl, alkaline phos phatase, ↓ serum Ca²⁺, Na⁺, K⁺, cholesterol **NIPE:** ↑ fluids, take other drugs 1 before or 6 h after

Ciclopirox (Loprox) **Uses:** *Tinea pedis, tinea cruris, tinea corporis, cuta neous candidiasis, tinea versicolor* **Action:** Antifungal antibiotic **Dose:** *Adults & Peds >10 y.* Massage into affected area bid **Caution:** [B, ?] **Contra:** Componen sensitivity **Supplied:** Cream; lotion 1% **SE:** Pruritus, local irritation, burning **Notes:** DC if irritation occurs; ⊘ occlusive dressings **Interactions:** None noted **NIPE:** Nail lacquer may take 6 mo to see improvement, cream/gel/lotion see im provement by 4 wk

Cidofovir (Vistide) **WARNING:** Renal impairment is the major toxicity Follow administration instructions **Uses:** *CMV retinitis in Pts w/ HIV* **Action:** Selective inhibition of viral DNA synthesis **Dose:** *Rx:* 5 mg/kg IV over 1 l once/wk for 2 wk; administered w/ probenecid. *Maint:* 5 mg/kg IV once/2 wk; ad ministered w/ probenecid. *Probenecid:* 2 g PO 3 h prior to cidofovir, & then 1 g PO at 2 h & 8 h after cidofovir; ↓ in renal impairment **Caution:** [C, –] SCr >1.5 mg/dL or CrCl = 55 mL/min or urine protein >100 mg/dL; other nephrotoxic drug: **Contra:** Hypersensitivity to probenecid or sulfa **Supplied:** Inj 75 mg/mL **SE:** Renal toxicity, chills, fever, HA, N/V/D, thrombocytopenia, neutropenia **Notes:** Hydrate w/ NS prior to each inf **Interactions:** ↑ Nephrotoxicity w/ aminoglyco sides, amphotericin B, foscarnet, IV pentamidine, NSAIDs, vancomycin; ↑ effects w/ zidovudine **Labs:** ↑ SCr, BUN, alkaline phosphatase, LFTs, urine protein, WBCs; monitor for hematuria, glycosuria, hypocalcemia, hyperglycemia, hypokalemia, hyperlipidemia **NIPE:** Coadminister oral probenecid w/ each dose, possible hair loss

Cilostazol (Pletal) **Uses:** *Reduce Sxs of intermittent claudication* **Action:** Phosphodiesterase III inhibitor; ↑s cAMP in plts & blood vessels, to inhibit plt aggregation & vasodilation **Dose:** 100 mg PO bid, ½ h before or 2 h after breakfast & dinner **Caution:** [C, +/–] ↓ dose when used w/ other drugs that inhibit CYP3A4 & CYP2C19 **Contra:** In CHF of any severity **Supplied:** Tabs 50, 100 mg **SE:** HA, palpitation, diarrhea **Interactions:** ↑ Effects with diltiazem, macrolides, omeprazole, fluconazole, itraconazole, ketoconazole, sertraline, grapefruit juice; ↑ effects of ASA; ↓ effects with cigarette smoking; **Labs:** ↑ BUN/creatinine, ↓ Hgb, Hct **NIPE:** Take on empty stomach; may take up to 12 wk to ↓ cramping pain; may cause headache

Cimetidine (Tagamet, Tagamet HB) [OTC] **Uses:** *Duodenal ulcer; ulcer prophylaxis in hypersecretory states, eg, trauma, burns, surgery; & GERD* **Action:** H₂ receptor antagonist **Dose:** *Adults.* Active ulcer: 2400 mg/d IV cont inf or 300 mg IV q6h; 400 mg PO bid or 800 mg hs. *Maint:* 400 mg PO hs. *GERD:* 300–600 mg PO q6h; maint 800 mg PO hs. *Peds.* Infants: 10–20 mg/kg/24 h PO or IV ÷ q6–12h. *Children:* 20–40 mg/kg/24 h PO or IV ÷ q6h; ↑ dosing interval w/ renal insufficiency; ↓ dose in the elderly **Caution:** [B, +] Many drug interactions (P-450 system) **Contra:** Component sensitivity **Supplied:** Tabs 200, 300, 400, 800 mg; liq 300 mg/5 mL; inj 300 mg/2 mL **SE:** Dizziness, HA, agitation, thrombocytopenia, gynecomastia **Notes:** Take 1 h before or 2 h after antacids; ⊗ excessive EtOH **Interactions:** ↑ Effects of benzodiazepines, disulfram, flecainide, INH, lidocaine, oral contraceptives, sulfonylureas, warfarin, theophylline, phenytoin, metronidazole, triamterene, procainamide, quinidine, propranolol, diazepam, nifedipine, TCAs, procainamide, tacrine, carbamazepine, valproic acid, xanthines; ↓ effects w/ antacids, tobacco; ↓ effects of digoxin, ketoconazole, cefpodoxime, indomethacin, tetracyclines **Labs:** ↑ Creatinine, LFTs, false + hemoccult **NIPE:** Take w/ meals, monitor for gynecomastia, breast pain, impotence

Cinacalcet (Sensipar) **Uses:** *Secondary hyperparathyroidism in CRF; hypercalcemia in parathyroid carcinoma* **Action:** ↓ PTH by ↑ Ca-sensing receptor sensitivity **Dose:** *Secondary hyperparathyroidism:* 30 mg PO bid. *Parathyroid carcinoma:* 30 mg PO daily; titrate q2–4wk based on Ca & PTH levels; swallow whole; take w/ food **Caution:** [C, ?/–] Dose adjust w/ addition/deletion of CYP3A4 inhibitors **Supplied:** Tabs 30, 60, 90 mg **SE:** N/V/D, myalgia, dizziness, hypocalcemia **Notes:** Monitor Ca²⁺, PO₄⁻², PTH **Labs:** Monitor serum Ca and serum P **NIPE:** Must take drug with vitamin D and/or phosphate binders

Ciprofloxacin (Cipro) **Uses:** *Rx lower resp tract, sinuses, skin & skin structure, bone/joints, & UTI infections including prostatitis* **Action:** Quinolone antibiotic; inhibits DNA gyrase. *Spectrum:* Broad-spectrum gram(+) & gram(–)

aerobics; little against streptococci; *Pseudomonas, E. coli, Bacteroides fragilis, Proteus mirabilis, Klebsiella pneumoniae, Campylobacter jejuni,* or *Shigella* **Dose: Adults.** 250–750 mg PO q12h; XR 500–1000 mg PO q24h; or 200–400 mg IV q12h; ↓ in renal impairment **Caution:** [C, ?/–] Children <18 y **Contra:** Component sensitivity **Supplied:** Tabs 100, 250, 500, 750 mg; Tabs XR 500, 1000 mg; susp 5 g/100 mL, 10 g/100 mL; inj 200, 400 mg **SE:** Restlessness, N/V/D, rash, ruptured tendons, ↑ LFTs **Notes:** ⊘ Antacids; reduce/restrict caffeine intake; interactions w/ theophylline, caffeine, sucralfate, warfarin, antacids **Interactions:** ↑ Effects w/ probenecid; ↑ effects of diazepam, theophylline, caffeine, metoprolol, propranolol, phenytoin, warfarin; ↓ effects w/ antacids, didanosine, Fe salts, Mg, sucralfate, Na bicarbonate, Zn **Labs:** ↑ LFTs, alkaline phosphatase, serum bilirubin, LDH, BUN, SCr, amylase, uric acid, K⁺, PT, triglycerides, cholesterol; ↓ Hmg, Hct; **NIPE:** ⊘ give to children <18 y, ↑ fluids to 2–3 L/d, may cause photosensitivity—use sunscreen

Ciprofloxacin, Ophthalmic (Ciloxan)
Uses: *Rx & prevention of ocular infections (conjunctivitis, blepharitis, corneal abrasions)* **Action:** Quinolone antibiotic; inhibits DNA gyrase **Dose:** 1–2 gtt in eye(s) q2h while awake for 2 d, then 1–2 gtt q4h while awake for 5 d **Caution:** [C, ?/–] **Contra:** Component sensitivity **Supplied:** Soln 3.5 mg/mL **SE:** Local irritation **Interactions:** None reported **NIPE:** Limited systemic absorption

Ciprofloxacin, Otic (Cipro HC Otic)
Uses: *Otitis externa* **Action:** Quinolone antibiotic; inhibits DNA gyrase **Dose: Adult & Peds >1 mo.** 1–2 gtt in ear(s) bid for 7 d **Caution:** [C, ?/–] **Contra:** Perforated tympanic membrane, viral infections of the external canal **Supplied:** Susp ciprofloxacin 0.2% & hydrocortisone 1% **SE:** HA, pruritus **NIPE:** W/ diabetics, first-choice therapy for otitis externa

Cisplatin (Platinol, Platinol AQ)
Uses: *Testicular, small-cell & non-small-cell lung, bladder, ovarian, breast, head & neck, & penile CAs; osteosarcoma; pediatric brain tumors* **Action:** DNA-binding; denatures double helix; intrastrand cross-linking; formation of DNA adducts **Dose:** 10–20 mg/m²/d for 5 d q3wk; 50–120 mg/m² q3–4wk; refer to specific protocols; ↓ dose in renal impairment **Caution:** [D, –] Cumulative renal toxicity may be severe; serum Mg²⁺, electrolytes, should be monitored before & w/in 48 h after cisplatin therapy **Contra:** Hypersensitivity to platinum-containing compounds; preexisting renal insufficiency, myelosuppression, hearing impairment **Supplied:** Inj 1 mg/mL **SE:** Allergic Rxns, N/V, nephrotoxicity (worse w/administration of other nephrotoxic drugs, minimize by NS inf & mannitol diuresis), high-frequency hearing loss in 30%, peripheral "stocking glove"-type neuropathy, cardiotoxicity (ST-, T-wave changes), ↓ Mg²⁺, mild myelosuppression, hepatotoxicity; renal impairment dose-related & cumulative **Notes:** Give taxanes before platinum derivatives **Interactions:** ↑ Effect of antineoplastic drugs and radiation therapy; ↑ ototoxicity w/ loop diuretics; ↑ nephrotoxicity w/ aminoglycosides, amphotericin B, vancomycin; ↓ effects w/ Na

thiosulfate; ↓ effects of phenytoin **Labs:** ↑ BUN, creatinine, serum bilirubin, AST; ↓ Ca²⁺, Mg²⁺, phosphate, Na⁺, K⁺ **NIPE:** Drug ineffective w/ Al needles or equipment, may cause infertility, ⊘ immunizations

Citalopram (Celexa) **WARNING:** Closely monitor for worsening depression or emergence of suicidality, particularly in pediatric Pts **Uses:** *Depression* **Action:** SSRI **Dose:** Initial 20 mg/d, may be ↑ to 40 mg/d; ↓ dose in elderly & hepatic/renal insufficiency **Caution:** [C, +/–] Hx of mania; Hx Szs & Pts at risk for suicide **Contra:** MOAI or w/in 14 d of MAOI use **Supplied:** Tabs 10, 20, 40 mg; Soln 10 mg/5 mL **SE:** Somnolence, insomnia, anxiety, xerostomia, diaphoresis; sexual dysfunction **Notes:** May cause hyponatremia/SIADH **Interactions:** ↑ Effects w/ azole antifungals, cimetidine, Li, macrolides, EtOH; ↑ effects of BBs, carbamazepine, warfarin; ↓ effects w/ carbamazepine; ↓ effects of phenytoin; may cause fatal Rxn w/ MAOIs **Labs:** ↑ LFTs, alkaline phosphatase **NIPE:** ⊘ PRG, breast-feeding, use barrier contraception

Cladribine (Leustatin) **Uses:** *HCL, CLL, NHLs, progressive MS* **Action:** Induces DNA strand breakage; interferes w/ DNA repair/synthesis; purine nucleoside analog **Dose:** 0.09–0.1 mg/kg/d cont IV inf for 1–7 d (refer to specific protocols) **Caution:** [D, ?/–] Observe for signs of neutropenia & infection **Contra:** Component sensitivity **Supplied:** Inj 1 mg/mL **SE:** Myelosuppression, T-lymphocyte suppression may be prolonged (26–34 wk), fever in 46% (possibly tumor lysis), infections (especially lung & IV sites), rash (50%), HA, fatigue **Notes:** Consider prophylactic allopurinol; **Interactions:** ↑ Risk of bleeding w/ anticoagulants, NSAIDs, salicylates, ↑ risk of nephrotoxicity w/ amphotericin B; **Labs:** Monitor CBC, LFTs, SCr; **NIPE:** ⊘ PRG, breast-feeding

Clarithromycin (Biaxin, Biaxin XL) **Uses:** *Upper/lower resp tract, skin/skin structure infections, H. pylori infections, & infections caused by nontuberculosis (atypical) Mycobacterium; prevention of MAC infections in HIV-infection* **Action:** Macrolide antibiotic; inhibits protein synthesis. *Spectrum: H. influenzae, M. catarrhalis, S. pneumoniae, Mycoplasma pneumoniae, H. pylori* **Dose:** *Adults.* 250–500 mg PO bid or 1000 mg (2 × 500 mg XR tab)/d. *Mycobacterium:* 500–1000 mg PO bid. *Peds >9 mo.* 7.5 mg/kg/dose PO bid; ↓ in renal/hepatic impairment **Caution:** [C, ?] Antibiotic-associated colitis; rare QT prolongation & ventricular arrhythmias, including torsades de pointes **Contra:** Hypersensitivity to macrolides; combo w/ ranitidine in Pts w/ Hx of porphyria or CrCl < 25 mL/min **Supplied:** Tabs 250, 500 mg; susp 125, 250 mg/5 mL; 500 mg XR tab **SE:** Prolongs QT interval, causes metallic taste, diarrhea, nausea, abdominal pain, HA, rash **Notes:** Multiple drug interactions, ↑s theophylline & carbamazepine levels; ⊘ refrigerate suspension **Interactions:** ↑ Effects w/ amprenavir, indinavir, nelfinavir, ritonavir; ↑ effects of atorvastatin, buspirone, clozapine, colchicine, diazepam, felodipine, itraconazole, lovastatin, simvastatin, methylprednisolone, theophylline, phenytoin, quinidine, digoxin, carbamazepine, triazolam, warfarin, ergotamine, alprazolam, valproic acid; ↓ effects w/ EtOH; ↓ effects of

penicillin, zafirlukast **Labs:** ↑ Serum AST, ALT, GTT, alkaline phosphatase, LDH, total bilirubin, BUN, creatinine, PT; ↓ WBC **NIPE:** May take w/f food

Clemastine Fumarate (Tavist, Tavist-1) [OTC]
Uses: *Allergic rhinitis & Sxs of urticaria* **Action:** Antihistamine **Dose:** *Adults & Peds >12 y.* 1.34 mg bid–2.68 mg tid; max 8.04 mg/d *<12 y:* 0.4 mg PO bid **Caution:** [C, M] Bladder neck obstruction, symptomatic BPH **Contra:** Narrow-angle glaucoma **Supplied:** Tabs 1.34, 2.68 mg; syrup 0.67 mg/5 mL **SE:** Drowsiness, dyscoordination, epigastric distress **Notes:** ⊘ EtOH **Interactions:** ↑ Effects w/ CNS depressants, MAOIs, EtOH; ↓ effects of heparin, sulfonylureas

Clindamycin (Cleocin, Cleocin-T)
Uses: *Rx aerobic & anaerobic infections; topical for severe acne & vaginal infections* **Action:** Bacteriostatic; interferes w/ protein synthesis. *Spectrum:* Streptococci, pneumococci, staphylococci, & gram(+) & gram(−) anaerobes; no activity against gram(−) aerobes & bacterial vaginosis **Dose:** *Adults.* *PO:* 150–450 mg PO q6–8h. *Intravenous:* 300–600 mg IV q6h or 900 mg IV q8h. *Vaginal:* 1 applicatorful hs for 7 d. *Topical:* Apply 1% gel, lotion, or soln bid. *Peds. Neonates:* ⊘ use; (contains benzyl EtOH) 10–15 mg/kg/24 h ÷ q8–12h. *Children >1 mo:* 10–30 mg/kg/24 h ÷ q6–8h, to a max of 1.8 g/d PO or 4.8 g/d IV. *Topical:* Apply 1%, gel, lotion, or soln bid; ↓ in severe hepatic impairment **Caution:** [B, +] Can cause fatal colitis **Contra:** Previous pseudomembranous colitis **Supplied:** Caps 75, 150, 300 mg; susp 75 mg/5 mL; inj 300 mg/2 mL; vaginal cream 2% **SE:** Diarrhea may be pseudomembranous colitis caused by *C. difficile*, rash, ↑ LFTs **Notes:** DC drug if significant diarrhea. **Interactions:** ↑ Effects of neuromuscular blockage w/ tubocurarine, pancuronium; ↓ effects w/ erythromycin, kaolin, foods w/ sodium cyclamate **Labs:** Monitor CBC, LFTs, BUN, creatinine; false ↑ serum theophylline **NIPE:** ⊘ Intercourse, tampons, douches while using vaginal cream; take oral meds w/ 8 oz water

Clofazimine (Lamprene)
Uses: *Leprosy & combination therapy for MAC in AIDS* **Action:** Bactericidal; inhibits DNA synthesis. *Spectrum:* Multibacillary dapsone-sensitive leprosy; erythema nodosum leprosum; *Mycobacterium avium-intracellulare* **Dose:** *Adults.* 100–300 mg PO daily. *Peds.* 1 mg/kg/d in combo w/ dapsone & rifampin; take w/ meals **Caution:** [C, +/−] In Pts w/ GI problems; use dosages >100 mg/d for as short a duration as possible **Contra:** Hypersensitivity to any component **Supplied:** Caps 50 mg **SE:** Pink to brownish-black discoloration of the skin & conjunctiva, dry skin, GI intolerance **Notes:** Orphan drug for the Rx of dapsone-resistant leprosy; monitor for GI complaints. **Interactions:** ↑ Effects w/ INH, food, ↓ effect w/ dapsone **Labs:** ↑ Effects of AST, serum bilirubin, albumin, glucose, ESR **NIPE:** Take w/ food

Clonazepam (Klonopin) [C-IV]
Uses: *Lennox–Gastaut syndrome akinetic & myoclonic Szs, absence Szs, panic attacks,* restless legs syndrome neuralgia, parkinsonian dysarthria, bipolar disorder **Action:** Benzodiazepine; anticonvulsant **Dose:** *Adults.* 1.5 mg/d PO in 3 ÷ doses; ↑ by 0.5–1 mg/d q3d PRN up to 20 mg/d. *Peds.* 0.01–0.03 mg/kg/24 h PO ÷ tid; ↑ to 0.1–0.2 mg/kg/24 h÷tid; ⊘

brupt withdrawal **Caution:** [D, M] Elderly Pts, resp Dz, CNS depression, severe epatic impairment, narrow-angle glaucoma **Contra:** Severe liver Dz, acute narrow-angle glaucoma **Supplied:** Tabs 0.5, 1, 2 mg **SE:** CNS side effects, including drowsiness, dizziness, ataxia, memory impairment **Notes:** Can cause retrograde amnesia; CYP3A4 substrate **Interactions:** ↑ Effects w/ anticonvulsants, antihistamines, cimetidine, ciprofloxacin, clarithromycin, clozapine, CNS depressants, diltiazem, disulfiram, digoxin, erythromycin, fluconazole, fluoxetine, INH, itraconazole, ketoconazole, labetalol, levodopa, metoprolol, opioids, ritonavir, valproic acid, verapamil, EtOH, kava kava, valerian; ↑ effects of phenytoin; ↓ effects w/ barbiturates, carbamazepine, phenytoin, rifampin, rifabutin; ↓ effects of levodopa **NIPE:** ⊘ DC abruptly

Clonidine, Oral (Catapres) Uses: *HTN*; opioid, EtOH, & tobacco withdrawal **Action:** Centrally acting α-adrenergic stimulant **Dose: Adults.** 0.1 mg PO bid adjust daily by 0.1- to 0.2-mg increments (max 2.4 mg/d). **Peds.** 5–10 μg/kg/d ÷ q8–12h (max 0.9 mg/d); ↓ dose in renal impairment **Caution:** [C, +/–] ⊘ w/ BBs; withdraw slowly **Contra:** Component sensitivity **Supplied:** Tabs 0.1, 0.2, 0.3 mg **SE:** Rebound HTN w/ abrupt cessation of doses >0.2 mg bid; drowsiness, orthostatic hypotension, xerostomia, constipation, bradycardia, dizziness **Notes:** More effective for HTN if combined w/ diuretics

Clonidine, Transdermal (Catapres TTS) Uses: *HTN* **Action:** Centrally acting α-adrenergic stimulant **Dose:** Apply 1 patch q7d to hairless area (upper arm/torso); titrate to effect; ↓ in severe renal impairment; ⊘ DC abruptly (rebound HTN) **Caution:** [C, +/–] ⊘ w/ BBs, withdraw slowly **Contra:** Component sensitivity **Supplied:** TTS-1, TTS-2, TTS-3 (delivers 0.1, 0.2, 0.3 mg, respectively, of clonidine/d for 1 wk) **SE:** Drowsiness, orthostatic hypotension, xerostomia, constipation, bradycardia **Notes:** Doses >2 TTS-3 usually not associated w/ ↑ efficacy; steady state in 2–3 d **Interactions:** ↑ Effects w/ BBs, neuroleptics, nitroprusside, EtOH; ↑ effects of barbiturates; ↓ effects w/ MAOIs, TCAs, tolazoline, antidepressants, prazosin, capsicum; ↓ effects of levodopa **Labs:** ↑ Glucose, phosphatase, CPK **NIPE:** Tolerance develops w/ long-term use

Clonidine, Transdermal (Catapres TTS) Uses: HTN **Action:** Centrally acting α-adrenergic stimulant **Dose:** Apply 1 patch q7–10d to hairless area (upper arm/torso); titrate to effect; ↓ in severe renal impairment, ⊘ DC abruptly (rebound HTN) **Caution:** [C, +/–] ⊘ w/ BBs **Supplied:** TTS-1, TTS-2, TTS-3 (delivers 0.1, 0.2, 0.3 mg, respectively, of clonidine/d for 1 wk) **Notes:** Doses >2 TTS-3 usually not associated w/ ↑ efficacy; steady state in 3 d **SE:** Drowsiness, orthostatic hypotension, xerostomia, constipation, bradycardia. See Clonidine. **NIPE:** Rotate transdermal site weekly

Clopidogrel (Plavix) Uses: *Reduction of atherosclerotic events* **Action:** Inhibits plt aggregation **Dose:** 75 mg/d **Caution:** [B, ?] Active bleeding; TTP; liver Dz **Contra:** Active pathologic bleeding; intracranial bleeding **Supplied:** Tabs 75 mg **SE:** Prolongs bleeding time, GI intolerance, HA, dizziness, rash, thrombocy-

topenia, leukopenia **Notes:** Use w/ caution in persons at risk of bleeding fro
trauma & other causes; plt aggregation returns to baseline ≈5 d after DC; plt tran
fusion reverses effects acutely; 300 mg PO × 1 dose can be used to load Pts **Inte
actions:** ↑ Risk of GI bleed w/ ASA, NSAIDs, heparin, warfarin, feverfew, garli
ginger, ginkgo biloba; ↑ effects of phenytoin, tamoxifen, tolbutamide **Labs:**
LFTs; ↓ plts, neutrophils **NIPE:** DC drug 1 wk prior to surgery

Clorazepate (Tranxene) [C-IV] **Uses:** *Acute anxiety disorders, acu
EtOH withdrawal Sxs, adjunctive therapy in partial Szs* **Action:** Benzodiazepin
antianxiety agent **Dose:** *Adults.* 15–60 mg/d PO single or ÷ doses. *Elderly & debi
itated Pts:* Start at 7.5–15 mg/d in ÷ doses. *EtOH withdrawal:* Day 1: Initially, 3
mg; then 30–60 mg in ÷ doses; Day 2: 45–90 mg in ÷ doses; Day 3: 22.5–45 mg
÷ doses; Day 4: 15–30 mg in ÷ doses. *Peds.* 3.75–7.5 mg/dose bid to 60 mg/d ma
÷ bid–tid **Caution:** [D, ?/–] ⊘ for <9 y of age; caution in elderly & w/ Hx depres
sion **Contra:** Narrow-angle glaucoma **Supplied:** Tabs 3.75, 7.5, 15 mg; Tabs-S
(once-daily) 11.25, 22.5 mg **SE:** CNS depressant effects (drowsiness, dizzines
ataxia, memory impairment), hypotension **Notes:** Monitor Pts w/ renal/hepatic im
pairment (drug may accumulate); may cause dependence **Interactions:** ↑ Effec
w/ antidepressants, antihistamines, barbiturates, MAOIs, narcotics, phenothiazine
cimetidine, disulfiram, EtOH; ↓ effects of levodopa; ↓ effects w/ ginkgo, tobacc
Labs: ↓ Hct, abnormal LFTs, BUN, creatinine **NIPE:** ⊘ DC abruptly

Clotrimazole (Lotrimin, Mycelex) [OTC] **Uses:** *Candidiasis &
tinea infections* **Action:** Antifungal; alters cell wall permeability. *Spectrum*
Oropharyngeal candidiasis, dermatophytoses, superficial mycoses, cutaneous can
didasis, & vulvovaginal candidiasis **Dose:** *PO: Prophylaxis:* One troche dissolve
in mouth TID *Rx:* One troche dissolved in mouth 5 ×/d for 14 d. *Vaginal 1*
Cream: 1 applicatorful hs for 7 d. *2% Cream:* 1 applicatorful hs for 3 d *Tabs:* 10
mg vaginally hs for 7 d or 200 mg (2 tabs) vaginally hs for 3 d or 500-mg tab
vaginally hs once. *Topical:* Apply bid for 10–14 d **Caution:** [B, (C if PO), ?] N
for systemic fungal infection; safety in children <3 y not established **Contra:** Hy
persensitivity to any component **Supplied:** 1% cream; soln; lotion; troche 10 mg
vaginal tabs 100, 500 mg; vaginal cream 1%, 2% **SE:** *Topical:* Local irritation
PO: N/V, ↑ LFTs **Notes:** PO prophylaxis used for immunosuppressed Pts **Interac
tions:** ↑ Effects of cyclosporine, tacrolimus; ↓ effects of spermicides

Clotrimazole & Betamethasone (Lotrisone) **Uses:** *Fungal ski
infections* **Action:** Imidazole antifungal & anti-inflammatory. *Spectrum:* Tine
pedis, cruris, & corpora **Dose:** *Pts ≥17 y.* Apply & massage into area bid for 2–
wk **Caution:** [C, ?] Varicella infection **Contra:** Children <12 y **Supplied:** Crea
15, 45 g; lotion 30 mL **SE:** Local irritation, rash **Notes:** ⊘ use for diaper dermatit
or under occlusive dressings

Clozapine (Clozaril) **WARNING:** Myocarditis, agranulocytosis, Szs, &
orthostatic hypotension have been associated w/ clozapine **Uses:** *Refractory se
vere schizophrenia*; childhood psychosis **Action:** Tricyclic "atypical" antipsy

hotic **Dose:** 25 mg daily–bid initial; ↑ to 300–450 mg/d over 2 wk. Maintain at he lowest dose possible; ⊘ DC abruptly **Caution:** [B, +/–] Monitor for psychosis & cholinergic rebound **Contra:** Uncontrolled epilepsy; comatose state; WBC ount ≤3500 cells/mm³ before Rx or <3000 cells/mm³ during Rx **Supplied:** Tabs 25, 100 mg **SE:** Tachycardia, drowsiness, weight gain, constipation, urinary incon- nence, rash, Szs, CNS stimulation **Notes:** Benign, self-limiting temperature ele- ations may occur during the 1st 3 wk of Rx, weekly CBC mandatory for 1st 6 mo, hen qowk **Interactions:** ↑ Effects w/ clarithromycin, cimetidine, erythromycin, luoxetine, paroxetine, quinidine, sertraline; ↑ depressant effects w/ CNS depres- ants, EtOH; ↑ effects of digoxin, warfarin; ↓ effects w/ carbamazepine, phenytoin, rimidone, phenobarbital, valproic acid, St. John's wort, nutmeg, caffeine; ↓ ef- ects of phenytoin **Labs:** Monitor WBCs **NIPE:** ↑ Risk of developing agranulocy- osis

Cocaine [C-II] **Uses:** *Topical anesthetic for mucous membranes* **Action:** Narcotic analgesic, local vasoconstrictor **Dose:** Apply lowest amount of topical oln that provides relief; 1 mg/kg max **Caution:** [C, ?] **Contra:** PRG **Supplied:** Topical soln & viscous preps 4, 10%; powder, soluble tabs (135 mg) for soln **SE:** CNS stimulation, nervousness, loss of taste/smell, chronic rhinitis **Notes:** Use only on mucous membranes of the PO, laryngeal, & nasal cavities; ⊘ use on extensive areas of broken skin **Interactions:** ↑ Effects w/ MAOIs, ↑ risk of HTN & arrhyth- mias w/ epinephrine

Codeine [C-II] **Uses:** *Mild/moderate pain; symptomatic relief of cough* **Action:** Narcotic analgesic; depresses cough reflex **Dose:** *Adults.* Analgesic: 15–60 mg PO or IM qid PRN. *Antitussive:* 10–20 mg PO q4h PRN; max 120 mg/d. *Peds.* Analgesic: 0.5–1 mg/kg/dose PO q4–6h PRN. *Antitussive:* 1–1.5 mg/kg/24 h PO ÷ q4h; max 30 mg/24 h; ↓ in renal/hepatic impairment **Caution:** [C, (D if pro- longed use or high doses at term), +] **Contra:** Component sensitivity **Supplied:** Tabs 15, 30, 60 mg; soln 15 mg/5 mL; inj 30, 60 mg/mL **SE:** Drowsiness, consti- pation **Notes:** Usually combined w/ APAP for pain or w/ agents (eg, terpin hydrate) as an antitussive; 120 mg IM = 10 mg IM morphine **Interactions:** ↑ CNS depres- sion w/ CNS depressants, antidepressants, MAOIs, TCAs, barbiturates, benzodi- azepines, muscle relaxants, phenothiazines, cimetidine, antihistamines, sedatives, EtOH; ↑ effects of digitoxin, phenytoin, rifampin; ↓ effects w/ nalbuphine, penta- zocine, tobacco **Labs:** False ↑ amylase, lipase, ↑ urine morphine

Colchicine **Uses:** *Acute gouty arthritis & prevention of recurrences; familial Mediterranean fever*; primary biliary cirrhosis **Action:** Inhibits migration of leukocytes; ↓ production of lactic acid by leukocytes **Dose:** *Initially:* 0.5–1.2 mg PO, then 0.5 mg q1–2h until relief or GI SE develop (max 8 mg/d); ⊘ repeat for 3 d. *IV:* 1–3 mg, then 0.5 mg q6h until relief (max 4 mg/d); ⊘ repeat for 7 d. *Prophylaxis:* PO: 0.5–0.6 mg/d or 3–4 d/wk; ↓ renal impairment; caution in elderly **Caution:** [D, +] Severe local irritation can occur following SQ/IM **Contra:** Seri- ous renal, GI, hepatic, or cardiac disorders; blood dyscrasias **Supplied:** Tabs 0.5,

0.6 mg; inj 1 mg/2 mL **SE:** N/V/D, abdominal pain, bone marrow suppression, he patotoxicity **Notes:** Colchicine 1–2 mg IV w/in 24–48 h of an acute attack diag nostic/therapeutic in monoarticular arthritis **Interactions:** ↑ GI effects w NSAIDs; ↑ effects of sympathomimetics, CNS depressants, bone marrow depres sants, radiation therapy; ↓ effects of vitamin B $_{12}$ **Labs:** Monitor CBC, BUN, crea tinine; false + urine Hgb & RBCs **NIPE:** ⊘ EtOH

Colesevelam (Welchol) **Uses:** *Reduction of LDL & total cholestero alone or in combination w/ an HMG-CoA reductase inhibitor* **Action:** Bile acic sequestrant **Dose:** 3 tabs PO bid w/ meals **Caution:** [B, ?] Severe GI motility dis orders; safety & efficacy not established in peds **Contra:** Bowl obstruction **Sup plied:** Tabs 625 mg **SE:** Constipation, dyspepsia, myalgia, weakness **Notes:** May decrease absorption of fat-soluble vitamins **Interactions:** ↓ Effects of verapamil **Labs:** Monitor lipids **NIPE:** Take w/ food and liquid

Colestipol (Colestid) **Uses:** *Adjunct to ↓ serum cholesterol in primary hypercholesterolemia* **Action:** Binds intestinal bile acids to form an insoluble complex **Dose:** Granules: 5–30 g/d ÷ 2–4 doses; tabs: 2–16 g/d daily–bid **Caution:** [C, ?] ⊘ w/ high triglycerides, GI dysfunction **Contra:** Bowl obstruction **Sup plied:** Tabs 1 g; granules 5, 300, 500 g **SE:** Constipation, abdominal pain, bloating HA **Notes:** ⊘ Use dry powder; mix w/ beverages, soups, cereals, etc; may decrease absorption of other medications; may decrease absorption of fat-soluble vitamins **Interactions:** ↓ Absorption of numerous drugs especially anticoagulants, cardiac glycosides, digitoxin, digoxin, phenobarbital, penicillin G, tetracycline, thiazide di uretics, thyroid drugs **Labs:** ↓ Serum cholesterol, ↑ PT **NIPE:** Take other meds 1 h before or 4 h after colestipol

Colfosceril Palmitate (Exosurf Neonatal) **Uses:** *Prophylaxis & Rx for RDS in infants* **Action:** Synthetic lung surfactant **Dose:** 5 mL/kg/dose through ET tube as soon after birth as possible & again at 12 & 24 h **Caution:** [?, ?] Pulmonary hemorrhaging **Supplied:** Inj 108 mg **SE:** Pulmonary hemorrhage possible in infants weighing <700 g at birth; mucous plugging **Notes:** Monitor pul monary compliance & oxygenation carefully; monitor ECG **Interactions:** None noted

Cortisone See Steroids, Tables 4 and 5 (pages 271 & 272)

Cromolyn Sodium (Intal, NasalCrom, Opticrom) **Uses:** *Ad junct to the Rx of asthma; prevent exercise-induced asthma; allergic rhinitis; ophth allergic manifestations*; food allergy **Action:** Antiasthmatic; mast cell stabilizer **Dose:** *Adults & Children >12 y.* Inhal: 20 mg (as powder in caps) inhaled qid or met-dose inhaler 2 puffs qid. *PO:* 200 mg qid 15–20 min ac, up to 400 mg qid. *Nasal instillation:* Spray once in each nostril 2–6×/d. *Ophth:* 1–2 gtt in each eye 4–6×/d. *Peds.* Inhal: 2 puffs qid of met-dose inhaler. *PO: Infants <2 y:* (⊘) 20 mg/kg/d in 4 ÷ doses. *2–12 y:* 100 mg qid ac **Caution:** [B, ?] **Contra:** Acute asth matic attacks **Supplied:** PO conc 100 mg/5 mL; soln for neb 20 mg/2 mL; met dose inhaler; nasal soln 40 mg/mL; ophth soln 4% **SE:** Unpleasant taste.

oarseness, coughing **Notes:** No benefit in acute Rx; 2–4 wk for maximal effect in erennial allergic disorders **Interactions:** None noted **Labs:** Monitor pulmonary xn tests

Cyanocobalamin [Vitamin B₁₂] **Uses:** *Pernicious anemia & other vitamin B₁₂ deficiency states; ↑d requirements due to PRG; thyrotoxicosis; liver or idney Dz* **Action:** Dietary suppl of vitamin B₁₂ **Dose:** *Adults.* 100 μg IM or SQ for 5–10 d, then 100 μg IM 2×/wk for 1 mo, then 100 μg IM monthly. *Peds.* 100 g/d IM or SQ for 5–10 d, then 30–50 μg IM q4wk **Caution:** [A (C if dose exeeds RDA), +] **Contra:** Hypersensitivity to Co; hereditary optic nerve atrophy; eber's Dz **Supplied:** Tabs 50, 100, 250, 500, 1000 μg; inj 100, 1000 μg/mL; gel 00 μg/0.1 mL **SE:** Itching, diarrhea, HA, anxiety **Notes:** PO absorption erratic, alered by many drugs & ⊘; for use w/ hyperalimentation **Interactions:** ↓ Effects w/ ninosalicylic acid, chloramphenicol, cholestyramine, cimetidine, colchicines, eomycin, amino salicylate, EtOH **Labs:** Antibiotics, MRX, pyrimethamine invalidate blood assays of vitamin B₁₂ and folic acid

Cyclobenzaprine (Flexeril) **Uses:** *Relief of muscle spasm* **Action:** Centrally acting skeletal muscle relaxant; reduces tonic somatic motor activity **Dose:** 10 mg PO 2–4×/d (2–3 wk max) **Caution:** [B, ?] Shares the toxic potential f the TCAs; urinary hesitancy or angle-closure glaucoma **Contra:** ⊘ Use conomitantly or w/in 14 days of MAOIs; hyperthyroidism; HF; arrhythmias **Supplied:** Tabs 10 mg **SE:** Sedation & anticholinergic side effects **Notes:** May inhibit mental alertness or physical coordination **Interactions:** ↑ Effects of CNS depresion w/ CNS depressants, TCAs, barbiturates, EtOH; ↑ risk of HTN & convulsions √/ MAOIs **NIPE:** ↑ Fluids & fiber for constipation

Cyclopentolate (Cyclogyl) **Uses:** *Diagnostic procedures requiring cycloplegia & mydriasis* **Action:** Cycloplegic & mydriatic agent (can last up to 24) **Dose:** 1 gt then another in 5 min **Caution:** [C, ?] **Contra:** Narrow-angle glaucoma **Supplied:** Soln, 0.5, 1, 2% **SE:** Blurred vision, ↑ sensitivity to light, tachycardia, restlessness **Interactions:** ↓ Effects of carbachol, cholinesterase inhibitors, ilocarpine **NIPE:** Burning sensation when instilled

Cyclophosphamide (Cytoxan, Neosar) **Uses:** *Hodgkin's & NHLs; multiple myeloma; small-cell lung, breast, & ovarian CAs; mycosis fungoides; neuroblastoma; retinoblastoma; acute leukemias; & allogeneic & ABMT in igh doses; severe rheumatologic disorders* **Action:** Converted to acrolein & phosphoramide mustard, the active alkylating moieties **Dose:** 500–1500 mg/m² as single dose at 2–4-wk intervals; 1.8 g/m² to 160 mg/kg (or ≈12 g/m² in a 75-kg ndividual) in the BMT setting (refer to specific protocols); adjust in renal/hepatic mpairment **Caution:** [D, ?] In bone marrow suppression **Contra:** Component sensitivity **Supplied:** Tabs 25, 50 mg; inj 100 mg **SE:** Myelosuppression (leukopenia & thrombocytopenia); hemorrhagic cystitis, SIADH, alopecia, anorexia; N/V; heatotoxicity & rarely interstitial pneumonitis; irreversible testicular atrophy possible; cardiotoxicity rare; 2nd malignancies (bladder CA & acute leukemias);

cumulative risk 3.5% at 8 y, 10.7% at 12 y **Notes:** Hemorrhagic cystitis prophy laxis: continuous bladder irrigation & mesna uroprotection; encourage adequa hydration **Interactions:** ↑ Effects w/ allopurinol, cimetidine, phenobarbital, r fampin; ↑ effects of succinylcholine, warfarin; ↓ effects of digoxin **Labs:** May in hibit + Rxns to skin tests for PPD, risk of false + Pap smear results **NIPE:** Ma cause sterility, hair loss, ⊘ PRG, breast-feeding, immunizations

Cyclosporine (Sandimmune, Neoral) Uses: *Organ rejection i kidney, liver, heart, & BMT w/ steroids; RA; psoriasis;* CA Rx; BMT **Action:** Im munosuppressant; reversible inhibition of immunocompetent lymphocytes **Dose** *Adults & Peds.* PO: 15 mg/ kg/d 12 h pretransplant; after 2 wk, taper by 5 mg/w to 5–10 mg/kg/d. IV: If NPO, give ⅓ PO dose IV; ↓ in renal/hepatic impairmen **Caution:** [C, ?] Dose-related risk of nephrotoxicity/hepatotoxicity; live, attenuate vaccines may be less effective **Contra:** Abnormal renal Fxn; uncontrolled HTI **Supplied:** Caps 25, 50, 100 mg; PO soln 100 mg/mL; inj 50 mg/mL **SE:** May BUN & creatinine & mimic transplant rejection; HTN; HA; hirsutism **Notes:** Ad minister in glass containers; many drug interactions; Neoral & Sandimmune not in terchangeable; interaction w/ St. John's wort. **Interactions:** ↑ Effects w/ azol antifungals, allopurinol, amiodarone, anabolic steroids, CCBs, cimetidine, chloro quine, clarithromycin, clonidine, diltiazem, macrolides, metoclopramide, nicardip ine, NSAIDs, oral contraceptives, ticlopidine, grapefruit juice; ↑ nephrotoxicity w aminoglycosides, amphotericin B, acyclovir, colchicine, enalapril, ranitidine, sul fonamides; ↑ risk digoxin toxicity; ↑ risk of hyperkalemia w/ diuretics, ACEIs; effects w/ barbiturates, carbamazepine, INH, nafcillin, pyrazinamide, phenytoin, ri fampin, sulfonamides, St. John's wort, alfalfa sprouts, astragalus, echinacea licorice; ↓ effects immunizations **Labs:** ↑ SCr, BUN, total bilirubin, K⁺, alkalin phosphatase, lipids **NIPE:** Monitor for hyperglycemia, hyperkalemia, hyper uricemia, risk of photosensitivity—use sunscreen

Cyproheptadine (Periactin) Uses: *Allergic Rxns; itching* **Action** Phenothiazine antihistamine; serotonin antagonist **Dose:** *Adults.* 4–20 mg PO q8h; max 0.5 mg/kg/d. *Peds.* 2–6 y: 2 mg bid–tid (max 12 mg/24 h). 7–14 y: 4 m bid–tid; ↓ dose in hepatic impairment **Caution:** [B, ?] Symptomatic BPH **Contra** Neonates or <2 y; narrow-angle glaucoma; bladder neck obstruction; acute asthma GI obstruction **Supplied:** Tabs 4 mg; syrup 2 mg/5 mL **SE:** Anticholinergic drowsiness, **Notes:** May stimulate appetite **Interactions:** ↑ Effects w/ CNS depres sants, MAOIs, EtOH; ↓ effects of epinephrine, fluoxetine **Labs:** False – skin test ing; false + urine TCA assay; ↑ serum amylase, prolactin; ↓ FBS **NIPE:** ↑ Ris photosensitivity—use sunscreen, take w/ food if GI distress

Cytarabine [ARA-C] (Cytosar-U) Uses: *Acute leukemias, CML NHL; IT administration for leukemic meningitis or prophylaxis* **Action:** An timetabolite; interferes w/ DNA synthesis **Dose:** 100–150 mg/m²/d for 5–10 d (lo dose); 3 g/m² q12h for 8–12 doses (high dose); 1 mg/kg 1–2/wk (SQ maintenance regimens); 5–70 mg/m² up to 3/wk IT (refer to specific protocols); ↓ in renal/he

patic impairment **Caution:** [D, ?] In marked bone marrow suppression, ↓ dosage by ↓ the number of days of administration **Contra:** Component sensitivity **Supplied:** Inj 100, 500 mg, 1, 2 g **SE:** Myelosuppression, N/V/D, stomatitis, flu-like syndrome, rash on palms/soles, hepatic dysfunction, cerebellar dysfunction, noncardiogenic pulmonary edema, neuropathy **Notes:** Of little use in solid tumors; toxicity of high-dose regimens (conjunctivitis) ameliorated by corticosteroid ophth soln **Interactions:** ↑ Effects w/ alkylating drugs and radiation therapy; ↓ effects of digoxin, gentamicin, MRX, flucytosine **Labs:** ↑ Uric acid, monitor CBC, BUN, creatinine, LFTs **NIPE:** ⊘ EtOH, NSAIDs, ASA, PRG, breast-feeding, immunizations

Cytarabine Liposome (DepoCyt) **Uses:** *Lymphomatous meningitis* **Action:** Antimetabolite; interferes w/ DNA synthesis **Dose:** 50 mg IT q14d for 5 doses, then 50 mg IT q28d for 4 doses; use dexamethasone prophylaxis **Caution:** [D, ?] May cause neurotoxicity; blockage to CSF flow may ↑ the risk of neurotoxicity; use in peds not established **Contra:** Active meningeal infection **Supplied:** IT inj 50 mg/5 mL **SE:** Neck pain/rigidity, HA, confusion, somnolence, fever, back pain, N/V, edema, neutropenia, thrombocytopenia, anemia **Notes:** Cytarabine liposomes are similar in microscopic appearance to WBCs; care must be taken in interpreting CSF examinations **Interactions:** None noted, perhaps because of limited systemic exposure **Labs:** May interfere w/ CSF interpretation **NIPE:** ⊘ PRG, use contraception

Cytomegalovirus Immune Globulin [CMV-IG IV] (CytoGam) **Uses:** *Attenuation of primary CMV Dz associated w/ transplantation* **Action:** Exogenous IgG antibodies to CMV **Dose:** 150 mg/kg/dose w/in 72 h of transplant, for 16 wk posttransplant; see insert for dosing schedule **Caution:** [C, ?] Anaphylactic Rxns; renal dysfunction **Contra:** Hypersensitivity to immunoglobulins; immunoglobulin A deficiency **Supplied:** Inj 50 mg/mL **SE:** Flushing, N/V, muscle cramps, wheezing, HA, fever **Notes:** IV use only; administer by separate line; ⊘ shake **Interactions:** ↓ Effects of live virus vaccines **NIPE:** Admin immunizations at least 3 mo after CMV-IG

Dacarbazine (DTIC) **Uses:** *Melanoma, Hodgkin's Dz, sarcoma* **Action:** Alkylating agent; antimetabolite as a purine precursor; inhibits protein synthesis, RNA, & especially DNA **Dose:** 2–4.5 mg/kg/d for 10 consecutive d or 250 mg/m²/d for 5 d (refer to specific protocols); ↓ in renal impairment **Caution:** [C, ?] In bone marrow suppression; renal/hepatic impairment **Contra:** Component sensitivity **Supplied:** Inj 100, 200, 500 mg **SE:** Myelosuppression, severe N/V, hepatotoxicity, flu-like syndrome, ↓ BP, photosensitivity, alopecia, facial flushing, facial paresthesias, urticaria, phlebitis at inj site **Notes:** ⊘ extravasation **Interactions:** ↑ Effects w/ amphotericin B, anticoagulants, ASA, bone-marrow suppressants; ↑ effects of phenobarbital, phenytoin **Labs:** ↑ AST, ALT **NIPE:** Risk of photosensitivity—use sunscreen, hair loss, infection

Daclizumab (Zenapax) **Uses:** *Prevent acute organ rejection* **Action:** IL-2 receptor antagonist **Dose:** 1 mg/kg/dose IV; 1st dose pretransplant, then 4

doses 14 d apart posttransplant **Caution:** [C, ?] **Contra:** Component sensitivity **Supplied:** Inj 5 mg/mL **SE:** Hyperglycemia, edema, HTN, hypotension, constipation, HA, dizziness, anxiety, nephrotoxicity, pulmonary edema, pain **Notes:** Administer w/in 4 h of prep **Interactions:** ⊘ Echinacea **NIPE:** ⊘ Immunizations, infections, ↑ fluid intake

Dactinomycin (Cosmegen) **Uses:** *Choriocarcinoma, Wilms' tumor, Kaposi's sarcoma, Ewing's sarcoma, rhabdomyosarcoma, testicular CA* **Action:** DNA intercalating agent **Dose:** 0.5 mg/d for 5 d; 2 mg/wk for 3 consecutive wk; 15 μg/kg or 0.45 mg/m²/d (max 0.5 mg) for 5 d q3–8wk in pediatric sarcoma (refer to specific protocols); ↓ in renal impairment **Caution:** [C, ?] **Contra:** Use w/ concurrent or recent chickenpox or herpes zoster; ⊘ in infants <6 mo **Supplied:** Inj 0.5 mg **SE:** Myelo- & immunosuppression, severe N/V, alopecia, acne, hyperpigmentation, radiation recall phenomenon, tissue damage w/ extravasation, hepatotoxicity **Interactions:** ↑ Effects bone marrow suppressants, radiation therapy; ↓ effects of vitamin K **Labs:** ↑ Uric acid; monitor CBC w/ differential & plts, LFTs, BUN, creatinine **NIPE:** ⊘ PRG, breast-feeding; risk of irreversible infertility, reversible hair loss, ↑ fluids to 2–3 L/d

Dalteparin (Fragmin) **Uses:** *Unstable angina, non-Q-wave MI, prevention of ischemic complications due to clot formation in Pts on concurrent ASA; prevention & Rx of DVT following surgery* **Action:** LMW heparin **Dose:** *Angina/MI:* 120 IU/kg (max 10,000 IU) SQ q12h w/ ASA. *DVT prophylaxis:* 2500–5000 IU SC 1–2 h preop, then qd for 5–10 d. *Systemic anticoagulation:* 200 IU/kg/d SQ or 100 IU/kg bid SQ; use w/ caution in renal/hepatic impairment **Caution:** [B, ?] Active hemorrhage, cerebrovascular Dz, cerebral aneurysm, severe uncontrolled HTN **Contra:** HIT; hypersensitivity to pork products; **Supplied:** Inj 2500 IU (16 mg/0.2 mL), 5000 IU (32 mg/0.2 mL), 10,000 IU (64 mg/mL) **SE:** Bleeding, pain at inj site, thrombocytopenia **Notes:** Predictable antithrombotic effects eliminate need for laboratory monitoring; not for IM or IV use **Interactions:** ↑ Bleeding w/ oral anticoagulants, plt inhibitors, penicillins, cephalosporins, garlic, ginger, ginkgo biloba, ginseng, chamomile, vitamin E **Labs:** ↑ AST, ALT, monitor CBC and plts **NIPE:** ⊘ Give PO or IM; give deep SC

Danaparoid (Orgaran) **Uses:** *Prophylaxis of DVT to prevent PE, in hip replacement surgery* **Action:** Antithrombotic; inhibits factor Xa & IIa **Dose:** 750 anti-Xa units bid SQ 1–4 h preop & starting no sooner than 2 h postop; ↓ dose in severe renal impairment **Caution:** [B, ?/–] **Contra:** Active major bleeding, hemophilia, ITP, type II thrombocytopenia w/ a + antiplt antibody test **Supplied:** Amps & prefilled syringes 0.6 mL (750 anti-Xa units) **SE:** Bleeding, fever, inj site pain, ↑d risk of epidural & spinal hematoma in Pts receiving epidural/spinal anesthesia **Notes:** aPTT monitoring not necessary

Dantrolene (Dantrium) **Uses:** *Rx clinical spasticity due to upper motor neuron disorders, eg, spinal cord injuries, strokes, CP, MS; Rx malignant hyperthermia* **Action:** Skeletal muscle relaxant **Dose:** *Adults.* Spasticity: Initially, 25

ng PO qd; ↑ to effect by 25 mg to a max dose of 100 mg PO qid PRN. **Peds.** Initially, 0.5 mg/kg/dose bid; ↑ by 0.5 mg/kg to effect to Rx to a max dose of 3 mg/kg/dose qid PRN. **Adults & Peds.** Malignant hyperthermia: **Rx:** Continuous rapid IV push, start at 1 mg/kg until Sxs subside or 10 mg/kg is reached. *Postcrisis follow-up:* 4–8 mg/kg/d in 3–4 ÷ doses for 1–3 d to prevent recurrence **Caution:**[C, ?] ↓ Cardiac Fxn or pulmonary Fxn **Contra:** Active hepatic Dz; should not be used where spasticity is used to maintain posture or balance **Supplied:** Caps 25, 50, 100 mg; powder for inj 20 mg/vial **SE:** Hepatotoxicity w/↑ LFTs, drowsiness, dizziness, rash, muscle weakness, pleural effusion w/ pericarditis, diarrhea, blurred vision, hepatitis **Notes:** Monitor transaminases; ⊘ sunlight/ EtOH /CNS depressants **Interactions:** ↑ effects w/ CNS depressants, antihistamines, opioids, EtOH; ↑ risk of hepatotoxicity w/ estrogens; ↑ risk of CV collapse & ventricular fib w/ CCBs; ↓ plasma protein binding w/ clofibrate, warfarin **Labs:** ↑ AST, ALT, alkaline phosphatase, LDH, BUN, total serum bilirubin **NIPE:** ↑ Risk of photosensitivity—use sunscreen

Dapsone (Avlosulfon) **Uses:** *Rx & prevent PCP; toxoplasmosis prophylaxis; leprosy* **Action:** Unknown; bactericidal **Dose:** *Adults.* PCP prophylaxis 50–100 mg/d PO; Rx PCP 100 mg/d PO w/ TMP 15–20 mg/kg/d for 21 d. *Peds.* Prophylaxis of PCP 1–2 mg/kg/24 h PO qd; max 100 mg/d **Caution:** [C, +] G6PD deficiency; severe anemia **Contra:** Component sensitivity **Supplied:** Tabs 25, 100 mg **SE:** Hemolysis, methemoglobinemia, agranulocytosis, rash, cholestatic jaundice **Notes:** Absorption ↑ by an acidic environment; w/ leprosy, combine w/ rifampin & other agents **Interactions:** ↑ Effects w/ probenecid, trimethoprim; ↓ effects w/ activated charcoal, rifampin **Labs:** Monitor CBC, LFTs **NIPE:** ↑ Risk of photosensitivity—use sunscreen

Darbepoetin Alfa (Aranesp) **Uses:** *Anemia associated w/ CRF* **Action:** Stimulates erythropoiesis, recombinant variant of erythropoietin **Dose:** 0.45 µg/kg single IV or SQ qwk; titrate dose, ⊘ exceed target Hgb of 12 g/dL; see insert if converting from Epogen **Caution:** [C, ?] May ↑ risk of CV &/or neurologic SE in renal failure; HTN; Hx of Szs **Contra:** Uncontrolled hypertension, allergy to components **Supplied:** 25, 40, 60, 100 µg/mL, in polysorbate or albumin excipient **SE:** May ↑ risk of cardiac events, CP, hypo-/hypertension, N/V/D, myalgia, arthralgia, dizziness, edema, fatigue, fever, ↑ risk infection **Notes:** Longer ½-life than Epogen; follow weekly CBC until stable **Interactions:** None noted **Labs:** Monitor CBC w/ differential & plts, BUN, creatinine, serum P, K+, Fe stores **NIPE:** Monitor BP & for Sz activity, shaking vial inactivates drug

Daunorubicin (Daunomycin, Cerubidine) **WARNING:** Cardiac Fxn must be monitored due to potential risk for cardiac toxicity & CHF **Uses:** *Acute leukemias* **Action:** DNA intercalating agent; inhibits topoisomerase II; generates oxygen free radicals **Dose:** 45–60 mg/m²/d for 3 consecutive d; 25 mg/m²/wk (refer to specific protocols); ↓ dose in renal/hepatic impairment **Caution:** [D, ?] **Contra:** Component sensitivity **Supplied:** Inj 20 mg **SE:** Myelosuppression, mucositis, N/V, alopecia, radiation recall phenomenon, hepatotoxicity (hyperbilirubinemia), tissue necrosis on extravascular extravasation, & cardiotoxicity (1–2% CHF risk w/ 550 mg/m² cumulative dose) **Notes:** Prevent cardiotoxicity w/ dexrazoxane; administer allopurinol prior to initiating Rx to prevent hyperuricemia **Interactions:** ↑ Risk of cardiotoxicity w/ cyclophosphamide; ↑ myelosuppression w/ antineoplastic agents; ↓ response to live virus vaccines **Labs:** Serum alkaline phosphatase, bilirubin, AST, monitor uric acid, CBC, LFTs **NIPE:** ⊘ ASA, NSAIDs, EtOH, PRG, breast-feeding, immunizations; risk of hair loss

Delavirdine (Rescriptor) **Uses:** *HIV infection* **Action:** Nonnucleoside RT inhibitor **Dose:** 400 mg PO tid **Caution:** [C, ?] CDC recommends HIV-infected mothers not breast-feed due to risk of HIV transmission to infant; use caution in renal/hepatic impairment **Contra:** Concomitant use w/ drugs highly dependent on CYP 3A for clearance (ie, alprazolam, ergot alkaloids, midazolam, pimozide, triazolam) **Supplied:** Tabs 100 mg **SE:** HA, fatigue, rash, ↑ serum transaminases N/V/D **Notes:** ⊘ Antacids; inhibits cytochrome P-450 enzymes; numerous drug interactions; monitor LFTs **Interactions:** ↑ Effects w/ fluoxetine; (up) benzodiazepines, cisapride, clarithromycin, dapsone, ergotamines, indinavir, lovastatin midazolam, nifedipine, quinidine, ritonavir, simvastatin, terfenadine, triazolam warfarin; ↓ effects w/ antacids, barbiturates, carbamazepine, cimetidine, famotidine, lansoprazole, nizatidine, phenobarbital, phenytoin, ranitidine, rifabutin, rifampin; ↓ effects of didanosine **Labs:** ↑ AST, ALT, ↓ neutrophil counts **NIPE:** Take w/o regard to food

Demeclocycline (Declomycin) **Uses:** SIADH **Action:** Antibiotic, antagonizes action of ADH on renal tubules **Dose:** 300–600 mg PO q12h on an empty stomach; ↓ in renal failure; ⊘ antacids **Caution:** [D, +] ⊘ in hepatic/renal dysfunction & children **Contra:** Hypersensitivity to tetracyclines **Supplied:** Tabs 150, 300 mg **SE:** Diarrhea, abdominal cramps, photosensitivity, DI **Notes:** ⊘ prolonged exposure to sunlight **Interactions:** Effects of digoxin, anticoagulants; ↓ effects w/ antacids, Bi salts, Fe, Na bicarbonate, barbiturates, carbamazepine, hydantoins, food; ↓ effects of oral contraceptives, penicillin **Labs:** False – urine glucose; monitor CBC, LFTs, BUN, creatinine **NIPE:** Risk of photosensitivity—use sunscreen

Desipramine (Norpramin) **Uses:** *Endogenous depression,* chronic pain, & peripheral neuropathy **Action:** TCA; ↑s synaptic conc of serotonin or norepinephrine in CNS **Dose:** 25–200 mg/d single or ÷ doses; usually a single hs dose (max 300 mg/d) **Caution:** [C, ?/–] Caution in CV Dz, Sz disorder, hypothyroidism **Contra:** Use of MAOIs w/in 14 d; during recovery phase of MI **Supplied:** Tabs 10, 25, 50, 75, 100, 150 mg; caps 25, 50 mg **SE:** Anticholinergic (blurred vision, urinary retention, xerostomia); orthostatic hypotension; prolongs QT interval, arrhythmias **Notes:** Numerous drug interactions; may cause urine to turn blue-green; ⊘ sunlight **Interactions:** ↑ Effects w/ cimetidine, diltiazem, fluoxetine, indinavir, MAOIs, paroxetine, propoxyphene, quinidine, ritonavir ranitidine, EtOH, grapefruit juice; ↑ effects of Li, sulfonylureas; ↓ effects w/ barbiturates, carbamazepine rifampin, tobacco **NIPE:** Full effect of drug may take 4 wk, risk of photosensitivity—use sunscreen

Desloratadine (Clarinex)
Uses: *Symptoms of seasonal & perennial allergic rhinitis; chronic idiopathic urticaria* **Action:** Active metabolite of Claritin, H_1-antihistamine, blocks inflammatory mediators **Dose: Adults & Peds >12 y.** 5 mg PO qd; in hepatic/renal impairment 5 mg PO qod **Caution:** [C, ?/–] RediTabs contain phenylalanine; safety not established for <12 y **Supplied:** Tabs & RediTabs (rapid dissolving) 5 mg **SE:** Hypersensitivity Rxns, anaphylaxis somnolence, HA, dizziness, fatigue, pharyngitis, xerostomia, nausea, dyspepsia, myalgia **Labs:** ↑ LFTs, bilirubin **NIPE:** Take w/o regard to food

Desmopressin (DDAVP, Stimate)
Uses: *DI (intranasal & parenteral); bleeding due to uremia, hemophilia A, & type I von Willebrand's Dz (parenteral), nocturnal enuresis* **Action:** Synthetic analog of vasopressin, a naturally occurring human ADH; ↑ factor VIII **Dose: DI: Intranasal: Adults.** 0.1–0.4 mL (10–40 µg/d) in 1–4 ÷ doses. **Peds 3 mo–12 y.** 0.05–0.3 mL/d in 1 or 2 doses. *Parenteral: Adults.* 0.5–1 mL (2–4 µg/d in 2 ÷ doses; if converting from nasal to parenteral, use ¹/₁₀ nasal dose. **PO: Adults.** 0.05 mg bid; ↑ to max of 1.2 mg. *Hemophilia A & von Willebrand's Dz (type I): Adults & Peds >10 kg.* 0.3 µg/kg in 50 mL NS, inf over 15–30 min. **Peds <10 kg.** As above w/ dilution to 10 mL w/ NS. *Nocturnal enuresis: Peds >6 y.* 20 µg intranasally hs **Caution:** [B, M] ⊘ overhydration **Contra:** Hemophilia B; severe classic von Willebrand's Dz; Pts w/ factor VIII antibodies **Supplied:** Tabs 0.1, 0.2 mg; inj 4 µg/mL; nasal soln 0.1, 1.5 mg/mL **SE:** Facial flushing, HA, dizziness, vulval pain, nasal congestion, pain at inj site, hyponatremia, water intoxication **Notes:** In very young & old Pts, ↓ fluid intake to ⊘ water intoxication & hyponatremia **Interactions:** ↑ Antidiuretic effects w/ carbamazepine, chlorpropamide, clofibrate; ↑ effects of vasopressors; ↓ antidiuretic effects w/ demeclocycline, Li, norepinephrine **NIPE:** Monitor I&O, ⊘ EtOH, overhydration

Dexamethasone, Nasal (Dexacort Phosphate Turbinaire)
Uses: *Chronic nasal inflammation or allergic rhinitis* **Action:** Antiinflammatory corticosteroid **Dose: Adult & Peds >12 y.** 2 sprays/nostril bid–tid, max 12 sprays/d. **Peds 6–12 y.** 1–2 sprays/nostril bid, max 8 sprays/d **Caution:** [C, ?] **Contra:** Untreated infection **Supplied:** Aerosol, 84 µg/activation **SE:** Local irritation **NIPE:** Use decongestant nose gtt 1st if nasal congestion

Dexamethasone, Ophthalmic (AK-Dex Ophthalmic, Decadron Ophthalmic)
Uses: *Inflammatory or allergic conjunctivitis* **Action:** Antiinflammatory corticosteroid **Dose:** Instill 1–2 gtt tid–qid **Caution:** [C, ?/–] **Contra:** Active untreated bacterial, viral, & fungal eye infections **Supplied:** Susp & soln 0.1%; oint 0.05% **SE:** Long-term use associated w/ cataract formation **NIPE:** Eval intraocular pressure and lens if prolonged use

Dexamethasone Systemic, Topical (Decadron)
See Steroids, Systemic, page 223, & Table 4, page 271, & Steroids, Topical, Table 5, page 272

Interactions: ↑ Effects w/ cyclosporine, estrogens, oral contraceptives, macrolides; ↑ effects of cyclosporine; ↓ effects w/ aminoglutethimide, antacids, barbiturates, carbamazepine, cholestyramine, colestipol, phenytoin, phenobarbital, rifampin; ↓ effects of anticoagulants, hypoglycemics, INH, toxoids, salicylates, vaccines **Labs:** False – allergy skin tests **NIPE:** ⊘ Vaccines, breast-feeding, use on broken skin

Dexpanthenol (Ilopan-Choline PO, Ilopan) Uses: *Minimize paralytic ileus, Rx postop distention* **Action:** Cholinergic agent **Dose:** *Adults. Relief of gas:* 2–3 tabs PO tid. *Prevent postop ileus:* 250–500 mg IM stat, repeat in 2 h, then q6h PRN. *Ileus:* 500 mg IM stat, repeat in 2 h, followed by doses q6h, PRN **Caution:** [C, ?] **Contra:** Hemophilia, mechanical obstruction **Supplied:** Inj; tabs 50 mg; cream **SE:** GI cramps

Dexrazoxane (Zinecard) Uses: *Prevent anthracycline-induced cardiomyopathy* **Action:** Chelates heavy metals; binds intracellular Fe & prevents anthracycline-induced free radicals **Dose:** 10:1 ratio dexrazoxane:doxorubicin 30 min prior to each dose **Caution:** [C, ?] **Contra:** Component sensitivity **Supplied:** Inj 10 mg/mL **SE:** Myelosuppression (especially leukopenia), fever, infection, stomatitis, alopecia, N/V/D; mild ↑ transaminase, pain at inj site **Interactions:** ↑ Length of muscle relaxation w/ succinylcholine

Dextran 40 (Rheomacrodex) Uses: *Shock, prophylaxis of DVT & thromboembolism, adjunct in peripheral vascular surgery* **Action:** Expands plasma volume; ↓ blood viscosity **Dose:** *Shock:* 10 mL/kg inf rapidly; 20 mL/kg max in the 1st 24 h; beyond 24 h 10 mL/kg max; DC after 5 d. *Prophylaxis of DVT & thromboembolism:* 10 mL/kg IV day of surgery, then 500 mL/d IV for 2–3 d, then 500 mL IV q2–3d based on risk for up to 2 wk **Caution:** [C, ?] Inf Rxns; Pts receiving corticosteroids **Contra:** Major hemostatic defects of all types; cardiac decompensation; renal Dz w/ severe oliguria/anuria **Supplied:** 10% dextran 40 in 0.9% NaCl or 5% dextrose **SE:** Hypersensitivity/anaphylactoid Rxn (observe closely during 1st min of inf), arthralgia, cutaneous Rxns, hypotension, fever **Notes:** Monitor Cr & electrolytes; Pts should be well hydrated **Interactions:** ↑ Bleeding times w/ antiplt agents or anticoagulants **Labs:** False ↑ serum glucose, urinary protein, bilirubin assays, & total protein assays **NIPE:** Draw blood before administration of drug, Pt should be well hydrated prior to inf

Dextromethorphan (Mediquell, Benylin DM, PediaCare 1, others) [OTC] Uses: *Controlling nonproductive cough* **Action:** Depresses the cough center in the medulla **Dose:** *Adults.* 10–30 mg PO q4h PRN (max 120 mg/24 h). *Peds. 7 mo–1 y:* 2–4 mg q6–8h. *2–6 y:* 2.5–7.5 mg q4–8h (max 30 mg/24 h). *7–12 y:* 5–10 mg q4–8h (max 60 mg/24/h) **Caution:** [C, ?/–] Not for persistent or chronic cough **Supplied:** Caps 30 mg; lozenges 2.5, 5, 7.5, 15 mg; syrup 15 mg/15 mL, 10 mg/5 mL; liq 10 mg/15 mL, 3.5, 7.5, 15 mg/5 mL; sustained-action liq 30 mg/5 mL **SE:** GI disturbances **Notes:** May be found in combination OTC products w/ guaifenesin **Interactions:** ↑ Effects w/ amiodarone, fluoxetin, quinidine, terbinafine; ↑ risk of serotonin syndrome w/ sibutramine, MAOIs; ↑ CNS depression w/ antihistamines, antidepressants, sedative, opioids, EtOH **NIPE:** ↑ Fluids, humidity to environment, stop MAOIs for 2 wk before administering drug

Dezocine (Dalgan) Uses: *Moderate to severe pain* **Action:** Narcotic agonist–antagonist **Dose:** 5–20 mg IM or 2.5–10 mg IV q2–4h PRN; ↓ in renal impairment **Caution:** [C, ?] **Contra:** Pts <18 y **Supplied:** Inj 5, 10, 15 mg/mL **SE:** Sedation, dizziness, vertigo, N/V, inj site Rxn **Notes:** Withdrawal possible in Pts dependent on narcotics **Interactions:** ↑ Effects w/ CNS depressants, ⊘ MAOIs **NIPE:** ↑ Resp depression greatest 1st h after admin

Diazepam (Valium) [C-IV] Uses: *Anxiety, EtOH withdrawal, muscle spasm, status epilepticus, panic disorders, amnesia, preoperative sedation* **Action:** Benzodiazepine **Dose:** *Adults.* Status epilepticus: 5–10 mg q10–20min to 30 mg max in 8-h period. *Anxiety, muscle spasm:* 2–10 mg PO bid–qid or IM/IV q3–4h PRN. *Preop:* 5–10 mg PO or IM 20–30 min or IV just prior to procedure. *EtOH withdrawal:* Initial 2–5 mg IV, then 5–10 mg q5–10min, 100 mg in 1 h max. May require up to 1000 mg in 24-h period for severe withdrawal. Titrate to agitation; ⊘ excessive sedation; may lead to aspiration or resp arrest. *Peds.* Status epilepticus: <5 y: 0.05–0.3 mg/kg/dose IV q15–30min up to a max of 5 mg. >5 y: Give up to max of 10 mg. *Sedation, muscle relaxation:* 0.04–0.3 mg/kg/dose q2–4h IM or IV to max of 0.6 mg/kg in 8 h, or 0.12–0.8 mg/kg/24 h PO + tid–qid; ↓ in hepatic impairment; ⊘ abrupt withdrawal **Caution:** [D, ?/–] **Contra:** Coma, CNS depression, resp depression, narrow-angle glaucoma, severe uncontrolled pain, PRG **Supplied:** Tabs 2, 5, 10 mg; soln 1, 5 mg/mL; inj 5 mg/mL; rectal gel 5 mg/mL **SE:** Sedation, amnesia, bradycardia, hypotension, rash, decreased resp rate **Notes:** ⊘ exceed 5 mg/min IV in adults or 1–2 mg/min in peds because resp arrest possible; IM absorption erratic **Interactions:** ↑ Effects w/ antihistamines, azole antifungals, BBs, CNS depressants, cimetidine, ciprofloxin, disulfiram, INH, oral contraceptives, omeprazole, phenytoin, valproic acid, verapamil, EtOH, kava kava, valerian; ↑ effects of digoxin, diuretics; ↓ effects w/ barbiturates, carbamazepine, theophylline, ranitidine, tobacco; ↓ effects of haloperidol, levodopa **Labs:** False – urine glucose; monitor LFTs, BUN, creatinine, CBC w/ long-term drug use **NIPE:** Risk ↑ Sz activity

Diazoxide (Hyperstat, Proglycem) Uses: *Hypoglycemia due to hyperinsulinism (Proglycem); hypertensive crisis (Hyperstat)* **Action:** Inhibits pancreatic insulin release; antihypertensive **Dose:** *Hypertensive crisis:* 1–3 mg/kg IV (150 mg max in a single inj); repeat in 5–15 min until BP controlled; repeat every 4–24 h; monitor BP closely. *Hypoglycemia: Adults & Peds.* 3–8 mg/kg/24 h PO ÷ q8–12h. *Neonates.* 8–15 mg/kg/24 h ÷ in 3 equal doses; maint 8–10 mg/kg/24 h PO in 2–3 equal doses **Caution:** [C, ?] ↓ effect w/ phenytoin; ↑ effect w/ diuretics, warfarin **Contra:** Hypersensitivity to thiazides or other sulfonamide-containing products; HTN associated w/ aortic coarctation, AV shunt, or pheochromocytoma

Supplied: Inj 15 mg/mL; caps 50 mg; PO susp 50 mg/mL **SE:** Hyperglycemia, hy
potension, dizziness, Na & water retention, N/V, weakness **Notes:** Can give false
insulin response to glucagons; treat extravasation w/ warm compress **Interactions**
↑ Effects w/ carboplatin, cisplatin, diuretics, phenothiazines; ↑ effects of anticoag
ulants; ↓ effects w/ sulfonylureas; ↓ effects of phenytoin, sulfonylureas; **Labs:**
Serum uric acid, AST, alkaline phosphatase, false – response to glucagon **NIPE**
Daily weights, ↑ reversible body hair growth

Dibucaine (Nupercainal) Uses: *Hemorrhoids & minor ski
conditions* **Action:** Topical anesthetic **Dose:** Insert PR w/ applicator bid & afte
each bowel movement; apply sparingly to skin **Caution:** [C, ?] **Contra:** Compo
nent sensitivity **Supplied:** 1% oint w/ rectal applicator; 0.5% cream **SE:** Local irri
tation, rash **Interactions:** None noted

Diclofenac (Cataflam, Voltaren) Uses: *Arthritis & pain* **Action**
NSAID **Dose:** 50–75 mg PO bid; w/ food or milk **Caution:** [B (3rd tri or nea
delivery), ?] CHF, HTN, renal/hepatic dysfunction, & Hx PUD **Contra:** Hypersen
sitivity to NSAIDs or ASA; porphyria **Supplied:** Tabs 50 mg; tabs DR 25, 50, 75
100 mg; XR tabs 100 mg; ophthalmic soln 0.1% **SE:** Abdominal cramps, hear
burn, GI ulceration, rash, interstitial nephritis **Notes:** Watch for GI bleed **Interac
tions:** ↑ Risk of bleeding w/ feverfew, garlic, ginger, ginkgo biloba; ↑ effects o
digoxin, MRX, cyclosporine, Li, insulin, sulfonylureas, K-sparing diuretics, war
farin; ↓ effects w/ ASA; ↓ effects of thiazide diuretics, furosemide, BBs **Labs:**
LFTs, serum glucose & cortisol, ↓ serum uric acid; **NIPE:** Risk of photosensitiv
ity—use sunscreen, monitor LFTs, CBC, BUN, creatinine, take w/ food, ⊘ crus
tablets

Dicloxacillin (Dynapen, Dycill) Uses: *Rx of pneumonia, skin & sof
tissue infections, & osteomyelitis caused by penicillinase-producing staphy
lococci* **Action:** Bactericidal; inhibits cell wall synthesis. *Spectrum: S. aureus &
Streptococcus* **Dose: Adults.** 250–500 mg qid **Peds <40 kg.** 12.5–25 mg/kg/d ÷ qid
take on empty stomach **Caution:** [B, ?] **Contra:** Component or PCN sensitivity
Supplied: Caps 125, 250, 500 mg; soln 62.5 mg/5 mL **SE:** Diarrhea, nausea, ab
dominal pain **Notes:** Monitor PTT if Pt concurrently on warfarin **Interactions:** ↑
Effects w/ disulfiram, probenecid; ↑ effects of MRX, ↓ effects w/ macrolides
tetracyclines, food; ↓ effects of oral contraceptives, warfarin **Labs:** False ↑ naf
cillin level, urine & serum proteins, uric acid **NIPE:** Take w/ water

Dicyclomine (Bentyl) Uses: *Functional IBSs* **Action:** Smooth muscle
relaxant **Dose: Adults.** 20 mg PO qid; ↑ to max dose of 160 mg/d or 20 mg IM q6h
Peds. Infants >6 mo: 5 mg/dose tid–qid. *Children:* 10 mg/dose tid–qid **Caution**
[B, –] **Contra:** Infants < 6 mo, narrow-angle glaucoma, MyG, severe UC, obstruc
tive uropathy **Supplied:** Caps 10, 20 mg; tabs 20 mg; syrup 10 mg/5 mL; inj 10
mg/mL **SE:** Anticholinergic side effects may limit use **Notes:** Take 30–60 min
before meal; **Interactions:** ↑ Anticholinergic effects w/ anticholinergics, antihista
mines, amantadine, MAOIs, TCAs, phenothiazides; ↑ effects of atenolol, digoxin;

↓ effects w/ antacids; ↓ effects of haloperidol, ketoconazole, levodopa, phenothiazines **NIPE:** ⊘ EtOH, CNS depressant; adequate hydration

Didanosine [ddI] (Videx) **WARNING:** Hypersensitivity manifested as fever, rash, fatigue, GI/resp Sxs reported; stop drug immediately & ⊘ rechallenge; lactic acidosis & hepatomegaly/steatosis reported **Uses:** *HIV infection in zidovudine-intolerant Pts* **Action:** Nucleoside antiretroviral agent **Dose:** *Adults.* >60 kg: 400 mg/d PO or 200 mg PO bid. *<60 kg:* 250 mg/d PO or 125 mg PO bid; adults should take 2 tabs/administration. *Peds.* Dose by following table; ↓ in renal impairment:

BSA (m²)	Tablets (mg)	Powder (mg)
1.1–1.4	100 bid	125 bid
0.8–1	75 bid	94 bid
0.5–0.7	50 bid	62 bid
<0.4	25 bid	31 bid

Caution: [B, –] CDC recommends HIV-infected mothers not breast-feed due to risk of transmission of HIV to their infant **Contra:** Component sensitivity **Supplied:** Chew tabs 25, 50, 100, 150, 200 mg; powder packets 100, 167, 250, 375 mg; powder for soln 2, 4 g **SE:** Pancreatitis, peripheral neuropathy, diarrhea, HA **Notes:** ⊘ Take w/ meals; thoroughly chew tablets, ⊘ mix w/ fruit juice or other acidic beverages; reconstitute powder w/ water **Interactions:** ↑ Effects w/ allopurinol, ganciclovir; ↓ effects w/ methadone, food; ↑ risk of pancreatitis w/ thiazide diuretics, IV pentamidine, EtOH; ↓ effects of azole antifungals, dapsone, delavirdine, ganciclovir, indinavir, quinolones, ranitidine, tetracyclines **Labs:** ↑ LFTs, uric acid, amylase, lipase, triglycerides **NIPE:** May cause hyperglycemia, take w/o food, chew or crush tabs

Diflunisal (Dolobid) **Uses:** *Mild to moderate pain; osteoarthritis* **Action:** NSAID **Dose:** *Pain:* 500 mg PO bid. *Osteoarthritis:* 500–1500 mg PO in 2–3 ÷ doses; ↓ in renal impairment, take w/ food/milk **Caution:** [C (D 3rd tri or near delivery), ?] CHF, HTN, renal/hepatic dysfunction, & Hx PUD. **Contra:** Hypersensitivity to NSAIDs or ASA, active GI bleed **Supplied:** Tabs 250, 500 mg **SE:** May prolong bleeding time; HA, abdominal cramps, heartburn, GI ulceration, rash, interstitial nephritis, fluid retention **Interactions:** ↑ Effects w/ probenecid; ↑ effects of acetaminophen, anticoagulants, digoxin, HCTZ, indomethacin, Li, MRX, phenytoin, sulfonamides, sulfonylureas; ↓ effects w/ antacids, ASA; ↓ effects of furosemide **Labs:** ↑ Salicylate levels, PT, ↓ uric acid, T_3, T_4; **NIPE:** Take w/ food, ⊘ chew or crush tabs

Digoxin (Lanoxin, Lanoxicaps) **Uses:** *CHF, AF & flutter, & PAT* **Action:** + Inotrope; ↑ AV node refractory period **Dose:** *Adults.* PO digitalization:

0.5–0.75 mg PO, then 0.25 mg PO q6–8h to total 1–1.5 mg. *IV or IM digitalization:* 0.25–0.5 mg IM or IV, then 0.25 mg q4–6h to total ≈1 mg. *Daily maint:* 0.125–0.5 mg/d PO, IM, or IV (average daily dose 0.125–0.25 mg). **Peds.** Preterm infants: Digitalization: 30 µg/kg PO or 25 µg/kg IV; give ½ of dose initially, then ¼ of dose at 8–12-h intervals for 2 doses. *Maint:* 5–7.5 µg/kg/24 h PO or 4–6 µg/kg/24 h IV ÷ q12h. *Term infants: Digitalization:* 25–35 µg/kg PO or 20–30 µg/kg IV; give ½ the dose initially, then ¼ at 8–12 h. *Maint:* 6–10 µg/kg/24 h PO or 5–8 µg/kg/24 h ÷ q12h. *1 mo–2 y: Digitalization:* 35–60 µg/kg PO or 30–50 µg/kg IV; give ½ the dose initially, then ¼ dose at 8–12-h intervals for 2 doses. *Maint:* 10–15 µg/kg/24 h PO or 7.5–15 µg/kg/24 h IV ÷ q12h. *2–10 y: Digitalization:* 30–40 µg/kg PO or 25 µg/kg IV; give ½ dose initially, then ¼ of the dose at 8–12-h intervals for 2 doses. *Maint:* 8–10 µg/kg/24 h PO or 6–8 µg/kg/24 h IV ÷ q12h. *7–10 y:* Same as for adults; ↓ in renal impairment, follow serum levels **Caution:** [C, +] **Contra** AV block; idiopathic hypertrophic subaortic stenosis; constrictive pericarditis **Supplied:** Caps 0.05, 0.1, 0.2 mg; tabs 0.125, 0.25, 0.5 mg; elixir 0.05 mg/mL; inj 0.1, 0.25 mg/mL **SE:** Can cause heart block; ↓ K⁺ potentiates toxicity; N/V, HA, fatigue, visual disturbances (yellow-green halos around lights), cardiac arrhythmias **Notes:** Multiple drug interactions; IM inj painful, has erratic absorption & should not be used; see Drug Levels, Table 2, page 265. **Interactions:** ↑ Effects w/ alprazolam, amiodarone, azole antifungals, BBs, carvedilol, cyclosporine, corticosteroids, diltiazem, diuretics, erythromycin, NSAIDs, quinidine spironolactone, tetracyclines, verapamil, goldenseal, hawthorn, licorice, quinine Siberian ginseng; ↓ effects w/ charcoal, cholestyramine, cisapride, neomycin, rifampin, sucralfate, thyroid hormones, psyllium, St. John's wort **Labs:** ↓ PT, monitor serum electrolytes, LFTs, BUN, creatinine **NIPE:** Different bioavailability in various brands

Digoxin Immune Fab (Digibind)   Uses: *Life-threatening digoxin intoxication* **Action:** Antigen-binding fragments bind & inactivate digoxin **Dose Adults & Peds.** Based on serum level & Pt's weight; see charts provided w/ the drug **Caution:** [C, ?] **Contra:** Hypersensitivity to sheep products **Supplied:** Inj 38 mg/vial **SE:** Worsening of cardiac output or CHF, hypokalemia, facial swelling, & redness **Notes:** Each vial binds ≈ 0.6 mg of digoxin; in renal failure may require redosing in several days because of breakdown of the immune complex **Interactions:** ↓ Effects of cardiac glycosides **NIPE:** Will take up to 1 wk for accurate serum digoxin levels after use of Digibind

Diltiazem (Cardizem, Cardizem CD, Cardizem SR, Cartia XT, Dilacor XR, Diltia XT, Tiamate, Tiazac)   Uses: *Angina, prevention of reinfarction, HTN, AF or flutter, & PAT* **Action:** CCB **Dose: PO:** Initially, 30 mg PO qid; ↑ to 180–360 mg/d in 3–4 ÷ doses PRN. *SR:* 60–120 mg PO bid; ↑ to 360 mg/d max. *CD or XR:* 120–360 mg/d (max 480 mg/d). *IV:* 0.25 mg/kg IV bolus over 2 min; may repeat in 15 min at 0.35 mg/kg; may begin inf of 5–15 mg/h **Caution:** [C, +] ↑ effect w/ amiodarone, cimetidine, fentanyl, Li, cyclosporine,

digoxin, BBss, cisapride, theophylline **Contra:** SSS, AV block, hypotension, AMI, pulmonary congestion **Supplied:** *Cardizem CD:* Caps 120, 180, 240, 300, 360 mg; *Cardizem SR:* caps 60, 90, 120 mg; *Cardizem:* Tabs 30, 60, 90, 120 mg; *Cartia XT:* Caps 120, 180, 240, 300 mg; *Dilacor XR:* Caps 180, 240 mg; *Diltia XT:* Caps 120, 180, 240 mg; *Tiazac:* Caps 120, 180, 240, 300, 360, 420 mg; *Tiamate (XR):* Tabs 120, 180, 240 mg; inj 5 mg/mL **SE:** Gingival hyperplasia, bradycardia, AV block, ECG abnormalities, peripheral edema, dizziness, HA **Notes:** Cardizem CD, Dilacor XR, & Tiazac not interchangeable **Interactions:** ↑ Effects w/ α-blockers, azole antifungals, BBs, erythromycin, H₂ receptor antagonists, nitroprusside, quinidine, EtOH, grapefruit juice; ↑ effects of carbamazepine, cyclosporine, digitalis glycosides, quinidine, phenytoin, prazosin, theophylline, TCAs; ↓ effects w/ NSAIDs, phenobarbital, rifampin **Labs:** False ↑ urine ketones, ↑ LFTs, BUN, creatinine **NIPE:** ⊘ Chew or crush SR or ER preps, risk of photosensitivity—use sunscreen

Dimenhydrinate (Dramamine, others) **Uses:** *Prevention & Rx of N/V, dizziness, or vertigo of motion sickness* **Action:** Antiemetic **Dose:** *Adults.* 50–100 mg PO q4–6h, max 400 mg/d; 50 mg IM/IV PRN. *Peds.* 5 mg/kg/24 h PO or IV ÷ qid (max 300 mg/d) **Caution:** [B, ?] **Contra:** Component sensitivity **Supplied:** Tabs 50 mg; chew tabs 50 mg; liq 12.5 mg/4 mL, 12.5 mg/5 mL, 15.62 mg/5 mL; inj 50 mg/mL **SE:** Anticholinergic side effects **Interactions:** ↑ Effects w/ CNS depressants, antihistamines, opioids, quinidine, MAOIs, TCAs, EtOH **Labs:** False ↑ allergy skin tests **NIPE:** ⊘ Drug 72 h prior to allergy skin testing, take before motion sickness occurs

Dimethyl Sulfoxide [DMSO] (Rimso 50) **Uses:** *Interstitial cystitis* **Action:** Unknown **Dose:** Intravesical, 50 mL, retain for 15 min; repeat q2wk until relief **Caution:** [C, ?] **Contra:** Component sensitivity **Supplied:** 50% soln in 50 mL **SE:** Cystitis, eosinophilia, GI, & taste disturbance **Interactions:** ↓ Effects of sulindac **Labs:** Monitor CBC, LFTs, BUN, creatinine levels **NIPE:** ↑ Taste & smell of garlic

Dinoprostone (Cervidil Vaginal Insert, Prepidil Vaginal Gel) **Uses:** *Induce labor; terminate PRG (12–28 wk); evacuate uterus in missed abortion or fetal death* **Action:** prostaglandin, changes consistency, dilatation, & effacement of the cervix; induces uterine contraction **Dose:** *Gel:* 0.5 mg; if no cervical/uterine response, repeat 0.5 mg q6h (max 24-h dose 1.5 mg). *Vaginal insert:* 1 insert (10 mg = 0.3 mg dinoprostone/h over 12 h); remove w/ onset of labor or 12 h after insertion. *Vaginal supp:* 20 mg repeated every 3–5 h; adjust PRN supp: 1 high in vagina, repeat at 3–5-h intervals until abortion (240 mg max) **Caution:** [X, ?] **Contra:** Ruptured membranes, hypersensitivity to prostaglandins, placenta previa or unexplained vaginal bleeding during PRG, when oxytocic drugs contraindicated or if prolonged uterine contractions are inappropriate (Hx C-section or major uterine surgery, presence of cephalopelvic disproportion, etc) **Supplied** *Gel, endocervical:* 0.5 mg in 3-g syringes (each package contains a 10-mm & 20-mm shielded catheter); *vaginal gel:* 0.5 mg/3 g; *vaginal supp:* 20 mg; *vagi-*

nal insert, CR: 0.3 mg/h **SE:** N/V/D, dizziness, flushing, headache, fever **Interactions:** ↑ Effects of oxytocics, ↓ effects w/ large amts EtOH **NIPE:** Pt supine after insertion of supp or gel up to ½ h

Diphenhydramine (Benadryl) [OTC] **Uses:** *Rx & prevent allergic Rxns, motion sickness, potentiate narcotics, sedation, cough suppression, & Rx of extrapyramidal Rxns* **Action:** Antihistamine, antiemetic **Dose:** *Adults.* 25–50 mg PO, IV, or IM bid–tid. *Peds.* 5 mg/kg/24 h PO or IM ÷ q6h (max 300 mg/d); ↑ dosing interval in moderate/severe renal failure **Caution:** [B, –] **Contra:** ⊘ Use in acute asthma attack **Supplied:** Tabs & caps 25, 50 mg; chew tabs 12.5 mg; elixir 12.5 mg/5 mL; syrup 12.5 mg/5 mL; liq 6.25 mg/5 mL, 12.5 mg/5 mL; inj 50 mg/mL **SE:** Anticholinergic side effects (xerostomia, urinary retention, sedation) **Interactions:** ↑ Effects w/ CNS depressants, antihistamines, opioids, MAOIs, TCAs, EtOH; ↑ effects of metoprolol **Labs:** ↓ Response to allergy skin testing **NIPE:** ↑ Risk of photosensitivity—use sunscreen

Diphenoxylate + Atropine (Lomotil) [C-V] **Uses:** *Diarrhea* **Action:** Constipating meperidine congener, reduces GI motility **Dose:** *Adults.* Initial, 5 mg PO tid–qid until under control, then 2.5–5.0 mg PO bid. *Peds >2 y:* 0.3–0.4 mg/kg/24 h (of diphenoxylate) bid–qid **Caution:** [C, +] **Contra:** Obstructive jaundice, diarrhea due to bacterial infection; children <2 y **Supplied:** Tabs 2.5 mg of diphenoxylate/0.025 mg of atropine; liq 2.5 mg diphenoxylate/0.025 mg atropine/5 mL **SE:** Drowsiness, dizziness, xerostomia, blurred vision, urinary retention, constipation **Interactions:** ↑ Effects w/ CNS depressants, opioids, EtOH, ↑ risk HTN crisis w/ MAOIs **NIPE:** ↓ Effectiveness w/ diarrhea caused by antibiotics

Diphtheria, Tetanus Toxoids, & Acellular pertussis adsorbed, Hepatitis B (recombinant), & Inactivated Poliovirus Vaccine [IPV] combined (Pediarix) **Uses:** *Vaccine against diphtheria, tetanus, pertussis, HBV, polio(types 1, 2, 3) as a three-dose primary series in infants & children <7, born to HBsAg-negative mothers* **Actions:** Active immunization **Dose:** Infants 3 0.5-mL doses IM, at 6–8-wk intervals, start at 2 mo; child given 1 dose of hep B vaccine, same; child previously vaccinated w/ one or more doses IPV, use to complete series **Caution:** [C, N/A] **Contra:** If HbsAG+ mother, adults, children >7 y, immunosuppressed, hypersensitivity to yeast, neomycin, or polymyxin B, Hx allergy to any component of the vaccine, encephalopathy, or progressive neurologic disorders; caution in bleeding disorders. **Supplied:** Single-dose vials 0.5 mL **SE:** Drowsiness, restlessness, fever, fussiness, ↓ appetite, nodule redness, pain, & swelling at inj site **Notes:** Give IM only **Interactions:** ↓ Effects w/ immunosuppressants, corticosteroids

Dipivefrin (Propine) **Uses:** *Open-angle glaucoma* **Action:** α-Adrenergic agonist **Dose:** 1 gt into eye q12h **Caution:** [B, ?] **Contra:** Closed-angle glaucoma **Supplied:** 0.1% soln **SE:** HA, local irritation, blurred vision, photophobia, hypertension **Interactions:** ↑ Effects w/ BBs, ophthalmic anhydrase inhibitors, osmotic drugs, sympathomimetics, ↑ risk of cardiac arrhythmias w/ digoxin, TCAs **NIPE:** Discard discolored solutions

Dipyridamole (Persantine) Uses: *Prevent postop thromboembolic disorders, often in combination w/ ASA or warfarin (eg, CABG, vascular graft); w/ warfarin after artificial heart valve; chronic angina; w/ ASA to prevent coronary artery thrombosis; dipyridamole IV used in place of exercise stress test for CAD* **Action:** Antiplt activity; coronary vasodilator **Dose:** *Adults.* 75–100 mg PO tid–qid; stress test 0.14 mg/kg/min (max 60 mg over 4 min). *Peds >12 y.* 3–6 mg/kg/d divided tid **Caution:** [B, ?/–] Caution w/ other drugs that affect coagulation **Contra:** Component sensitivity **Supplied:** Tabs 25, 50, 75 mg; inj 5 mg/mL **SE:** HA, hypotension, nausea, abdominal distress, flushing rash, dyspnea **Notes:** IV use can worsen angina **Interactions:** ↑ Effects w/ anticoagulants, heparin, evening primrose oil, feverfew, garlic, ginger, ginkgo biloba, ginseng, grapeseed extract; ↑ effects of adenosine; ↑ bradycardia w/ BBs; ↓ effects w/ aminophylline **NIPE:** ⊘ EtOH or tobacco because of vasoconstriction effects; + effects may take several mo

Dipyridamole & Aspirin (Aggrenox) Uses: *↓ Reinfarction after MI; prevent occlusion after CABG; ↓ risk of stroke* **Action:** ↓ Plt aggregation (both agents) **Dose:** 1 cap PO bid **Caution:** [C, ?] **Contra:** Ulcers, bleeding diathesis **Supplied:** Dipyridamole (XR) 200 mg/ASA 25 mg **SE:** ASA component: allergic Rxns, skin Rxns, ulcers/GI bleed, bronchospasm; dipyridamole component: dizziness, HA, rash **Notes:** Swallow capsule whole

Dirithromycin (Dynabac) Uses: *Bronchitis, community-acquired pneumonia, & skin & skin structure infections* **Action:** Macrolide antibiotic. Spectrum: *M. catarrhalis, Streptococcus pneumoniae, Legionella, H. influenzae, S. pyogenes, Staphylococcus aureus* **Dose:** 500 mg/d PO; take w/ food **Caution:** [C, M] **Contra:** Use w/ pimozide **Supplied:** Tabs 250 mg **SE:** Abdominal discomfort, HA, rash, hyperkalemia **Notes:** Swallow whole **Interactions:** ↑ Effects w/ antacids, H₂ antagonists, food; ↑ effects of theophylline; ↓ effects of penicillins **NIPE:** Take w/ food, ⊘ crush or chew

Disopyramide (Norpace, NAPamide) Uses: *Suppression & prevention of VT* **Action:** Class 1A antiarrhythmic **Dose:** *Adults.* 400–800 mg/d ÷ q6h for regular & q12h for SR. *Peds. <1 y:* 10–30 mg/kg/24 h PO (÷ qid). *1–4 y:* 10–20 mg/kg/24 h PO (÷ qid). *4–12 y:* 10–15 mg/kg/24 h PO (÷ qid). *12–18 y:* 6–15 mg/kg/24 h PO (÷ qid); ↓ in renal/hepatic impairment **Caution:** [C, +] **Contra:** AV block, cardiogenic shock **Supplied:** Caps 100, 150 mg; SR caps 100, 150 mg **SE:** Anticholinergic side effects; negative inotropic properties may induce CHF **Notes:** See Drug Levels, Table 2, page 265. **Interactions:** ↑ Effects w/ cimetidine, clarithromycin, erythromycin, quinidine; ↑ effects of digoxin, hypoglycemics, insulin, warfarin; ↑ risk of arrhythmias w/ pimozide; ↓ effects w/ barbiturates, phenytoin, phenobarbital, rifampin **Labs:** ↑ LFTs, lipids, BUN, creatinine; ↓ serum glucose, Hmg, Hct **NIPE:** Risk of photosensitivity—use sun screen, daily weights

Dobutamine (Dobutrex) Uses: *Short-term use in cardiac decompensation secondary to depressed contractility* **Action:** + inotropic agent **Dose:** *Adults & Peds.* Cont IV inf of 2.5–15 µg/kg/min; rarely, 40 µg/kg/min may be required titrate to response **Caution:** [C, ?] **Contra:** Sensitivity to sulfites, idiopathic hypertrophic subaortic stenosis **Supplied:** Inj 250 mg/20 mL **SE:** Chest pain, HTN, dyspnea **Notes:** Monitor PWP & cardiac output if possible; check ECG for ↑ heart rate, ectopic activity; follow BP **Interactions:** ↑ Effects w/ furazolidone, methyldopa, MAOIs, TCAs; ↓ effects w/ BBs, NaHCO₃; ↓ effects of guanethidine **Labs:** ↓ K; **NIPE:** Eval for adequate hydration; monitor I&O, cardiac output, ECG, BP during inf

Docetaxel (Taxotere) Uses: *Breast (anthracycline-resistant), ovarian, lung cancers, & CAP* **Action:** Antimitotic agent; promotes microtubular aggregation; semisynthetic taxoid **Dose:** 100 mg/m² over 1 h IV q3wk (refer to specific protocols); start dexamethasone 8 mg bid prior to docetaxel & continue for 3–4 d; ↓ dose w/ ↑ bilirubin levels **Caution:** [D, –] **Contra:** Component sensitivity **Supplied:** Inj 20, 40, 80 mg/mL **SE:** Myelosuppression, neuropathy, N/V, alopecia, fluid retention syndrome; cumulative doses of 300–400 mg/m² w/o steroid prep & posttreatment & 600–800 mg/m² w/ steroid prep; hypersensitivity Rxns possible, but rare w/ steroid prep **Interactions:** ↑ Effects w/ cyclosporine, ketoconazole, erythromycin, terfenidine **Labs:** ↑ AST, ALT, alkaline phosphatase **NIPE:** ↑ Fluids to 2–3 L/d, ↑ risk of hair loss, ↑ susceptibility to infection, urine may become reddish-brown

Docusate Calcium (Surfak)/Docusate Potassium (Dialose)/ Docusate Sodium (DOS, Colace) Uses: *Constipation; adjunct to painful anorectal conditions (hemorrhoids)* **Action:** Stool softener **Dose:** *Adults.* 50–500 mg PO ÷ daily–qid. *Peds.* Infants–3 y: 10–40 mg/24 h ÷ daily–qid. *3–6 y:* 20–60 mg/24 h ÷ daily–qid. *6–12 y:* 40–150 mg/24 h ÷ daily–qid **Caution:**[C, ?] **Contra:** Concomitant use of mineral oil; intestinal obstruction, acute abdominal pain, N/V **Supplied:** *Ca:* Caps 50, 240 mg. *K:* Caps 100, 240 mg. *Na:* Caps 50, 100 mg; syrup 50, 60 mg/15 mL; liq 150 mg/15 mL; soln 50 mg/mL **SE:** No significant side effects, rare abdominal cramping, diarrhea; no laxative action **Notes:** Take w/ full glass of water; ⊘ use >1 wk **Interactions:** ↑ Absorption of mineral oil **Labs:** ↓ K⁺ Cl **NIPE:** Short-term use, take w/ juices or milk to mask bitter taste

Dofetilide (Tikosyn) WARNING: To minimize the risk of induced arrhythmia, Pts initiated or reinitiated on Tikosyn should be placed for a minimum of 3 d in a facility that can provide calculations of CrCl, continuous ECG monitoring, & cardiac resuscitation Uses: *Maintain normal sinus rhythm in AF/A flutter after conversion* **Action:** Type III antiarrhythmic **Dose:** 125–500 µg PO bid based on CrCl & QTc (see insert) **Caution:** [C, –] **Contra:** Baseline QTc is > 440 ms (500 ms w/ ventricular conduction abnormalities) or CrCl < 20 mL/min; concomitant use of verapamil, cimetidine, trimethoprim, or ketoconazole **Supplied:** Caps 125, 250, 500 µg **SE:** Ventricular arrhythmias, HA, CP, dizziness **Notes:** ⊘ w/ other drugs that prolong the QT interval; hold class I or III antiarrhythmics for at least 3 ½-lives prior to dofetilide; amiodarone level should be < 0.3 mg/L prior to dofetilide **Interactions:** ↑ Effects w/ amiloride, amiodarone, azole antifungals, cimetidine, diltiazem, macrolides, metformin, megestrol, nefazodone, norfloxacin, SSRIs, TCAs, triamterene, trimethoprim, verapamil, zafirlukast, quinine, grapefruit juice **NIPE:** Take w/o regard to food; monitor LFTs, BUN, creatinine

Dolasetron (Anzemet) **Uses:** *Prevent chemotherapy-associated N/V* **Action:** 5-HT$_3$ receptor antagonist **Dose:** *Adults & Peds.* IV: 1.8 mg/kg IV as single dose 30 min prior to chemotherapy. *Adults.* PO: 100 mg PO as a single dose 1 h prior to chemotherapy. *Peds.* PO: 1.8 mg/kg PO to max 100 mg as single dose **Caution:** [B, ?] **Contra:** Component sensitivity **Supplied:** Tabs 50, 100 mg; inj 20 mg/mL **SE:** Prolongs QT interval, HTN, HA, abdominal pain, urinary retention, transient ↑ LFTs **Interactions:** ↑ Effects w/ cimetidine; ↑ risk of arrhythmias w/ diuretics; ↓ effects w/ rifampin **Labs:** ↑ ALT, AST, alkaline phosphatase, PTT **NIPE:** Monitor LFTs, PTT, CBC, plts, & alkaline phosphatase w/ prolonged use

Dopamine (Intropin) **Uses:** *Short-term use in cardiac decompensation secondary to decreased contractility; ↑s organ perfusion (at low dose)* **Action:** + Inotropic agent w/ dose response: 2–10 µg/kg/min β-effects (↑ CO & renal perfusion); 10–20 µg/kg/min β-effects (peripheral vasoconstriction, pressor). >20 µg/kg/min peripheral & renal vasoconstriction **Dose:** *Adults & Peds.* 5 µg/kg/min by cont inf, ↑ increments of 5 µg/kg/min to 50 µg/kg/min max based on effect **Caution:** [C, ?] **Contra:** Pheochromocytoma, VF, sulfite sensitivity **Supplied:** Inj 40, 80, 160 mg/mL **SE:** Tachycardia, vasoconstriction, hypotension, HA, N/V, dyspnea **Notes:** Dosage >10 µg/kg/min may ↓ renal perfusion; monitor urinary output; monitor ECG for ↑ in heart rate, BP, & ectopic activity; monitor PCWP & cardiac output if possible **Interactions:** ↑ Effects w/ α-blockers, diuretics, ergot alkaloids, MAOIs, BBs, anesthetics, phenytoin; ↓ effects w/ guanethidine **Labs:** False ↑ urine catecholamines, urine amino acids; false ↓ SCr **NIPE:** Maintain adequate hydration

Dornase Alfa (Pulmozyme) **Uses:** *↓ Frequency of resp infections in CF* **Action:** Enzyme that selectively cleaves DNA **Dose:** Inhal 2.5 mg/d **Caution:** [B, ?] **Contra:** Hypersensitivity to Chinese hamster ovary cell products **Supplied:** Soln for inhal 1 mg/mL **SE:** Pharyngitis, voice alteration, CP, rash **Notes:** Use w/ recommended nebulizer **Interactions:** None noted **NIPE:** ⊘ Mix or dilute w/ other drugs

Dorzolamide (Trusopt) **Uses:** *Glaucoma* **Action:** Carbonic anhydrase inhibitor **Dose:** 1 gt in eye(s) tid **Caution:** [C, ?] **Contra:** Component sensitivity **Supplied:** 2% soln **SE:** Local irritation, bitter taste, superficial punctate keratitis, ocular allergic Rxn **Interactions:** ↑ Effects w/ oral carbonic anhydrase inhibitors, salicylates **NIPE:** ⊘ Wear soft contact lenses

Dorzolamide & Timolol (Cosopt) Uses: *Glaucoma* Action: Carbonic anhydrase inhibitor w/ β-adrenergic blocker Dose: 1 gt in eye(s) bid Caution: [C, ?] Contra: Component sensitivity Supplied: Soln dorzolamide 2% & timolol 0.5% SE: Local irritation, bitter taste, superficial punctate keratitis, ocular allergic Rxn

Doxazosin (Cardura) Uses: *HTN & symptomatic BPH* Action: α_1-Adrenergic blocker; relaxes bladder neck smooth muscle Dose: *HTN:* Initial 1 mg/d PO; may be ↑ to 16 mg/d PO. *BPH:* Initial 1 mg/d PO, may be ↑ to 8 mg/d PO Caution: [B, ?] Contra: Component sensitivity Supplied: Tabs 1, 2, 4, 8 mg SE: Dizziness, HA, drowsiness, sexual dysfunction, doses >4 mg ↑ likelihood of postural hypotension Notes: Take first dose hs; syncope may occur w/in 90 min of initial dose Interactions: ↑ effects w/ nitrates, antihypertensives, EtOH; ↓ effects w/ NSAIDs, butcher's broom; ↓ effects of clonidine NIPE: May be taken w/ food

Doxepin (Sinequan, Adapin) Uses: *Depression, anxiety, chronic pain* Action: TCA; ↑s the synaptic CNS concs of serotonin or norepinephrine Dose: 25–150 mg/d PO, usually hs but can be in ÷ doses; ↓ in hepatic impairment Caution: [C, ?/–] Contra: Narrow-angle glaucoma Supplied: Caps 10, 25, 50, 75, 100, 150 mg; PO conc 10 mg/mL SE: Anticholinergic side effects, hypotension, tachycardia, drowsiness, photosensitivity Interactions: ↑ Effects w/ fluoxetine, MAOIs, albuterol, CNS depressants, anticholinergics, cimetidine, oral contraceptives, propoxyphene, quinidine, EtOH, grapefruit juice; ↑ effects of carbamazepine, anticoagulants, amphetamines, thyroid drugs, sympathomimetics; ↓ effects w/ ascorbic acid, cholestyramine, tobacco; ↓ effects of bretylium, guanethidine, levodopa Labs: ↑ Serum bilirubin, alkaline phosphatase, glucose NIPE: Risk of photosensitivity—use sunscreen, urine may turn blue-green, may take 4–6 wk for full effect

Doxepin, Topical (Zonalon) Uses: *Short-term Rx pruritus (atopic dermatitis or lichen simplex chronicus)* Action: Antipruritic; H_1- & H_2-receptor antagonism Dose: Apply thin coating qid for max 8 d Caution: [C, ?/–] Contra: Component sensitivity Supplied: 5% cream SE: ↓ BP, tachycardia, drowsiness, photosensitivity Notes: Limit application area to ⊘ systemic toxicity

Doxorubicin (Adriamycin, Rubex) Uses: *Acute leukemias; Hodgkin's & NHLs; breast CA; soft tissue & osteosarcomas; Ewing's sarcoma; Wilms' tumor; neuroblastoma; bladder, ovarian, gastric, thyroid, & lung CAs* Action: Intercalates DNA; inhibits DNA topoisomerases I & II Dose: 60–75 mg/m^2 q3wk; ↑ cardiotoxicity w/ weekly (20 mg/m^2/wk) or cont inf (60–90 mg/m^2 over 96 h); refer to specific protocols Caution: [D, ?] Contra: Severe CHF, cardiomyopathy, preexisting myelosuppression, ↓ cardiac Fxn, Pts who received previous Rx w/ complete cumulative doses of doxorubicin, idarubicin, daunorubicin Supplied: Inj 10, 20, 50, 75, 200 mg SE: Myelosuppression, venous streaking & phlebitis, N/V/D, mucositis, radiation recall phenomenon, cardiomyopathy rare but dose-related; limit of 550 mg/m^2 cumulative dose (400 mg/m^2 if prior mediastinal irradiation) **Notes:** Dexrazoxane may limit cardiac toxicity; extravasation leads to tissue damage; discolors urine red/orange **Interactions:** ↑ Effects w/ streptozocin, verapamil, green tea; ↑ bone-marrow depression w/ antineoplastic drugs and radiation; ↓ effects w/ phenobarbital; ↓ effects of digoxin, phenytoin, live virus vaccines **Labs:** ↑ Urine and plasma uric acid levels **NIPE:** ⊘ PRG, use contraception at least 4 mo after drug Rx

Doxycycline (Vibramycin) **Uses:** *Broad-spectrum antibiotic activity* **Action:** Tetracycline; interferes w/ protein synthesis. *Spectrum: Rickettsia* sp, *Chlamydia*, & *M. pneumoniae* **Dose:** *Adults.* 100 mg PO q12h on 1st day, then 100 mg PO qd–bid or 100 mg IV q12h. *Peds >8y.* 5 mg/kg/24 h PO, to a max of 200 mg/d ÷ daily–bid **Supplied:** Tabs 50, 100 mg; caps 20, 50, 100 mg; syrup 50 mg/5 mL; susp 25 mg/5 mL; inj 100, 200 mg/vial **Caution:** [D, +] **Contra:** Children <8 y, severe hepatic dysfunction **SE:** Diarrhea, GI disturbance, photosensitivity **Notes:** Useful for chronic bronchitis; ↓ effect w/ antacids containing Al, Ca, Mg; tetracycline of choice in renal impairment **Interactions:** ↑ Effects of digoxin, warfarin; ↓ effects w/ antacids, Fe, barbiturates, carbamazepine, phenytoins, food; ↓ effects of penicillins **Labs:** False – urine glucose, false ↑ urine catecholamines; false ↓ urine urobilinogen **NIPE:** ↑ Risk of superinfection, ⊘ PRG, use barrier contraception

Dronabinol (Marinol) [C-II] **Uses:** *N/V associated w/ CA chemotherapy; appetite stimulation* **Action:** Antiemetic; inhibits the vomiting center in the medulla **Dose:** *Adults & Peds.* Antiemetic: 5–15 mg/m²/dose q4–6h PRN. *Adults.* Appetite stimulant: 2.5 mg PO before lunch & dinner **Caution:** [C, ?] **Contra:** Should not be used in Pts w/ Hx schizophrenia **Supplied:** Caps 2.5, 5, 10 mg **SE:** Drowsiness, dizziness, anxiety, mood change, hallucinations, depersonalization, orthostatic hypotension, tachycardia **Notes:** Principal psychoactive substance present in marijuana **Interactions:** ↑ Effects w/ anticholinergics, CNS depressants, EtOH; ↓ effects of theophylline **Labs:** ↓ FSH, LH, growth hormone, testosterone

Droperidol (Inapsine) **Uses:** *N/V; anesthetic premedication* **Action:** Tranquilizer, sedation, & antiemetic **Dose:** *Adults.* Nausea: 2.5–5 mg IV or IM q3–4h PRN. *Premed:* 2.5–10 mg IV, 30–60 min preop. *Peds.* Premed: 0.1–0.15 mg/kg/dose **Caution:** [C, ?] **Contra:** Component sensitivity **Supplied:** Inj 2.5 mg/mL **SE:** Drowsiness, moderate hypotension, occasional tachycardia & extrapyramidal Rxns, QT interval prolongation, arrhythmias **Notes:** Give IVP slowly over 2–5 min **Interactions:** ↑ Effects w/ CNS depressants, fentanyl, EtOH; ↑ hypotension w/ antihypertensives, nitrates

Drotrecogin Alfa (Xigris) **Uses:** *Reduce mortality in adults w/ severe sepsis (associated w/ acute organ dysfunction) at high risk of death (eg, as determined by APACHE II)* **Action:** Recombinant of human activated protein C; mechanism unknown **Dose:** 24 µg/kg/h for a total of 96 h **Caution:** [C, ?] **Contra:** Active bleeding, recent stroke or CNS surgery, head trauma, epidural catheter, CNS lesion at risk for herniation **Supplied:** 5-, 20-mg vials for reconstitution **SE:**

Bleeding most common SE **Notes:** For percutaneous procedures stop inf 2 h before the procedure & resume 1 h after; major surgery stop inf 2 h before surgery & resume 12 h after surgery in absence of bleeding **Interactions:** ↑ Risk of bleeding w/ plt inhibitors, anticoagulants **Labs:** ↑ aPTT **NIPE:** DC drug 2 h before invasive procedures

Dutasteride (Avodart)   **Uses:** *Symptomatic BPH* **Action:** 5α-reductase inhibitor **Dose:** 0.5 mg PO qd **Caution:** [X, –] Caution in hepatic impairment; PRG women should ⊘ handling pills **Contra:** Women & children **Supplied:** Caps 0.5 mg **SE:** ↓ PSA levels, impotence, ↓ libido, gynecomastia **Notes:** ⊘ Donate blood until 6 mo after discontinuation of this drug **Interactions:** ↑ Effects w/ cimetidine, ciprofloxacin, diltiazem, ketoconazole, ritonavir, verapamil **Labs:** ↓ PSA levels **NIPE:** ⊘ Handling by PRG women, take w/o regard to food

Echothiophate Iodine (Phospholine Ophthalmic)   **Uses:** *Glaucoma* **Action:** Cholinesterase inhibitor **Dose:** 1 gt eye(s) bid w/ one dose hs **Caution:** [C, ?] **Contra:** Active uveal inflammation or any inflammatory Dz of iris/ciliary body; glaucoma associated w/ iridocyclitis **Supplied:** Powder to reconstitute 1.5 mg/0.03%; 3 mg/ 0.06%; 6.25 mg/0.125%; 12.5 mg/0.25% **SE:** Local irritation, myopia, blurred vision, hypotension, bradycardia **Interactions:** ↑ Effects w/ cholinesterase inhibitors, pilocarpine, succinylcholine, carbamate or organophosphate insecticides; ↑ effects of cocaine; ↓ effects w/ anticholinergics, atropine, cyclopentolate, ophthalmic adrenocorticoids **NIPE:** ⊘ Drug 2 wk before surgery if succinylcholine to be administered, keep drug refrigerated, monitor for lens opacities

Econazole (Spectazole)   **Uses:** *Tinea, cutaneous Candida, & tinea versicolor infections* **Action:** Topical antifungal **Dose:** Apply to areas bid (daily for tinea versicolor) for 2–4 wk **Caution:** [C, ?] **Contra:** Component sensitivity **Supplied:** Topical cream 1% **SE:** Local irritation, pruritus, erythema **Notes:** Symptom/clinical improvement seen early in Rx, must carry out course of therapy to ⊘ recurrence **Interactions:** ↓ Effects w/ corticosteroids **NIPE:** Topical use only, ⊘ eye area

Edrophonium (Tensilon)   **Uses:** *Diagnosis of MyG; acute MyG crisis; curare antagonist* **Action:** Anticholinesterase **Dose:** *Adults.* Test for MyG: 2 mg IV in 1 min; if tolerated, give 8 mg IV; + test is brief ↑ in strength. *Peds.* Test for MyG: Total dose 0.2 mg/kg; 0.04 mg/kg test dose; if no Rxn, give remainder in 1 mg increments to 10 mg max; ↓ in renal impairment **Caution:** [C, ?] **Contra:** GI or GU obstruction; hypersensitivity to sulfite **Supplied:** Inj 10 mg/mL **SE:** N/V/D, excessive salivation, stomach cramps, ↑ aminotransferases **Notes:** Can cause severe cholinergic effects; keep atropine available **Interactions:** ↑ Effects w/ tacrine; ↑ cardiac effects w/ digoxin; ↑ effects of neostigmine, pyridostigmine, succinylcholine, jaborandi tree, pill-bearing spurge; ↓ effects w/ corticosteroids, procainamide, quinidine **Labs:** ↑ AST, ALT, serum amylase **NIPE:** ↑ Risk uterine irritability & premature labor in PRG Pts near term

Efalizumab (Raptiva) **WARNING:** Associated w/ serious infections, malignancy, thrombocytopenia **Uses:** Chronic moderate to severe plaque psoriasis **Action:** Monoclonal antibody **Dose:** *Adults.* 0.7 mg/kg SQ conditioning dose, followed by 1 mg/kg/wk; single doses should not exceed 200 mg **Caution:** [C, +/–] **Contra:** Admin of most vaccines **Supplied:** 125-mg vial **SE:** First-dose Rxn, HA, worsening psoriasis, ↑ LFT, immunosuppressive-related Rxns (see warning) **Notes:** Minimize first-dose Rxn by administering conditioning dose; monitor plts monthly, then every 3 mo & Rx progresses; Pts may be trained in self-admin **Interactions:** ↑ Risk of infection & malignancy with immunosuppressive agents; ↓ immune response with live virus vaccines; **Labs:** ↑ Lymphocytes **NIPE:** Reconstituted soln may be stored for 8 h; monitor for bleeding gums & bruising

Efavirenz (Sustiva) **Uses:** *HIV infections* **Action:** Antiretroviral; nonnucleoside RTI **Dose:** *Adults.* 600 mg/d PO q hs. *Peds.* See insert; ⊘ high-fat meals **Caution:** [C, ?] CDC recommends HIV-infected mothers not breast-feed due to risk of transmission of HIV to infant **Contra:** Component sensitivity **Supplied:** Caps 50, 100, 200 mg **SE:** Somnolence, vivid dreams, dizziness, rash, N/V/D **Notes:** Monitor LFT, cholesterol **Interactions:** ↑ Effects w/ ritonavir; ↑ effects of CNS depressants, ergot derivatives, midazolam, ritonavir, simvastatin, triazolam, warfarin; ↓ effects w/ carbamazepine, phenobarbital, rifabutin, rifampin, saquinavir, St. John's wort; ↓ effects of amprenavir, carbamazepine, clarithromycin, indinavir, phenobarbital, saquinavir, warfarin; may alter effectiveness of oral contraceptive **Labs:** ↑ AST, ALT, amylase, total cholesterol, triglycerides; false + urine cannabinoid test **NIPE:** ⊘ High–fat foods, take w/o regard to food, use barrier contraception

Emedastine (Emadine) **Uses:** *Allergic conjunctivitis* **Action:** Antihistamine; selective H₁-antagonist **Dose:** 1 gt in eye(s) up to qid **Caution:** [B, ?] **Contra:** Hypersensitivity to ingredients (preservatives benzalkonium, tromethamine) **Supplied:** 0.05% soln **SE:** HA, blurred vision, burning/stinging, corneal infiltrates/staining, dry eyes, foreign body sensation, hyperemia, keratitis, tearing, pruritus, rhinitis, sinusitis, asthenia, bad taste, dermatitis, discomfort **Notes:** ⊘ Use contact lenses if eyes are red **NIPE:** ⊘ Wear soft contact lens for 15 min after use

Emtricitabine (Emtriva) **WARNING:** Class warning for lipodystrophy, lactic acidosis, & severe hepatomegaly **Uses:** HIV-1 infection **Action:** Nucleoside RT inhibitor (NRTI) **Dose:** 200 mg PO daily; ↓ dose for renal impairment. **Caution:** [B, –] **Contra:** Component sensitivity **Supplied:** 200 mg caps **SE:** HA, diarrhea, nausea, rash **Notes:** Rare hyperpigmentation of feet & hands; posttreatment exacerbation of hepatitis; first NRTI w/ once-daily dosing **Interactions:** None noted w/ additional NRTIs **NIPE:** Take w/o regard to food, causes redistribution and accumulation of body fat; take w/ other antiretrovirals; not a cure for HIV or prevention of opportunistic infections

Enalapril (Vasotec) **Uses:** *HTN, CHF, LVD,* DN **Action:** ACEI **Dose:** *Adults.* 2.5–40 mg/d PO; 1.25 mg IV q6h. *Peds.* 0.05–0.08 mg/kg/dose PO q12–24h; ↓ dose in renal impairment **Caution** [C (1st tri; D 2nd & 3rd tri), +] Use w/ NSAIDs, K suppls **Contra:** Bilateral renal artery stenosis, angioedema **Supplied:** Tabs 2.5, 5, 10, 20 mg; IV 1.25 mg/mL (1, 2 mL) **SE:** Symptomatic ↓ BP w/ initial dose (especially w/ concomitant diuretics), ↑ K⁺, nonproductive cough, angioedema **Notes:** Monitor Cr; DC diuretic for 2–3 d prior to initiation **Interactions:** ↑ Effects w/ loop diuretics; ↑ risk of cough w/ capsaicin; ↑ effects of α-blockers, insulin, Li; ↑ risk of hyperkalemia w/ K suppl, K-sparing diuretics, salt substitutes, trimethoprim; ↓ effects w/ ASA, NSAIDs, rifampin **Labs:** May cause ↑ serum K⁺, direct Coombs' test, false + urine acetone **NIPE:** Several weeks needed for full hypotensive effect

Enfuvirtide (Fuzeon) **WARNING:** Rarely causes hypersensitivity; never rechallenge Pt **Uses:** *Combination w/ antiretroviral agents for Rx of HIV-1 infection in Rx-experienced Pts w/ evidence of viral replication despite ongoing antiretroviral therapy* **Action:** Fusion inhibitor **Dose:** 90 mg (1 mL) SQ bid in upper arm, anterior thigh, or abdomen **Caution:** [B, –] **Contra:** Previous hypersensitivity to drug **Supplied:** 90 mg/mL on reconstitution; dispensed as Pt convenience kit w/ monthly supplies **SE:** Inj site Rxns (in nearly all Pts); pneumonia, diarrhea, nausea, fatigue, insomnia, peripheral neuropathy **Notes:** Rotate inj site; available only via restricted drug distribution system; must be immediately administered on reconstitution or refrigerated for up to 24 h prior to use **Interactions:** None noted w/ other antiretrovirals **NIPE:** Does not cure HIV; does not ↓ risk of transmission or prevent opportunistic infections; take w/o regard to food

Enoxaparin (Lovenox) **WARNING:** Recent or anticipated epidural/spinal anesthesia ↑s risk of spinal/epidural hematoma w/ subsequent paralysis **Uses:** *Prevention & Rx of DVT; Rx PE; unstable angina & non-Q-wave MI* **Action:** LMW heparin **Dose:** *Adults.* Prevention: 30 mg SQ bid or 40 mg SQ q24h. *DVT/PE Rx:* 1 mg/kg SQ q12h or 1.5 mg/kg SQ q24h. *Angina:* 1 mg/kg SQ q12h. *Peds.* Prevention: 0.5 mg/kg SQ q12h. *DVT/PE Rx:* 1mg/kg SQ q12h; ↓ or ⊘ w/ severe renal impairment **Caution:** [B, ?] ⊘ for thromboprophylaxis in prosthetic heart valves **Contra:** Active bleeding, HIT antibody + **Supplied:** Inj 10 mg/0.1 mL (30-, 40-, 60-, 80-, 100-, 120-, & 150-mg syringes) **SE:** Bleeding, hemorrhage, bruising, thrombocytopenia, pain/hematoma at inj site, ↑ AST/ALT **Notes:** Does not significantly affect bleeding time, plt Fxn, PT, or aPTT; monitor plts, bleeding; may monitor anti-factor Xa **Interactions:** ↑ Bleeding effects w/ ASA, anticoagulants, cephalosporins, NSAIDs, penicillin, chamomile, garlic, ginger, ginkgo biloba, feverfew, horse chestnut **Labs:** ↑ AST, ALT **NIPE:** No need to monitor aPTT, admin deep SQ ⊘ IM

Entacapone (Comtan) **Uses:** *Parkinson's Dz* **Action:** Selective & reversible carboxymethyl transferase inhibitor **Dose:** 200 mg w/ each levodopa/carbidopa dose; max 1600 mg/d; ↓ levodopa/carbidopa dose by 25% if levodopa dose >800 mg **Caution:** [C, ?] Hepatic impairment **Contra:** Concurrent use w/ nonselective MAOI **Supplied:** Tabs 200 mg **SE:** Dyskinesia, hyperkinesia, nausea, dizziness, hallucinations, orthostatic hypotension, brown-orange urine, diarrhea **Notes:** Monitor LFT; **Interactions:** ↑ Effects w/ ampicillin, choramphenicol, cholestyramine, erythromycin, MAOIs, probenecid, rifampin; ↑ risk of arrhythmias & HTN w/ bitolterol, dopamine, dobutamine, epinephrine, isoetharine, methyldopa, norepinephrine **NIPE:** ⊘ DC abruptly, breast-feed

Ephedrine Uses: *Acute bronchospasm, bronchial asthma, nasal congestion,* ↓ BP, narcolepsy, enuresis, & MyG **Action:** Sympathomimetic; stimulates α- & β-receptors; bronchodilator **Dose:** *Adults.* 25–50 mg IM or IV q10min to a max of 150 mg/d or 25–50 mg PO q3–4h PRN. *Peds.* 0.2–0.3 mg/kg/dose IM/IV q4–6h PRN **Caution:** [C, ?/–] **Contra:** Cardiac arrhythmias; angle-closure glaucoma **Supplied:** Inj 50 mg/mL; caps 25 mg; nasal spray 0.25% **SE:** CNS stimulation (nervousness, anxiety, trembling), tachycardia, arrhythmia, HTN, xerostomia, painful urination **Notes:** Protect from light; monitor BP, HR, urinary output; can cause false + amphetamine EMIT; take last dose 4–6h before hs **Interactions:** ↑ Effects w/ acetazolamide, antacids, MAOIs, TCAs, urinary alkalinizers; ↑ effects of sympathomimetics; ↓ response w/ diuretics, methyldopa, reserpine, urinary acidifiers; ↓ effects of antihypertensives, BBs, dexamethasone, guanethidine **Labs:** False ↑ urine amino acids **NIPE:** ⊘ EtOH, store away from light/heat

Epinephrine (Adrenalin, Sus-Phrine, EpiPen, others) Uses: *Cardiac arrest, anaphylactic Rxn, bronchospasm, open-angle glaucoma* **Action:** β-adrenergic agonist, some α-effects **Dose:** *Adults.* ACLS: 0.5–1 mg (5–10 mL of 1:10,000) IV q 5 min to response. *Anaphylaxis:* 0.3–0.5 mL SQ of 1:1000 dilution, may repeat q5–15min to a max of 1 mg/dose & 5 mg/d. *Asthma:* 0.1–0.5 mL SQ of 1:1000 dilution, repeated at 20–min–4h intervals or 1 inhal (met-dose) repeat in 1–2 min or susp 0.1–0.3 mL SQ for extended effect. *Peds.* ACLS: 1st dose 0.1 mL/kg IV of 1:10,000 dilution, then 0.1 mL/kg IV of 1:1000 dilution q3–5min to response. *Anaphylaxis:* 0.001mg/kg SQ q15min ×2 doses, then q4h PRN. *Asthma:* 0.01 mL/kg SQ of 1:1000 dilution q8–12h. **Caution:** [C, ?] ↓ bronchodilation w/ BBs **Contra:** Cardiac arrhythmias, angle-closure glaucoma **Supplied:** Inj 1:1000, 1:2000, 1:10,000, 1:100,000; susp for inj 1:200; aerosol 220 μg/spray; soln for inhal 1% **SE:** CV (tachycardia, HTN, vasoconstriction), CNS stimulation (nervousness, anxiety, trembling), ↓ renal blood flow **Notes:** Can give via ET tube if no central line (2–2.5 × IV dose) **Interactions:** ↑ HTN effects w/ α-blockers, BBs, ergot alkaloids, furazolidone, MAOIs; ↑ cardiac effects w/ antihistamines, cardiac glycosides, levodopa, thyroid hormones, TCAs; ↑ effects of sympathomimetics; ↓ effects of diuretics, guanethidine, hypoglycemics, methyldopa **Labs:** ↑ Serum bilirubin, glucose, & uric acid, urine catecholamines **NIPE:** ⊘ OTC inhalation drugs

Epirubicin (Ellence) Uses: *Adjuvant therapy w/ evidence of axillary node tumor involvement following resection of primary breast CA* **Actions:** An anthracycline cytotoxic agent **Dose:** Refer to specific protocols; ↓ dose w/ hepatic impairment. **Caution:** [D, –] **Contra:** Baseline neutrophil count < 1500 cells/mm³, severe myocardial insufficiency, recent MI, severe arrhythmias, severe hepatic dysfunction, previous Rx w/ anthracyclines up to max cumulative dose **Supplied:** In 50 mg/25 mL, 200 mg/100 mL **SE:** Mucositis, N/V/D, alopecia, myelosuppression, cardiotoxicity, secondary AML, severe tissue necrosis if extravasation occurs **Interactions:** ↑ Effects with cimetidine; ↑ effects of cytotoxic drugs, radiation therapy; ↑ risk of HF with CCBs, trastuzumab; incompatible chemically with fluorouracil, heparin **Labs:** Monitor before & after treatment AST, total bilirubin, creatinine, CBC, LVEF **NIPE:** ⊘ Handle if PRG breast-feeding; urine reddish up to 2 d after treatment, use contraception during treatment, burning at inj site indicates infiltration, menstruation may cease permanently

Eplerenone (Inspra)   **Uses:** *HTN* **Action:** Selective aldosterone antagonist **Dose: Adults:** 50 mg PO daily–bid, doses >100 mg/d no benefit w/ ↑ hyperkalemia; ↓ dose to 25 mg PO qd if giving w/ weak CYP3A4 inhibitors **Caution:** [B, +/–] Use of CYP3A4 inhibitors (ketoconazole, itraconazole, erythromycin, fluconazole, verapamil, saquinavir); monitor K⁺ w/ ACEIs, ARBs, NSAIDs, K-sparing diuretics; grapefruit juice, St. John's wort **Contra:** K⁺ >5.5 mEq/L; NIDDM w/ microalbuminuria; SCr >2 mg/dL (males), >1.8 mg/dL (females); CrCl <50 mL/min; concurrent K suppls/K-sparing diuretics **Supplied:** Tabs 25, 50, 100 mg **SE:** Hypertriglyceridemia, ↑ K⁺, HA, dizziness, gynecomastia, hypercholesterolemia, diarrhea, orthostatic hypotension **Notes:** May take 4 wk to see full effect **Interactions:** ↑ Risk hyperkalemia w/ ACEIs; ↑ risk of toxic effects w/ azole antifungals, erythromycin, saquinavir, verapamil, ↑ effects of Li; ↓ effects w/ NSAIDs **NIPE:** ⊘ High-K foods, may cause reversible breast pain or enlargement w/ use

Epoetin Alfa [Erythropoietin, EPO] (Epogen, Procrit)   **Uses:** *Anemia associated w/ CRF,* zidovudine Rx in HIV-infected Pts, CA chemotherapy; reduction in transfusions associated w/ surgery **Action:** Induces erythropoiesis **Dose: Adults & Peds.** 50–150 units/kg IV/SQ 3×/wk; adjust the dose q4–6wk PRN. *Surgery:* 300 units/kg/d × 10 d prior to surgery to 4 d after; decrease dose if Hct approaches 36%/Hgb, or ↑ >4 points in 2-wk period **Caution:** [C, +] **Contra:** Uncontrolled HTN **Supplied:** Inj 2000, 3000, 4000, 10,000, 20,000, 40,000 units/mL **SE:** HTN, HA, fatigue, fever, tachycardia, N/V **Notes:** Store in refrigerator; monitor baseline & posttreatment Hct/Hgb, BP, ferritin **Interactions:** None noted **Labs:** ↑ WBCs, plts **NIPE:** Monitor for access line clotting, ⊘ shake vial

Epoprostenol (Flolan)   **Uses:** *Pulmonary HTN* **Action:** Dilates pulmonary & systemic arterial vascular beds; inhibits plt aggregation **Dose:** Initial 2 ng/kg/min; ↑ by 2 ng/kg/min q15min until dose-limiting SE (CP, dizziness, N/V, HA, hypotension, flushing); IV cont inf 4 ng/kg/min less than maximum-tolerated rate; adjustments based on response: see package insert guidelines **Caution:** [B, ?] ↑ toxicity w/diuretics, vasodilators, acetate in dialysis fluids, anticoagulants **Contra:** Chronic use in CHF 2nd-deg severe LVSD **Supplied:** Inj 0.5, 1.5 mg **SE:** Flushing, tachycardia, CHF, fever, chills, nervousness, HA, N/V/D, jaw pain, flu-like Sxs **Notes:** Abrupt DC can cause rebound pulmonary HTN; monitor bleeding if using other antiplt/anticoagulants; watch hypotensive effects w/ other vasodilators/diuretics **Interactions:** ↑ Risk of bleeding w/ anticoagulants, antiplts; ↑ effects of digoxin; ↓ BP w/ antihypertensives, diuretics, vasodilators **NIPE:** ⊘ Mix or administer w/ other drugs

Eprosartan (Teveten) Uses: *HTN,* DN, CHF **Action:** ARB **Dose:** 400–800 mg/d single dose or bid **Caution:** [C (1st tri); D (2nd & 3rd tri), –] Li, ↑ K⁺ w/ K-sparing diuretics/suppls/high-dose trimethoprim **Contra:** Bilateral renal artery stenosis, 1st-deg aldosteronism **Supplied:** Tabs 400, 600 mg **SE:** Fatigue, depression, hypertriglyceridemia, URI, UTI, abdominal pain, rhinitis/pharyngitis/cough **Interactions:** ↑ Risk of hyperkalemia w/ K-sparing diuretics, K suppls, trimethoprim; ↑ effects of Li **Labs:** ↑ ALT, AST, alkaline phosphatase, BUN, creatinine; ↓ Hmg **NIPE:** Monitor LFTs, CBC & differential, renal Fxn; ⊘ PRG, breast-feeding

Eptifibatide (Integrilin) Uses: *ACS, PCI* **Action:** Glycoprotein IIb/IIIa inhibitor **Dose:** 180 µg/kg IV bolus, then 2 µg/kg/min cont inf; ↓ dose in renal impairment (SCr >2 mg/dL, <4 mg/dL: 135 µg/kg bolus & 0.5 µg/kg/min inf) **Caution:** [B, ?] Monitor bleeding w/ other anticoagulants **Contra:** Other GPIIb/IIIa inhibitors, Hx abnormal bleeding, hemorrhagic stroke (w/in 30 d), severe HTN, major surgery (w/in 6 wk), plt count <100,000 cells/mm³, renal dialysis **Supplied:** Inj 0.75, 2 mg/mL **SE:** Bleeding, hypotension, inj site Rxn, thrombocytopenia **Notes:** Monitor bleeding, coags, plts, SCr, activated coagulation time (ACT) w/ prothrombin consumption index (maintain ACT between 200–300 s) **Interactions:** ↑ Bleeding w/ ASA, cephalosporins, clopidogrel, heparin, NSAIDs, thrombolytics, ticlopidine, warfarin, evening primrose oil, feverfew, garlic, ginger, ginkgo biloba, ginseng, grapeseed extract

Ertapenem (Invanz) Uses: *Complicated intraabdominal, acute pelvic, & skin infections, pyelonephritis, community-acquired pneumonia* **Action:** A carbapenem; β-lactam antibiotic, inhibits cell wall synthesis. *Spectrum:* Good gram(+/–) & anaerobic coverage, but not *Pseudomonas*, penicillin-resistant pneumococci, MRSA, *Enterococcus*, β-lactamse(+) *H. influenza, Mycoplasma, Chlamydia* **Dose:** *Adults.* 1 g IM/IV daily; 500 mg/d in CrCl <30 mL/min **Caution:** [C, ?/–] Probenecid ↓ renal clearance of ertapenem **Contra:** <18 y, penicillin allergy **Supplied:** Inj 1 g/vial **SE:** HA, N/V/D, inj site Rxns, thrombocytosis, ↑ LFTs **Notes:** Can give IM × 7 d, IV × 14 d; 137 mg Na⁺(6 mEq)/g ertapenem **Interactions:** ↑ Effects w/ probenecid; **Labs:** ↑ AST, ALT, serum alkaline phosphatase, bilirubin, glucose, creatinine, PT, RBCs, urine WBCs **NIPE:** Monitor for superinfection

Erythromycin (E-Mycin, E.E.S., Ery-Tab) Uses: *Bacterial infections; bowel decontamination*; GI motility; *acne vulgaris* **Action:** Bacteriostatic; interferes w/ protein synthesis. *Spectrum:* Group A streptococci (S. pyogenes), *S. pneumoniae, N. meningitides, N. gonorrhea* (in penicillin-allergic Pts), *Legionella, M. pneumoniae* **Dose:** *Adults.* Base 250–500 mg PO q6–12h or ethylsuccinate 400–800 mg q6–12h; 500 mg–1 g IV q6h. *Prokinetic:* 250 mg PO tid 30 mins ac. **Peds.** 30–50 mg/kg/d PO ÷ q6–8h or 20–40 mg/kg/d IV ÷ q6h, max 2 g/d **Caution:** [B, +] ↑ toxicity of carbamazepine, cyclosporine, digoxin, methylprednisolone, theophylline, felodipine, warfarin, simvastatin/lovastatin **Contra:** Hepatic impairment, preexisting liver Dz (estolate), use w/ pimozide **Supplied:** *Powder for inj as lactobionate:* 500 mg, 1 g. *Base:* Tabs 250, 333, 500 mg; caps 250 mg. *Estolate:* Susp 125, 250 mg/5 mL. *Stearate:* Tabs 250, 500 mg. *Ethylsuccinate:* Chew tabs 200 mg; tabs 400 mg; susp 200, 400 mg/5 mL **SE:** HA, abdominal pain, N/V/D; [QT prolongation, torsades de pointes, ventricular arrhythmias/tachycardias (rarely)]; cholestatic jaundice (estolate) **Notes:** 400 mg ethylsuccinate = 250 mg base/state/estolate; take w/ food to minimize GI upset; lactobionate salt contains benzyl EtOH (caution in neonates) **Interactions:** ↑ Effects w/ amprenavir, indinavir, ritonavir, saquinavir, grapefruit juice; ↑ effects of alprazolam, benzodiazepines, buspirone, carbamazepine, clozapine, colchicines, cyclosporine, digoxin, felodipine, lovastatin, midazolam, quinidine, sildenafil, simvastatin, tacrolimus, theophylline, triazolam, valproic acid; ↑ QT w/ astemizole, cisapride; ↓ effects of penicillin, zafirlukast **Labs:** False ↑ AST, ALT, serum bilirubin, urine amino acids, false ↓ folate assay **NIPE:** Take w/ food if GI upset, monitor for superinfection & ototoxicity

Erythromycin & Benzoyl Peroxide (Benzamycin)
Uses: Topical Rx of *acne vulgaris* **Action:** Macrolide antibiotic w/ keratolytic **Dose:** Apply bid (AM & PM) **Caution:** [C, ?] **Contra:** Component sensitivity **Supplied:** Gel erythromycin 30 mg/benzoyl peroxide 50 mg/g **SE:** Local irritation, dryness

Erythromycin & Sulfisoxazole (Eryzole, Pediazole)
Uses: *Upper & lower resp tract; bacterial infections; otitis media in children due to H. influenzae*; infections in penicillin-allergic Pts **Action:** Macrolide antibiotic w/ sulfonamide **Dose:** Based on erythromycin content. *Adults.* 400 mg erythromycin/1200 mg sulfisoxazole PO q6h. **Peds.** >2 mo. 40–50 mg/kg/d erythromycin & 150 mg/kg/d sulfisoxazole PO ÷ q6h; max 2 g/d erythromycin or 6 g/d sulfisoxazole × 10 d; ↓ in renal impairment **Caution:** [C (D if given near term), +] PO anticoagulants, MRX, hypoglycemics, phenytoin, cyclosporine **Contra:** Infants <2 mo **Supplied:** Susp erythromycin ethylsuccinate 200 mg/sulfisoxazole 600 mg/5 mL (100, 150, 200 mL) **SE:** GI disturbance **Additional Interactions:** ↑ Effects of sulfonamides w/ ASA, diuretics, NSAIDs, probenecid **Labs:** False + urine protein **NIPE:** ↑ Risk of photosensitivity—use sunscreen, ↑ fluid intake

Erythromycin, Ophthalmic (Ilotycin Ophthalmic)
Uses: *Conjunctival/corneal infections* **Action:** Macrolide antibiotic **Dose:** ½ in. 2–6 ×/d **Caution:** [B, +] **Contra:** Hypersensitivity to erythromycin **Supplied:** 0.5% oint **SE:** Local irritation **NIPE:** May cause burning, stinging, blurred vision

Erythromycin, Topical (A/T/S, Eryderm, Erycette, T-Stat)
Uses: *Acne vulgaris* **Action:** Macrolide antibiotic **Dose:** Wash & dry area, apply

2% product over area bid **Caution:** [B, +] **Contra:** Component sensitivity **Supplied:** Soln 1.5%, 2%; gel 2%; impregnated pads & swabs 2% **SE:** Local irritation

Escitalopram (Lexapro) **WARNING:** Closely monitor for worsening depression or emergence of suicidality, particularly in pediatric Pts **Uses:** Depression, anxiety **Action:** SSRI **Dose:** *Adults.* 10–20 mg PO daily; 10 mg/d in elderly & hepatic impairment **Caution:** [C, +/–] ↑ Risk of serotonin syndrome w/ other SSRI, tramadol, linezolid, sumatriptan **Contra:** W/ or w/in 14 d of MAOI **Supplied:** Tabs 5, 10, 20 mg; soln 1 mg/mL **SE:** N/V/D, sweating, insomnia, dizziness, xerostomia, sexual dysfunction **Interactions:** ↑ Risk of serotonin syndrome w/ linezolid; ↑ risk of bleeding w/ anticoagulants, ASA, NSAIDs; may ↑ CNS effects w/ CNS depressants **NIPE:** ⊘ DC abruptly; may take up to 2–4 wk for full effects; take w/o regard to food

Esmolol (Brevibloc) **Uses:** *SVT & noncompensatory sinus tachycardia, AF/flutter* **Action:** β_1-Adrenergic blocker; class II antiarrhythmic **Dose:** *Adults & Peds.* Initiate Rx w/ 500 µg/kg load over 1 min, then 50 µg/kg/min × 4 min; if inadequate response, repeat the loading dose & maint inf of 100 µg/kg/min × 4 min; titrate by repeating load, then incremental ↑ in the maint dose of 50 µg/kg/min for 4 min until desired heart rate reached or hypotension; average dose 100 µg/kg/min **Caution:** [C (1st tri; D 2nd or 3rd tri), ?] **Contra:** Sinus bradycardia, heart block, uncompensated CHF, cardiogenic shock, hypotension **Supplied:** Inj 10, 250 mg/mL; premix inf 10 mg/mL **SE:** Hypotension (↓ or discontinuing inf reverses hypotension in 30 min); bradycardia, diaphoresis, dizziness, pain on inj **Notes:** Hemodynamic effects back to baseline w/in 20–30 mins after DC inf **Interaction:** ↑ Effects w/ verapamil; ↑ effects of digoxin, antihypertensives, nitrates; ↑ HTN w/ amphetamines, cocaine, ephedrine, epinephrine, MAOIs, norepinephrine, phenylephrine, pseudoephedrine; ↓ effects of glucagons, insulin, hypoglycemics, theophylline; ↓ effects w/ NSAIDs, thyroid hormones **Labs:** ↑ Glucose, cholesterol **NIPE:** Monitor BS of Pts w/ DM

Esomeprazole (Nexium) **Uses:** *Short-term (4–8 wk) Rx of erosive esophagitis/GERD; Rx of H. pylori infection in combination w/ antibiotics* **Action:** Proton pump inhibitor, ↓ gastric acid production **Dose:** *Adults.* GERD/erosive gastritis: 20–40 mg/d PO × 4–8 wk; *Maint:* 20 mg/d PO. *H. pylori infection:* 40 mg/d PO, plus clarithromycin 500 mg PO bid & amoxicillin 1000 mg/bid for 10 d **Caution:** [B, ?/–] **Contra:** Component sensitivity **Supplied:** Caps 20, 40 mg **SE:** HA, diarrhea, abdominal pain **Notes:** ⊘ Chew; may open capsule & sprinkle on applesauce; take on empty stomach 1 h ac

Estazolam (ProSom) [C-IV] **Uses:** *Short-term management of insomnia* **Action:** Benzodiazepine **Dose:** 1–2 mg PO qhs PRN; ↓ in hepatic impairment/elderly/debilitated **Caution:** [X, –] ↑ effects w/ CNS depressants **Contra:** PRG **Supplied:** Tabs 1, 2 mg **SE:** Somnolence, weakness, palpitations **Notes:** May cause psychological/physical dependence; ⊘ abrupt DC after prolonged use **Inter-**

actions: ↑ Effects w/ amoxicillin, clarithromycin; ↑ effects of diazepam, phenytoin, warfarin; ↓ effects w/ food; ↓ effects of azole antifungals, digoxin **Labs:** ↑ LFTs, bilirubin, SCr, uric acid, TSH; ↓ Hgb, WBC, plts, K⁺, Na⁺, thyroxine **NIPE:** Take at least 1 h ac

Esterified Estrogens (Estratab, Menest)   WARNING: ⊘ Use in the
prevention of CV Dz **Uses:** *Vasomotor Sxs or vulvar/vaginal atrophy associated w/ menopause*; female hypogonadism **Action:** Estrogen suppl **Dose:** *Menopause:* 0.3–1.25 mg/d, cyclically 3 wk on, 1 wk off. *Hypogonadism:* 2.5–7.5 mg/d PO × 20 d, off × 10 d **Caution:** [X, –] **Contra:** Genital bleeding of unknown cause, breast CA, estrogen-dependent tumors, thromboembolic disorders, thrombophlebitis, recent MI, PRG, severe hepatic Dz **Supplied:** Tabs 0.3, 0.625, 1.25, 2.5 mg **SE:** Nausea, HA, bloating, breast enlargement/tenderness, edema, venous thromboembolism, hypertriglyceridemia, gallbladder Dz **Notes:** Use at lowest dose for shortest time; refer to Women's Health Initiatives (WHI) data **Interactions:** ↑ Effects of corticosteroids, cyclosporine, TCAs, theophylline, caffeine, tobacco; ↓ effects w/ barbiturates, phenytoin, rifampin; ↓ effects of anticoagulants, hypoglycemics, insulin, tamoxifen **Labs:** ↑ Prothrombin & factors VII, VIII, IX, X, plt aggregability, thyroid-binding globulin, T₄, triglycerides; ↓ antithrombin III, folate **NIPE:** ⊘ PRG, breast-feeding

Esterified Estrogens + Methyltestosterone (Estratest, Estratest HS)   **Uses:** *Vasomotor Sxs*; postpartum breast engorgement **Action:** Estrogen & androgen suppl **Dose:** 1 tab/d × 3 wk, 1 wk off **Caution:** [X, –] **Contra:** Genital bleeding of unknown cause, breast CA, estrogen-dependent tumors, thromboembolic disorders, thrombophlebitis, recent MI, PRG **Supplied:** Tabs (estrogen/methyltestosterone) 0.625 mg/1.25 mg (hs), 1.25 mg/2.5 mg **SE:** Nausea, HA, bloating, breast enlargement/tenderness, edema, ↑ triglycerides, venous thromboembolism, gallbladder Dz **Notes:** Use at lowest dose for shortest time. See Esterified Estrogens, page 110. **Additional Interactions:** ↑ Effects of insulin; ↓ effects of oral anticoagulants

Estradiol (Estrace)   **Uses:** *Atrophic vaginitis, vasomotor Sxs associated w/ menopause, osteoporosis* **Action:** Estrogen suppl **Dose:** *PO:* 1–2 mg/d, adjust PRN to control Sxs. *Vaginal cream:* 2–4 g/d × 2 wk, then 1 g 1–3×/wk **Caution:** [X, –] **Contra:** Genital bleeding of unknown cause, breast CA, estrogen-dependent tumors, thromboembolic disorders, thrombophlebitis; recent MI; hepatic impairment **Supplied:** Tabs 0.5, 1, 2 mg; vaginal cream 0.1 mg/g **SE:** Nausea, HA, bloating, breast enlargement/tenderness, edema, ↑ triglycerides, venous thromboembolism, gallbladder Dz **Interactions:** ↑ Effects w/ grapefruit juice; ↑ effects of corticosteroids, cyclosporine, TCAs, theophylline, caffeine, tobacco; ↓ effects w/ barbiturates, carbamazepine, phenytoin, primidone, rifampin; ↓ effects of clofibrate, hypoglycemics, insulin, tamoxifen, warfarin **Labs:** ↑ Prothrombin & factors VII, VIII, IX, X, plt aggregability, thyroid-binding globulin, T₄, triglycerides; ↓ antithrombin III, folate **NIPE:** ⊘ PRG, breast-feeding

Estradiol Cypionate & Medroxyprogesterone Acetate (Lunelle) Warning: Cigarette smoking ↑ risk of serious CV side effects from contraceptives containing estrogen. This risk ↑ w/ age & w/ heavy smoking (> 15 cigarettes/d) & is quite marked in women > 35 y. Women who use Lunelle should be strongly advised not to smoke Uses: *Contraceptive* Action: Estrogen & progestin Dose: 0.5 mL IM (deltoid, ant thigh, buttock) monthly, ⊘ exceed 33 d Caution: [X, M] HTN, gallbladder Dz, ↑ lipids, migraines, sudden HA, valvular heart Dz w/ complications Contra: PRG, heavy smokers >35 y, DVT, PE, cerebro-/CV Dz, estrogen-dependent neoplasm, undiagnosed abnormal uterine bleeding, hepatic tumors, cholestatic jaundice Supplied: Estradiol cypionate (5 mg), medroxyprogesterone acetate (25 mg) single-dose vial or prefilled syringe (0.5 mL) SE: Arterial thromboembolism, HTN, cerebral hemorrhage, MI, amenorrhea, acne, breast tenderness Notes: Start w/in 5 d of menstruation. Eee Estradiol. **Additional Interactions:** ↓ Effects w/ aminoglutethimide

Estradiol, Transdermal (Estraderm, Climara, Vivelle) Uses: *Severe menopausal vasomotor Sxs; female hypogonadism* Action: Estrogen suppl Dose: 0.1 mg/d patch 1–2×/wk depending on product; adjust PRN to control Sxs Caution: [X, –] (See estradiol) Contra: PRG, undiagnosed genital bleeding, carcinoma of breast, estrogen-dependent tumors, Hx of thrombophlebitis, thrombosis, thromboembolic disorders associated w/ estrogen use Supplied: TD patches (deliver mg/24 h) 0.025, 0.0375, 0.05, 0.075, 0.1 SE: Nausea, bloating, breast enlargement/tenderness, edema, HA, hypertriglyceridemia, gallbladder Dz Notes: ⊘ Apply to breasts, place on trunk of body & rotate sites. See Estradiol. **Additional NIPE:** Rotate application sites

Estramustine Phosphate (Estracyt, Emcyt) Uses: *Advanced CAP* Action: Antimicrotubule agent; weak estrogenic & antiandrogenic activity Dose: 14 mg/kg/d in 3–4 ÷ doses; take on empty stomach, ⊘ take w/ milk/milk products Caution: [NA, not used in females] Contra: Active thrombophlebitis or thromboembolic disorders Supplied: Caps 140 mg SE: N/V, exacerbation of preexisting CHF, thrombophlebitis, MI, PE, gynecomastia in 20–100% Interactions: ↓ Effects w/ antacids, Ca suppls, Ca-containing foods; ↓ effects of anticoagulants NIPE: Take on empty stomach, several wk may be needed for full effects, store in refrigerator

Estrogen, Conjugated (Premarin) WARNING: Should not be used for the prevention of CV Dz. The WHI reported ↑ risk of MI, stroke, breast CA, PE & DVT when combined w/ methoxyprogesterone over 5 y of Rx; ↑ risk of endometrial CA Uses: *Moderate to severe menopausal vasomotor Sxs; atrophic vaginitis; palliative therapy of advanced prostatic carcinoma; prevention & Rx of estrogen deficiency-induced osteoporosis* Action: Hormonal replacement Dose: 0.3–1.25 mg/d PO cyclically; prostatic carcinoma requires 1.25–2.5 mg PO tid; Caution: [X, –] Contra: Severe hepatic impairment, genital bleeding of unknown cause, breast CA, estrogen-dependent tumors, thromboembolic disorders, thrombosis, thrombophlebitis, recent MI **Supplied:** Tabs 0.3, 0.625, 0.9, 1.25, 2.5 m; inj 25 mg/mL **SE:** ↑ Risk of endometrial carcinoma, gallbladder Dz, thromboen bolism, HA, & possibly breast CA; generic products not equivalent **Interaction** ↑ Effects of corticosteroids, cyclosporine, TCAs, theophylline, tobacco; ↓ effec of anticoagulants, clofibrate; ↓ effects w/ barbiturates, carbamazepine, phenytoi rifampin **Labs:** ↑ Prothrombin & factors VII, VIII, IX, X, plt aggregability, thy roid-binding globulin, T_4, triglycerides; ↓ antithrombin III, folate **NIPE:** ⊘ PR(breast-feeding

Estrogen, Conjugated-Synthetic (Cenestin)　Uses: *Rx of mode ate to severe vasomotor Sxs associated w/ menopause* **Action:** Hormonal replac ment **Dose:** 0.625–1.25 mg PO qd **Caution:** [X, –] **Contra:** See estroge conjugated **Supplied:** Tabs 0.625, 0.9, 1.25 mg **SE:** Associated w/ an ↑ risk of e dometrial CA, gallbladder Dz, thromboembolism, & possibly breast CA. See E trogen, Conjugated, page 111

Estrogen, Conjugated + Medroxyprogesterone (Prempro Premphase)　**WARNING:** Should not be used for the prevention of CV D. the WHI study reported ↑ risk of MI, stroke, breast CA, PE, & DVT over 5 y of R **Uses:** *Moderate to severe menopausal vasomotor Sxs; atrophic vaginitis; preven tion of postmenopausal osteoporosis* **Action:** Hormonal replacement **Dose:** Prem pro 1 tab PO qd; Premphase 1 tab PO qd **Caution:** [X, –] **Contra:** Severe hepat impairment, genital bleeding of unknown cause, breast CA, estrogen-dependent tu mors, thromboembolic disorders, thrombosis, thrombophlebitis **Supplied:** (e) pressed as estrogen/medroxyprogesterone) Prempro: tabs 0.625/2.5, 0.625/5 m; Premphase: tabs 0.625/0 (days 1–14) & 0.625/5 mg (days 15–28) **SE:** Gallbladd(Dz, thromboembolism, HA, breast tenderness. See Estrogen, Conjugated. **Add** **tional Interactions:** ↓ Effects w/ aminoglutethimide

Estrogen, Conjugated + Methylprogesterone (Premarin Methylprogesterone)　**Uses:** *Menopausal vasomotor Sxs; osteoporosi* **Action:** Estrogen & androgen combination **Dose:** 1 tab/d **Caution:** [X, –] **Contra** Severe hepatic impairment, genital bleeding of unknown cause, breast CA, estro gen-dependent tumors, thromboembolic disorders, thrombosis, thrombophlebit **Supplied:** Tabs 0.625 mg estrogen, conjugated, & 2.5 or 5 mg of methylproges terone **SE:** Nausea, bloating, breast enlargement/tenderness, edema, HA, hype triglyceridemia, gallbladder Dz. See Estrogen, Conjugated, page 111

Estrogen, Conjugated + Methyltestosterone (Premarin Methyltestosterone)　**Uses:** *Moderate to severe menopausal vasomoto Sxs*; postpartum breast engorgement **Action:** Estrogen & androgen combinatio **Dose:** 1 tab/d × 3 wk, then 1 wk off **Caution:** [X, –] **Contra:** Severe hepatic im pairment, genital bleeding of unknown cause, breast CA, estrogen-dependent tu mors, thromboembolic disorders, thrombosis, thrombophlebitis **Supplied:** Tab (estrogen/methyltestosterone) 0.625 mg/5 mg, 1.25 mg/10 mg **SE:** Nausea, bloa ng, breast enlargement/tenderness, edema, HA, hypertriglyceridemia, gallbladder Dz. See Estrogen, Conjugated **Additional Interactions:** ↑ Effects of insulin

Etanercept (Enbrel) Uses: *Reduces Sxs of RA in Pts who have failed other DMARD (Dz-modifying antirheumatic drug),* Crohn's Dz **Action:** Binds TNF **Dose:** *Adults.* 25 mg SQ 2×/wk (separated by at least 72–96 h). *Peds 4–17 y.* 0.4 mg/kg SQ 2×/wk (max 25 mg) **Caution:** [B, ?] **Contra:** Active infection; caution in conditions that predispose to infection (ie, DM) **Supplied:** Inj 25 mg/vial **SE:** HA, rhinitis, inj site Rxn, URI, rhinitis **Interactions:** ↓ Response to live virus vaccine **NIPE:** Rotate inj sites, ⊘ live vaccines

Ethambutol (Myambutol) Uses: *Pulmonary TB* & other mycobacterial infections, MAC **Action:** Inhibits RNA synthesis **Dose:** *Adults & Peds.* >12 y: 15–25 mg/kg/d PO as a single dose; ↓ dose in renal impairment, take w/ food, ⊘ antacids **Caution:** [B, +] **Contra:** Optic neuritis **Supplied:** Tabs 100, 400 mg **SE:** HA, hyperuricemia, acute gout, abdominal pain, ↑ LFTs, optic neuritis, GI upset **Interactions:** ↑ Neurotoxicity w/ neurotoxic drugs; ↓ effects w/ Al salts **NIPE:** Monitor visual acuity

Ethinyl Estradiol (Estinyl, Feminone) Uses: *Menopausal vasomotor Sxs; female hypogonadism* **Action:** Estrogen suppl **Dose:** 0.02–1.5 mg/d ÷ daily–tid **Caution:** [X, –] **Contra:** Severe hepatic impairment; genital bleeding of unknown cause, breast CA, estrogen-dependent tumors, thromboembolic disorders, thrombosis, thrombophlebitis **Supplied:** Tabs 0.02, 0.05, 0.5 mg **SE:** Nausea, bloating, breast enlargement/tenderness, edema, HA, hypertriglyceridemia, gallbladder Dz **Interactions:** ↑ Effects of corticosteroids; ↓ effects w/ barbiturates, carbamazepine, hypoglycemics, insulin, phenytoin, primidone, rifampin, ↓ effects of anticoagulants, tamoxifen; **Labs:** ↑ Prothrombin & factors VII, VIII, IX, X, plt aggregability, thyroid-binding globulin, T_4, triglycerides; ↓ antithrombin III, folate **NIPE:** ⊘ PRG, breast-feeding

Ethinyl Estradiol & Levonorgestrel (Preven) Uses: *Emergency contraceptive* ("morning-after pill"); prevent PRG after contraceptive failure or unprotected intercourse **Actions:** Estrogen & progestin; interferes w/ implantation **Dose:** 4 tabs, take 2 tabs q12h × 2 (w/in 72 h of intercourse) **Caution:** [X, M] **Contra:** Known/suspected PRG, abnormal uterine bleeding **Supplied:** Kit ethinyl estradiol (0.05), levonorgestrel (0.25) blister pack w/ 4 pills & urine PRG test **SE:** Peripheral edema, N/V/D, bloating, abdominal pain, fatigue, HA, & menstrual changes **Notes:** Will not induce abortion; may ↑ risk of ectopic PRG. See Ethinyl Estradiol, page 113. **Additional Interactions:** ↑ Effects of ASA, benzodiazepines, metoprolol, TCAs **NIPE:** Monitor for vision changes or ↓ tolerance of contact lens

Ethinyl Estradiol & Norelgestromin (Ortho Evra) Uses: *Contraceptive patch* **Action:** Estrogen & progestin **Dose:** Apply patch to abdomen, buttocks, upper torso (not breasts), or upper outer arm at the beginning of the menstrual cycle; new patch is applied weekly for 3 wk; week 4 is patch-free **Caution:** [X, M] **Contra:** Thrombophlebitis, undiagnosed vaginal bleeding, PRG, carcinoma of breast, estrogen-dependent tumor **Supplied:** 20 cm^2 patch (6 mg norelgestromin (active metabolite norgestimate) & 0.75 mg of ethinyl estradiol) **SE:** Breast discomfort, HA, application site Rxns, nausea, menstrual cramps; thrombosis risks similar to OCP **Notes:** Less effective in women >90 kg. See Ethinyl Estradiol. **Additional Labs:** ↑ Serum amylase, Na, Ca, protein

Ethosuximide (Zarontin) Uses: *Absence (petit mal) Szs* **Action:** Anticonvulsant; ↑ Sz threshold **Dose:** *Adults.* Initial, 250 mg PO ÷ bid; ↑ by 250 mg/d q4–7d PRN (max 1500 mg/d). *Peds.* 3–6 y. *Initial:* 15 mg/kg/d PO ÷ bid. *Maint* 15–40 mg/kg/d ÷ bid, max 1500 mg/d; use w/ caution in renal/hepatic impairment **Caution:** [C, +] **Contra:** Component sensitivity **Supplied:** Caps 250 mg; syrup 250 mg/5 mL **SE:** Blood dyscrasias, GI upset, drowsiness, dizziness, irritability **Interactions:** ↑ Effects w/ INH, phenobarbital, EtOH; ↑ effects of CNS depressants, phenytoin; ↓ effects w/ carbamazepine, valproic acid, ginkgo biloba; ↓ effects of phenobarbital **NIPE:** Take w/ food, ⊘ EtOH

Etidronate Disodium (Didronel) Uses: *Hypercalcemia of malignancy, Paget's Dz, & heterotopic ossification* **Action:** Inhibits normal & abnormal bone resorption **Dose:** *Paget's:* 5–10 mg/kg/d PO ÷ doses (for 3–6 mo). *Hypercalcemia:* 7.5 mg/kg/d IV inf over 2 h × 3 d, then 20 mg/kg/d PO on last day of inf × 1–3 mo **Caution:** [B PO (C parenteral), ?] **Contra:** SCr >5 mg/dL **Supplied:** Tabs 200, 400 mg; inj 50 mg/mL **SE:** GI intolerance (↓ by dividing daily doses); hypophosphatemia, hypomagnesemia, bone pain, abnormal taste, fever, convulsions, nephrotoxicity **Notes:** Take PO on empty stomach 2 h before any meal **Interactions:** ↓ Effects w/ antacids, foods that contain Ca **NIPE:** ⊘ Take w/ food, improvement may take 3 mo

Etodolac (Lodine) Uses: *Osteoarthritis & pain,* RA **Action:** NSAID **Dose:** 200–400 mg PO bid–qid (max 1200 mg/d) **Caution:** [C (D 3rd tri), ?] ↑ bleeding risk w/ ASA, warfarin; ↑ nephrotoxicity w/ cyclosporine; Hx CHF, HTN, renal/hepatic impairment, PUD **Contra:** Active GI ulcer **Supplied:** Tabs 400, 500 mg; ER tabs 400, 500, 600 mg; caps 200, 300 mg **SE:** N/V/D, gastritis, abdominal cramps, dizziness, HA, depression, edema, renal impairment **Notes:** ⊘ Crush tabs **Interactions:** ↑ Risk of bleeding w/ anticoagulants, antiplts; ↑ effects of Li, MRX digoxin, cyclosporine; ↓ effects w/ ASA; ↓ effects of antihypertensives **Labs:** False + of urine ketones & bilirubin **NIPE:** Take w/ food

Etonogestrel/Ethinyl Estradiol (NuvaRing) Uses: *Contraceptive* **Action:** Estrogen & progestin combination **Dose:** Rule out PRG first; insert ring vaginally for 3 wk, remove for 1 wk; insert new ring 7 d after last removed (even if still bleeding) at same time of day ring removed. First day of menses is day 1, insert prior to day 5 even if still bleeding. Use other contraception for first 7 d of starting therapy. See insert if converting from other contraception; after delivery or 2nd-tri abortion, insert 4 wk postpartum (if not breast-feeding) **Caution:** [X, ?/–

HTN, gallbladder Dz, ↑ lipids, migraines, sudden HA **Contra**: PRG, heavy smokers >35 y, DVT, PE, cerebro-/CV Dz, estrogen-dependent neoplasm, undiagnosed abnormal genital bleeding, hepatic tumors, cholestatic jaundice **Supplied**: Intravaginal ring: ethinyl estradiol 0.015 mg/d & etonogestrel 0.12 mg/d **Notes**: If accidentally removed, rinse w/ cool/lukewarm water (not hot) & reinsert ASAP; if not reinserted w/in 3h, effectiveness decreased; ⊘ use w/ diaphragm. See Ethinyl Estradiol

Etoposide [VP-16] (VePesid, Toposar) Uses: *Testicular CA, non-small-cell lung CA, Hodgkin's & NHLs, pediatric ALL, & allogeneic/autologous BMT in high doses* **Action**: Topoisomerase II inhibitor **Dose**: 50 mg/m²/d IV for 3–5 d; 50 mg/m²/d PO for 21 d (PO bioavailability = 50% of the IV form); 2–6 g/m² or 25–70 mg/kg used in BMT (refer to specific protocols); ↓ in renal/hepatic impairment **Caution**: [D, –] **Contra**: IT administration **Supplied**: Caps 50 mg; inj 20 mg/mL **SE**: Myelosuppression, N/V, alopecia, hypotension if infused too rapidly, anorexia, anemia, leukopenia, potential for secondary leukemias **Notes**: Emetic potential low (10–30%) **Interactions**: ↑ Bleeding w/ ASA, NSAIDs, warfarin; ↑ bone marrow suppression w/ antineoplastics & radiation; ↑ effects of cisplatin; ↓ effects of live vaccines **Labs**: ↑ Uric acid **NIPE**: ⊘ EtOH, immunizations, PRG, breast-feeding; use contraception, 2–3 L/d fluids

Exemestane (Aromasin) Uses: *Rx of advanced breast CA in postmenopausal women whose Dz has progressed following tamoxifen therapy* **Action**: An irreversible, steroidal aromatase inhibitor; ↓ circulating estrogens **Dose**: 25 mg PO qd after a meal **Caution**: [D, ?/–] **Contra**: Component sensitivity **Supplied**: Tabs 25 mg **SE**: Hot flashes, nausea, fatigue **Interactions**: ↓ Effects with erythromycin, ketoconazole, phenobarbital, rifampin, other drugs that inhibit P4503A4, St John's wort, black cohosh, dong quai **Labs**: ↑ Alkaline phosphatase, AST, ALT **NIPE**: ⊘ PRG, breast-feeding; take pc and same time each day; monitor BP

Ezetimibe (Zetia) Uses: *Primary hypercholesterolemia alone or in combination w/ an HMG-CoA reductase inhibitor* **Action**: Inhibits intestinal absorption of cholesterol & phytosterols **Dose**: *Adults & Peds.* >10 y. 10 mg/d PO **Caution**: [C, +/–] Bile acid sequestrants ↓ bioavailability **Contra**: Hepatic impairment **Supplied**: Tabs 10 mg **SE**: HA, diarrhea, abdominal pain, ↑ transaminases in combination w/ an HMG-CoA reductase inhibitor **Interactions**: ↑ Effects w/ cyclosporine; ↓ effects w/ cholestyramine, fenofibrate, gemfibrozil **NIPE**: If used w/ fibrates ↑ risk of cholethiasis

Famciclovir (Famvir) Uses: *Acute herpes zoster (shingles) & genital herpes* **Action**: Inhibits viral DNA synthesis **Dose**: *Zoster*: 500 mg PO q8h ×7 d. *Simplex*: 125–250 mg PO bid; ↓ in renal impairment **Caution**: [B, –] **Contra**: Component sensitivity **Supplied**: Tabs 125, 250, 500 mg **SE**: Fatigue, dizziness, HA, pruritus, nausea, diarrhea **Interactions**: ↑ Effects w/ cimetidine, probenecid, theophylline; ↑ effects of digoxin **NIPE**: Not affected by food, therapy most effective if taken w/in 72 h of rash

Famotidine (Pepcid)   Uses: *Short-term Rx of active duodenal ulcer & be
nign gastric ulcer; maint for duodenal ulcer, hypersecretory conditions, GERD,
heartburn* **Action:** H₂-antagonist; inhibits gastric acid secretion **Dose:** *Adult*
Ulcer: 20 mg IV q12h or 20–40 mg PO qhs × 4–8 wk. *Hypersecretion:* 20–160 m
PO q6h. *GERD:* 20 mg PO bid ×6 wk; maint: 20 mg PO hs. *Heartburn:* 10 mg PO
PRN q12h. **Peds.** 0.5–1 mg/kg/d; ↓ dose in severe renal insufficiency **Caution:** [E
M] **Contra:** Component sensitivity **Supplied:** Tabs 10, 20, 40 mg; chew tabs 1
mg; susp 40 mg/5 mL; inj 10 mg/2 mL **SE:** Dizziness, HA, constipation, diarrhea
thrombocytopenia **Notes:** Chewable tablets contain phenylalanine **Interactions:**
Effects of glipizide, glyburide, nifedipine, nitrendipine, nisoldipine, tolbutamide;
effects w/ antacids; ↓ effects of azole antifungals, cefuroxime, enoxacin, diazepam
NIPE: ⊘ ASA, EtOH, tobacco, caffeine; take hs

Felodipine (Plendil)   Uses: *HTN & CHF* **Action:** CCB **Dose:** 2.5–10 m
PO qd; ↓ in hepatic impairment **Caution:** [C, ?] ↑ effects w/ azole antifungals, ery
thromycin, bioavailability ↑ w/ grapefruit juice **Contra:** Component sensitivi
Supplied: ER tabs 2.5, 5, 10 mg **SE:** Peripheral edema, flushing, tachycardia, HA
gingival hyperplasia **Notes:** Follow BP in elderly & in ↓ hepatic Fxn; swallow
whole **Interactions:** ↑ Effects w/ azole antifungals, cimetidine, cyclosporine, ran
tidine, propranolol, EtOH, grapefruit juice; ↑ effects of digoxin, erythromycin;
effects w/ barbiturates, carbamazepine, nafcillin, oxcarbazepine, phenytoin; ri
fampin; ↓ effects of theophylline **NIPE:** ↑ effects of theophylline

Fenofibrate (Tricor)   Uses: *Hypertriglyceridemia* **Action:** Inhibit
triglyceride synthesis **Dose:** 54–160 mg qd; ↓ in renal impairment, take w/ meal
Caution: [C, ?] **Contra:** Hepatic/severe renal insufficiency, 1st-deg biliary cirrho
sis, unexplained persistent ↑ LFTs, gallbladder Dz **Supplied:** Tabs 54, 160 mg **SE:**
GI disturbances, cholecystitis, arthralgia, myalgia, dizziness **Notes:** Monitor LFT
Interactions: ↑ Effects of anticoagulants; ↓ effects w/ BBs, cholestyramine
colestipol, estrogens, resins, rifampin, thiazide diuretics **Labs:** ↑ LFTs, BUN, crea
tinine; ↓ Hgb, Hct, WBCs, uric acid

Fenoldopam (Corlopam)   Uses: *Hypertensive emergency* **Action:**
Rapid vasodilator **Dose:** Initial 0.03–0.1 μg/kg/min IV inf, titrate q15min i
0.05–0.1 μg/kg/min increments **Caution:** [B, ?] Hypotension w/ BBs **Contra:** Hy
persensitivity to sulfites **Supplied:** Inj 10 mg/mL **SE:** Hypotension, edema, facia
flushing, N/V/D, atrial flutter/fibrillation, ↑ intraocular pressure **Notes:** ⊘ Concur
rent BBs **Interactions:** ↑ Effects w/ acetaminophen ↑ hypotension w/ BBs **Labs**
↑ Serum urea nitrogen, creatinine, LFTs, LDH; ↑ K⁺

Fenoprofen (Nalfon)   Uses: *Arthritis & pain* **Action:** NSAID **Dose**
200–600 mg q4–8h, to 3200 mg/d max; take w/ food **Caution:** [B (D 3rd tri), +/–
CHF, HTN, renal/hepatic impairment, Hx PUD **Contra:** NSAID sensitivity **Sup
plied:** Caps 200, 300 mg; tabs 600 mg **SE:** GI disturbance, dizziness, HA, rash
edema, renal impairment, hepatitis **Notes:** Take w/ food, swallow whole **Interac
tions:** ↑ Effects w/ ASA, anticoagulants; ↑ hyperkalemia w/ K-sparing diuretics;

ffects of aminoglycoside, anticoagulants, Li, MRX, phenytoin, sulfonamides, sulonylureas; ↓ effects w/ phenobarbital; ↓ effects of antihypertensives **Labs:** False free and total T_3 levels, false + urine barbiturates & benzodiazepines; ↑ serum Na & Cl **NIPE:** ⊘ ASA, EtOH, OTC drugs

entanyl (Sublimaze) [C-II] Uses: *Short-acting analgesic* in anesthesia & PCA **Action:** Narcotic analgesic **Dose:** *Adults.* 25–100 μg/kg/dose IV/IM ttrated to effect. *Peds.* 1–2 μg/kg IV/IM q1–4h titrated to effect; ↓ in renal impairnent **Caution:** [B, +] ↑d ICP, resp depression, severe renal/hepatic imairment **Supplied:** Inj 0.05 mg/mL **SE:** Sedation, hypotension, bradycardia, onstipation, nausea, resp depression, miosis **Notes:** 0.1 mg of fentanyl = 10 mg of orphine IM **Interactions:** ↑ Effects w/ CNS depressants, cimetidine, phenothazines, ritonavir, TCAs, EtOH, grapefruit juice; ↑ risks of HTN crisis w/ MAOIs; ∕ effects w/ buprenorphine, dezocine, nalbuphine, pentazocine **Labs:** False ↑ erum amylase, lipase

entanyl, Transdermal (Duragesic) [C-II] Uses: *Chronic pain* **Action:** Narcotic **Dose:** Apply patch to upper torso q72h; dose calculated from arcotic requirements in previous 24 h; ↓ in renal impairment **Caution:** [B, +] **Contra:** ↑ ICP, resp depression, severe renal/hepatic impairment **Supplied:** TD atches 25, 50, 75, 100 μg/h **SE:** Sedation, ↓ BP, bradycardia, constipation, nauea, resp depression, miosis **Notes:** 0.1 mg of fentanyl = 10 mg of morphine IM. ee Fentanyl. **NIPE:** ↑ Risk of ↑ absorption w/ elevated temperature; cleanse skin nly w/ water, ⊘ soap, lotions, or EtOH because they may ↑ absorption; ⊘ use in hildren <110 lb

entanyl, Transmucosal System (Actiq) [C-II] Uses: *Induction f anesthesia; breakthrough CA pain* **Action:** Narcotic analgesic **Dose:** *Adults.* Anesthesia: 5–15 μg/kg. *Pain:* 200 μg over 15 min, titrate to effect; ↓ in renal imairment **Caution:** [B, +] **Contra:** ↑ ICP, resp depression, severe renal/hepatic imairment **Supplied:** Lozenges on stick 200, 400, 600, 800, 1200, 1600 μg **SE:** ;edation, ↓ BP, bradycardia, constipation, nausea, resp depression, miosis **Notes:**).1 mg of fentanyl = 10 mg of morphine IM See Fentanyl. **Additional NIPE:** ⊘ Jse for children <33 lb and <2 y old

errous Gluconate (Fergon) Uses: *Fe deficiency anemia* & Fe suppl **Action:** Dietary suppl **Dose:** *Adults.* 100–200 mg of elemental Fe/d ÷ doses. *Peds.* 4–6 mg/kg/d ÷ doses; take on empty stomach (OK w/ meals if GI upset occurs); ⊘ antacids **Caution:** [A, ?] **Contra:** Hemochromatosis, hemolytic anemia **Supplied:** Tabs 300 (34 mg Fe), 325 mg (36 mg Fe) **SE:** GI upset, constipation, dark stools, discoloration of urine, may stain teeth **Notes:** 12% elemental Fe **Interactions:** ↑ Effects w/ chloramphenicol, citrus fruits or juices; ↓ effects w/ antacids, cimetidine, black cohosh, chamomile, feverfew, gossypol, hawthorn, nettle, plantain, St. John's wort, whole-grain breads, cheese, eggs, milk, coffee, tea, yogurt; ↓ effects of fluoroquinolones, levodopa **Labs:** False + guaiac test **NIPE:** ⊘ Antacids, tetracyclines, take liq form in liquids and through a straw to prevent teeth staining

Ferrous Gluconate Complex (Ferrlecit) Uses: *Fe deficiency ar mia or suppl to erythropoietin therapy* **Action:** Suppl Fe **Dose:** Test dose: 2 m (25 mg Fe) infused over 1 h. If no Rxn, 125 mg (10 mL) IV over 1 h. Usual cum lative dose 1 g Fe over 8 sessions (until favorable Hct achieved) **Caution:** [B, **Contra:** Anemia not caused by Fe deficiency; CHF; Fe overload **Supplied:** 12.5 mg/mL Fe **SE:** Hypotension, serious hypersensitivity Rxns, GI disturbanc inj site Rxn **Notes:** Dose expressed as mg Fe; may be infused during dialysis. S Ferrous Gluconate

Ferrous Sulfate Uses: *Fe deficiency anemia & Fe suppl* **Action:** Dieta suppl**Dose:** *Adults.* 100–200 mg of elemental Fe/d in ÷ doses. *Peds.* 1–6 mg/kg/d daily–tid; take on empty stomach (OK w/ meals if GI upset occurs); ⊗ antaci **Caution:** [A, ?] ↑ absorption w/ vitamin C; ↓ absorption w/ tetracycline, fluor quinolones, antacids, H₂ blockers, proton pump inhibitors **Contra:** Hemochr matosis, hemolytic anemia **Supplied:** Tabs 187 (60 mg Fe), 200 (65 mg Fe), 32 (65 mg Fe), 325 mg (65 mg Fe); SR caplets & tabs 160 mg (50 mg Fe), 200 mg (6 mg Fe); gtt 75 mg/0.6 mL (15 mg Fe/0.6 mL); elixir 220 mg/5 mL (44 mg Fe mL); syrup 90 mg/5 mL (18 mg Fe/5 mL) **SE:** GI upset, constipation, dark stoo discolored urine. See Ferrous Gluconate

Fexofenadine (Allegra, Allegra-D) Uses: *Allergic rhinitis* **Actio** Antihistamine **Dose:** *Adults & Peds.* >12 y. 60 mg PO bid or 180 mg/d; ↓ in ren impairment **Caution:** [C, ?] **Contra:** Component sensitivity **Supplied:** Caps 6 mg; tabs 30, 60, 180 mg; Allegra-D (60 mg fexofenadine/120 mg pse doephedrine) **SE:** Drowsiness (uncommon) **Interactions:** ↑ Effects w/ er thromycin, ketoconazole; ↓ effects w/ antacids **NIPE:** ⊗ EtOH or CN depressants

Filgrastim [G-CSF] (Neupogen) Uses: *↓ Incidence of infection febrile neutropenic Pts; Rx chronic neutropenia* **Action:** Recombinant G-CS **Dose:** *Adults & Peds.* 5 μg/kg/d SQ or IV single daily dose; DC therapy whe ANC >10,000 **Caution:** [C, ?] Drug interactions w/ drugs that potentiate release neutrophils (eg, Li) **Contra:** Hypersensitivity to *E. coli*-derived proteins or G-CS **Supplied:** Inj 300 μg/mL **SE:** Fever, alopecia, N/V/D, splenomegaly, bone pai HA, rash **Notes:** Monitor CBC & plt; monitor for cardiac events; no benefit w ANC >10,000/mm³ **Interactions:** ↑ Interference w/ cytotoxic drugs; ↑ release neutrophils w/ Li **NIPE:** Monitor CBC & plts

Finasteride (Proscar, Propecia) Uses: *BPH & androgenet alopecia* **Action:** Inhibits 5α-reductase **Dose:** *BPH:* 5 mg/d PO. *Alopecia:* 1 mg PO; food may reduce absorption **Caution:** [X, –] Caution in hepatic impairme **Contra:** PRG women should ⊗ handling pills **Supplied:** Tabs 1 mg (Propecia), mg (Proscar) **SE:** ↓ PSA levels; ↓ libido, impotence (rare) **Notes:** Reestablish PS baseline at 6 mo; 3–6 mo for effect on urinary Sxs; continue therapy to maintai new hair **Interactions:** ↑ Effects w/ saw palmetto; ↓ effects w/ anticholinergic adrenergic bronchodilators, theophylline

lavoxate (Urispas) Uses: *Symptomatic relief of dysuria, urgency, nocuria, suprapubic pain, urinary frequency, & incontinence* **Action:** Antispasmodic **Dose:** 100–200 mg PO tid–qid **Caution:** [B, ?] **Contra:** Pyloric or duodenal obstruction, GI hemorrhage, GI obstruction, ileus, achalasia, BPH **Supplied:** Tabs 100 mg **SE:** Drowsiness, blurred vision, xerostomia **Interactions:** ↑ Effects of CNS depressants **NIPE:** ↑ Risk of heat stroke w/ exercise and in hot weather

lecainide (Tambocor) Uses: *Prevent AF/flutter & PSVT, *prevent/suppress life-threatening ventricular arrhythmias* **Action:** Class 1C antiarrhythmic **Dose:** *Adults.* 100 mg PO q12h; ↑ by 50 mg q12h q4d to max 400 mg/d. *Peds.* 3–6 mg/kg/d in 3 ÷ doses; ↓ in renal impairment, monitor in hepatic impairment **Caution:** [C, +] ↑ conc w/ amiodarone, digoxin, quinidine, ritonavir/amprenavir, BB, verapamil **Contra:** 2nd-/3rd-degree AV block, RBBB w/ bifascicular or trifascicular block, cardiogenic shock, CAD, ritonavir/amprenavir, alkalinizing agents **Supplied:** Tabs 50, 100, 150 mg **SE:** Dizziness, visual disturbances, dyspnea, palpitations, edema, tachycardia, CHF, HA, fatigue, rash, nausea **Notes:** May cause new/worsened arrhythmias; initiate Rx in hospital; dose q8h if Pt is intolerant/condition is uncontrolled at 12-h intervals **Interactions:** ↑ Effects w/ alkalinizing drugs, amiodarone, cimetidine, propranolol, quinidine; ↑ effects of digoxin; ↑ risk of arrhythmias w/ CCBs, antiarrhythmics, disopyramide; ↓ effects w/ acidifying drugs, tobacco **Labs:** ↑ Alkaline phosphatase **NIPE:** Full effects may take 3–5 d

Floxuridine (FUDR) Uses: *GI adenoma, liver, renal cell carcinoma*; colon & pancreatic CAs **Action:** Inhibitor of thymidylate synthase; interferes w/ DNA synthesis (S-phase specific) **Dose:** 0.1–0.6 mg/kg/d for 1–6 wk (refer to specific protocols) **Caution:** [D, –] Drug intoxication w/ live & rotavirus vaccine **Contra:** Bone marrow suppression, poor nutritional status, potentially serious infection **Supplied:** Inj 500 mg **SE:** Myelosuppression, anorexia, abdominal cramps, N/V/D, mucositis, alopecia, skin rash, & hyperpigmentation; rare neurotoxicity (blurred vision, depression, nystagmus, vertigo, & lethargy); intraarterial catheter-related problems (ischemia, thrombosis, bleeding, & infection) **Notes:** Need effective birth control; palliative Rx for inoperable/incurable Pts **Interactions:** ↑ Effects w/ metronidazole **Labs:** ↑ LFTs, 5-HIAA urine excretion; ↓ plasma albumin **NIPE:** ↑ Risk of photosensitivity—use sunscreen

Fluconazole (Diflucan) Uses: *Candidiasis (esophageal, oropharyngeal, urinary tract, vaginal, prophylaxis); cryptococcal meningitis* **Action:** Antifungal; inhibits fungal cytochrome P-450 sterol demethylation. *Spectrum:* All *Candida* sp except *C. krusei* **Dose:** *Adults.* 100–400 mg/d PO or IV. *Vaginitis:* 150 mg PO daily. *Cryptococcal meningitis:* 400 mg day 1, then 200 mg × 10–12 wk after CSF (–). *Peds.* 3–6 mg/kg/d PO or IV; ↓ in renal impairment **Caution:** [C, –] **Contra:** Use w/ terfenadine **Supplied:** Tabs 50, 100, 150, 200 mg; susp 10, 40 mg/mL; inj 2 mg/mL **SE:** HA, rash, GI upset, hypokalemia, ↑ LFTs **Notes:** PO use produces the same blood levels as IV; PO preferred when possible **Interactions:** ↑ Effects w/ HCTZ, benzodiazepines, anticoagulants; ↑ effects of amitriptyline, carbamazepine, cyclosporine, hypoglycemics, losartan, methadone, phenytoin, quinidine, tacrolimus, TCAs, theophylline, caffeine, zidovudine; ↓ effects w/ cimetidine, rifampin **Labs:** ↑ LFTs

Fludarabine Phosphate (Flamp, Fludara) **Uses:** *Autoimmune hemolytic anemia, CLL, cold agglutinin hemolysis,* low-grade lymphoma, mycosis fungoides **Action:** Inhibits ribonucleotide reductase; blocks DNA polymerase-induced DNA repair **Dose:** 18–30 mg/m²/d for 5 d, as a 30-min inf (refer to specific protocols) **Caution:** [D, –] Give cytarabine before fludarabine (↓ its metabolism) **Contra:** Severe infections **Supplied:** Inj 50 mg **SE:** Myelosuppression, N/V/D, LFT, edema, CHF, fever, chills, fatigue, dyspnea, nonproductive cough, pneumonitis, severe CNS toxicity rare in leukemia **Notes:** ⊘ in CrCl <30 mL/min **Interactions:** ↑ Effects w/ other myelosuppressive drugs; ↑ risk of pulmonary effects w/ pentostatin **NIPE:** May take several weeks for full effect, use barrier contraception

Fludrocortisone Acetate (Florinef) **Uses:** *Adrenocortical insufficiency, Addison's Dz, salt-wasting syndrome* **Action:** Mineralocorticoid replacement **Dose:** *Adults.* 0.1–0.2 mg/d PO. *Peds.* 0.05–0.1 mg/d PO **Caution:** [C, ?] **Contra:** Systemic fungal infections; known hypersensitivity **Supplied:** Tabs 0.1 mg **SE:** HTN, edema, CHF, HA, dizziness, convulsions, acne, rash, bruising, hyperglycemia, HPA suppression, cataracts **Notes:** For adrenal insufficiency, must use w/ glucocorticoid suppl; dosage changes based on plasma renin activity **Interactions:** ↑ Risk of hypokalemia w/ amphotericin B, thiazide diuretics, loop diuretics; ↓ effects w/ rifampin, barbiturates, hydantoins; ↓ effects of ASA, INH **Labs:** ↑ Serum K⁺ **NIPE:** Eval for fluid retention

Flumazenil (Romazicon) **Uses:** *Reverse sedative effects of benzodiazepines & general anesthesia* **Action:** Benzodiazepine receptor antagonist **Dose:** *Adults.* 0.2 mg IV over 15 s; repeat PRN, to 1 mg max (3 mg max in benzodiazepine OD). *Peds.* 0.01 mg/kg (0.2 mg/dose max) IV over 15 s; repeat 0.005 mg/kg at 1-min intervals to max 1 mg total; ↓ in hepatic impairment **Caution:** [C, ?] **Contra:** In TCA OD; if Pts given benzodiazepines to control life-threatening conditions (ICP/status epilepticus) **Supplied:** Inj 0.1 mg/mL **SE:** N/V, palpitations, HA, anxiety, nervousness, hot flashes, tremor, blurred vision, dyspnea, hyperventilation, withdrawal syndrome **Notes:** Does not reverse narcotic Sx or amnesia **Interactions:** ↑ Risk of Szs and arrhythmias when benzodiazepine action is reduced **NIPE:** Food given during IV administration will reduce drug serum level

Flunisolide (AeroBid, Nasalide) **Uses:** *Bronchial asthma in Pts requiring chronic steroid therapy; relief of seasonal/perennial allergic rhinitis* **Action:** Topical steroid **Dose:** *Adults.* Met-dose inhal: 2 inhal bid (max 8/d). *Nasal:* 2 sprays/nostril bid (max 8/d). *Peds.* >6 y. *Met-dose inhal:* 2 inhal bid (max 4/d). *Nasal:* 1–2 sprays/nostril bid (max 4/d) **Caution:** [C, ?] **Contra:** Status asthmaticus **Supplied:** Aerosol 250 mg/actuation; nasal spray 0.025% **SE:** tachycardia, bitter taste, local effects, oral candidiasis **Notes:** Not for acute asthma **NIPE:** Shake well before use

Fluorouracil [5-FU] (Adrucil) Uses: *Colorectal, gastric, pancreatic, reast, basal cell,* head, neck, bladder, CAs* **Action:** Inhibitor of thymidylate syn-hetase (interferes w/ DNA synthesis, S-phase specific) **Dose:** 370–1000 mg/m²/d or 1–5 d IV push to 24-h cont inf; protracted venous inf of 200–300 mg/m²/d refer to specific protocol) **Caution:** [D, ?] ↑ toxicity w/ allopurinol; ⊘ give MRX efore 5-FU **Contra:** Poor nutritional status, depressed bone marrow Fxn, throm-ocytopenia, major surgery w/in past mo, DPD enzyme deficiency, PRG, serious nfection, bilirubin >5 mg/dL **Supplied:** Inj 50 mg/mL **SE:** Stomatitis, sophagopharyngitis, N/V/D, anorexia, myelosuppression (leukocytopenia, throm-ocytopenia, & anemia), rash/dry skin/photosensitivity, tingling in hands/feet v/pain (palmar–plantar erythrodysesthesia), phlebitis/discoloration at inj sites Notes: ↑ thiamine intake; sun sensitivity; daily doses > 800 mg ⊘ **Interactions:** ↑ ffects w/ leucovorin, Ca **Labs:** ↑ LFTs **NIPE:** ⊘ EtOH, ↑ risk of photosensitiv-ty—use sunscreen, ↑ fluids 2–3 L/d, use barrier contraception

Fluorouracil, Topical [5-FU] (Efudex) Uses: *Basal cell carcinoma; ctinic/solar keratosis* **Action:** Inhibitor of thymidylate synthetase (inhibits DNA ynthesis, S-phase specific) **Dose:** Apply 5% cream bid × 3–6 wk **Caution:** [D, ?] rritant chemotherapy **Contra:** Component sensitivity **Supplied:** Cream 1, 5%; oln 1, 2, 5% **SE:** Rash, dry skin, photosensitivity **Notes:** Complete healing may ot be evident for 1–2 mo; ⊘ overuse. See Fluorouracil. **Additional NIPE:** ⊘ Use cclusive dressing; wash hands immediately after application

Fluoxetine (Prozac, Sarafem) WARNING: Closely monitor for wors-ning depression or emergence of suicidality, particularly in pediatric Pts Uses: *Depression, OCD, panic disorder, bulimia, PMDD* (Sarafem) **Action:** SSRI Dose: 20 mg/d PO (max 80 mg ÷); weekly regimen 90 mg/wk after 1–2 wk of tandard dose. *Bulimia:* 60 mg q AM. *Panic disorder:* 20 mg/d. *OCD:* 20–80 mg/d. PMDD: 20 mg/d or 20 mg intermittently starting 14 d prior to menses, repeat w/ ach cycle; ↓ dose in hepatic failure **Caution:** [B, ?/–] Risk of serotonin syndrome v/ MAOI, SSRI, serotonin agonists, linezolid; risk of QT prolongation w/ phenoth-azines **Contra:** MAOI/thioridazine (wait 5 wk after DC before starting MAOI) **Supplied:** *Prozac:* Caps 10, 20, 40 mg; scored tabs 10 mg; SR cap 90 mg; soln 20 ng/5 mL. *Sarafem:* Caps 10, 20 mg **SE:** Nausea, nervousness, weight loss, HA, in-omnia **Interactions:** ↑ Effects w/ CNS depressants, MAOIs, EtOH, St. John's vort; ↑ effects of alprazolam, BBs, carbamazepine, clozapine, cardiac glycosides, iazepam, dextromethorphan, loop diuretics, haloperidol, phenytoin, Li, ritonavir, hioridazine, tryptophan, warfarin, sympathomimetic drugs; ↓ effects w/ cyprohep-adine; ↓ effects of buspirone, statins **Labs:** ↑ LFTs, BUN, creatinine, urine albu-nin **NIPE:** Stop MAOIs 14 d before start of this drug

Fluoxymesterone (Halotestin) Uses: *Androgen-responsive metastatic breast CA, hypogonadism* **Action:** Inhibits secretion of LH & FSH by feedback nhibition **Dose:** *Breast CA:* 10–40 mg/d ÷ × 1–3 mo *Hypogonadism:* 5–20 mg/d Caution: [X, ?/–] ↑ effect w/ anticoagulants, cyclosporine, insulin, Li, narcotics

Contra: Serious cardiac, liver, or kidney Dz; PRG **Supplied:** Tabs 2, 5, 10 mg S█ Virilization, amenorrhea & menstrual irregularities, hirsutism, alopecia, acne, na sea, & cholestasis. *Hematologic toxicity:* Suppression of clotting factors II, V, V▪ & X & polycythemia; ↑ libido, HA, & anxiety **Notes:** ↓ total T₄ levels **Intera tions:** ↑ Effects w/ narcotics, EtOH, echinacea; ↑ effects of anticoagulants, c closporine, insulin, hypoglycemics, tacrolimus; ↓ effects w/ anticholinergic barbiturates **Labs:** ↑ Creatinine, creatinine clearance; ↓ thyroxine-binding glob lin, serum total T₄ **NIPE:** Radiographic studies of skeletal maturation (hand/wris q6mo in prepubertal children; monitor fluid retention

Fluphenazine (Prolixin, Permitil) **Uses:** *Schizophrenia* **Actio** Phenothiazine antipsychotic; blocks postsynaptic mesolimbic dopaminergic bra receptors **Dose:** 0.5–10 mg/d in ÷ doses PO q6–8h, average maint 5 mg/d; or 1.2 mg IM, then 2.5–10 mg/d in ÷ doses q6–8h PRN; ↓ dose in elderly **Caution:** [(?/–] **Contra:** Severe CNS depression, coma, subcortical brain damage, bloc dyscrasias, hepatic Dz **Supplied:** Tabs 1, 2.5, 5, 10 mg; conc 5 mg/mL; elixir 2 mg/5 mL; inj 2.5 mg/mL; depot inj 25 mg/mL **SE:** Drowsiness, extrapyramidal e fects **Notes:** Monitor LFTs; less sedative/hypotensive than chlorpromazine; ⊘ a minister conc w/ caffeine, tannic acid, or pectin-containing products **Interactions** ↑ Effects w/ antimalarials, BBs, CNS depressants, EtOH, kava kava; ↑ effects anticholinergics, BBs, nitrates; ↓ effects w/ antacids, caffeine, tobacco; ↓ effects anticonvulsants, guanethidine, levodopa, sympathomimetics **Labs:** False + urit PRG test; ↑ serum cholesterol, glucose, LFTs, ↓ uric acid **NIPE:** Photosensiti ity—use sunscreen, urine may turn pink or red in color, ↑ risk of heatstroke in h weather

Flurazepam (Dalmane) [C-IV] **Uses:** *Insomnia* **Action:** Benzo▢ azepine **Dose:** *Adults & Peds.* >15 y. 15–30 mg PO qhs PRN; ↓ in elderly **Cau tion:** [X, ?/–] Caution in elderly, low albumin, hepatic impairment **Contra** Narrow-angle glaucoma; PRG **Supplied:** Caps 15, 30 mg **SE:** "Hangover" due accumulation of metabolites, apnea **Notes:** May cause dependency

Flurbiprofen (Ansaid) **Uses:** *Arthritis* **Action:** NSAID **Dose:** 50–3█ mg/d ÷ bid–qid, max 300 mg/d **Caution:** [B (D in 3rd tri), +] **Contra:** PRG (3r tri); ASA allergy **Supplied:** Tabs 50, 100 mg **SE:** Dizziness, GI upset, peptic ulce Dz **Notes:** Take w/ food to ↓ GI upset **Interactions:** ↑ Effects w/ amprenavir, ant▪ convulsants, azole antifungals, BBs, CNS depressants, cimetidine, ciprofloxi▪ clozapine, digoxin, disulfiram, diltiazem, INH, levodopa, macrolides, oral contra ceptives, rifampin, ritonavir, SSRIs, valproic acid, verapamil, EtOH, grapefru▪ juice, kava kava, valerian; ↓ effects w/ aminophylline, carbamazepine, rifampin, r▪ fabutin, theophylline; ? ↓ effects of levodopa **Labs:** ↑ LFTs, false − urine glucos▪ **NIPE:** ⊘ PRG, breast-feeding

Flutamide (Eulexin) **WARNING:** Liver failure & death reported. Measur▪ LFT before, monthly, & periodically after; DC immediately if ALT 2× upper limi of normal or jaundice develops **Uses:** Advanced *CAP* (in combination w/ LHR▨

gonists, (eg, leuprolide or goserelin); w/ radiation & GnRH for localized CAP **Action:** Nonsteroidal antiandrogen **Dose:** 250 mg PO tid (750 mg total) **Caution:** [D, – Contra:** Severe hepatic impairment **Supplied:** Caps 125 mg **SE:** Hot flashes, ess of libido, impotence, diarrhea, N/V, gynecomastia **Interactions:** ↑ Effects w/ nticoagulants **Labs:** ↑ LFTs, BUN **NIPE:** Urine amber/yellow-green in color

luticasone, Nasal (Flonase) **Uses:** *Seasonal allergic rhinitis* **Action:** Topical steroid **Dose:** *Adults & Adolescents.* Nasal: 2 sprays/nostril/d. *Peds.* -11 y. Nasal: 1–2 sprays/nostril/d **Caution:** [C, M] **Contra:** Primary Rx of status thmaticus **Supplied:** Nasal spray 50 μg/actuation **SE:** HA, dysphonia, oral candiasis **Interactions:** ↑ Effects w/ ketoconazole **Labs:** ↑ Cholesterol **NIPE:** Clear ares of exudate before use

luticasone, Oral (Flovent, Flovent Rotadisk) **Uses:** Chronic asthma* **Action:** Topical steroid **Dose:** *Adults & Adolescents.* 2–4 puffs bid. *eds.* 4–11 y. 50 μg bid **Caution:** [C, M] **Contra:** Primary Rx of status asthmati-s **Supplied:** Met-dose inhal 44, 110, 220 μg/activation; Rotadisk dry powder: 0, 100, 250 μg/activation **SE:** HA, dysphonia, oral candidiasis **Notes:** Risk of rush; counsel Pts on use of device **Interactions:** ↑ Effects w/ ketoconazole **abs:** ↑ Cholesterol **NIPE:** Rinse mouth after use, ⊘ & report exposure to easles & chickenpox

luticasone Propionate & Salmeterol Xinafoate (Advair iskus) **Uses:** *Maint therapy for asthma* **Action:** Corticosteroid w/ long-act-g bronchodilator **Dose:** *Adults & Peds.* >12 y. 1 inhal bid q 12 h **Caution:** [C, M] **ontra:** Not for acute attack or in conversion from PO steroids; status asthmaticus **upplied:** Met-dose inhal powder(fluticasone/salmeterol in μg) 100/50, 250/50, 00/50 **SE:** Upper resp infection, pharyngitis, HA **Notes:** Combination of Flovent & Serevent; ⊘ use w/ spacer, ⊘ wash mouthpiece, ⊘ exhale into device **Interac-ons:** ↑ Bronchospasm w/ BBs; ↑ hypokalemia w/ loop and thiazide diuretics; ↑ ffects w/ ketoconazole, MAOIs, TCAs **Labs:** ↑ Cholesterol **NIPE:** ⊘ & report xposure to measles & chickenpox, rinse mouth after use

luvastatin (Lescol) **Uses:** *Atherosclerosis, primary hyperchole-rolemia, hypertriglyceridemia* **Action:** HMG-CoA reductase inhibitor **Dose:** 0–80 mg PO qhs; ↓ dose w/ hepatic impairment **Caution:** [X, –] **Contra:** Active ver Dz, ↑ LFTs, PRG, breast-feeding **Supplied:** Caps 20, 40 mg; XL 80 mg **SE:** A, dyspepsia, nausea, diarrhea, abdominal pain **Interactions:** ↑ Effects w/ azole ntifungals, cimetidine, danazol, glyburide, macrolides, phenytoin, ritonavir, tOH, grapefruit juice; ↑ effects of diclofenac, glyburide, phenytoin, warfarin; ↓ ffects w/ cholestyramine, colestipol, isradipine, rifampin **Labs:** ↑ LFTs, CPK, yroid Fxn **NIPE:** Take hs, ↑ photosensitivity—use sunscreen

luvoxamine (Luvox) **WARNING:** Closely monitor for worsening de-ression or emergence of suicidality, particularly in pediatric Pts **Uses:** *OCD* **Ac-on:** SSRI **Dose:** Initial 50 mg as single qhs dose, ↑ to 300 mg/d in ÷ doses; ↓ ose in elderly/hepatic impairment, titrate slowly **Caution:** [C, ?/–] Numerous in-

teractions (MAOIs, phenothiazines, SSRIs, serotonin agonists) Supplied: Tabs
50, 100 mg SE: HA, nausea, diarrhea, somnolence, insomnia Notes: ÷ doses >1
mg Interactions: ↑ Effects w/ melatonin, MAOIs; ↑ effects of BBs, benzo
azepines, methadone, carbamazepine, haloperidol, Li, phenytoin, TCAs, the
phylline, warfarin, St. John's wort; ↑ risks of serotonin syndrome w/ buspiro
dexfenfluramine, fenfluramine, tramadol, nefazodone, sibutramine, tryptophan;
effects w/ buspirone, cyproheptadine, tobacco; ↓ effects of buspirone, HMG-C
reductase inhibitors NIPE: ⊘ MAOIs for 14 d before start of drug; ⊘ EtOH

Folic Acid Uses: *Megaloblastic anemia; folate deficiency* Action: Dieta
suppl Dose: *Adults.* Suppl: 0.4 mg/d PO. *PRG:* 0.8 mg/d PO. *Folate deficiency.*
mg PO daily–tid. *Peds.* Suppl: 0.04–0.4 mg/24 h PO, IM, IV, or SQ. *Folate de
ciency:* 0.5–1 mg/24 h PO, IM, IV, or SQ Caution: [A, +] Contra: Pernicio
aplastic, normocytic anemias Supplied: Tabs 0.4, 0.8, 1 mg; inj 5 mg/mL SE: W
tolerated Notes: Recommended for all women of childbearing age; ↓ fetal neu
tube defects by 50%; no effect on normocytic anemias Interactions: ↓ Effects
anticonvulsants, sulfasalazine, aminosalicyclic acid, chloramphenicol, MRX, o
contraceptives, pyrimethamine, triamterene, trimethoprim; ↓ effects of phenobar
tal, phenytoin

Fondaparinux (Arixtra) WARNING: When epidural/spinal anesthe
or spinal puncture is used, Pts anticoagulated or scheduled to be anticoagulate
LMW heparins, heparinoids, or fondaparinux for prevention of thromboembo
complications are at risk for epidural or spinal hematoma, which can result in lon
term or permanent paralysis Uses: *DVT prophylaxis* in hip fracture or replac
ment or knee replacement Action: Synthetic, specific inhibitor of activated fac
X; an LMW heparin Dose: 2.5 mg SQ daily, up to 5–9 d; start at least 6 h post
Caution: [B, ?] ↑ bleeding risk w/ anticoagulants, antiplts, drotrecogin al
NSAIDs Contra: Wt <50 kg, CrCl <30 mL/min, active bleeding, bacterial end
carditis, thrombocytopenia associated w/ antiplt antibody Supplied: Prefilled s
ringes 2.5 mg/0.5mL SE: Thrombocytopenia, anemia, fever, nausea Notes: DC
plts <100,000 mm³; only give SQ; may monitor anti-factor Xa levels Interaction
↑ Effects w/ anticoagulants, cephalosporins, NSAIDs, penicillins, salicylat
Labs: ↑ LFTs

Formoterol (Foradil Aerolizer) Uses: Maint Rx of *asthma & preve
tion of bronchospasm* w/ reversible obstructive airway Dz; exercise-induced bro
chospasm Action: Long-acting β₂-adrenergic agonist, bronchodilator Dose: *Adu
& Peds.* >5 y. Asthma: Inhale one 12-μg cap q12h w/ aerolizer, 24 μg/d ma
Adults & Peds. > 12 y. Exercise-induced bronchospasm: 1 inhal 12-μg cap 15 m
before exercise Caution: [C, ?] Contra: Need for acute bronchodilation; use w
2 wk of MAOI Supplied: 12-μg blister pack for use in aerolizer SE: Paradoxic
bronchospasm; URI, pharyngitis, back pain Notes: ⊘ swallow caps—for use or
w/ inhaler; ⊘ start w/ significantly worsening or acutely deteriorating asthm
which may be life-threatening Interactions: ↑ Effects w/ adrenergics; ↑ effects

Bs; ↑ risk of hypokalemia w/ corticosteroids, diuretics, xanthines; ↑ risk of arythmias w/ MAOIs, TCAs

osamprenavir (Lexiva) **WARNING:** ⊘ Use w/ severe liver dysfunction, duce dose w/ mild–moderate liver impairment (fosamprenavir 700 mg bid **w/o** ritonir) **Uses:** HIV infection **Action:** Protease inhibitor **Dose:** 1400 mg bid w/o ritonavir; given w/ ritonavir, fosamprenavir 1400 mg + ritonavir 200 mg qd or fosamprenavir 0 mg + ritonavir 100 mg bid. If given w/ efavirenz & ritonavir, then fosamprenavir 400 mg + ritonavir 300 mg qd **Caution:** [C, ?/–]; **Contra:** Cannot be given w/ ergot kaloids, midazolam, triazolam, or pimozide; ⊘ if sulfa allergy **Supplied:** Tabs 700 g **SE:** N/V/D, HA, fatigue, rash **Notes:** Numerous drug interactions because of hetic metabolism **Interactions:** ↑ Effects with indinavir, nelfinavir; ↑ effects of antiarythmics, amitriptyline, atorvastatin, benzodiazepine, bepridil, CCBs, cyclosporine, gotamine, ethinyl estradiol, imipramine, itraconazole, ketoconazole, midazolam, orethindrone, rapamycin, rifabutin, sildenafil, tacrolimus, TCA, vardenafil, warfarin; effects with antacids, carbamazepine, dexamethasone, didanosine, efavirenz, H₂-reptor antagonists, nevirapine, phenobarbital, phenytoin, proton pump inhibitors, rimpin St. John's wort; ↓ effects of methadone; **Labs:** ↑ ALT, AST, triglycerides, ucose, lipase **NIPE:** Take w/o regard to food, use barrier contraception, monitor for oportunistic infection, inform about fat redistribution/accumulation

oscarnet (Foscavir) **Uses:** *CMV retinitis*; acyclovir-resistant *herpes* fections* **Action:** Inhibits viral DNA polymerase & RT **Dose:** *CMV retinitis: Induction:* 60 mg/kg IV q8hr or 100 mg/kg q12h × 14–21 d. *Maint:* 90–120 mg/kg/d V (Monday–Friday). *Acyclovir-resistant HSV induction:* 40 mg/kg IV q8–12h × 4–21 d; ↓ w/ renal impairment **Caution:** [C, –] ↑ Sz potential w/ flouroinolones; ⊘ nephrotoxic Rx (cyclosporine, aminoglycosides, ampho B, protease hibitors) **Contra:** Significant renal impairment (CrCl <0.4 mL/min/kg) **Suplied:** Inj 24 mg/mL **SE:** Nephrotoxicity, causes electrolyte abnormalities **Notes:** la loading (500 mL 0.9% NaCl) before & after helps minimize nephrotoxicity; onitor ionized Ca; administer through central line **Interactions:** ↑ Risks of Sz w/ uinolones; ↑ risks of nephrotoxicity w/ aminoglycosides, amphotericin B, didanoine, pentamidine, vancomycin **Labs:** ↓ LFTs, CPK, BUN, SCr; ↓ Hmg, Hct, Ca²⁺, g²⁺, K⁺, P **NIPE:** ↑ Fluids; perioral tingling, extremity numbness & paresthesia dicates electrolyte imbalance

osfomycin (Monurol) **Uses:** *Uncomplicated UTI* **Action:** Inhibits acterial cell wall synthesis. **Spectrum:** Gram(+) (staph, pneumococci); gram(–) *E. coli, Enterococcus, Salmonella, Shigella, H. influenzae, Neisseria,* indole-negave *Proteus, Providencia*); *B. fragilis* & anaerobic gram(–) cocci are resistant **ose:** 3 g PO dissolved in 90–120 mL of water single dose; ↓ in renal impairment **aution:** [B, ?] ↓ absorption w/ antacids/Ca salts **Contra:** Component sensitivity **upplied:** Granule packets 3 g **SE:** HA, GI upset **Notes:** May take 2–3 d for Sxs to nprove **Interactions:** ↓ Effects w/ antacids, metoclopramide **Labs:** ↑ LFTs; ↓ mg, Hct **NIPE:** May take w/o regard to food

Fosinopril (Monopril) Uses: *HTN, CHF,* DN Action: ACEI Dose: mg/d PO initial; max 40 mg/d PO; ↓ dose in elderly; ↓ in renal impairment Caution [D, +] ↑ K⁺ w/ K suppls, ARBs, K-sparing diuretics; ↑ renal AE w/ NSAII diuretics, hypovolemia Contra: Hereditary/idiopathic angioedema or angioede. w/ ACEI, bilateral renal artery stenosis Supplied: Tabs 10, 20, 40 mg SE: Nonpr ductive cough, dizziness, angioedema, hyperkalemia Interactions: ↑ Effects antihypertensives, diuretics; ↑ effects of Li; ↑ risk of hyperkalemia w/ K-sparing diuretics, salt substitutes; ↑ cough w/ capsaicin; ↓ effects w/ antacids, AS NSAIDs Labs: ↓ Hmg, Hct NIPE: ⊘ PRG, breast-feeding

Fosphenytoin (Cerebyx) Uses: *Status epilepticus* Action: Inhibits spread in motor cortex Dose: Dosed as phenytoin equivalents (PE). Load: 15– mg PE/kg. Maint: 4–6 mg PE/kg/d; ↓ dosage monitor levels in hepatic impairme Caution: [D, +] May ↑ phenobarbital Contra: Sinus bradycardia, SA block, 2r /3rd-degree AV block, Adams–Stokes syndrome, rash during Rx Supplied: Inj mg/mL SE: ↓ BP, dizziness, ataxia, pruritus, nystagmus Notes: 15 min to conve fosphenytoin to phenytoin; admin <150 mg PE/min to prevent hypotension; admi ister w/ BP monitoring Interactions: ↑ Effects w/ amiodarone, chloramphenic cimetidine, diazepam, disulfiram, estrogens, INH, omeprazole, phenothiazines, s icylates, sulfonamides, tolbutamide; ↓ effects w/ TCAs, antituberculosis dru carbamazepine, EtOH, nutritional suppls, ginkgo biloba; ↓ effects of anticoag lants, corticosteroids, digitoxin, doxycycline, oral contraceptives, folic acid, Ca, tamin D, rifampin, quinidine, theophylline Labs: ↑ Serum glucose, alkali phosphatase; ↓ serum thyroxine, Ca NIPE: Breast-feeding, for short-term use

Frovatriptan (Frova) See Table 11, page 283

Fulvestrant (Faslodex) Uses: Hormone receptor-+ metastatic *brea CA* in postmenopausal women w/ Dz progression following antiestrogen thera Action: Estrogen receptor antagonist Dose: 250 mg IM monthly, either a single mL inj or two concurrent 2.5-mL IM inj into buttocks Caution: [X, ?/–] ↑ effec w/ CYP3A4 inhibitors (amiodarone, clarithromycin, fluoxetine, grapefruit juic ketoconazole, ritonavir, etc), w/ hepatic impairment Contra: PRG Supplied: Pr filled syringes 50 mg/mL (single 5 mL, dual 2.5 mL) SE: N/V/D, constipation, a dominal pain, HA, back pain, hot flushes, pharyngitis, inj site Rxns Notes: On use IM; caution in hepatic impairment Interactions: ↑ Risk of bleeding w/ antic agulants NIPE: ⊘ PRG, breast-feeding; use barrier contraception

Furosemide (Lasix) Uses: *CHF, HTN, edema,* ascites Action: Loop c uretic; inhibits Na & Cl reabsorption in ascending loop of Henle & distal tubu Dose: Adults. 20–80 mg PO or IV daily bid. Peds. 1 mg/kg/dose IV q6–12h; mg/kg/dose PO q12–24h (max 6 mg/kg/dose) Caution: [C, +] Hypokalemia m ↑ risk of digoxin toxicity; ↑ risk of ototoxicity w/ aminoglycosides, cisplatin (esp in renal dysfunction) Contra: Hypersensitivity to sulfonylureas; anuria; h patic coma/severe electrolyte depletion Supplied: Tabs 20, 40, 80 mg; soln mg/mL, 40 mg/5 mL; inj 10 mg/mL SE: Hypotension, hyperglycemia, h kalemia **Notes:** Monitor electrolytes, renal Fxn; high doses IV may cause oto-xicity **Interactions:** ↑ Nephrotoxic effects w/ cephalosporins; ↑ ototoxicity w/ minoglycosides, cisplatin; ↑ risk of hypokalemia w/ antihypertensives, carbenox-one, corticosteroids, digitalis glycosides, terbutaline; ↓ effects w/ barbiturates, olestyramine, colestipol, NSAIDs, phenytoin, dandelion, ginseng; ↓ effects of poglycemics **Labs:** ↑ BUN, serum amylase, cholesterol, glucose, triglycerides, ic acid, ↓ serum K+, Na+, Ca2+, Mg2+ **NIPE:** Risk of photosensitivity—use sun-

abapentin (Neurontin) **Uses:** Adjunct therapy in the Rx of *partial s; postherpetic neuralgia (PHN)*; chronic pain syndromes **Action:** Anticonvul-nt **Dose:** *Anticonvulsant:* 300–1200 mg PO tid (max 3600 mg/d). *PHN:* 300 mg y 1, 300 mg bid day 2, 300 mg tid day 3, titrate (1800–3600 mg/d); ↓ in renal pairment **Caution:** [C, ?] **Contra:** Component sensitivity **Supplied:** Caps 100, 0, 400 mg; soln 250 mg/5mL; tab 600, 800 mg **SE:** Somnolence, dizziness, axia, fatigue **Notes:** Not necessary to monitor levels **Interactions:** ↑ Effects w/ metidine, CNS depressants; ↑ effects of phenytoin; ↓ effects w/ antacids, ginkgo oba **Labs:** False + urinary protein **NIPE:** Take w/o regard to food

alantamine (Reminyl) **Uses:** *Alzheimer's Dz* **Action:** Acetyl-olinesterase inhibitor **Dose:** 4 mg PO bid, ↑ to 8 mg bid after 4 wk; may ↑ to 12 g bid in 4 wk **Caution:** [B, ?] ↑ effect w/ succinylcholine, amiodarone, dilti-em, verapamil, NSAIDs, digoxin; ↓ effect w/ anticholinergics **Contra:** Severe nal/hepatic impairment **Supplied:** Tabs 4, 8, 12 mg; soln 4 mg/mL **SE:** GI distur-nces, weight loss, sleep disturbances, dizziness, HA **Notes:** Caution w/ urinary tflow obstruction, Parkinson's; severe asthma/COPD, severe heart Dz or hy-otension **Interactions:** ↑ Effects w/ amitriptyline, cimetidine, erythromycin, flu-xetine, fluvoxamine, ketoconazole, paroxetine, quinidine **Labs:** ↑ Alkaline osphatase **NIPE:** ↑ Dosage q4wk, if DC several days then restart at lowest dose; ke w/ food and maintain adequate fluid intake

allium Nitrate (Ganite) **Uses:** *Hypercalcemia of malignancy*; blad-r CA **Action:** Inhibits bone resorption of Ca2+ **Dose:** *Hypercalcemia:* 200 g/m2/day × 5 d. *CA:* 350 mg/m2 cont inf × 5 d to 700 mg/m2 rapid IV inf q2wk in tineoplastic settings (refer to specific protocols) **Caution:** [C, ?] ⊘ give w/ live ccines or rotavirus vaccine **Contra:** SCr >2.5 mg/dL **Supplied:** Inj 25 mg/mL **E:** Renal insufficiency, ↓ Ca2+, hypophosphatemia, <1% acute otic neuritis **Notes:** Bladder CA: use in combination w/ vinblastine & ifosfamide **teractions:** ↑ Risks of nephrotoxicity w/ amphotericin B, aminoglycosides, van-omycin **NIPE:** Monitor SCr, adequate fluids

anciclovir (Cytovene, Vitrasert) **Uses:** *Rx & prevent CMV retini-, prevent CMV Dz* in transplant recipients **Action:** Inhibits viral DNA synthesis ose: *Adults & Peds.* IV: 5 mg/kg IV q12h for 14–21 d, then maint 5 mg/kg/d IV 7 d/wk or 6 mg/kg/d IV × 5 d/wk. *Ocular implant:* One implant q5–8mo. *Adults.* D: Following induction, 1000 mg PO tid. *Prevention:* 1000 mg PO tid; take w/

food; ↓ in renal impairment **Caution:** [C, –] ↑ effect w/ immunosuppressi
imipenem/cilastatin, zidovudine, didanosine, other nephrotoxic Rx **Contra:** N
tropenia (ANC <500), thrombocytopenia (plt <25,000), intravitreal implant **S
plied:** Caps 250, 500 mg; inj 500 mg; ocular implant 4.5 mg **S**
Granulocytopenia & thrombocytopenia, fever, rash, GI upset **Notes:** Not a cure
CMV; inj should be handled w/ cytotoxic cautions; implant confers no syste
benefit **Interactions:** ↑ Effects w/ cytotoxic drugs, immunosuppressive dru
probenecid; ↑ risks of nephrotoxicity w/ amphotericin B, cyclosporine ; ↑ effe
w/ didanosine **Labs:** ↑ LFTs; ↓ blood glucose **NIPE:** Take w/ food, ⊘ PI
breast-feeding, EtOH, NSAIDs; photosensitivity—use sunscreen

Gatifloxacin (Tequin) **Uses:** *Bronchitis, sinusitis, community-acqui
pneumonia, UTI, uncomplicated skin/soft tissue infection* **Action:** Quinolone
tibiotic, inhibits DNA-gyrase. *Spectrum:* Gram(+) (except MRSA, *Lister
gram(–) (not *Pseudomonas*), atypicals, some anaerobes (*Clostridium*, not *C. d
cile*) **Dose:** 400 mg/d PO or IV; ↓ in renal impairment **Caution:** [C, M] **Cont
Prolongation of QT interval, uncorrected hypokalemia, use w/ other Rx that p
long QT interval (Class Ia & III antiarrhythmics, erythromycin, antipsychot
TCA); children <18 y or in PRG/lactating women **Supplied:** Tabs 200, 400 mg;
10 mg/mL; premixed infuse D₅W 200 mg, 400 mg **SE:** Prolonged QT inter
HA, nausea & diarrhea, tendon rupture, photosensitivity **Notes:** Reliable activ
against *S. pneumoniae*; take 4 h after antacids containing Mg, Al, Fe, or Zn a
drink plenty of fluids; ⊘ direct sunlight **Interactions:** ↑ Effects w/ antiarrhy
mics, antipsychotics, cimetidine, erythromycin, loop diuretics, probenecid, TC
↑ CNS effects and Szs w/ NSAIDs; ↓ effects of digoxin, warfarin; ↓ effects
antacids, didanosine, H₂ antagonists, proton pump inhibitors, Fe

Gefitinib (Iressa) **Uses:** *Rx locally advanced or metastatic non-small-c
lung CA after failure of both platinum-based & docetaxel chemotherapies* **Acti
Inhibits intracellular phosphorylation of tyrosine kinases **Dose:** 250 mg/d PO **C
tion:** [D, –] **Supplied:** Tabs 250 mg **SE:** Diarrhea, rash, acne, dry skin, N/V, inter
tial lung Dz, ↑d liver transaminases **Notes:** Follow LFTs **Interactions:** ↑ Effects
ketoconazole, itraconazole, and other CYP3A4 inhibitors; ↑ risk of bleeding w/ w
farin; ↓ effects w/ cimetidine, ranitidine and other H₂ receptor antagonists; ↓ effe
w/ phenytoin, rifampin, and other CYP3A4 inducers **Labs:** ↑ ALT, AST, PT **NII
⊘ PRG or breast-feeding; take w/o regard to food; ↑ risk of corneal erosion/ulcer

Gemcitabine (Gemzar) **Uses:** *Pancreatic CA, brain mets, NSCLC
gastric CA* **Action:** Antimetabolite; inhibits ribonucleotide reductase; produ
false nucleotide base-inhibiting DNA synthesis **Dose:** 1000 mg/m² over 30 mi
h IV inf/wk × 3–4 wk or 6–8 wk; dose modifications based on hematologic F
(refer to specific protocol) **Caution:** [D, ?/–] **Contra:** PRG **Supplied:** Inj 200 m
1 g **SE:** Myelosuppression, N/V/D, drug fever, skin rash **Notes:** Reconstituted s
has concn of 38 mg/mL (not 40 mg/mL as earlier labeling); monitor hepatic
renal Fxn prior & during Rx **Interactions:** ↑ Bone marrow depression w/ radiati

therapy, antineoplastic drugs; ↓ live virus vaccines **Labs:** ↑ LFTs, BUN, SCr **IPE:** ⊘ EtOH, NSAIDs, immunizations, PRG?

Gemfibrozil (Lopid) **Uses:** *Hypertriglyceridemia, coronary heart Dz* **Action:** Fibric acid **Dose:** 1200 mg/d PO ÷ bid 30 min ac AM & PM **Caution:** [C, ?] enhances the effect of warfarin, sulfonylureas; ↑ risk of rhabdomyopathy w/ HMG-CoA reductase inhibitors; ↓ effects w/ cyclosporine **Contra:** Renal/hepatic impairment (SCr >2.0 mg/dL), gallbladder Dz, primary biliary cirrhosis **Supplied:** Tabs 600 mg **SE:** Cholelithiasis, GI upset **Notes:** ⊘ Concurrent use w/ the HMG-CoA reductase inhibitors; monitor LFTs & serum lipids **Interactions:** ↑ Effects of anticoagulants, sulfonylureas; ↓ effects w/ rifampin; ↓ effects of cyclosporine **Labs:** ↑ LFTs, + ANA, ↓ Hmg, Hct, WBCs

Gemtuzumab Ozogamicin (Mylotarg) **WARNING:** Can cause severe hypersensitivity Rxns & other inf-related Rxns including severe pulmonary events; hepatotoxicity, including severe hepatic venoocclusive Dz (VOD) reported **Uses:** *Relapsed CD33+ AML in Pts > 60 who are poor candidates for chemotherapy* **Action:** Monoclonal antibody linked to calicheamicin; selective for myeloid cells **Dose:** Refer to specific protocol **Caution:** [D,?/–] **Contra:** Component sensitivity **Supplied:** 5 mg/20 mL vial **SE:** Myelosuppression, hypersensitivity (including anaphylaxis), inf Rxns (chills, fever, N/V, HA), pulmonary events, hepatotoxicity **Notes:** Only use as single-agent chemo & not in combination w/ other agents; premedicate w/ diphenhydramine & acetaminophen **Interactions:** ↑ Risk for allergic or hypersensitive reaction and thrombocytopenia w/ abciximab; ↓ effects with abciximab **Labs:** Monitor before & after therapy CBC, ALT, AST, electrolytes **NIPE:** Mmonitor for bleeding, myelosuppression, BP; ⊘ ASA, PRG, breast-feeding

Gentamicin (Garamycin, G-Mycitin, others) **Uses:** *Serious infections* caused by Pseudomonas, Proteus, E. coli, Klebsiella, Enterobacter, & Serratia & initial Rx of gram(–) sepsis **Action:** Bactericidal; inhibits protein synthesis. *Spectrum:* Synergy w/ penicillins; gram(–) (not Neisseria, Legionella, Acinetobacter) **Dose: Adults.** 3–7 mg/kg/24h IV ÷ q8–24h. Synergy: 1 mg/kg q8h. **Peds. Infants** <7 d <1200 g: 2.5 mg/kg/dose q18–24h. **Infants >1200 g:** 2.5 mg/kg/dose q12–18h. **Infants >7 d:** 2.5 mg/kg/dose IV q8–12h. **Children:** 2.5 mg/kg/d IV q8h; ↓ w/ renal insufficiency **Caution:** [C, +/–] ⊘ other nephrotoxic Rxs **Contra:** Aminoglycoside sensitivity **Supplied:** Premixed infus 40, 60, 70, 80, 90, 100, 120 mg; ADD-Vantage inj vials 10 mg/mL; inj 40 mg/mL; IT preservative-free 2 mg/mL **SE:** Nephrotoxic/ototoxic/neurotoxic **Notes:** Follow CrCl & serum conc for dosage adjustments (see Table 2, page 265); once daily dosing becoming popular; follow SCr; use IBW to dose (use adjusted if obese >30% IBW) **Interactions:** ↑ Ototoxicity, neurotoxicity, nephrotoxicity w/ aminoglycosides, amphotericin B, cephalosporins, loop diuretics, penicillins; ↑ effects w/ NSAIDs; ↓ effects w/ carbenicillin; **Labs:** False ↑ AST, urine protein; ↑ urine amino acids **NIPE:** Photosensitivity—use sunscreen

Gentamicin & Prednisolone, Ophthalmic (Pred-G Op thalmic) **Uses:** *Steroid-responsive ocular & conjunctival infections* sensiti to gentamicin (eg, *Staphylococcus, E. coli, H. influenzae, Klebsiella, Neisser Pseudomonas, Proteus,* & *Serratia* sp) **Action:** Bactericidal; inhibits protein sy thesis plus antiinflammatory **Dose:** *Oint:* ½ in. in conjunctival sac qd–tid. *Susp gt* bid–qid, up to 1 gt/h for severe infections **Contra:** Aminoglycoside sensitiv **Caution:** [C, ?] **Supplied:** *Oint, ophth:* Prednisolone acetate 0.6% & gentamic sulfate 0.3% (3.5 g). *Susp, ophth:* Prednisolone acetate 1% & gentamicin sulfa 0.3% (2, 5, 10 mL) **SE:** Local irritation. See Gentamicin. **Additional NIPE:** Sy temic effects w/ long-term use

Gentamicin, Ophthalmic (Garamycin, Genoptic, Gentacidi Gentak, others) **Uses:** *Conjunctival infections* **Action:** Bactericidal; i hibits protein synthesis **Dose:** *Oint:* Apply ½ in. bid–tid. *Soln:* 1–2 gtt q2–4h, up 2 gtt/h for severe infection **Caution:** [C, ?] **Contra:** Aminoglycoside sensitiv **Supplied:** Soln & oint 0.3% **SE:** Local irritation **Notes:** ⊘ Use of other eye dro w/in 5–10 mins; ⊘ touch dropper to eye. See Gentamicin. **NIPE:** ⊘ Other e drops for 10 min after administering this drug

Gentamicin, Topical (Garamycin, G-Mycitin) **Uses:** *Skin infe tions* caused by susceptible organisms **Action:** Bactericidal; inhibits protein sy thesis **Dose:** *Adults & Peds.* >1 y: Apply tid–qid **Caution:** [C, ?] **Contr** Aminoglycoside sensitivity **Supplied:** Cream & oint 0.1% **SE:** Irritation. See Ge tamicin. **NIPE:** ⊘ Apply to large denuded areas

Glimepiride (Amaryl) **Uses:** *Type 2 DM* **Action:** Sulfonylurea; stim lates pancreatic insulin release; ↑ peripheral insulin sensitivity; ↓ hepatic gluco output & production **Dose:** 1–4 mg/d, max 8 mg **Caution:** [C, –] **Contra:** DK **Supplied:** Tabs 1, 2, 4, mg **SE:** HA, nausea, hypoglycemia **Notes:** Give w/ 1st me of day **Interactions:** ↑ Effects w/ ACEIs, adrenergic antagonists, BBs, chloran phenicol, MAOIs, NSAIDs, probenecid, salicylates, sulfonamides, warfarin, gi seng, garlic; ↓ effects w/ corticosteroids, estrogens, INH, oral contraceptive nicotinic acid, phenytoin, sympathomimetics, thiazide diuretics, thyroid hormone **NIPE:** Antabuse-like effect w/ EtOH

Glipizide (Glucotrol, Glucotrol XL) **Uses:** *Type 2 DM* **Action:** Su fonylurea; stimulates pancreatic insulin release; ↑ peripheral insulin sensitivity; hepatic glucose output & production; ↓ intestinal absorption of glucose **Dose:** mg initial, ↑ by 2.5–5 mg/d; XL max 20 mg **Caution:** [C, ?/–] se vere liver Dz **Contra:** DKA, Type 1 DM, sensitivity to sulfonamides **Supplie** Tabs 5, 10 mg; XL tabs 2.5, 5, 10 mg **SE:** HA, anorexia, N/V/D, constipation, ful ness, rash, urticaria, photosensitivity **Notes:** Counsel Pt about diabetes manage ment; wait several days before adjusting dose; monitor glucose; give 30 min befo meal; hold dose if Pt NPO **Interactions:** ↑ Effects w/ azole antifungals, anabol steroids, chloramphenicol, cimetidine, clofibrate, MAOIs, NSAIDs, probenecid salicylates, sulfonamides, TCAs, warfarin, celery, coriander, dandelion root, fenu reek, ginseng, garlic, juniper berries; ↓ effects w/ amphetamines, corticosteroids, pinephrine, estrogens, glucocorticoids, oral contraceptives, phenytoin, rifampin, ympathomimetics, thiazide diuretics, thyroid hormones, tobacco **NIPE:** ntabuse-like effect w/ EtOH

Glucagon Uses: Severe *hypoglycemic* Rxns in DM w/ sufficient liver lycogen stores or BB OD **Action:** Accelerates liver gluconeogenesis **Dose:** *dults.* 0.5–1 mg SQ, IM, or IV; repeat in 20 min PRN. *BB OD:* 3–10 mg IV; re-eat in 10 min PRN; may give as cont infus 1–5 mg/h. *Peds.* Neonates: 0.3 ng/kg/dose SQ, IM, or IV; repeat in 20 min PRN. *Children:* 0.025–0.1 mg/kg/dose SQ, IM, or V; repeat in 20 min PRN **Caution:** [B, M] **Contra:** Known pheochromocytoma **supplied:** Inj 1 mg **SE:** N/V, hypotension **Notes:** Administration of glucose IV ecessary; ineffective in states of starvation, adrenal insufficiency, or chronic hypo-lycemia **Interactions:** ↑ Effect w/ epinephrine, phenytoin; ↑ effects of anticoagu-ants; **Labs:** ↑ Serum K+; **NIPE:** Response w/in 20 min after inj

Glyburide (DiaBeta, Micronase, Glynase) Uses: *Type 2 DM* **Action:** Sulfonylurea; stimulates pancreatic insulin release; ↑ peripheral insulin ensitivity; ↓ hepatic glucose output & production; ↓ intestinal absorption of glu-ose **Dose:** 1.25–10 mg qd–bid, max 20 mg/d. *Micronized:* 0.75–6 mg qd–bid, max 2 mg/d **Caution:** [C, ?] Renal impairment **Contra:** DKA, Type I DM **Supplied:** abs 1.25, 2.5, 5 mg; micronized tabs 1.5, 3, 6 mg **SE:** HA, hypoglycemia **Notes:** for CrCl <50 mL/min; hold dose if Pt NPO **Interactions:** ↑ Effects w/ anticoag-lants, anabolic steroids, BBs, chloramphenicol, cimetidine, clofibrate, MAOIs, NSAIDs, probenecid, salicylates, sulfonamides, TCAs, EtOH, celery, coriander, landelion root, fenugreek, ginseng, garlic, juniper berries; ↓ effects w/ amphe-amines, corticosteroids, baclofen, epinephrine, glucocorticoids, oral contraceptives, phenytoin, rifampin, sympathomimetics, thiazide diuretics, thyroid hormones, to-acco **Labs:** False ↑ urine protein **NIPE:** Antabuse-like effect w/ EtOH

Glyburide/Metformin (Glucovance) Uses: *Type 2 DM* **Action:** *Sulfonylurea:* Stimulates pancreatic insulin release *Metformin:* ↑ Peripheral in-sulin sensitivity; ↓ hepatic glucose output & production; ↓ intestinal absorption of glucose **Dose:** 1st line (naive Pts) 1.25/250 mg PO qd–bid; 2nd line, 2.5/500 mg or 5/500 mg bid (max 20/2000 mg); take w/ meals, ↑ dose gradually **Caution:** [C, –] **Contra:** SCr >1.4 in females or >1.5 in males; hypoxemic conditions (CHF, sepsis, recent MI); alcoholism; metabolic acidosis; liver Dz; hold dose prior to & 48 h after ionic contrast media **Supplied:** Tabs 1.25/250 mg, 2.5/500 mg, 5/500 mg **SE:** HA, hypoglycemia, lactic acidosis, anorexia, N/V, rash **Notes:** ⊘ EtOH; hold dose f NPO; monitor folate levels for megaloblastic anemia. See Glyburide. **Addi-ional Interactions:** ↑ Effects w/ amiloride, ciprofloxacin cimetidine, digoxin, mi-conazole, morphine, nifedipine, procainamide, quinidine, quinine, ranitidine, riamterene, trimethoprim, vancomycin; ↓ effects w/ CCBs, INH, phenothiazines

Glycerin Suppository Uses: *Constipation* **Action:** Hyperosmolar laxa-ive **Dose:** *Adults.* 1 adult supp PR PRN. *Peds.* 1 infant supp PR qd–bid PRN **Cau-**

tion: [C, ?] **Supplied:** Supp (adult, infant); liq 4 mL/applicatorful **SE:** Can cau diarrhea **Interactions:** ↑ Effects w/ diuretics **Labs:** ↑ Serum triglycerides, pho phatidylglycerol in amniotic fluid; ↓ serum Ca **NIPE:** Insert and retain for 15 mi

Gonadorelin (Lutrepulse) Uses: *Primary hypothalamic amenorrhe **Action:** Stimulates the pituitary to release the gonadotropins LH & FSH **Dose:** μg IV q 90 min × 21 d using Lutrepulse pump kit **Caution:** [B, M] ↑ levels w/ a drogens, estrogens, progestins, glucocorticoids, spironolactone, levodopa; ↓ leve w/ OCP, digoxin, dopamine antagonists **Contra:** Any condition exacerbated PRG, ovarian cysts, causes of anovulation other than hypothalamic, conditio worsened by reproductive hormones, hormone-dependent tumor **Supplied:** Inj 10 μg **SE:** Risk of multiple pregnancies; inj site pain **Notes:** Monitor LH, FSH **Inte actions:** ↑ Effects w/ androgens, estrogens, glucocorticoids, levodopa, progestir spironolactone; ↓ effects w/ digoxin, dopamine antagonists, oral contraceptive phenothiazines

Goserelin (Zoladex) Uses: Advanced *CAP* & w/ radiation for localize CAP, *endometriosis, breast CA* **Action:** LHRH agonist, ↓initially LH, resulting ↓ testosterone **Dose:** 3.6 mg SQ (implant) q 28d or 10.8 mg SQ q3mo; usually in lower abdominal wall **Caution:** [X, –] **Contra:** PRG, breast-feeding, 10.8-mg in plant not for women **Supplied:** Subcutaneous implant 3.6 (1 mo), 10.8 mg (3 m **SE:** Hot flashes, ↓ libido, gynecomastia, & transient exacerbation of CA-relate bone pain ("flare Rxn" 7–10 d after 1st dose) **Notes:** Inject SQ into fat in abdom nal wall; ⊘ aspirate; females must use contraception **Interactions:** None note **Labs:** ↑ Alkaline phosphatase, estradiol, HDL, LDL, triglycerides; initial ↑ then ↓ after 1–2 wk FSH, LH, testosterone

Granisetron (Kytril) Uses: *Prevention of N/V* **Action:** Serotonin recep tor antagonist **Dose:** *Adults & Peds.* 10 μg/kg/dose IV 30 min prior to initiation c chemotherapy *Adults.* 2 mg PO 1 h prior to chemotherapy, then 12 h later. *Posto N/V:* 1 mg IV before end of operative case **Caution:** [B, +/–] St. John's wort may levels **Contra:** Liver Dz, children <2 y **Supplied:** Tabs 1 mg; inj 1 mg/mL; soln mg/10 mL **SE:** HA, constipation **Interactions:** ↑ Serotonergic effects w/ hore hound; ↑ extrapyramidal Rxns w/ drugs causing these effects **Labs:** ↑ ALT, AS **NIPE:** May cause anaphylactic Rxn

Guaifenesin (Robitussin, others) Uses: *Symptomatic relief of dr nonproductive cough* **Action:** Expectorant **Dose:** *Adults.* 200–400 mg (10–2 mL) PO q4h (max 2.4 g/d). *Peds.* <2 y: 12 mg/kg/d in 6 ÷ doses. *2–5 y:* 50–100 m (2.5–5 mL) PO q4h (max 600 mg/d). *6–11 y:* 100–200 mg (5–10 mL) PO q4 (max 1.2 g/d) **Caution:** [C, ?] **Supplied:** Tabs 100, 200; SR tabs 600, 1200 mg caps 200 mg; SR caps 300 mg; liq 100 mg/5 mL **SE:** GI upset **Notes:** Give w large amount of water; some dosage forms contain EtOH **Interactions:** ↑ Bleedin w/ heparin **Labs:** False results of urine 5-HIAA, VMA **NIPE:** ↑ Fluid intake

Guaifenesin & Codeine (Robitussin AC, Brontex, others) [C V] Uses: *Symptomatic relief of dry, nonproductive cough* **Action:** Antitussiv w/ expectorant **Dose:** *Adults.* 5–10 mL or 1 tab PO q6–8h (max 60 mL/24 h). *Peds.* 2–6 y: 1–1.5 mg/kg codeine/d ÷ dose q4–6h (max 30 mg/24 h). *6–12 y:* 5 mL q4h (max 30 mL/24 h) **Caution:** [C, +] **Supplied:** Brontex tab 10 mg codeine/300 mg guaifenesin; liq 2.5 mg codeine/75 mg guaifenesin/5 mL; others 10 mg codeine/100 mg guaifenesin/5 mL **SE:** Somnolence **Interactions:** ↑ CNS depression w/ barbiturates, antihistamines, glutethimide, methocarbamol, cimetidine, EtOH; ↓ effects w/ quinidine **Labs:** ↑ Urine porphobilin; false ↑ amylase, lipase **NIPE:** Take w/ food

Guaifenesin & Dextromethorphan (many OTC brands)
Uses: *Cough* due to upper resp tract irritation **Action:** Antitussive w/ expectorant **Dose:** *Adults & Peds.* >12 y: 10 mL PO q6–8h (max 40 mL/24 h). *Peds.* 2–6 y: Dextromethorphan 1–2 mg/kg/24 h ÷ 3–4 × d (max 10 mL/d). *6–12 y:* 5 mL q6–8h (max 20 mL/d) **Caution:** [C, +] **Contra:** Administration w/ MAOI **Supplied:** Many OTC formulations **SE:** Somnolence **Notes:** Give w/ plenty of fluids **Interactions:** ↑ Effects w/ quinidine, terbinafine; ↑ effects of isocarboxazid, MAOIs, phenelzine; ↑ risk of serotonin syndrome w/ sibutramine

Haemophilus B Conjugate Vaccine (ActHIB, HibTITER, PedvaxHIB, Prohibit, others)
Uses: Routine *immunization* of children against *H. influenzae* type B Dzs **Action:** Active immunization against *Haemophilus* B **Dose:** *Peds.* 0.5 mL (25 mg) IM in deltoid or vastus lateralis **Caution:** [C, +] **Contra:** Febrile illness, immunosuppression, hypersensitivity to thimerosal **Supplied:** Inj 7.5, 10, 15, 25 μg/0.5 mL **SE:** Observe for anaphylaxis; edema, ↑ risk of *Haemophilus* B infection in the week after vaccination **Notes:** Booster not required; report all serious adverse Rxn to VAERS: 1-800-822-7967 **Interactions:** ↓ effects w/ immunosuppressives, steroids

Haloperidol (Haldol)
Uses: *Psychotic disorders, agitation, Tourette's disorders, & hyperactivity in children* **Action:** Antipsychotic, neuroleptic **Dose:** *Adults.* Moderate Sxs: 0.5–2.0 mg PO bid–tid. Severe Sxs/agitation: 3–5 mg PO bid–tid or 1–5 mg IM q4h PRN (max 100 mg/d). *Peds.* 3–6 y: 0.01–0.03 mg/kg/24 h PO qd. *6–12 y:* Initially, 0.5–1.5 mg/24 h PO; ↑ by 0.5 mg/24 h to maintenance of 2–4 mg/24 h (0.05–0.1 mg/kg/24 h) or 1–3 mg/dose IM q4–8h to a max of 0.1 mg/kg/24 h; Tourette's may require up to 15 mg/24 h PO; ↓ dose in elderly **Caution:** [C, ?] ↑ effects w/ SSRIs, CNS depressants, TCA, indomethacin, metoclopramide; ↑ levodopa (inhibits antiparkinsonian effects of levodopa) **Contra:** Narrow-angle glaucoma, severe CNS depression, Parkinson's, bone marrow suppression, severe cardiac/hepatic Dz, coma **Supplied:** Tabs 0.5, 1, 2, 5, 10, 20 mg; conc liq 2 mg/mL; inj 5 mg/mL; decanoate inj 50, 100 mg/mL **SE:** Extrapyramidal Sxs (EPS), hypotension, anxiety, dystonias **Notes:** ⊘ administer decanoate IV; dilute PO conc liq w/ water/juice; monitor for EPS **Interactions:** ↑ Effects w/ CNS depressants, quinidine, EtOH; ↑ hypotension w/ antihypertensives, nitrates; ↑ anticholinergic effects w/ antihistamines, antidepressants, atropine, phenothiazines, quinidine, disopyramide; ↓ effects w/ antacids, carbamazepine, Li, nutmeg, to-

bacco; ↓ effects of anticoagulants, levodopa, guanethidine **Labs:** False + PRG test, ↓ serum cholesterol **NIPE:** ↑ Risk of photosensitivity—use sunscreen

Haloprogin (Halotex) **Uses:** *Topical Rx of tinea pedis, tinea cruris, tinea corporis, tinea manus* **Action:** Topical antifungal **Dose:** *Adults.* Apply bid for up to 2 wk; intertriginous Sxs may require up to 4 wk **Caution:** [B, ?] **Contra:** Component sensitivity **Supplied:** 1% cream; soln **SE:** Local irritation **Notes:** ⊘ Contact w/ eyes; improvement should occur w/in 4 wk

Heparin **Uses:** *Rx & prevention of DVT & PE,* unstable angina, AF w/ emboli formation, & acute arterial occlusion **Action:** Acts w/ antithrombin III to inactivate thrombin & inhibit thromboplastin formation **Dose:** *Adults.* Prophylaxis: 3000–5000 units SQ q8–12h. *Thrombosis Rx:* Loading dose 50–80 units/kg IV, then 10–20 units/kg IV qh (adjust based on PTT). *Peds.* Infants: Loading dose 50 units/kg IV bolus, then 20 units/kg/h IV by cont inf. *Children:* Loading dose 50 units/kg IV, then 15–25 units/kg cont inf or 100 units/kg/dose q4h IV intermittent bolus (adjust based on PTT) **Caution:** [B, +] ↑ risk of hemorrhage w/ anticoagulants, ASA, antiplts, cephalosporins that contain MTT side chain **Contra:** Uncontrolled bleeding, severe thrombocytopenia, suspected ICH **Supplied:** Inj 10, 100, 1000, 2000, 2500, 5000, 7500, 10,000, 20,000, 40,000 units/mL **SE:** Bruising, bleeding, thrombocytopenia **Notes:** Follow PTT, thrombin time, or activated clotting time to assess effectiveness; little effect on the PT; therapeutic PTT is 1.5–2 × control for most conditions; monitor for thrombocytopenia (HIT); follow plt counts **Interactions:** ↑ Effects w/ anticoagulants, antihistamines, ASA, clopidogrel, cardiac glycosides, cephalosporins, pyridamole, NSAIDs, quinine, tetracycline, ticlopidine, feverfew, ginkgo biloba, ginger, valerian; ↓ effects w/ nitroglycerine, ginseng, goldenseal, ↓ effects of insulin **Labs:** ↑ LFTs, TFTs

Hepatitis A Vaccine (Havrix, Vaqta) **Uses:** *Prevent hepatitis A* in high-risk individuals (eg, travelers, certain professions, or high-risk behaviors) **Action:** Provides active immunity **Dose:** (Expressed as ELISA units [EL. U.]) *Havrix: Adults.* 1440 EL. U. single IM dose. *Peds.* >2 y: 720 EL. U. single IM dose. *Vaqta: Adults.* 50 units single IM dose. *Peds.* 25 units single IM dose **Caution:** [C, +] **Contra:** Hypersensitivity to any component of formulation **Supplied:** Inj 720 EL.U./0.5 mL, 1440 EL.U./1 mL.; 50 units/mL **SE:** Fever, fatigue, pain at inj site, HA **Notes:** Booster recommended 6–12 mo after primary vaccination; report all serious adverse Rxns to VAERS: 1-800-822-7967 **Interactions:** None noted **NIPE:** ⊘ if Pt febrile

Hepatitis A (Inactivated) & Hepatitis B (Recombinant) Vaccine (Twinrix) **Uses:** *Active immunization against hepatitis A/B* **Action:** Active immunity **Dose:** 1 mL IM at 0, 1, & 6 mo **Caution:** [C, +] **Contra:** Component sensitivity **Supplied:** Single-dose vials, syringes **SE:** Fever, fatigue, pain at inj site, HA **Notes:** Booster recommended 6–12 mo after primary vaccination; report all serious adverse Rxns to VAERS: 1-800-822-7967 **Interactions:** ↓ Immune reponse w/ corticosteroids, immunosuppressants **NIPE**: ↑ Response if inj in deltoid s gluteus

Hepatitis B Immune Globulin (HyperHep, H-BIG) Uses: *Exposure to HBsAg+ materials,* eg, blood, plasma, or serum (accidental needle-stick, mucous membrane contact, or PO ingestion) **Action**: Passive immunization **Dose**: *Adults & Peds.* 0.06 mL/kg IM to a max of 5 mL; w/in 24 h of needle-stick or percutaneous exposure; w/in 14 d of sexual contact; repeat 1 & 6 mo after exposure **Caution**: [C, ?] **Contra**: Allergies to γ-globulin or antiimmunoglobulin antibodies; allergies to thimerosal, IgA deficiency **Supplied**: Inj **SE**: Pain at site, dizziness **Notes**: Administered IM in gluteal or deltoid; if exposure continues, Pt should also receive the hepatitis B vaccine **Interactions**: ↓ Immune response if given w/ live virus vaccines

Hepatitis B Vaccine (Engerix-B, Recombivax HB) Uses: *Prevention of hepatitis B* **Action**: Active immunization **Dose**: *Adults.* 3 IM doses of 1 mL each, the 1st 2 doses given 1 mo apart, the 3rd 6 mo after the 1st. *Peds.* 0.5 mL IM given on the same schedule as for adults **Caution**: [C, +] **Contra**: Yeast hypersensitivity **Supplied**: *Engerix-B:* Inj 20 μg/mL; peds inj 10 μg/0.5 mL. *Recombivax HB:* Inj 10 & 40 μg/mL; peds inj 5 μg/0.5 mL **SE**: Fever, inj site soreness **Notes**: IM inj for adults & older peds in the deltoid; in other peds, administer in the anterolateral thigh; derived from recombinant DNA technology **Interactions**: ↓ Immune response w/ corticosteroids, immunosuppressants **NIPE**: ↑ Response inj in deltoid vs gluteus

Hetastarch (Hespan) Uses: *Plasma volume expansion* as adjunct in the Rx of shock & leukapheresis **Action**: Synthetic colloid w/ actions similar to albumin **Dose**: *Volume expansion:* 500–1000 mL (1500 mL/d max) IV at a rate not to exceed 20 mL/kg/h. *Leukapheresis:* 250–700 mL; ↓ in renal failure **Caution**: [C, +] **Contra**: Severe bleeding disorders, CHF, or renal failure w/ oliguria or anuria **Supplied**: Inj 6 g/100 mL **SE**: Bleeding side effect (prolongs PT, PTT, bleed time, etc) **Notes**: Not a substitute for blood or plasma **NIPE**: Monitor CBC, PT, PTT; observe for anaphylactic Rxns

Hydralazine (Apresoline, others) Uses: *Moderate to severe HTN; CHF* (w/ Isordil) **Action**: Peripheral vasodilator **Dose**: *Adults.* Begin at 10 mg PO qid, then ↑ to 25 mg qid to max of 300 mg/d. *Peds.* 0.75–3 mg/kg/24 h PO ÷ q6–12h; ↓ in renal impairment; check CBC & ANA before starting **Caution**: [C, +] ↓ hepatic Fxn & CAD; ↑ toxicity w/ MAOI, indomethacin, BBs **Contra**: Dissecting aortic aneurysm, mitral valve rheumatic heart Dz **Supplied**: Tabs 10, 25, 50, 100 mg; inj 20 mg/mL **SE**: Chronically high doses cause SLE-like syndrome; SVT following IM administration, peripheral neuropathy **Notes**: Compensatory sinus tachycardia eliminated w/ use of a BB **Interactions**: ↑ Effects w/ antihypertensives, diazoxide, diuretics, MAOIs, nitrates, EtOH; ↓ pressor response w/ epinephrine; ↓ effects w/ NSAIDs; **NIPE**: Take w/ food

Hydrochlorothiazide (HydroDIURIL, Esidrix, others) Use ***Edema, HTN* Action:** Thiazide diuretic; inhibits Na reabsorption in the dist tubule **Dose:** *Adults.* 25–100 mg/d PO in single or ÷ doses. *Peds.* <6 mo: 2– mg/kg/d in 2 ÷ doses. *>6 mo:* 2 mg/kg/d in 2 ÷ doses **Caution:** [D, +] **Contra** Anuria, sulfonamide allergy, renal decompensation **Supplied:** Tabs 25, 50, 100 m caps 12.5 mg; PO soln 50 mg/5 mL **SE:** ↓ K⁺, hyperglycemia, hyperuricemia, hy ponatremia **Interactions:** ↑ Hypotension w/ ACEIs, antihypertensives, carbeno olone, ↑ hypokalemia w/ carbenoxolone, corticosteroids; ↑ hypergylcemia w/ BB diazoxide, hypoglycemic drugs; ↑ effects of Li, MRX; ↓ effects w/ amphetamine cholestyramine, colestipol, NSAIDs, quinidine, dandelion **Labs:** False ↓ urine estrie **NIPE:** Monitor uric acid, take w/ food, ↑ risk of photosensitivity—use sunscreen

Hydrochlorothiazide & Amiloride (Moduretic) **Uses:** *HTN **Action:** Combined effects of a thiazide diuretic & a K-sparing diuretic **Dose:** 1– tabs/d PO **Caution:** [D, ?] **Contra:** ⊘ Give to Pts w/ renal failure, sulfonamide a lergy **Supplied:** Tabs (amiloride/HCTZ) 5 mg/50 mg **SE:** Hypotension, photoser sitivity, hyper-/hypokalemia, hyperglycemia, hyponatremia, hyperlipidemi hyperuricemia

Hydrochlorothiazide & Spironolactone (Aldactazide) Uses *Edema, HTN* **Action:** Combined thiazide diuretic & a K-sparing diuretic **Dose** 25–200 mg each component/d in ÷ doses **Caution:** [D, +] **Contra:** Sulfonamic allergy **Supplied:** Tabs (HCTZ/spironolactone) 25 mg/25 mg, 50 mg/50 mg **SE** Photosensitivity, hypotension, hyper-/hypokalemia, hyperglycemia, hyponatremi hyperlipidemia, hyperuricemia. See Hydrochlorothiazide **Additional Interaction** ↑ Risk of hyperkalemia w/ ACEIs, K-sparing diuretics, K suppls, salt substitutes; effects of digoxin **NIPE:** DC drug 3 d before glucose tolerance test

Hydrochlorothiazide & Triamterene (Dyazide, Maxzide) **Uses:** *Edema & HTN* **Action:** Combined thiazide diuretic & a K-sparing d uretic **Dose:** *Dyazide:* 1–2 caps PO qd–bid. *Maxzide:* 1 tab/d PO **Caution:** [D, +/– **Contra:** Sulfonamide allergy **Supplied:** (Triamterene/HCTZ) 37.5 mg/25 mg, 5(mg/25 mg, 75 mg/50 mg **SE:** Photosensitivity, hypotension, hyper-/hypokalemia hyperglycemia, hyponatremia, hyperlipidemia, hyperuricemia **Notes:** HCTZ com ponent in Maxzide more bioavailable than in Dyazide. See Hydrochlorothiazide **Additional Interactions:** ↑ Risk of hyperkalemia w/ ACEIs, K-sparing diuretics K suppls, salt substitutes; ↑ effects w/ cimetidine, licorice root, ↓ effects of digoxi **Labs:** ↑ Serum glucose, BUN, creatinine K⁺, Mg²⁺, uric acid, urinary Ca²⁺; inter ference w/ assay of quinidine & lactic dehydrogenase **NIPE:** Urine may turn blue

Hydrocodone & Acetaminophen (Lorcet, Vicodin, others [C-III] Uses: *Moderate to severe pain*; hydrocodone has antitussive propertie **Action:** Narcotic analgesic w/ nonnarcotic analgesic **Dose:** 1–2 caps or tabs PC q4–6h PRN **Caution:** [C, M] **Contra:** CNS depression, severe resp depression **Supplied:** Many different combinations; specify hydrocodone/APAP dose; cap 5/500; tabs 2.5/500, 5/400, 5/500, 7.5/400, 10/400, 7.5/500, 7.5/650, 7.5/750

10/325, 10/400, 10/500, 10/650; elixir & soln (fruit punch flavor) 2.5 mg hydrocodone/167 mg APAP/mL **SE:** GI upset, sedation, fatigue **Notes:** ⊘ Exceed >4 g acetaminophen/d **Interactions:** ↑ Effects w/ antihistamines, cimetidine, CNS depressants, dextroamphetamines, glutethimide, MAOIs, protease inhibitors, TCAs, EtOH, St. John's wort; ↑ effects of warfarin; ↓ effects w/ phenothiazines **Labs:** False ↑ amylase, lipase **NIPE:** Take w/ food, ↑ fluid intake

Hydrocodone & Aspirin (Lortab ASA, others) [C-III]
Uses: *Moderate to severe pain* **Action:** Narcotic analgesic w/ NSAID **Dose:** 1–2 PO q4–6h PRN **Caution:** [C, M] ↓ renal Fxn, gastritis/PUD, ⊘ use in children for chickenpox (Reye's syndrome) **Contra:** Component sensitivity **Supplied:** 5 mg hydrocodone/500 mg ASA/tab **SE:** GI upset, sedation, fatigue **Notes:** Give w/ food/milk; monitor for GI bleed. See Hydrocodone and Acetaminophen

Hydrocodone & Guaifenesin (Hycotuss Expectorant, others) [C-III]
Uses: *Nonproductive cough* associated w/ resp infection **Action:** Expectorant plus cough suppressant **Dose:** *Adults & Peds.* >12 y: 5 mL q4h pc & hs. *Peds.* < 2 y: 0.3 mg/kg/d ÷ qid. *2–12 y:* 2.5 mL q4h pc & hs **Caution:** [C, M] **Contra:** Component sensitivity **Supplied:** Hydrocodone 5 mg/guaifenesin 100 mg/5 mL **SE:** GI upset, sedation, fatigue. See Hydrocodone and Acetaminophen. **Additional Interactions:** ↑ Bleeding w/ heparin **Labs:** False results of urine 5-HIAA, VMA

Hydrocodone & Homatropine (Hycodan, Hydromet, others) [C-III]
Uses: *Relief of cough* **Action:** Combination antitussive **Dose:** (Dose based on hydrocodone) *Adults.* 5–10 mg q4–6h. *Peds.* 0.6 mg/kg/d ÷ tid–qid **Caution:** [C, M] **Contra:** Narrow-angle glaucoma, ↑ ICP, depressed ventilation **Supplied:** Syrup 5 mg hydrocodone/5 mL; tabs 5 mg hydrocodone **SE:** Sedation, fatigue, GI upset **Notes:** ⊘ Give >q4h; see individual Rx monographs. See Hydrocodone and Acetaminophen. **Additional Labs:** ↑ ALT, AST

Hydrocodone & Ibuprofen (Vicoprofen) [C-III]
Uses: *Moderate to severe pain (<10 d)* **Action:** Narcotic w/ NSAID **Dose:** 1–2 tabs q4–6h PRN **Caution:** [C, M] Renal insufficiency; ↓ effect w/ ACEIs & diuretics; ↑ effect w/ CNS depressants, EtOH, MAOI, ASA, TCA, anticoagulants **Contra:** Component sensitivity **Supplied:** Tabs 7.5 mg hydrocodone/200 mg ibuprofen **SE:** Sedation, fatigue, GI upset. See Hydrocodone and Acetaminophen **Additional Interactions:** ↓ Effects of ACEIs, diuretics

Hydrocodone & Pseudoephedrine (Detussin, Histussin-D, others) [C-III]
Uses: *Cough & nasal congestion* **Action:** Narcotic cough suppressant w/ decongestant **Dose:** 5 mL qid, PRN **Caution:** [C, M] **Contra:** MAOIs **Supplied:** 5 mg hydrocodone/60 mg pseudoephedrine/5 mL **SE:** ↑ BP, GI upset, sedation, fatigue. See Hydrocodone and Acetaminophen **Additional Interactions:** ↑ Effects w/ sympathomimetics

Hydrocodone, Chlorpheniramine, Phenylephrine, Acetaminophen, & Caffeine (Hycomine Compound)[C-III]
Uses:

Cough & Sxs of URI **Action:** Narcotic cough suppressant w/ decongestants & analgesic **Dose:** 1 tab PO q4h PRN **Caution:** [C, M] **Contra:** Narrow-angle glaucoma **Supplied:** Hydrocodone 5 mg/chlorpheniramine 2 mg/phenylephrine 10 mg/APAP 250 mg/caffeine 30 mg **SE:** ↑ BP, GI upset, sedation, fatigue. See Hydrocodone and Acetaminophen

Hydrocortisone, Rectal (Anusol-HC Suppository, Cortifoam Rectal, Proctocort, others)

Uses: *Painful anorectal conditions,* radiation proctitis, management of ulcerative colitis **Action:** Antiinflammatory steroid **Dose:** *Adults. Ulcerative colitis:* 10–100 mg PR 1–2×/d for 2–3 wk **Caution:** [B, ?/–] **Contra:** Component sensitivity **Supplied:** *Hydrocortisone acetate:* Rectal aerosol 90 mg/applicator; supp 25 mg. *Hydrocortisone base:* Rectal 1%; rectal susp 100 mg/60 mL **SE:** Minimal systemic effect **NIPE:** Administer after BM, insert supp blunt end first, admin enema w/ Pt lying on side and retain for 1 h

Hydrocortisone, Topical & Systemic (Cortef, Solu-Cortef)

Caution: [B, –] **Contra:** Viral, fungal, or tubercular skin lesions; serious infections (except septic shock or tuberculous meningitis) **SE:** Systemic forms: ↑d appetite, insomnia, hyperglycemia, bruising **Notes:** May cause HPA axis suppression **Interactions:** ↑ Effects w/ cyclosporine, estrogens; ↑ effects of cardiac glycosides, cyclosporine; ↑ risk of GI bleed w/ NSAIDs; ↓ effects w/ aminoglutethimide, antacids, barbiturates, cholestyramine, colestipol, ephedrine, phenobarbital, phenytoin, rifampin; ↓ effects of anticoagulants, hypoglycemics, insulin, INH, salicylates **Labs:** False – in skin allergy tests **NIPE:** ⊘ EtOH, live virus vaccines, abrupt DC of drug; take w/ food; may mask S/Sxs infection

Hydromorphone (Dilaudid) [C–II]

Uses: *Moderate/severe pain* **Action:** Narcotic analgesic **Dose:** 1–4 mg PO, IM, IV, or PR q4–6h PRN; 3 mg PR q6–8h PRN; ↓ w/ hepatic failure **Caution:** [B (D if prolonged use or high doses near term), ?] ↑ effects w/ CNS depressants, phenothiazines, TCA **Contra:** Component sensitivity **Supplied:** Tabs 1, 2, 3, 4, 8 mg; liq 5 mg/mL; inj 1, 2, 4, 10 mg/mL; supp 3 mg **SE:** Sedation, dizziness, GI upset **Notes:** Morphine 10 mg IM = hydromorphone 1.5 mg IM **Interactions:** ↑ Effects w/ CNS depressants, phenothiazines, TCAs, EtOH, St. John's wort; ↓ effects w/ nalbuphine, pentazocine **Labs:** ↑ Serum amylase, lipase **NIPE:** Take w/ food, ↑ fluids & fiber to prevent constipation

Hydroxyurea (Hydrea, Droxia)

Uses: *CML, head & neck, ovarian & colon CA, melanoma, acute leukemia, sickle cell anemia, polycythemia vera, HIV* **Action:** Inhibitor of the ribonucleotide reductase system **Dose:** (Refer to individual protocols) 50–75 mg/kg for WBC counts of >100,000 cells/mL; 20–30 mg/kg in refractory CML. *HIV:* 1000–1500 mg/d in single or ÷ doses; ↓ in renal insufficiency **Caution:** [D, –] ↑ effects w/ zidovudine, zalcitabine, didanosine, stavudine, fluorouracil **Contra:** Severe anemia, severe bone marrow suppression, WBC <2500 or plt <100,000, PRG **Supplied:** Caps 200, 300, 400, 500 mg, tabs

1000 mg **SE:** Myelosuppression (primarily leukopenia), N/V, rashes, facial erythema, radiation recall Rxns, & renal dysfunction **Notes:** Capsules can be opened & emptied into water **Interactions:** ↑ Risk of pancreatitis w/ didanosine, indinavir, stavudine; ↑ bone marrow depression w/ antineoplastic drugs or radiation therapy **Labs:** ↑ Serum uric acid, BUN, creatinine **NIPE:** ↑ Fluids 10–12 glasses/d, use barrier contraception, ↑ risk of infertility

Hydroxyzine (Atarax, Vistaril) Uses: *Anxiety, sedation, itching* **Action:** Antihistamine, antianxiety **Dose:** *Adults.* Anxiety or sedation: 50–100 mg PO or IM qid or PRN (max 600 mg/d). *Itching:* 25–50 mg PO or IM qid-qid. *Peds.* 0.5–1.0 mg/kg/24 h PO or IM q6h; ↓ in hepatic failure **Caution:** [C, +/–] ↑ effects w/ CNS depressants, anticholinergics, EtOH **Contra:** Component sensitivity **Supplied:** Tabs 10, 25, 50, 100 mg; caps 25, 50, 100 mg; syrup 10 mg/5 mL; susp 25 mg/5 mL; inj 25, 50 mg/mL **SE:** Drowsiness & anticholinergic effects **Notes:** Useful in potentiating effects of narcotics; not for IV/SQ use due to thrombosis & digital gangrene **Interactions:** ↑ Effects w/ antihistamines, anticholinergics, CNS depressants, EtOH **Labs:** False – skin allergy tests; false ↑ in urinary 17-hydroxycorticosteroid levels

Hyoscyamine (Anaspaz, Cystospaz, Levsin, others) Uses: *Spasm associated w/ GI & bladder disorders* **Action:** Anticholinergic **Dose:** *Adults.* 0.125–0.25 mg (1–2 tabs) SL/PO tid–qid, ac & hs; 1 SR cap q12h **Caution:** [C, +] ↑ effects w/ amantadine, antihistamines, antimuscarinics, haloperidol, phenothiazines, TCA, MAOI **Contra:** Obstructive uropathy, GI obstruction, glaucoma, MyG, paralytic ileus, severe ulcerative colitis, MI **Supplied:** (Cystospaz-M, Levsinex): cap timed release 0.375 mg; elixir (EtOH); soln 0.125 mg/5 mL; inj 0.5 mg/mL; tab 0.125 mg; tab (Cystospaz) 0.15 mg; XR tab (Levbid): 0.375 mg; SL (Levsin SL) 0.125 mg **SE:** Dry skin, xerostomia, constipation, anticholinergic SE **Notes:** Administer tabs ac/food; heat prostration may occur in hot weather **Interactions:** ↑ Effects w/ amantadine, antimuscarinics, haloperidol, phenothiazines, quinidine, TCAs, MAOIs; ↓ effects w/ antacids, antidiarrheals; ↓ effects of levodopa **NIPE:** ↑ Risk of heat intolerance, photophobia

Hyoscyamine, Atropine, Scopolamine, & Phenobarbital (Donnatal, others) Uses: *Irritable bowel, spastic colitis, peptic ulcer, spastic bladder* **Action:** Anticholinergic, antispasmodic **Dose:** 0.125–0.25 mg (1–2 tabs) tid–qid, 1 cap q12h (SR), 5–10 mL elixir tid–qid or q8h **Caution:** [D, M] **Contra:** Narrow-angle glaucoma **Supplied:** Many combinations/manufacturers available; *Cap* (Donnatal, others): Hyoscyamine 0.1037 mg/atropine 0.0194 mg/scopolamine 0.0065 mg/phenobarbital 16.2 mg. *Tabs* (Donnatal, others): Hyoscyamine 0.1037 mg/atropine 0.0194 mg/scopolamine 0.0065 mg/phenobarbital 16.2 mg. *Long-acting* (Donnatal): Hyoscyamine 0.311 mg/atropine 0.0582 mg/scopolamine 0.0195 mg/phenobarbital 48.6 mg. *Elixirs* (Donnatal, others): Hyoscyamine 0.1037 mg/atropine 0.0194 mg/scopolamine 0.0065 mg/phenobarbital 16.2 mg/5 mL **SE:** Sedation, xerostomia, constipation **Interactions:** ↑ Effects w/ anticoagulants, amantadine, antihistamines, antidiarrheals, anticonvulsants, CNS depressants, corticosteroids, digitalis, griseofulvin, MAOIs, phenothiazines, tetracyclines, TCAs **NIPE:** ↑ Risk of photophobia, constipation, urinary hesitancy

Ibuprofen (Motrin, Rufen, Advil, others) [OTC] **Uses:** *Arthritis & pain* **Action:** NSAID **Dose:** *Adults.* 200–800 mg PO bid–qid (max 2.4 g/d) *Peds.* 30–40 mg/kg/d in 3–4 ÷ doses (max 40 mg/kg/d); best taken w/ food, caution when combined w/ other NSAIDs **Caution:** [B, +] **Contra:** Severe hepatic impairment, hypersensitivity to NSAIDs, UGI bleed, or ulcers, 3rd tri PRG **Supplied:** Tabs 100, 200, 400, 600, 800 mg; chew tabs 50, 100 mg; caps 200 mg; susp 100 mg/2.5 mL, 100 mg/5 mL, 40 mg/mL (200 mg is OTC prep) **SE:** Dizziness, peptic ulcer, plt inhibition, worsening of renal insufficiency **Interactions:** ↑ Effects w/ ASA, corticosteroids, probenecid, EtOH; ↑ effects of aminoglycosides, anticoagulants, digoxin, hypoglycemics, Li, MRX; ↑ risks of bleeding w/ abciximab, cefotetan, valproic acid, thrombolytic drugs, warfarin, ticlopidine, garlic, ginger, ginkgo biloba; ↓ effects w/ feverfew; ↓ effects of antihypertensives **Labs:** ↑ BUN, creatinine; ↓ Hmg, Hct, BS, plts **NIPE:** Take w/ food

Ibutilide (Corvert) **Uses:** *Rapid conversion of AF or flutter* **Action:** Class III antiarrhythmic agent **Dose:** 0.01 mg/kg (max 1 mg) IV inf over 10 min; may be repeated once **Caution:** [C, –] ⊘ administer class I or III antiarrhythmics concurrently or w/in 4 h of ibutilide inf **Contra:** QTc > 440 ms **Supplied:** Inj 0.1 mg/mL **SE:** Arrhythmias, HA **Notes:** Observe Pt w/ continuous ECG monitoring **Interactions:** ↑ Refractory effects w/ amiodarone, disopyramide, procainamide, quinidine, sotalol; ↑ QT interval w/ antihistamines, antidepressants, erythromycin, phenothiazines, TCAs

Idarubicin (Idamycin) **Uses:** *Acute leukemias* (AML, ALL, ANLL), *CML in blast crisis, breast CA* **Action:** DNA intercalating agent; inhibits DNA topoisomerases I & II **Dose:** (Refer to individual protocols) 10–12 mg/m^2/d for 3–4 d; ↓ in renal/hepatic dysfunction **Caution:** [D, –] **Contra:** Bilirubin >5 mg/dL, PRG **Supplied:** Inj 1 mg/mL (5-, 10-, 20-mg vials) **SE:** Myelosuppression, cardiotoxicity, N/V, mucositis, alopecia, & irritation at sites of IV administration, rare changes in renal/hepatic Fxn **Notes:** ⊘ Extravasation—potent vesicant; only given IV **Interactions:** ↑ Myelosuppression w/ antineoplastic drugs and radiation therapy; ↓ effects of live virus vaccines **NIPE:** ↑ Fluids to 2–3 L/d

Ifosfamide (Ifex, Holoxan) **Uses:** *Lung, breast, pancreatic & gastric CA, HL/NHL, soft tissue sarcoma* **Action:** Alkylating agent **Dose:** (Refer to individual protocols) 1.2 g/m^2/d for 5 d by bolus or cont inf; 2.4 g/m^2/d for 3 d; w/ mesna uroprotection; ↓ in renal/hepatic impairment **Caution:** [D, M] ↑ effect w/ phenobarbital, carbamazepine, phenytoin; St. John's wort may ↓ levels **Contra:** Severely depressed bone marrow Fxn, PRG **Supplied:** Inj 1, 3 g **SE:** Hemorrhagic cystitis, nephrotoxicity, N/V, mild to moderate leukopenia, lethargy & confusion, alopecia, & ↑ hepatic enzyme **Notes:** Administer w/ mesna to prevent hemorrhagic cystitis **Interactions:** ↑ Effects w/ allopurinol, chloral hydrate, phenobarbital, phenytoin, grapefruit juice; ↑ myelosuppression w/ antineoplastic drugs and radiation therapy; ↓ effects of live virus vaccines **NIPE:** ↑ Fluids to 2–3 L/d

Imatinib (Gleevec) **Uses:** *Rx of CML, blast crisis, gastrointestinal stromal tumors (GIST)* **Action:** Inhibits BCL-ABL tyrosine kinase (signal transduction) **Dose:** *Chronic phase CML:* 400–600 mg PO qd. *Accelerated/blast crisis:* 600–800 mg PO qd. *GIST:* 400–600 mg PO qd **Caution:** [D, ?/–] Metabolized by CYP3A4 (caution w/ warfarin, cyclosporine, azole antifungals, erythromycin, phenytoin, rifampin, carbamazepine) **Contra:** Component sensitivity **Supplied:** Caps 100 mg **SE:** GI upset, fluid retention, muscle cramps, musculoskeletal pain arthralgia, rash, HA, neutropenia, thrombocytopenia **Notes:** Follow CBCs & LFTs baseline & monthly **Additional Interactions:** ↓ Effects w/ St. John's wort **NIPE:** Take w/ food, ↑ fluids, use barrier contraception

Imipenem–Cilastatin (Primaxin) **Uses:** *Serious infections* caused by a wide variety of susceptible bacteria **Action:** Bactericidal; interferes w/ cell wall synthesis. *Spectrum:* Gram(+) (inactive against *S. aureus*, group A & B streptococci), gram(–) (not *Legionella*), anaerobes **Dose:** *Adults.* 250–1000 mg (imipenem) IV q6–8h. *Peds.* 60–100 mg/kg/24 h IV ÷ q6h; ↓ in renal Dz if calculated CrCl is <70 mL/min **Caution:** [C, +/–] Probenecid may ↑ risk for toxicity **Contra:** Pediatric Pts w/ CNS infection (↑ Sz risk) & <30 kg w/ renal impairment **Supplied:** Inj (imipenem/cilastatin) 250/250 mg, 500/500 mg **SE:** Szs may occur if drug accumulates, GI upset, thrombocytopenia **Interactions:** ↑ Risks of Szs w/ ganciclovir, theophylline; ↓ effects w/ aztreonam, cephalosporins, chloramphenicol, penicillins, probenicid **Labs:** ↑ LFTs, BUN, creatinine; ↓ Hmg, Hct **NIPE:** Eval for superinfection

Imipramine (Tofranil) **Uses:** *Depression, enuresis,* panic attack, chronic pain **Action:** TCA; ↑ synaptic conc of serotonin or norepinephrine in the CNS **Dose:** *Adults.* Hospitalized: Initial 100 mg/24 h PO in ÷ doses; can ↑ over several wks to max 300 mg/d. *Outpatient:* Maint 50–150 mg PO hs, 300 mg/24 h max. *Peds.* Antidepressant: 1.5–5 mg/kg/24 h ÷ qd–qid. *Enuresis:*>6 y: 10–25 mg PO qhs; ↑ by 10–25 mg at 1–2-wk intervals (max 50 mg for 6–12 y, 75 mg for >12 y); treat for 2–3 mo, then taper **Caution:** [D, ?/–] **Contra:** Use w/ MAOIs, narrow-angle glaucoma, acute recovery phase of MI, PRG, CHF, angina, CVD, arrhythmias **Supplied:** Tabs 10, 25, 50 mg; caps 75, 100, 125, 150 mg **SE:** CV Sxs, dizziness, xerostomia, discolored urine **Notes:** Less sedation than w/ amitriptyline **Interactions:** ↑ Effects w/ amiodarone, anticholinergics, BBs, cimetidine, diltiazem, Li, oral contraceptives, quinidine, phenothiazines, ritonavir, verapamil, EtOH, evening primrose oil; ↑ effects of CNS depressants, hypoglycemics, warfarin; ↑ risk of serotonin syndrome w/ MAOIs; ↓ effects w/ carbamazepine, phenobarbital, rifampin, tobacco; ↓ effects of clonidine, guanethidine, methyldopa, reserpine **Labs:** ↑ Serum glucose, bilirubin, alkaline phosphatase **NIPE:** DC 48 h before surgery, DC MAOIs 2 wk before admin this drug, 4–6 wk for full effects, take w/ food

Imiquimod Cream, 5% (Aldara) Uses: *Anogenital warts, HPV, condylomata acuminata* Action: Unknown; may induce cytokines Dose: Applied 3×/wk, leave on skin for 6–10 h & wash off w/ soap & water, continue therapy for a max of 16 wk Caution: [B, ?] Contra: Component sensitivity Supplied: Single-dose packets 5% (250 mg of the cream) SE: Local skin Rxns common Notes: Not a cure; wash hands before & after application of cream NIPE: Condoms & diaphragms may be weakened—⊝ contact

Immune Globulin, IV (Gamimune N, Sandoglobulin, Gammar IV) Uses: *IgG antibody deficiency Dz states, (eg, congenital agammaglobulinemia, CVH, & BMT), HIV, hepatitis A prophylaxis, ITP* Action: IgG supplation Dose: Adults & Peds. Immunodeficiency: 100–200 mg/kg/mo IV at rate of 0.01–0.04 mL/kg/min to a max of 400 mg/kg/dose. ITP: 400 mg/kg/dose IV qd × 5 d. BMT: 500 mg/kg/wk; ↓ in renal insufficiency Caution: [C, ?] Separate administration of live vaccines by 3 mo Contra: Isolated immunoglobulin A deficiency w/ antibodies to IgA, severe thrombocytopenia or coagulation disorders Supplied: Inj SE: Adverse effects associated mostly w/ rate of inf, GI upset Interactions: ↓ Effects of live virus vaccines NIPE: Give live virus vaccines 3 mo after this drug; rapid inf can cause anaphylactoid Rxn

Inamrinone [Amrinone] (Inocor) Uses: *Acute CHF, ischemic cardiomyopathy* Action: + inotrope w/ vasodilator activity Dose: Initial IV bolus 0.75 mg/kg over 2–3 min, then maint dose 5–10 μg/kg/min; 10 mg/kg max; ↓ if ClCr <10 mL/min Caution: [C, ?] Contra: Hypersensitivity to bisulfites Supplied: Inj 5 mg/mL SE: Monitor for fluid, electrolyte, & renal changes Notes: Incompatible w/ dextrose-containing solns Interactions: Precipitates form if contact made with furosemide; diuretics cause significant hypovolemia; ↑ effects of digitalis Labs: Monitor ALT, AST, BUN, creatinine, plts NIPE: Monitor I&O, daily weights, BP, pulse

Indapamide (Lozol) Uses: *HTN, edema, CHF* Action: Thiazide diuretic; enhances Na, Cl, & water excretion in the proximal segment of the distal tubule Dose: 1.25–5 mg/d PO Caution: [D, ?] ↑ effect w/ loop diuretics, ACEIs, cyclosporine, digoxin, Li Contra: Anuria, thiazide/sulfonamide allergy, renal decompensation, PRG Supplied: Tabs 1.25, 2.5 mg SE: Hypotension, dizziness photosensitivity Notes: Doses >5 mg do not have additional effects on ↓ BP; take early in day to avoid nocturia; use sunscreen; may take w/ food/milk Interactions: ↑ Effects w/ antihypertensives, diazoxide, nitrates, EtOH; ↑ effects of ACEIs, Li; ↑ risk of gout w/ cyclosporine, thiazides; ↑ risk of hypokalemia w/ amphotericin B, corticosteroids, mezlocillin, piperacillin, ticarcillin; ↓ effects w/ cholestyramine colestipol, NSAIDs; ↓ effects of hypoglycemics Labs: ↑ Serum glucose, uric acid, ↓ K⁺, Na, Cl NIPE: ↑ Risk photosensitivity—use sunscreen, take w/ food

Indinavir (Crixivan) Uses: *HIV infection* Action: Protease inhibitor, inhibits maturation of immature noninfectious virions to mature infectious virus Dose: 800 mg PO q8h; use in combination w/ other antiretroviral agents; take on an empty stomach; ↓ in hepatic impairment **Caution:** [C, ?] Numerous drug interactions **Contra:** Concomitant use w/ triazolam, midazolam, pimozide, ergot alkaloids; ⊘ use simvastatin, lovastatin, sildenafil, St. John's wort **Supplied:** Caps 100, 200, 333, 400 mg **SE:** Nephrolithiasis, dyslipidemia, lipodystrophy, GI effects **Interactions:** ↑ Effects w/ aldesleukin, azole antifungals, clarithromycin, delavirdine, interleukins, quinidine, zidovudine; ↑ effects of amiodarone, cisapride, clarithromycin, ergot alkaloids, fentanyl, HMG-CoA reductase inhibitors, INH, oral contraceptives, phenytoin, rifabutin, ritonavir, sildenafil, stavudine, zidovudine; ↓ effects w/ efavirenz, fluconazole, phenytoin, rifampin, St. John's wort, high-fat/protein meals, grapefruit juice; ↓ effects of midazolam, triazolam **Labs:** ↑ Serum glucose, LFTs, ↓ Hmg, plts, neutrophils **NIPE:** ↑ Fluids 1–2 L/d, capsules moisture sensitive—keep dessicant in container

Indomethacin (Indocin) **Uses:** *Arthritis; closure of the ductus arteriosus; ankylosing spondylitis* **Action:** Inhibits prostaglandins **Dose:** *Adults.* 25–50 mg PO bid–tid, max 200 mg/d. *Infants.* 0.2–0.25 mg/kg/dose IV; may repeat in 12–24 h up to 3 doses; take w/ food **Caution:** [B, +] **Contra:** ASA/NSAID sensitivity, peptic ulcer Dz/active GI bleed, precipitation of asthma/urticaria/rhinitis by NSAIDs/ASA, premature neonates w/ necrotizing enterocolitis, ↓ renal Fxn, active bleeding, thrombocytopenia, 3rd tri PRG **Supplied:** Inj 1 mg/vial; caps 25, 50 mg; SR caps 75 mg; susp 25 mg/5 mL **SE:** GI bleeding or upset, dizziness, edema **Notes:** Monitor renal Fxn; must swallow SR caps whole **Interactions:** ↑ Effects w/ acetaminophen, antiinflammatories, gold compounds, diflunisal, probenecid; ↑ effects of aminoglycosides, anticoagulants, digoxin, hypoglycemics, Li, MRX, nifedipine, phenytoin, penicillamine, verapamil; ↓ effects w/ ASA; ↓ effects of antihypertensives **Labs:** ↑ Serum K+, BUN, creatinine, AST, ALT, urine glucose, protein, PT; ↓ Hmg, Hct, leukocytes, plts **NIPE:** Take w/ food

Infliximab (Remicade) **WARNING:** TB, invasive fungal infections, and other opportunistic infections reported, some fatal; TB skin testing must be performed prior to therapy **Uses:** *Moderate/severe Crohn's Dz; fistulizing Crohn's Dz; RA (combination w/ MTX)* **Action:** IgG1K neutralizes TNFα (human and murine regions) **Dose:** *Crohn's: Induction:* 5 mg/kg IV inf, follow w/doses at 2 and 6 wk after. *Maint:* 5 mg/kg IV inf q8wk. *RA:* 3 mg/kg IV inf at 0, 2, 6 wk, then q8wk **Caution:** [B, ?/–] Active infection **Contra:** Murine hypersensitivity, moderate–severe CHF **Supplied:** Inj **SE:** hypersensitivity Rxns,; Pts are predisposed to infection (especially TB); HA, fatigue, GI upset, inf Rxns **Interactions:** May ↓ effects of live virus vaccines; **Labs:** May ↑ + ANA **NIPE:** ↑ Susceptibility to infection

Influenza Vaccine (Fluzone, FluShield, Fluvirin) **Uses:** *Prevent influenza*; all adults >50 y, children 6–23 mo, PRG women (2nd/3rd tri during flu season), nursing home residents, chronic Dzs, health care workers and household contacts of high-risk Pts, children < 9 y receiving vaccine for the first time **Action:** Active immunization **Dose:** *Adults.* 0.5 mL/dose IM. *Peds.* ≥ 3 y: 0.5-mL IM;

6–35 mo: 0.25 mL IM; 6 mo–< 9 y (first-time vaccination): 2 doses > 4 wk apart 2nd dose before Dec if possible **Caution:** [C, +] **Contra:** Egg, gentamicin, thimerosal allergy, infection at site; high risk of anaphylaxis complications, Hx of Guillain–Barré, asthma, children 5–17 y on ASA **Supplied:** Based on specific manufacturer, 0.25- and 0.5- mL prefilled syringes **SE:** Soreness at inj site, fever, myalgia, malaise, Guillain–Barré syndrome (controversial) **Notes:** Optimal in U.S.: Oct–Nov, protection begins 1-2 wk after, lasts up to 6 mo; each year, vaccines manufactured based on predictions of flu active in flu season (December–Spring in U.S.); whole or split virus given to adults; Peds <13 y split virus or purified surface antigen to ↓ febrile Rxns **Interactions:** ↑ Effects of theophylline, warfarin; ↓ effects w/ corticosteroids, immunosuppressants; ↓ effects of aminopyrine, phenytoin

Influenza Virus Vaccine Live, Intranasal (FluMist)
Uses: *Prevention of influenza* **Action:** Live-attenuated vaccine **Dose:** *Adults 9–49 y.* 1 dose (0.5 mL) per season **Caution:** [C,?/–] **Contra:** Egg allergy, PRG, Hx Guillain–Barré syndrome, known/suspected immune deficiency, asthma or reactive airway Dz **Supplied:** Prefilled, single-use, intranasal sprayer **SE:** Runny nose, nasal congestion, HA, cough **Notes:** 0.25 mL into each nostril; ⊘ administer concurrently w/ other vaccines; ⊘ contact w/ immunocompromised individuals for 21 days **NIPE:** ⊘ Take w/ antivirals, ASA, NSAIDs, immunosuppressants, corticosteroids, radiation therapy

Insulin
Uses: *Type 1 or type 2 DM refractory to diet change or PO hypoglycemic agents; management of acute life-threatening hyperkalemia* **Action:** Insulin suppl **Dose:** Based on serum glucose levels; usually SQ but can be given IV (only regular)/IM; typical starting dose for type 1 0.5–1 U/kg/d; type 2 0.3–0.4 Units/kg/d; renal failure may ↓ insulin needs **Caution:** [B, +] **Contra:** Hypoglycemia **Supplied:** See Table 6, page 275 **SE:** Highly purified insulins ↑ free insulin; monitor Pts closely for several wks when changing doses/agents **Interactions:** ↑ Hypoglycemic effects w/ α-blockers, anabolic steroids, BBs, clofibrate, fenfluramine, guanethidine, MAOIs, NSAIDs, pentamidine, phenylbutazone salicylates, sulfinpyrazone, tetracyclines, EtOH, celery, coriander, dandelion root fenugreek, ginseng, garlic, juniper berries; ↓ hypoglycemic effects w/ corticosteroids, dextrothyroxine, diltiazem, dobutamine, epinephrine, niacin, oral contraceptives, protease inhibitor antiretrovirals, rifampin, thiazide diuretics, thyroid preps, marijuana, tobacco **NIPE:** If mixing insulins, draw up short-acting preps first in syringe

Interferon Alfa (Roferon-A, Intron A)
Uses: *Hairy cell leukemia, Kaposi's sarcoma, melanoma, CML, chronic hepatitis C, follicular NHL, condylomata acuminata,* multiple myeloma, renal cell carcinoma, and bladder CA **Action:** Antiproliferative against tumor cells; modulation of the host immune response **Dose:** See specific protocols. *Adults.* Hairy cell leukemia: Alfa-2a (Roferon-A): 3 MUNITS/d for 16–24 wk SQ or IM. Alfa-2b (Intron A): 2

MUNITS/m² IM or SQ 3×/wk for 2–6 mo **Peds. CML:** Alfa-2a (Roferon-A): 2.5–5 MUNITS/m² IM qd. *Chronic hepatitis B:* Alfa-2b (Intron A): 3–10 MUNITS/m² SQ 3×/wk **Contra:** Benzyl EtOH sensitivity, decompensated liver Dz, autoimmune Dz, rapidly progressing AIDS-related Kaposi's sarcoma **Supplied:** Injectable forms **SE:** Flu-like Sxs; fatigue common; anorexia in 20–30%; neurotoxicity at high doses; neutralizing antibodies in up to 40% of Pts receiving prolonged systemic therapy **Interactions:** ↑ Effects of antineoplastics, CNS depressants, doxorubicin, theophylline; ↓ effects of live virus vaccine **Labs:** ↑ LFTs, BUN, SCr, glucose, phosphorus, ↓ Hmg, Hct, Ca **NIPE:** ASA & EtOH use may cause GI bleed, ↑ fluids to 2–3 L/d

Interferon Alfa-2b and Ribavirin Combination (Rebetron)
WARNING: Contraindicated in PRG females and their male partners **Uses:** *Chronic hepatitis C in Pts w/ compensated liver Dz who have relapsed following α-interferon therapy* **Action:** Combination antiviral agents **Dose:** 3 MUNITS Intron A SQ 3×/wk w/ 1000–1200 mg of Rebetron PO ÷ bid dose for 24 wk. **Pts <75 kg:** 1000 mg of Rebetron/d **Caution:** [X, ?] **Contra:** PRG, males w/ PRG female partner, autoimmune hepatitis, creatinine clearance < 50 mL/min **Supplied:** **Pts <75 kg:** Combination packs: 6 vials Intron A (3 MUNITS/0.5 mL) w/ 6 syringes and EtOH swabs, 70 Rebetron caps; one 18 MUNITS multidose vial of Intron A inj (22.8 MUNITS/3.8 mL; 3 MUNITS/0.5 mL) and 6 syringes and swabs, 70 Rebetron caps; one 18 MUNITS Intron A inj multidose pen (22.5 MUNITS/1.5 mL; 3 MUNITS/0.2 mL) and 6 disposable needles and swabs, 70 Rebetron caps. **Pts <75 kg:** Identical except 84 Rebetron caps/pack **SE:** Flu-like syndrome, HA, anemia **Notes:** Negative PRG test required monthly; instruct Pts in self-administration of SQ Intron A. See Interferon Alfa **Additional Labs:** ↑ Uric acid

Interferon Alfacon-1 (Infergen)
Uses: *Management of chronic hepatitis C* **Action:** Biologic response modifier **Dose:** 9 µg SQ 3×/wk × 24 wk **Caution:** [C, M] **Contra:** Hypersensitivity to *E. coli*-derived products **Supplied:** Inj 9, 15 µg **SE:** Flu-like syndrome, depression, blood dyscrasias **Notes:** Allow at least 48 h between inj **Interactions:** ↑ Effects of theophylline **Labs:** ↑ Triglycerides, TSH; ↓ Hmg, Hct **NIPE:** Refrigerate, ⊘ shake, use barrier contraception

Interferon β-1b (Betaseron)
Uses: *MS, relapsing-remitting and secondary progressive* **Action:** Biologic response modifier **Dose:** 0.25 mg SQ qod **Caution:** [C, ?] **Contra:** Hypersensitivity to human albumin products **Supplied:** Powder for inj 0.3 mg **SE:** Flu-like syndrome, depression, blood dyscrasias **Interactions:** ↑ Effects of theophylline, zidovudine **Labs:** ↑ LFTs, BUN, urine protein **NIPE:** ↑ Risk of photosensitivity—use sunscreen, abortion; ↑ fluid intake, use barrier contraception

Interferon γ-1b (Actimmune)
Uses: *↓ incidence of serious infections in chronic granulomatous Dz (CGD), osteopetrosis* **Action:** Biologic response modifier **Dose:** *Adults.* CGD: 50 µg/m² SQ (1.5 MU/m²) BSA >0.5 m²; if BSA <0.5 m², give 1.5 µg/kg/dose; given 3×/wk. *Peds.* BSA ≤ 0.5 m²: 1.5 µg/kg/ SQ tid;

BSA > 0.5 m^2: 50 μg/m^2 SQ tid **Caution:** [C, ?] **Contra:** Hypersensitivity to *E. coli*-derived products **Supplied:** Inj 100 μg (2 MU) **SE:** Flu-like syndrome, depression, blood dyscrasias

Ipecac Syrup **Uses:** *Drug OD and certain cases of poisoning* **Action:** Irritation of the GI mucosa; stimulation of the chemoreceptor trigger zone **Dose:** *Adults.* 15–30 mL PO, followed by 200–300 mL of water; if no emesis in 20 min, repeat once. *Peds. 6–12 y:* 5–10 mL PO followed by 10–20 mL/kg of water; if no emesis in 20 min, repeat once. *1–12 y:* 15 mL PO followed by 10–20 mL/kg of water; if no emesis in 20 min, repeat once **Caution:** [C, ?] **Contra:** Ingestion of petroleum distillates, strong acid, base, or other caustic agents; in comatose or unconscious Pts **Supplied:** Syrup 15, 30 mL (OTC) **SE:** Lethargy, diarrhea, cardiotoxicity, protracted vomiting **Notes:** Caution in CNS depressant OD; usage is falling out of favor and is no longer recommended by some groups (www.clintox.org/Pos_Statements/Ipecac.html) **Interactions:** ↑ Effects of muscle-suppressives, theophylline, zidovudine **NIPE:** ↑ Fluids to 2–3 L/d, ⊘ EtOH, CNS depressants

Ipratropium (Atrovent) **Uses:** *Bronchospasm w/ COPD, rhinitis, and rhinorrhea* **Action:** Synthetic anticholinergic agent similar to atropine **Dose:** *Adults & Peds.* >12 y. 2–4 puffs qid. *Nasal:* 2 sprays/nostril bid–tid **Caution:** [B, +/–] **Contra:** Hypersensitivity to soya lecithin or related foods **Supplied:** Metdose inhaler 18 μg/dose; soln for inhal 0.02%; nasal spray 0.03%, 0.06%; nasal inhaler 20 μg/dose **SE:** Nervousness, dizziness, HA, cough, bitter taste, nasal dryness **Notes:** Not for acute bronchospasm **Interactions:** ↑ Effects w/ albuterol; ↑ effects of anticholinergics, antimuscarinics; ↓ effects w/ jaborandi tree, pill-bearing spurge **NIPE:** Adequate fluids, separate inhalation of other drugs by 5 min

Irbesartan (Avapro) **Uses:** *HTN*, DN, CHF **Action:** Angiotensin II receptor antagonist **Dose:** 150 mg/d PO, may ↑ to 300 mg/d **Caution:** [C (1st tri; D 2nd/3rd), ?/–] **Supplied:** Tabs 75, 150, 300 mg **SE:** Fatigue, hypotension **Interactions:** ↑ Risk of hyperkalemia w/ K-sparing diuretics, trimethoprim, K suppls; ↑ effects of Li **Labs:** ↑ BUN, SCr; ↓ Hmg **NIPE:** ⊘ PRG, breast-feeding

Irinotecan (Camptosar) **Uses:** *Colorectal* and lung CA **Action:** Topoisomerase I inhibitor; interferes w/ DNA synthesis **Dose:** Per protocol; 125–350 mg/m^2 weekly to every 3 wk (↓ hepatic dysfunction, as tolerated per toxicities) **Caution:** [D, –] **Contra:** Hypersensitivity to component **Supplied:** Inj 20 mg/mL **SE:** Myelosuppression, N/V/D, abdominal cramping, alopecia; diarrhea is dose-limiting; Rx acute diarrhea w/ atropine; Rx subacute diarrhea w/ loperamide **Notes:** Diarrhea correlated to levels of metabolite SN-38 **Interactions:** ↑ Effects of antineoplastics; ↑ risk of akathisia w/ prochlorperazine **Labs:** ↑ LFTs **NIPE:** Use barrier contraception, ⊘ exposure to infection

Iron Dextran (Dexferrum, INFeD) **Uses:** *Fe deficiency when PO suppl not possible* **Action:** Parenteral Fe suppl **Dose:** Estimate Fe deficiency, given IM/IV. A 0.5-mL test dose. Total replacement dose (mL) = 0.0476 × weight (kg) ×

[desired hemoglobin (g/dL) – measured hemoglobin (g/dL)] + 1 mL/5 kg weight (max 14 mL). **Adults.** Max daily dose: 100 mg Fe. **Peds.** Max daily dose: <5 kg: 25 mg Fe. *5–10 kg:* 50 mg Fe. *10–50 kg:* 100 mg Fe **Caution:** [C, M] **Contra:** Anemia w/o Fe deficiency. **Supplied:** Inj 50 mg (Fe)/mL **SE:** Anaphylaxis, flushing, dizziness, inj site and inf Rxns, metallic taste **Notes:** Give deep IM using "Z-track" technique; IV route preferred **Interactions:** ↓ Effects w/ chloramphenicol, ↓ absorption of oral Fe **Labs:** False ↓ serum Ca; false ↑ guaiac test **NIPE:** ⊘ Take oral Fe

Iron Sucrose (Venofer) Uses: *Fe deficiency anemia in chronic hemodialysis in those receiving erythropoietin* **Actions:** Fe replacement. **Dose:** 5 mL (100 mg) IV during dialysis, no faster than 1 mL (20 mg)/min. **Caution:** [C, M] **Contra:** Anemia w/o Fe deficiency **Supplied:** 20 mg elemental Fe per mL, 5-mL vials. **SE:** Anaphylaxis, hypotension, cramps, N/V/D, HA **Notes:** Most Pts require cumulative doses of 1000 mg; ensure drug administered at slow rate

Isoniazid (INH) Uses: *Rx and prophylaxis of TB* **Action:** Bactericidal; interferes w/ mycolic acid synthesis (disrupts cell wall) **Dose:** *Adults.* Active TB: 5 mg/kg/24 h PO or IM (usually 300 mg/d). *Prophylaxis:* 300 mg/d PO for 6–12 mo. *Peds.* Active TB: 10–20 mg/kg/24 h PO or IM to a max of 300 mg/d. *Prophylaxis:* 10 mg/kg/24 h PO; ↓ in hepatic/renal dysfunction **Caution:** [C, +] Liver Dz, dialysis; ⊘ EtOH **Contra:** Acute liver Dz, Hx INH hepatitis **Supplied:** Tabs 100, 300 mg; syrup 50 mg/5 mL; inj 100 mg/mL **SE:** Hepatitis, peripheral neuropathy, GI upset, anorexia, dizziness, skin Rxn **Notes:** Give w/ 2–3 other drugs for active TB, based on INH resistance patterns when TB acquired and sensitivity results; prophylaxis generally is INH alone. IM route rarely used. To prevent peripheral neuropathy, give pyridoxine 50–100 mg/d. Check CDC guidelines (in MMWR) for specific Rx recommendations **Interactions:** ↑ Effects of acetaminophen, anticoagulants, carbamazepine, cycloserine, diazepam, meperidine, hydantoins, theophylline, valproic acid, EtOH; ↑ effects w/ rifampin; ↓ effects w/ Al salts; ↓ effects of anticoagulants, ketoconazole **Labs:** False + urine glucose; false ↑ AST, uric acid, false ↓ serum glucose **NIPE:** Only take w/ food if GI upset

Isoproterenol (Isuprel) Uses: *Shock, bronchospasm, cardiac arrest, and AV nodal block* **Action:** β₁- and β₂-receptor stimulant **Dose:** *Adults.* 2–10 μg/min IV inf; titrate to effect. *Inhal:* 1–2 inhal 4–6×/d. *Peds.* 0.2–2 μg/kg/min IV inf; titrate to effect. *Inhal:* 1–2 inhal 4–6×/d **Caution:** [C, ?] **Contra:** Angina, tachyarrhythmias (digitalis-induced or others) **Supplied:** Met-inhaler; soln for neb 0.5%, 1%; inj 0.02 mg/mL, 0.2 mg/mL **SE:** Insomnia, arrhythmias, HA, trembling, dizziness **Notes:** Pulse > 130 bpm may induce ventricular arrhythmias **Interactions:** ↑ Eeffects w/ albuterol, guanethidine, oxytocic drugs, sympathomimetics, TCAs; ↑ risk of arrhythmias w/ amitriptyline, bretylium, cardiac glycosides, K-depleting drugs, theophylline; ↓ effects w/ BBs **Labs:** False ↑ serum AST, bilirubin, glucose **NIPE:** Saliva may turn pink in color, ↑ fluids to 2–3 L/d

Isosorbide Dinitrate (Isordil, Sorbitrate, Dilatrate-SR) Uses: *Rx and prevention of angina,* CHF (w/ hydralazine) **Action:** Relaxes vascular smooth muscle **Dose:** *Acute angina:* 5–10 mg PO (chew tabs) q2–3h or 2.5–10 mg SL PRN q5–10min; >3 doses should not be given in a 15630- min period. *Angina prophylaxis:* 5–40 mg PO q6h; ⊘ give nitrates on a chronic q6h or qd basis >7–10 d because tolerance may develop; provide 10–12-h drug-free intervals **Caution:** [C, ?] Sildenafil, tadalafil, vardenafil **Contra:** Severe anemia, closed-angle glaucoma, postural hypotension, cerebral hemorrhage, head trauma (can ↑ ICP), w/ sildenafil, tadalafil, vardenafil **Supplied:** Tabs 5, 10, 20, 30, 40 mg; SR tabs 40 mg; SL tabs 2.5, 5, 10 mg; chew tabs 5, 10 mg **SE:** HA, ↓ BP, flushing, tachycardia, dizziness **Notes:** Higher PO dose usually needed to achieve same results as SL forms **Interactions:** ↑ Hypotension w/ antihypertensives, ASA, CCBs, phenothiazides, sildenafil, EtOH **Labs:** False ↓ serum cholesterol **NIPE:** ⊘ Nitrates for a 8–12-h period/d to avoid tolerance

Isosorbide Mononitrate (Ismo, Imdur) Uses: *Prevention/Rx of angina pectoris* Action: Relaxes vascular smooth muscle Dose: 20 mg PO bid, w/ the 2 doses 7 h apart or XR (Imdur) 30–120 mg/d PO Caution: [C, ?] ⊘ coadminister w/ sildenafil Contra: Head trauma or cerebral hemorrhage (can ↑ ICP), w/ sildenafil, tadalafil, vardenafil Supplied: Tabs 10, 20 mg; XR 30, 60, 120 mg SE: HA, dizziness, ↓ BP Interactions: ↑ Hypotension w/ ASA, nitrates, sildenafil, EtOH Labs: False ↓ serum cholesterol

Isotretinoin [13-cis Retinoic Acid] (Accutane, Amnesteem, Claravis, Sotret) WARNING: Must not be used by PRG females; Pt must be capable of complying w/ mandatory contraceptive measures; prescribed according to product-specific risk management system Uses: *Refractory severe acne* Action: Retinoic acid derivative Dose: 0.5–2 mg/kg/d PO ÷ bid (↓ in hepatic Dz, take w/ food) Caution: [X, –] ⊘ tetracyclines Contra: Retinoid sensitivity, PRG Supplied: Caps 10, 20, 40 mg SE: Isolated reports of depression, psychosis, suicidal thoughts; dermatologic sensitivity, xerostomia, photosensitivity, ↑ LFTs, ↑ triglycerides Notes: Risk management program requires 2 – PRG tests before therapy and use of 2 forms of contraception 1 mo before, during, and 1 mo after therapy; informed consent recommended; monitor LFTs and lipids Interactions: ↑ Effects w/ corticosteroids, phenytoin, vitamin A ; ↑ risk of pseudotumor cerebri w/ tetracyclines; ↑ triglyceride levels w/ EtOH; ↓ effects of carbamazepine NIPE: ↑ Risk of photosensitivity—use sunscreen, take w/ food, ⊘ PRG

Isradipine (DynaCirc) Uses: *HTN* Action: CCB Dose: Adults. 2.5–10 mg PO bid. Peds. 0.05–0.15 mg/kg PO tid–qid, up to 20 mg/d (⊘ crush or chew) Caution: [C, ?] Contra: Severe heart block sinus bradycardia, CHF, dosing w/in several hours of IV BBs Supplied: Caps 2.5, 5 mg; tabs CR 5, 10 mg SE: HA, edema, flushing, fatigue, dizziness, palpitations Interactions: ↑Effects w/ azole antifungals, BBs, cimetidine; ↑ effects of carbamazepine, cyclosporine, digitalis glycosides, prazosin, quinidine; ↓ effects w/ Ca, rifampin; ↓ effects of lovastatin Labs: ↑ LFTs NIPE: ⊘ DC abruptly

Itraconazole (Sporanox) **WARNING:** Potential for negative inotropic effects on the heart; if signs Sxs of CHF occur during administration, continued use should be assessed **Uses:** *Fungal infections (aspergillosis, blastomycosis, histoplasmosis, candidiasis)* **Action:** Inhibits synthesis of ergosterol **Dose:** 200 mg PO or IV qd–bid (capsule w/ meals or cola/grapefruit juice); PO soln on empty stomach; ⊘ antacids **Caution:** [C, ?] Numerous drug interactions **Contra:** CrCl <30 mL/min, Hx of CHF or ventricular dysfunction, or w/ H₂-antagonist, omeprazole **Supplied:** Caps 100 mg; soln 10 mg/mL; inj 10 mg/mL **SE:** nausea, rash, hepatitis, hypokalemia, CHF **Notes:** PO soln and caps not interchangeable; useful in Pts who cannot take amphotericin B; watch for signs/Sxs of CHF w/ IV use **Interactions:** ↑ Effects w/ clarithromycin, erythromycin; ↑ effects of alprazolam, anticoagulants, atevirdine, atorvastatin, buspirone, cerivastatin, chlordiazepoxide, cyclosporine, diazepam, digoxin, felodipine, fluvastatin, indinavir, lovastatin, methadone, methylprednisolone, midazolam, nelfinavir, pravastatin, ritonavir, saquinavir, simvastatin, tacrolimus, tolbutamide, triazolam, warfarin; ↑ QT prolongation w/ astemizole, cisapride, pimozide, quinidine, terfenadine; ↓ effects w/ antacids, Ca, cimetidine, didanosine, famotidine, lansoprazole, Mg, nizatidine, omeprazole, phenytoin, rifampin, sucralfate, grapefruit juice **Labs:** ↑ LFTs, BUN, SCr **NIPE:** Take capsule w/ food & soln w/o food, ⊘ PRG or breast-feeding, ↑ risk of disulfiram-like response w/ EtOH

Kaolin-Pectin (Kaodene, Kao-Spen, Kapectolin, Parepectolin) **Uses:** *Diarrhea* **Action:** Absorbent demulcent **Dose:** *Adults.* 60–120 mL PO after each loose stool or q3–4h PRN. *Peds.* 3–6 y: 15–30 mL/dose PO PRN. *6–12 y:* 30–60 mL/dose PO PRN **Caution:** [C, +] **Contra:** Diarrhea secondary to pseudomembranous colitis **Supplied:** Multiple OTC forms; also available w/ opium (Parepectolin) **SE:** Constipation, dehydration **Interaction:** ↓ Effects of ciprofloxacin, clindamycin, digoxin, lincomycin, lovastatin, penicillamine, quinidine, tetracycline **NIPE:** Take other meds 2–3 h before or after this drug

Ketoconazole (Nizoral, Nizoral AD Shampoo) [OTC] **Uses:** *Systemic fungal infections; topical for local fungal infections due to dermatophytes and yeast; shampoo for dandruff,* short term in CAP when rapid reduction of testosterone needed (ie, cord compression) **Action:** Inhibits fungal cell wall synthesis **Dose:** *Adults.* PO: 200 mg PO qd; ↑ to 400 mg PO qd for serious infection; CAP 400 mg PO tid (short term). *Topical:* Apply to area qd (cream or shampoo). *Peds.* >2 y: 5–10 mg/kg/24 h PO ÷ q12–24h (↓ in hepatic Dz) **Caution:** [C, +/–] Any agent ↑ gastric pH prevents absorption; may enhance PO anticoagulants; w/ EtOH (disulfiram-like Rxn; numerous drug interactions) **Contra:** CNS fungal infections (poor CNS penetration), concurrent astemizole, cisapride, PO triazolam **Supplied:** Tabs 200 mg; topical cream 2%; shampoo 2% **SE:** Monitor LFTs w/ systemic use; can cause nausea **Notes:** PO form multiple drug interactions **Interactions:** ↑ Effects of alprazolam, anticoagulants, atevirdine, atorvastatin, buspirone, chlordiazepoxide, cyclosporine, diazepam, felodipine, fluvastatin, indinavir, lovastatin, methadone, methylprednisolone, midazolam, nelfinavir, pravastatin, ritonavir, saquinavir, simvastatin, tacrolimus, tolbutamide, triazolam warfarin; ↑ QT prolongation w/ astemizole, cisapride, quinidine, terfenadine; ↓ effects w/ antacids, Ca, cimetidine, didanosine, famotidine, lansoprazole, Mg, nizatidine, omeprazole, phenytoin, rifampin, sucralfate **Labs:** ↑ LFTs **NIPE:** Take tabs w/ citrus juice, take w/ food; shampoo wet hair 1 min, rinse, repeat for 3 min; ⊘ PRG or breast-feeding

Ketoprofen (Orudis, Oruvail) Uses: * Arthritis, pain* **Action:** NSAID; inhibits prostaglandins **Dose:** 25–75 mg PO tid–qid, 300 mg/d/max; take w/ food **Caution** [B (D 3rd tri), ?] **Contra:** NSAID/ASA sensitivity **Supplied:** Tabs 12.5 mg; caps 25, 50, 75 mg; caps, SR 100, 150, 200 mg **SE:** GI upset, peptic ulcers, dizziness, edema, rash **Interactions:** ↑ Effects w/ ASA, corticosteroids NSAIDs, probenicid, EtOH; ↑ effects of antineoplastics, hypoglycemics, insulin, Li, MRX; ↑ risk of nephrotoxicity w/ aminoglycosides, cyclosporines; ↑ risk of bleeding w/ anticoagulants, defamandole, cefotetan, cefoperazone, clopidogrel, eptifibatide, plicamycin, thrombolytics, tirofiban, valproic acid, dong quai, feverfew, garlic, ginkgo biloba, ginger, horse chestnut, red clover; ↓ effects of antihypertensives, diuretics **Labs:** ↑ LFTs, BUN, serum Na$^+$, creatinine, Cl$^-$, K$^+$, PT; ↑ or ↓ glucose; ↓ Hmg, Hct, plts, leukocytes **NIPE:** ↑ Risk of photosensitivity—use sunscreen, take w/ food

Ketorolac (Toradol) **WARNING:** Indicated for short-term (≥ 5 d) Rx of moderately severe acute pain that requires analgesia at opioid level **Uses:** *Pain* **Action:** NSAID; inhibits prostaglandins **Dose:** 15–30 mg IV/IM q6h or 10 mg PO qid; max IV/IM 120 mg/d, max PO 40 mg/d; ⊘ use for > 5 d; ↓ for age and renal dysfunction **Caution:** [B (D 3rd tri), –] **Contra:** Peptic ulcer Dz, NSAID sensitivity, advanced renal Dz, CNS bleeding, anticipated major surgery, labor and delivery, nursing mothers **Supplied:** Tabs 10 mg; inj 15 mg/mL, 30 mg/mL **SE:** Bleeding, peptic ulcer Dz, renal failure, edema, dizziness, hypersensitivity **Notes:** PO only as continuation of IM/IV therapy **Interactions:** ↑ Effects w/ ASA, corticosteroids, NSAIDs, probenicid, EtOH; ↑ effects of antineoplastics, hypoglycemics, insulin, Li, MRX; ↑ risk of nephrotoxicity w/ aminoglycosides, cyclosporines; ↑ risk of bleeding w/ anticoagulants, defamandole, cefotetan, cefoperazone, clopidogrel, eptifibatide, plicamycin, thrombolytics, tirofiban, valproic acid, dong quai, feverfew, garlic, ginkgo biloba, ginger, horse chestnut, red clover; ↓ effects of antihypertensives, diuretics **Labs:** ↑ LFTs, PT, BUN, SCr, Na$^+$, Cl$^-$, K$^+$ **NIPE:** 30-mg dose equals comparative analgesia of meperidine 100 mg or morphine 12 mg

Ketorolac Ophthalmic (Acular) Uses: *Ocular itching caused by seasonal allergies* **Action:** NSAID **Dose:** 1 gt qid **Caution:** [C, +] **Supplied:** Soln 0.5% **SE:** Local irritation. See Ketorolac **NIPE:** ⊘ Soft contact lenses

Ketotifen (Zaditor) Uses: *Allergic conjunctivitis* **Action:** H_1-receptor antagonist and mast cell stabilizer **Dose: *Adults & Peds.*** 1 gt in eye(s) q8–12h **Caution:** [C,?/–] **Supplied:** Soln 0.025%/5 mL **SE:** Local irritation, HA, rhinitis **NIPE:** Insert soft contact lenses 10 min after drug use

Labetalol (Trandate, Normodyne) Uses: *HTN* and hypertensive emergencies **Action:** α- and β-Adrenergic blocking agent **Dose: *Adults.*** HTN: Initial, 100 mg PO bid, then 200–400 mg PO bid. *Hypertensive emergency:* 20–80 mg IV bolus, then 2 mg/min IV inf, titrate to effect. ***Peds.*** PO: 3–20 mg/kg/d in ÷ doses. *Hypertensive emergency:* 0.4–1.5 mg/kg/h IV cont inf **Caution:** [C (D in 2nd or 3rd tri), +] **Contra:** Asthma/COPD, cardiogenic shock, uncompensated CHF, heart block **Supplied:** Tabs 100, 200, 300 mg; inj 5 mg/mL **SE:** Dizziness, nausea, ↓ BP, fatigue, CV effects **Interactions:** ↑ Effects w/ cimetidine, diltiazem, nitroglycerine, quinidine, paroxetine, verapamil; ↑ tremors w/ TCAs; ↓ effects w/ glutethimide, NSAIDs, salicylates; ↓ effects of antihypertensives, β-adrenergic bronchodilators, sulfonylureas **Labs:** False + urine catecholamines **NIPE:** May have transient tingling of scalp

Lactic Acid & Ammonium Hydroxide [Ammonium Lactate] (Lac-Hydrin) Uses: *Severe xerosis and ichthyosis* **Action:** Emollient moisturizer **Dose:** Apply bid **Caution:** [B, ?] **Supplied:** Lactic acid 12% w/ ammonium hydroxide **SE:** Local irritation

Lactobacillus (Lactinex Granules) [OTC] Uses: Control of diarrhea, especially after antibiotic therapy **Action:** Replaces normal intestinal flora **Dose: *Adults & Peds.*** >3 y: 1 packet, 2 caps, or 4 tabs tid–qid (w/ meals or liq) **Caution:** [A, +] **Contra:** Milk/lactose allergy **Supplied:** Tabs; caps; EC caps; powder in packets (all OTC) **SE:** Flatulence

Lactulose (Chronulac, Cephulac, Enulose) Uses: *Hepatic encephalopathy; constipation* **Action:** Acidifies the colon, drawing ammonia to diffuse into the colon **Dose:** *Acute hepatic encephalopathy:* 30–45 mL PO q1h until soft stools, then tid–qid. *Chronic laxative therapy:* 30–45 mL PO tid–qid; adjust q1–2d to produce 2–3 soft stools/d. *Rectally:* 200 g in 700 mL of water PR. ***Peds.*** Infants: 2.5–10 mL/24 h ÷ tid–qid. ***Peds:*** 40–90 mL/24 h ÷ tid–qid **Caution:** [B, ?] **Contra:** Galactosemia **Supplied:** Syrup 10 g/15 mL, soln 10 g/15 mL, 10 g/packet **SE:** Severe diarrhea, flatulence; may cause severe diarrhea and life-threatening electrolyte disturbances **Interactions:** ↓ Effects w/ antacids, neomycin **Labs:** ↓ Serum ammonia **NIPE:** May take 24–48 h for results

Lamivudine (Epivir, Epivir-HBV) WARNING: Lactic acidosis and severe hepatomegaly w/ steatosis reported w/ nucleoside analogs **Uses:** *HIV infection, chronic hepatitis B* **Action:** Inhibits HIV RT and hepatitis B viral polymerase, resulting in viral DNA chain termination **Dose:** HIV: *Adults & Peds.* >12 y: 150 mg PO bid. *Peds.* <12 y: 4 mg/kg bid. HBV: *Adults.* 100 mg/d. *Peds.* 2–17 y: 3 mg/kg/d PO, 100 mg max; ↓ in renal impairment **Caution:** [C, ?] **Con-**

tra: Hypersensitivity to any component **Supplied:** Tabs 100, 150 mg (HBV); soln 5 mg/mL, 10 mg/mL **SE:** HA, pancreatitis, anemia, GI upset, lactic acidosis **Interactions:** ↑ Effects w/ co-trimoxazole, trimethoprim/sulfamethoxazole; ↑ risk of lactic acidosis w/ antiretrovirals, reverse transcriptase inhibitors **Labs:** ↑ LFTs

Lamotrigine (Lamictal)   **WARNING:** Serious rashes requiring hospitalization and DC of Rx reported; rash less frequent in adults Uses: *Partial Szs, bipolar disorder, Lennox–Gastaut syndrome* **Action:** Phenyltriazine antiepileptic **Dose:** *Adults.* Szs: Initial 50 mg/d PO, then 50 mg PO bid for 2 wk, then maint 300–500 mg/d in 2 ÷ doses. *Bipolar:* Initial 25 mg/d PO, then 50 mg PO qd for 2 wk, then 100 mg PO qd for 1 wk; maint 200 mg/d. *Peds.* 0.15 mg/kg in 1–2 ÷ doses for wk 1 and 2, then 0.3 mg/kg for wk 3 and 4, then maint 1 mg/kg/d in 1–2 ÷ doses (↓ in hepatic Dz or if w/ enzyme inducers or valproic acid) **Caution:** [C, –] Interactions w/ other antiepileptics **Supplied:** Tabs 25, 100, 150, 200 mg; chew tabs 5, 25 mg **SE:** HA, GI upset, dizziness, ataxia, rash (potentially life-threatening in children > adults) **Notes:** Value of therapeutic monitoring not established **Interactions:** ↑ Effects valproic acid; ↑ effects of carbamazepine; ↓ effects w/ phenobarbital, phenytoin, primidone; **NIPE:** ↑ Risk of photosensitivity—use sunscreen

Lansoprazole (Prevacid)   Uses: *Duodenal ulcers, prevent and Rx NSAID gastric ulcers,* *H. pylori* infection, erosive esophagitis, and hypersecretory conditions **Action:** Proton pump inhibitor **Dose:** 15–30 mg/d PO; NSAID ulcer prevention 15 mg/d PO ≤ 12 wk, NSAID ulcers 30 mg/d PO, ×8 wk; ↓ in severe hepatic impairment **Caution:** [B, ?/–] **Supplied:** Caps 15, 30 mg **SE:** HA, fatigue **Interactions:** ↑ Effects of hypoglycemics, nifedipine; ↓ effects w/ sucralfate; ↓ effects of ampicillin, cefpodoxime, cefuroxime, digoxin, enoxacin, ketoconazole, theophylline **Labs:** ↑ LFTs, SCr, LDH, gastrin, lipids **NIPE:** Take ac

Latanoprost (Xalatan)   Uses: *Refractory glaucoma* **Action:** Prostaglandin **Dose:** 1 gt q(h)s hs **Caution:** [C, ?] **Supplied:** 0.005% soln **SE:** May darken light irises; blurred vision, ocular stinging, and itching **Interactions:** ↑ Risk of precipitation if mixed w/ eye drops w/ thimerosal

Leflunomide (Arava)   **WARNING:** PRG must be excluded prior to start of Rx Uses: *Active RA* **Action:** Inhibits pyrimidine synthesis **Dose:** Initial 100 mg/d PO for 3 d, then 10–20 mg/d **Caution:** [X, –] **Contra:** PRG **Supplied:** Tabs 10, 20, 100 mg **SE:** Monitor LFTs during initial therapy; diarrhea, infection, HTN, alopecia, rash, nausea, joint pain, hepatitis **Interactions:** ↑ Effects w/ rifampin; ↑ risk of hepatotoxicity w/ hepatotoxic drugs, MRX; ↑ effects of NSAIDs; ↓ effects w/ activated charcoal, cholestyramine **Labs:** ↑ LFTs **NIPE:** ⊘ PRG, breast-feeding, live virus vaccines

Lepirudin (Refludan)   Uses: *Heparin-induced thrombocytopenia* **Action:** Direct inhibitor of thrombin **Dose:** Bolus 0.4 mg/kg IV, then 0.15 mg/kg inf (↓ dose and inf rate if CrCl <60 mL/min) **Caution:** [B, ?/–] Hemorrhagic event or severe HTN **Contra:** Active major bleeding **Supplied:** Inj 50 mg **SE:** Bleeding, anemia, hematoma **Notes:** Adjust dose based on aPTT ratio, maintain aPTT ratio of 1.5–2.0 **Interactions:** ↑ Risk of bleeding w/ antiplt drugs, cephalosporins, NSAIDs, thrombolytics, salicylates, feverfew, ginkgo biloba, ginger, valerian

Letrozole (Femara) Uses: *Advanced breast CA* **Action:** Nonsteroidal aromatase inhibitor **Dose:** 2.5 mg/d PO **Caution:** [D, ?] **Contra:** PRG **Supplied:** Tabs 2.5 mg **SE:** Requires periodic CBC, thyroid Fxn, electrolyte, LFT, and renal monitoring; anemia, nausea, hot flashes, arthralgia **Interactions:** ↑ Risk of interference w/ action of drug w/ estrogens and oral contraceptives **Labs:** ↑ LFTs, cholesterol, Ca, ↓ lymphocytes

Leucovorin (Wellcovorin) Uses: *OD of folic acid antagonist; augmentation of 5-FU, ↓ MTX elimination* **Action:** Reduced folate source; circumvents action of folate reductase inhibitors (eg, MTX) **Dose:** *Adults & Peds.* MTX rescue: 10 mg/m²/dose IV or PO q6h for 72 h until MTX level <10⁻⁸. *5-FU:* 200 mg/m²/d IV 1–5 d during daily 5-FU Rx or 500 mg/m²/wk w/ weekly 5-FU therapy. *Adjunct to antimicrobials:* 5–15 mg/d PO **Caution:** [C, ?/–] **Contra:** Pernicious anemia **Supplied:** Tabs 5, 15, 25 mg; inj **SE:** Allergic Rxn, N/V/D, fatigue **Notes:** Many dosing schedules for leucovorin rescue following MTX Rx; should not be administered intrathecally/intraventricularly **Interactions:** ↑ Effects of fluorouracil; ↓ effects of MRX, phenobarbital, phenyotin, primidone, trimethoprim/sulfamethoxazole **NIPE:** ↑ Fluids to 3 L/d

Leuprolide (Lupron, Lupron DEPOT, Lupron DEPOT-Ped, Viadur, Eligard) Uses: *Advanced CAP (all products), endometriosis (Lupron), uterine fibroids (Lupron), and CPP (Lupron-Ped)* **Action:** LHRH agonist; paradoxically inhibits release of gonadotropin, resulting in ↓ pituitary gonadotropins (↓ LH); in men ↓ testosterone **Dose:** *Adults.* CAP: 7.5 mg IM q28d or 22.5 mg IM q3mo or 30 mg IM q4mo of depot; Viadur implant (CAP only); insert in inner upper arm using local anesthesia, replace q12mo. *Endometriosis (Lupron DEPOT):* 3.75 mg IM qmo ×6. *Fibroids:* 3.75 mg IM qmo ×3. *Peds.* CPP (Lupron-Ped): 50 µg/kg/d daily SQ inj; ↑ by 10 µg/kg/d until total down-regulation achieved. *DEPOT:* <25 kg: 7.5 mg IM q4wk. >25–37.5 kg: 11.25 mg IM q4wk. >37.5 kg: 15 mg IM q4wk **Caution:** [X, ?] **Contra:** Undiagnosed vaginal bleeding, implant dosage form in women and peds; PRG **Supplied:** Inj 5 mg/mL; Lupron DEPOT 3.75 (1 mo for fibroids, endometriosis); Lupron DEPOT for CAP: 7.5 mg (1 mo), 22.5 (3 mo), 30 mg (4 mo); Eligard depot for CAP: 7.5 mg (1 mo); Viadur 12-mo SQ implant, Lupron-Ped 7.5, 11.25, 15 mg **SE:** Hot flashes, gynecomastia, N/V, alopecia, anorexia, dizziness, HA, insomnia, paresthesias, depression exacerbation, peripheral edema, and bone pain (transient "flare Rxn" at 7–14 d after the 1st dose due to LH and testosterone surge before suppression) **Notes:** Nonsteroidal antiandrogen can block flare **Interactions:** ↓ Effects w/ androgens, estrogens **Labs:** ↑ LFTs, BUN, serum Ca, uric acid, glucose, lipids, WBC, PT; ↓ serum K⁺, plts

Levalbuterol (Xopenex) Uses: *Asthma (Rx and prevention of bronchospasm)* **Action:** Sympathomimetic bronchodilator **Dose:** 0.63 mg neb q6–8h

Caution: [C, ?] **Supplied:** Soln for inhal 0.63, 1.25 mg/3 mL **SE:** Tachycardia, nervousness, trembling, flu syndrome **Notes:** *R*-isomer of albuterol; potential for lower incidence of CV side effects compared with albuterol **Interactions:** ↑ Effects w/ MAOIs, TCAs; ↑ risk of hypokalemia w/ loop & thiazide diuretics; ↓ effects w/ BBs; ↓ effects of digoxin **Labs:** ↑ Serum glucose, ↓ serum K⁺ **NIPE:** Use other inhalants 5 min after this drug

Levamisole (Ergamisol) **Uses:** *Adjuvant therapy of Dukes C colon CA (in combination w/ 5-FU)* **Action:** Poorly understood immunostimulatory effects **Dose:** 50 mg PO q8h for 3 d q14d during 5-FU therapy; ↓ in hepatic dysfunction **Caution:** [C, ?/–] **Supplied:** Tabs 50 mg **SE:** N/V/D, abdominal pain, taste disturbance, anorexia, hyperbilirubinemia, disulfiram-like Rxn on EtOH ingestion, minimal bone marrow depression, fatigue, fever, conjunctivitis **Interactions:** ↑ Effects of phenytoin, warfarin **NIPE:** ⊘ Exposure to infection

Levetiracetam (Keppra) **Uses:** *Partial onset Szs* **Action:** Unknown **Dose:** *Adults.* 500 mg PO bid, may ↑ to max 3000 mg/d; *Peds.* 4–16 y: 10–20 mg/kg/d ÷ in 2 doses, up to 60 mg/kg/d(↓ in renal insufficiency) **Caution:** [C, ?/–] **Contra:** Component hypersensitivity **Supplied:** Tabs 250, 500, 750 mg **SE:** May cause dizziness and somnolence; may impair coordination **Interactions:** ↑ Effects w/ antihistamines, TCAs, benzodiazepines, narcotics, EtOH **NIPE:** May take w/ food

Levobunolol (A-K Beta, Betagan) **Uses:** *Glaucoma* **Action:** β-Adrenergic blocker **Dose:** 1–2 gtt/d 0.5% or 1–2 gtt 0.25% bid **Caution:** [C, ?] **Supplied:** Soln 0.25, 0.5% **SE:** Ocular stinging or burning **Notes:** Possible systemic effects if absorbed **Interactions:** ↑ Effects w/ BBs; ↑ risk of hypotension & bradycardia w/ quinidine, verapamil; ↓ intraocular pressure w/ carbonic anhydrase inhibitors, epinephrine, pilocarpine **NIPE:** Night vision and acuity may be decreased

Levocabastine (Livostin) **Uses:** *Allergic seasonal conjunctivitis* **Action:** Antihistamine **Dose:** 1 gt in eye(s) qid ≤ 4 wk **Caution:** [C, +/–] **Supplied:** 0.05% drops **SE:** Ocular discomfort **NIPE:** ⊘ Insert soft contact lenses

Levofloxacin (Levaquin, Quixin Ophthalmic) **Uses:** *Lower resp tract infections, sinusitis, UTI; topical for bacterial conjunctivitis, skin infections* **Action:** Quinolone antibiotic, inhibits DNA gyrase. *Spectrum:* Excellent gram(+) except MRSA and *E. faecium;* excellent gram(–) except *S. maltophilia* and *Acinetobacter* sp; poor anaerobic **Dose:** 250–500 mg/d PO or IV; community-acquired pneumonia 750 mg/day for 5 days; ophth 1–2 gtt in eye(s) q2h while awake for 2 d, then q4h while awake for 5 d; ↓ in renal insufficiency, ⊘ antacids if PO **Caution:** [C, –] Interactions w/ cation-containing products (eg antacids) **Contra:** Quinolone sensitivity **Supplied:** Tabs 250, 500 mg; premixed IV 250, 500 mg; Leva-Pak 750 mg × 5 days; ophth 0.5% soln **SE:** N/D, dizziness, rash, GI upset, photosensitivity **Interactions:** ↑ Effects of cyclosporine, digoxin, theophylline, warfarin, caffeine; ↑ risk of Szs w/ foscarnet, NSAIDs; ↑ risk of hyper- or hypoglycemia w/ hypoglycemic drugs; ↓ effects w/ antacids, antineoplastics, Ca, cimetidine, didanosine, famotidine, Fe, lansoprazole, Mg, nizatidine, omeprazole, phenytoin, ranititdine, NaHCO₃, sucralfate, Zn **NIPE:** Risk of tendon rupture & tendonitis—DC if pain or inflammation; ↑ fluids, use sunscreen, antacids 2 h before or after this drug

Levonorgestrel (Plan B) Uses: *Emergency contraceptive ("morning-after pill")*; prevents PRG if taken < 72 h after unprotected sex (contraceptive fails or if no contraception used) **Action:** Progestin **Dose:** 1 pill q12h × 2 **Caution:** [X, M] **Contra:** Known/suspected PRG, abnormal uterine bleeding **Supplied:** Tab, 0.75 mg, 2 blister pack **SE:** N/V, abdominal pain, fatigue, HA, menstrual changes. **Notes:** Will not induce abortion; may ↑ risk of ectopic PRG **Interactions:** ↓ Effects w/ barbiturates, carbamazepine, modafinil, phenobarbital, phenytoin, pioglitazone, rifabutin, rifampin, ritonavir, topiramate

Levonorgestrel Implant (Norplant) Uses: *Contraceptive* **Action:** Progestin **Dose:** Implant 6 caps in the midforearm **Caution:** [X, +/−] **Contra:** Undiagnosed abnormal uterine bleeding, hepatic Dz, thromboembolism, Hx of intracranial HTN, breast CA, renal impairment **Supplied:** Kits containing 6 implantable caps, each containing 36 mg **SE:** Uterine bleeding, HA, acne, nausea **Notes:** Prevents PRG for up to 5 y; removed if PRG desired **Interactions:** ↓ Effects w/ barbiturates, carbamazepine, modafinil, phenobarbital, phenytoin, pioglitazone, rifabutin, rifampin, ritonavir, topiramate **Labs:** ↑ uptake of T_3, ↑ T_4 sex hormone-binding globulin levels **NIPE:** Menstrual irregularities 1st y after implant, use barrier contraception if taking anticonvulsants, may cause vision changes or contact lens tolerability

Levorphanol (Levo-Dromoran) [C-II] Uses: *Moderate/severe pain; chronic pain* **Action:** Narcotic analgesic **Dose:** 2 mg PO or SQ PRN q6–8h (↓ in hepatic failure) **Caution:** [B/D (prolonged use or high doses at term), ?] **Contra:** Component hypersensitivity **Supplied:** Tabs 2 mg; inj 2 mg/mL **SE:** Tachycardia, hypotension, drowsiness, GI upset, constipation, resp depression, pruritus **Interactions:** ↑ CNS effects w/ antihistamines, cimetidine, CNS depressants, glutethimide, methocarbamol, EtOH, St. John's wort **Labs:** False ↑ amylase, lipase **NIPE:** ↑ Fluids & fiber, take w/ food

Levothyroxine (Synthroid, Levoxyl, others) Uses: *Hypothyroidism, myxedema coma* **Action:** Suppl of L-thyroxine **Dose:** *Adults.* Initial, 25–50 µg/d PO or IV; ↑ by 25–50 µg/d every mo; usual 100–200 µg/d. *Peds.* 0–1 y: 8–10 µg/kg/24 h PO or IV. 1–5 y: 4–6 µg/kg/24 h PO or IV. >5 y: 3–4 µg/kg/24 h PO or IV; titrate based on response and thyroid tests; dosage can ↑ more rapidly in young to middle-aged Pts **Caution:** [A, +] **Contra:** Recent MI, uncorrected adrenal insufficiency **Supplied:** Tabs 25, 50, 75, 88, 100, 112, 125, 137, 150, 175, 200, 300 µg; inj 200, 500 µg **SE:** Insomnia, weight loss, alopecia, arrhythmia **Interactions:** ↑ Effects of anticoagulants, sympathomimetics, TCAs, warfarin; ↓ effects w/ antacids, BBs, carbamazepine, cholestyramine, estrogens, Fe salts, phenytoin, phenobarbital, rifampin, simethicone, sucralfate, ↓ effects of digoxin, hypoglycemics, theophylline **Labs:** False ↑ serum T₃; drug alters thyroid uptake of radioactive I—DC drug 4 wk before studies **NIPE:** ⊘ Switch brands due to different bioavailabilities

Lidocaine (Anestacon Topical, Xylocaine, others)
Uses: Local anesthetic; Rx cardiac arrhythmias **Action:** Anesthetic; class IB antiarrhythmic **Dose: Adults.** Antiarrhythmic, ET: 5 mg/kg; follow w/ 0.5 mg/kg in 10 min if effective. *IV load:* 1 mg/kg/dose bolus over 2–3 min; repeat in 5–10 min; 200–300 mg/h max; cont inf 20–50 µg/kg/min or 1–4 mg/min. **Peds.** Antiarrhythmic, ET load: 1 mg/kg; repeat in 10–15 min max total 5 mg/kg, then IV inf 20–50 µg/kg/min. *Topical:* Apply max 3 mg/kg/dose. *Local inj anesthetic:* Max 4.5 mg/kg (see Table 2, page 265) **Caution:** [C, +] **Contra:** ⊘ Use lidocaine w/ epinephrine on the digits, ears, or nose because vasoconstriction may cause necrosis; heart block **Supplied:** *Inj local:* 0.5, 1, 1.5, 2, 4, 10, 20%. *Inj IV:* 1% (10 mg/mL), 2% (20 mg/mL); admixture 4, 10, 20%. *IV inf:* 0.2%, 0.4%; cream 2%; gel 2, 2.5%; oint 2.5, 5%; liq 2.5%; soln 2, 4%; viscous 2% **SE:** Dizziness, paresthesias and convulsions associated w/ toxicity **Notes:** 2nd line to amiodarone in ECC; dilute ET dose 1–2 mL w/ NS; epinephrine may be added for local anesthesia to ↑ effect and ↓ bleeding; for IV forms, ↓ w/ liver Dz or CHF; see Table 2, page 265 for drug levels **Interactions:** ↑ Effects w/ amprenavir, BBs, cimetidine; ↑ neuromuscular blockade w/ aminoglycosides, tubocurarine, pareira; ↑ cardiac depression w/ procainamide, tocainide; ↑ effects of succinylcholine **Labs:** False ↑ SCr, ↑ CPK for 48 h after IM inj **NIPE:** Oral spray/soln may impair swallowing

Lidocaine/Prilocaine (EMLA, LMX)
Uses: *Topical anesthetic*; adjunct to phlebotomy or dermal procedures **Action:** Topical anesthetic **Dose: Adults.** EMLA cream, anesthetic disc (1 g/10 cm²): Thick layer 2–2.5 g to intact skin and cover w/ occlusive dressing (eg, Tegaderm) for at least 1 h. *Anesthetic disc:* 1 g/10 cm² for at least 1 h. **Peds.** Max dose: <3 mo or <5 kg: 1 g/10 cm² for 1 h. *3–12 mo and >5 kg:* 2 g/20 cm² for 4 h. *1–6 y and >10 kg:* 10 g/100 cm² for 4 h. *7–12 y and >20 kg:* 20 g/200 cm² for 4 h **Caution:** [B, +] Methemoglobinemia **Contra:** Use on mucous membranes, broken skin, eyes; hypersensitivity to amide-type anesthetics **Supplied:** Cream 2.5% lidocaine/2.5% prilocaine; anesthetic disc (1 g) **SE:** Burning, stinging, methemoglobinemia **Notes:** Longer contact time gives greater effect.See Lidocaine **NIPE:** Low risk of systemic adverse effects

Lindane (Kwell)
Uses: *Head lice, crab lice, scabies* **Action:** Ectoparasiticide and ovicide **Dose: Adults & Peds.** Cream or lotion: Thin layer after bathing, leave for 8–12 h, pour on laundry. *Shampoo:* Apply 30 mL, develop a lather w/ warm water for 4 min, comb out nits **Caution:** [C, +/–] **Contra:** Open wounds, Sz disorder **Supplied:** Lotion 1%; shampoo 1% **SE:** Arrhythmias, Szs, local irritation, GI upset **Notes:** Caution w/ overuse; may be absorbed into blood; may repeat Rx in 7 days **Interactions:** Oil-based hair creams ↑ drug absorption **NIPE:** Apply to dry hair/dry, cool skin

inezolid (Zyvox) Uses: *Infections caused by gram(+) bacteria (including ancomycin-resistant enterococcus, VRE), pneumonia, skin infections* **Action:** nique, binds ribosomal bacterial RNA; bactericidal for strep, bacteriostatic for nterococci and staph. *Spectrum:* Excellent gram(+) activity including VRE and 1RSA **Dose:** *Adults.* 400–600 mg IV or PO q12h. *Peds.* 10 mg/kg IV or PO q8h. q12h in preterm neonates) **Caution:** [C, ?/–] W/ reversible MAOI, ⊘ foods containing tyramine and cough and cold products containing pseudoephedrine; myelouppression **Supplied:** Inj 2 mg/mL; tabs 400, 600 mg; susp 100 mg/5 mL **SE:** iTN, N/D, HA, insomnia, GI upset **Notes:** Follow weekly CBC **Interactions:** ↑ risk of serotonin syndrome w/ SSRIs, sibutramine, trazodone, venlafaxine; ↑ HTN v/ amphetamines, dextromethorphan, dopamine, epinephrine, levodopa, MAOIs, neperidine, metaraminol, phenylephrine, phenylpropanolamine, pseudoephedrine, yramine, ginseng, ephedra, ma huang, tyramine containing foods; ↑ risk of bleeding w/ antiplts **NIPE:** Take w/o regard to food, ⊘ tyramine-containing foods

iothyronine (Cytomel) Uses: *Hypothyroidism, goiter, myxedema oma, thyroid suppression therapy* **Action:** T_3 replacement **Dose:** *Adults.* Initial '5 μg/24 h, titrate q1–2wk to response w/ maint of 25–100 μg/d PO. *Myxedema coma:* 25–50 μg IV. *Peds.*Initial dose of 5 μg/24 h, then titrate by 5-g/24 h increments at 1–2-wk intervals; maint 25–75 μg/24 h PO qd; ↓ dose in el-erly **Caution:** [A, +] **Contra:** Recent MI, uncorrected adrenal insufficiency, ncontrolled HTN **Supplied:** Tabs 5, 12.5, 25, 50 μg; inj 10 μg/mL **SE:** Alopecia, rrhythmias, CP, HA, sweating **Notes:** Monitor TFT pain **Interactions:** ↑ Effects f anticoagulants; ↓ effects w/ bile acid sequestrants, carbamazepine, estrogens, henytoin, rifampin; ↓ effects of hypoglycemics, theophylline **NIPE:** Monitor car-iac status, take in AM

isinopril (Prinivil, Zestril) Uses: *HTN, CHF, prevent DN and AMI* **Action:** ACEI **Dose:** 5–40 mg/24 h PO qd–bid. *AMI:* 5 mg w/in 24 h of MI, fol-owed by 5 mg after 24 h, 10 mg after 48 h, then 10 mg/d; ↓ in renal insufficiency **Caution:** [D, –] **Contra:** ACEI sensitivity **Supplied:** Tabs 2.5, 5, 10, 20, 30, 40 ng **SE:** Dizziness, HA, cough, hypotension, angioedema, hyperkalemia **Notes:** To revent DN, start when urinary microalbuminemia begins **Interactions:** ↑ Effects v/ α-blockers, diuretics ↑ risk of hyperkalemia w/ K-sparing diuretics, trimetho-rim, salt substitutes; ↑ risk of cough w/ capsaicin; ↑ effects of insulin, Li; ↓ ef-ects w/ ASA, indomethacin, NSAIDs **Labs:** ↑ Serum K^+, creatinine, BUN **NIPE:** Maximum effect may take several weeks

Lithium Carbonate (Eskalith, Lithobid, others) Uses: *Manic pisodes of bipolar illness* **Action:** Effects shift toward intraneuronal metabolism f catecholamines **Dose:** *Adults.* Acute mania: 600 mg PO tid or 900 mg SR bid. *Maint:* 300 mg PO tid–qid *Peds.* 6–12 y: 15–60 mg/kg/d in 3–4 ÷ doses; must be itrated; follow serum levels; ↓ in renal insufficiency, elderly **Caution:** [D, –] Many drug interactions **Contra:** Severe renal impairment or CV Dz, lactation **Sup-**

plied: Caps 150, 300, 600 mg; tabs 300 mg; SR tabs 300, 450 mg; syrup 300 mg/mL **SE:** Polyuria, polydipsia, nephrogenic DI, tremor; Na retention or diuretic us may potentiate toxicity; arrhythmias, dizziness **Notes:** See Table 2, page 265, fo drug levels **Interactions:** ↑ Effects of TCA; ↑ effects w/ ACEIs, bumetanide, car bamazepine, ethacrynic acid, fluoxetine, furosemide, methyldopa, NSAIDs, pheny toin, phenothiazines, probenecid, tetracyclines, thiazide diuretics, dandelion juniper; ↓ effects w/ acetazolamide, antacids, mannitol, theophyllines, urea, vera pamil, caffeine **Labs:** False + urine glucose, ↑ serum glucose, creatinine kinase TSH, I-131 uptake; ↓ uric acid, T_3, T_4 **NIPE:** Several weeks before full effects o med, ↑ fluid intake to 2–3 L/d

Lodoxamide (Alomide) Uses: *Seasonal allergic conjunctivitis* Action Stabilizes mast cells **Dose:** *Adults & Peds.* >2 y: 1–2 gtt in eye(s) qid ≤ 3 mo **Caution:** [B, ?] **Supplied:** Soln 0.1% **SE:** Ocular burning, stinging, HA

Lomefloxacin (Maxaquin) Uses: *UTI, acute exacerbation of chroni bronchitis; prophylaxis in transurethral procedures* **Action:** Quinolone antibiotic inhibits DNA gyrase. *Spectrum:* Good gram(–) activity including *H. influenzae* ex cept *Stenotrophomonas maltophilia, Acinetobacer* sp, and some *P. aeruginos* **Dose:** 400 mg/d PO; ↓ in renal insufficiency; ⊘ antacids **Caution:** [C, –] Interac tions w/ cation-containing products **Contra:** Hypersensitivity to other quinolones children < 18 y **Supplied:** Tabs 400 mg **SE:** Photosensitivity, Szs, HA, dizziness **Interactions:** ↑ Effects w/ cimetidine, probenecid; ↑ effects of cyclosporine, war farin, caffeine; ↓ effects w/ antacids **Labs:** ↑ LFTs, ↑ K⁺ **NIPE:** ↑ Risk of photo sensitivity—use sunscreen, ↑ fluids to 2 L/d

Loperamide (Imodium) Uses: *Diarrhea* **Action:** Slows intestina motility **Dose:** *Adults.* Initially 4 mg PO, then 2 mg after each loose stool, up to 1₆ mg/d. *Peds.* 2–5 y, 13–20 kg: 1 mg PO tid. *6–8 y, 20–30 kg:* 2 mg PO bid. *8–12 y >30 kg:* 2 mg PO tid **Caution:** [B, +] ⊘ use in acute diarrhea caused by *Salmo nella, Shigella,* or *C. difficile* **Contra:** Pseudomembranous colitis, bloody diarrhea **Supplied:** Caps 2 mg; tabs 2 mg; liq 1 mg/5 mL (OTC) **SE:** Constipation, sedation dizziness **Interactions:** ↑ Effects w/ antihistamines, CNS depressants, phenoth iazines, TCAs, EtOH

Lopinavir/Ritonavir (Kaletra) Uses: *HIV infection* **Action:** Pro tease inhibitor **Dose:** *Adults.* 3 caps or 5 mL PO bid. *Peds.* 7–15 kg: 12/3 mg/kg PO bid. *15–40 kg:* 10/2.5 mg/kg PO bid. *>40 kg:* Adult dose (w/ food) **Caution:** [C, ?/–] Numerous drug interactions **Contra:** Concomitant drugs dependent o₁ CYP3A or CYP2D6 **Supplied:** Caps 133.3 mg/33.3 mg (lopinavir/ritonavir); soln 400 mg/100 mg/5 mL **SE:** Soln has EtOH, ⊘ disulfiram and metronidazole; G upset, asthenia, ↑ cholesterol and triglycerides, pancreatitis; protease metabolic syndrome **Interactions:** ↑ Effects w/ clarithromycin, erythromycin; ↑ effects o amiodarone, amprenavir, azole antifungals, bepridil, cisapride, cyclosporine CCBs, ergot alkaloids, flecainide, flurazepam, HMG-CoA reductase inhibitors, in dinavir, lidocaine, meperidine, midazolam, pimozide, propafenone, propoxyphene inidine, rifabutin, saquinavir, sildenafil, tacrolimus, terfenadine, triazolam, olpidem; ↓ effects w/ barbiturates, carbamazepine, dexamethasone, didanosine, favirenz, nevirapine, phenytoin, rifabutin, rifampin, St. John's wort; ↓ effects of al contraceptives, warfarin **NIPE:** Take w/ food, use barrier contraception

oracarbef (Lorabid) Uses: *Upper and lower resp tract, skin, bone, uriary tract, abdomen, and gynecologic system bacterial infections* **Action:** 2nden cephalosporin; inhibits cell wall synthesis. *Spectrum:* Weaker than 1st-gen gainst gram(+), enhanced activity against some gram(−) **Dose:** *Adults.* 200–400 g PO bid. *Peds.* 7.5–15 mg/kg/d PO ÷ bid; on empty stomach; ↓ in severe renal isufficiency **Caution:** [B, +] **Supplied:** Caps 200, 400 mg; susp 125, 250 mg/5 L **SE:** diarrhea **Interactions:** ↑ Effects w/ probenecid; ↑ effects of warfarin; ↑ ephrotoxicity w/ aminoglycosides, furosemide **NIPE:** Take w/o food

oratadine (Claritin, Alavert) Uses: *Allergic rhinitis, chronic idio-athic urticaria* **Action:** Nonsedating antihistamine **Dose:** *Adults.* 10 mg/d PO *eds.* 2–5 y: 5 mg PO qd. >6 y: Adult dose; take on an empty stomach; ↓ in he-atic insufficiency **Caution:** [B, +/−] **Contra:** Component hypersensitivity **Sup-lied:** Tabs 10 mg (OTC); rapidly disintegrating Reditabs 10 mg; syrup 1 mg/mL **E:** HA, somnolence, xerostomia **Interactions:** ↑ Effects w/ CNS depressants, rythromycin, ketoconazole, MAOIs, protease inhibitors, procarbazine, EtOH **IPE:** Take w/o food

orazepam (Ativan, others) [C-IV] Uses: *Anxiety and anxiety w/ epression; preop sedation; control of status epilepticus*; EtOH withdrawal; ntiemetic **Action:** Benzodiazepine; antianxiety agent **Dose:** *Adults.* Anxiety: 1–10 g/d PO in 2–3 ÷ doses. *Preop:* 0.05 mg/kg to 4 mg max IM 2 h before surgery. *nsomnia:* 2–4 mg PO hs. *Status epilepticus:* 4 mg dose IV PRN q10–15 min; sual total dose 8 mg. *Antiemetic:* 0.5–2 mg IV or PO q4–6h PRN. *EtOH with-rawal:* 2–5 mg IV or 1–2 mg PO initial depending on severity; subsequent based n response **Peds.** Status epilepticus: 0.05 mg/kg/dose IV, repeat at 1–20 min inter-als × 2 PRN. *Antiemetic, 2–15 y:* 0.05 mg/kg (to 2 mg/dose) prechemotherapy; ↓ n elderly; ⊘ administer IV >2 mg/min or 0.05 mg/kg/min **Caution:** [D, ?/−] **Con-ra:** Severe pain, severe hypotension, sleep apnea, narrow-angle glaucoma, hyper-ensitivity to propylene glycol or benzyl EtOH **Supplied:** Tabs 0.5, 1, 2 mg; soln, O conc 2 mg/mL; inj 2, 4 mg/mL **SE:** Sedation, ataxia, tachycardia, constipation, esp depression **Notes:** Up to 10 min for effect if IV **Interactions:** ↑ Effects w/ imetidine, disulfiram, probenecid, calendula, catnip, hops, lady's slipper, passion-lower, kava kava, valerian; ↑ effects of phenytoin; ↑ CNS depression w/ anticon-ulsants, antihistamines, CNS depressants, MAOIs, scopolamine, EtOH; ↓ effects // caffeine, tobacco; ↓ effects of levodopa **Labs:** ↑ LFTs **NIPE:** ⊘ DC abruptly

osartan (Cozaar) Uses: *HTN,* CHF, DN **Action:** Angiotensin II antag-nist **Dose:** 25–50 mg PO qd–bid; ↓ dose in elderly or hepatic impairment **Cau-on:** [C (1st tri), D 2nd and 3rd tri), ?/−] **Supplied:** Tabs 25, 50, 100 mg **SE:** ↓ BP n Pts on diuretics; GI upset, angioedema **Interactions:** ↑ Risk of hyperkalemia w/

K-sparing diuretics, K suppls, trimethoprim; ↑ effects of Li; ↓ effects w/ diltiazem, fluconazole, phenobarbital, rifampin **NIPE:** ⊘ PRG, breast-feeding

Lovastatin (Mevacor, Altocor) Uses: *Hypercholesterolemia* Action: HMG-CoA reductase inhibitor **Dose:** 20 mg/d PO w/ PM meal; may ↑ at 4-wk intervals to 80 mg/d max; taken w/ meals; ⊘ grapefruit juice **Caution:** [X, –] ⊘ w/gemfibrozil. **Contra:** Active liver Dz **Supplied:** Tabs 10, 20, 40 mg **SE:** HA and GI intolerance common; Pt should promptly report any unexplained muscle pain, tenderness, or weakness (myopathy) **Notes:** Must maintain cholesterol-lowering diet; monitor LFT q12wk × 1 y, then q6mo **Interactions:** ↑ Effects w/ grapefruit juice; ↑ risk of severe myopathy w/ azole antifungals, cyclosporine, erythromycin, gemfibrozil, HMG-CoA inhibitors, niacin; ↑ effects of warfarin; ↓ effects w/ isradipine, pectin **Labs:** ↑ LFTs **NIPE:** ⊘ PRG, take drug in evening, periodic eye exams

Lymphocyte Immune Globulin [Antithymocyte Globulin, ATG] (Atgam) Uses: *Allograft rejection in transplant Pts; aplastic anemia if not candidates for BMT* Action: ↓ Circulating T lymphocytes **Dose:** *Adults.* Prevent rejection: 15 mg/kg/day IV ×14 d, then qod ×7; initial w/in 24 h before/after transplant. *Treat rejection:* Same except use 10–15 mg/kg/day. *Peds.* 5–25 mg/kg/day IV. **Caution:** [C, ?] **Contra:** Hx Rxn to other equine γ-globulin prep, leukopenia, thrombocytopenia **Supplied:** Inj 50 mg/mL **SE:** DC w/ severe thrombocytopenia/leukopenia; rash, fever, chills, hypotension, HA, ↑ K⁺ **Notes:** *Test dose:* 0.1 mL 1:1000 dilution in NS **Interactions:** ↑ Immunosuppression w/ azathioprine, corticosteroids, immunosuppressants **Labs:** ↑ LFTs **NIPE:** Risk of febrile Rxn

Magaldrate (Riopan, Lowsium) Uses: *Hyperacidity associated w/ peptic ulcer, gastritis, and hiatal hernia* Action: Low-Na antacid **Dose:** 5–10 mL PO between meals and hs **Caution:** [B, ?] **Contra:** Ulcerative colitis, diverticulitis, ileostomy/coleostomy, renal insufficiency due to Mg content **Supplied:** Susp (OTC) **SE:** GI upset **Notes:** <0.3 mg Na/tab or tsp **Interactions:** ↑ Effects of levodopa quinidine; ↓ effects of allopurinol, anticoagulants, cefpodoxime, ciprofloxacin, clindamycin, digoxin, indomethacin, INH, ketoconazole, lincomycin, phenothiazines quinolones, tetracyclines **NIPE:** ⊘ Other meds w/in 1–2 h

Magnesium Citrate (various) [OTC] Uses: *Vigorous bowel prep* constipation Action: Cathartic laxative **Dose:** *Adults.* 120–240 mL PO PRN *Peds.* 0.5 mL/kg/dose, to a max of 200 mL PO; take w/ a beverage **Caution:** [B, +] **Contra:** Severe renal Dz, heart block, N/V, rectal bleeding **Supplied:** Effervescen soln (OTC) **SE:** Abdominal cramps, gas **Interactions:** ↓ Effects of anticoagulants digoxin, fluoroquinolones, ketoconazole, nitrofurantoin, phenothiazines, tetracy clines **Labs:** ↑ Mg²⁺; ↓ protein, Ca²⁺, K⁺ **NIPE:** ⊘ Other meds w/in 1–2 h

Magnesium Hydroxide (Milk of Magnesia) [OTC] Uses: *Con stipation* Action: NS laxative **Dose:** *Adults.* 15–30 mL PO PRN. *Peds.* 0. mL/kg/dose PO PRN (follow dose w/ 8 oz of water) **Caution:** [B, +] **Contra** Renal insufficiency or intestinal obstruction, ileostomy/colostomy **Supplied:** Tab

11 mg; liq 400, 800 mg/5 mL (OTC) **SE:** Diarrhea, abdominal cramps **Interactions:** ↓ Effects of chlordiazepoxide, dicumarol, digoxin, indomethacin, INH, quinolones, tetracyclines **Labs:** ↑ Mg^{2+}, ↓ protein, Ca^{2+}, K^+ **NIPE:** ⊘ Other meds w/in 1–2 h

Magnesium Oxide (Mag-Ox 400, others) **Uses:** *Replacement for low Mg levels* **Action:** Mg suppl **Dose:** 400–800 mg/d ÷ qd–qid w/ full glass of water **Caution:** [B, +] **Contra:** Ulcerative colitis, diverticulitis, ileostomy/colostomy, heart block, renal insufficiency **Supplied:** Caps 140 mg; tabs 400 mg (OTC) **SE:** Diarrhea, nausea **Interactions:** ↓ Effects of chlordiazepoxide, dicumarol, digoxin, indomethacin, INH, quinolones, tetracyclines **Labs:** ↑ Mg^{2+}, ↓ protein, Ca^{2+}, K^+ **NIPE:** ⊘ Other meds w/in 1–2 h

Magnesium Sulfate (various) **Uses:** *Replacement for low Mg levels; preeclampsia and premature labor*; refractory hypokalemia and hypocalcemia **Action:** Mg suppl **Dose:** *Adults.* Suppl: 1–2 g IM or IV; repeat PRN. *Preeclampsia/premature labor:* 4 g load then 1–4 g/h IV inf. *Peds.* 25–50 mg/kg/dose IM or IV q4–6h for 3–4 doses; repeat if ↓ Mg persists; ↓ dose w/ low urine output or renal insufficiency **Caution:** [B, +] **Contra:** Heart block, renal failure **Supplied:** Inj 100, 125, 250, 500 mg/mL; PO soln 500 mg/mL; granules 40 mEq/5 g **SE:** CNS depression, diarrhea, flushing, heart block **Interactions:** ↑ CNS depression w/ antidepressants, antipsychotics, anxiolytics, barbiturates, hypnotics, narcotics; EtOH; ↑ neuromuscular blockade w/ aminoglycosides, atracurium, galamine, pancuronium, tubocurarine, vecuronium **Labs:** ↑ Mg^{2+}; ↓ protein, Ca^{2+}, K^+ **NIPE:** Check for absent patellar reflexes

Mannitol (various) **Uses:** *Cerebral edema, intraocular pressure, renal impairment, poisonings* **Action:** Osmotic diuretic **Dose:** *Diuresis: Adults.* 0.2 g/kg/dose IV over 3–5 min; if no diuresis w/in 2 h, DC. *Peds.* 0.75 g/kg/dose IV over 3–5 min; if no diuresis w/in 2 h, DC. *Cerebral edema: Adults & Peds.* 0.25 g/kg/dose IV push, repeated at 5-min intervals PRN; ↑ slowly to 1 g/kg/dose PRN for ↑ ICP **Caution:** [C, ?] w/ CHF or volume overload **Contra:** Anuria, dehydration, HF, PE **Supplied:** Inj 5, 10, 15, 20, 25% **SE:** Initial volume ↑ may exacerbate CHF; monitor for volume depletion, N/V/D **Interactions:** ↑ Effects of cardiac glycosides; ↓ effects of barbiturates, imipramine, Li, salicylates **Labs:** ↑ / ↓ Serum phosphate

Mechlorethamine (Mustargen) **WARNING:** Highly toxic agent, handle w/ care **Uses:** *Hodgkin's and NHL, cutaneous T-cell lymphoma (mycosis fungoides), lung CA, CML, malignant pleural effusions,* and CLL **Action:** Alkylating agent (bifunctional) **Dose:** 0.4 mg/kg single dose or 0.1 mg/kg/d for 4 d; 6 mg/m² 1–2 ×/mo **Caution:** [D, ?] **Contra:** Presence of known infectious Dz **Supplied:** Inj 10 mg **SE:** Myelosuppression, thrombosis, or thrombophlebitis at inj site; tissue damage w/ extravasation (Na thiosulfate may be used topically to treat); N/V, skin rash, amenorrhea, and sterility (especially in men) and secondary leukemia in Pts treated for Hodgkin's Dz **Notes:** Highly volatile; administer w/in

30–60 min of prep **Interactions:** ↑ Risk of blood dyscrasias w/ amphotericin B; risk of bleeding w/ anticoagulants, NSAIDs, plt inhibitors, salicylates; ↑ myelo suppression w/ antineoplastic drugs, radiation therapy; ↓ effects of live virus vac cines **Labs:** ↑ Serum uric acid **NIPE:** ⊘ Fluids to 2–3 L/d; ⊘ PRG, breast-feeding vaccines, exposure to infection; ↑ risk of tinnitus

Meclizine (Antivert) Uses: *Motion sickness; vertigo* Action: Ant emetic, anticholinergic, and antihistaminic properties **Dose:** *Adults & Peds.* >12 y 25 mg PO tid–qid PRN **Caution:** [B, ?] **Supplied:** Tabs 12.5, 25, 50 mg; chew tab 25 mg; caps 25, 30 mg (OTC) **SE:** Drowsiness, xerostomia, and blurred visio common **Interactions:** ↑ Sedation w/ antihistamines, CNS depressants, neurolep tics, EtOH; ↑ anticholinergic effects w/ anticholinergics, atropine, disopyramide haloperidol, phenothiazines, quinidine **NIPE:** Use prophylactically

Medroxyprogesterone (Provera, Depo-Provera) Uses: *Con traception; secondary amenorrhea, and abnormal uterine bleeding (AUB) cause by hormonal imbalance; endometrial CA* **Action:** Progestin suppl **Dose:** *Contra ception:* 150 mg IM q3mo or 450 mg IM q6mo. *Secondary amenorrhea:* 5–1 mg/d PO for 5–10 d. *AUB:* 5–10 mg/d PO for 5–10 d beginning on the 16th or 21s d of menstrual cycle. *Endometrial CA:* 400–1000 mg/wk IM; ↓ in hepatic insuf ciency **Caution:** [X, +] **Contra:** Hx of thromboembolic disorders, hepatic Dz PRG **Supplied:** Tabs 2.5, 5, 10 mg; depot inj 100, 150, 400 mg/mL **SE:** Break through bleeding, spotting, altered menstrual flow, anorexia, edema, thromboen bolic complications, depression, weight gain **Notes:** Perform breast exam and Pa smear before therapy; as contraceptive obtain PRG test if last inj > 3 mo earlier **In teractions:** ↓ Effects w/ aminoglutethimide, phenytoin, carbamazepine, phenobar bital, rifampin, rifabutin **NIPE:** Sunlight exposure may cause melasma, if GI upse take w/ food

Megestrol Acetate (Megace) Uses: *Breast and endometrial CAs; ap petite stimulant in CA and HIV-related cachexia* **Action:** Hormone; progesteron analogue **Dose:** *CA:* 40–320 mg/d PO in ÷ doses. *Appetite:* 800 mg/d PO ÷ **Cau tion:** [X, –] Thromboembolism **Contra:** PRG **Supplied:** Tabs 20, 40 mg; soln 4 mg/mL **SE:** May induce DVT; ⊘ DC therapy abruptly; edema, menstrual bleeding photosensitivity, insomnia, rash, myelosuppression **Interactions:** ↑ Effects of wa farin **Labs:** ↑ LDH **NIPE:** ↑ Risk of photosensitivity—use sunscreen

Meloxicam (Mobic) Uses: *Osteoarthritis* **Action:** NSAID w/ ↑ COX-activity **Dose:** 7.5–15 mg/d PO; ↓ in renal insufficiency; take w/food **Caution:** [C ?/–] Peptic ulcer, NSAID, or ASA sensitivity **Supplied:** Tabs 7.5 mg **SE:** HA dizziness, GI upset, GI bleeding, edema **Interactions:** ↑ Effects of ASA, anticoag ulants, corticosteroids, Li, EtOH, tobacco; ↓ effects w/ cholestyramine; ↓ effects c antihypertensives **Labs:** False + guaiac test, ↑ LFTs **NIPE:** Take w/ food, ma take several days for full effect

Melphalan [L-PAM] (Alkeran) WARNING: Severe bone marrow de pression, leukemogenic, and mutagenic Uses: *Multiple myeloma, ovarian CAs, east, testicular, and, melanoma; allogenic and ABMT in high doses **Action:** kylating agent (bifunctional) **Dose:** (Per protocols) 6 mg/d or 0.25 mg/kg/d for ~7 d, repeated at 4–6-wk intervals, or 1-mg/kg single dose once q4–6wk; 0.15 g/kg/d for 5 d q6wk. *High-dose high-risk multiple myeloma:* Single dose 140 g/m². *ABMT:* 140–240 mg/m² IV; ↓ in renal insufficiency **Caution:** [D, ?] **Contra:** Hypersensitivity or resistance **Supplied:** Tabs 2 mg; inj 50, 100 mg **SE:** yelosuppression (leukopenia and thrombocytopenia), secondary leukemia, alope a, dermatitis, stomatitis, and pulmonary fibrosis; very rare hypersensitivity Rxns **Notes:** Take on empty stomach **Interactions:** ↑ Risk of nephrotoxicity w/ cis latin, cyclosporine; ↓ effects w/ cimetidine, interferon alfa **Labs:** ↑ Uric acid, rine 5-HIAA **NIPE:** ↑ Fluids, ⊘ PRG, breast-feeding

Memantine (Namenda) Uses: Moderate/severe Alzheimer's **Action:** *N*-methyl-D-aspartate receptor antagonist **Dose:** Target 20 mg/d, start 5 mg/d, ↑ 5 g/d to 20 mg/d, wait > 1 wk before ↑ dose; use + doses above 5 mg/d **Caution:** [B, ?/–] Hepatic/mild–moderate renal impairment **Supplied:** Tabs 5, 10 mg **E:** Dizziness **Notes:** Renal clearance ↓ by alkaline urine pH (↓ 80% at urine pH) **Interactions:** ↑ Effects with amantadine, carbonic anhydrase inhibitors, dex omethorphan, ketamine, sodium bicarbonate; ↑ effects with any drug, herb, food at alkalinizes urine **Labs:** Monitor BUN, SCr **NIPE:** Take w/o regard to food, tOH ↑ adverse effects & ↓ effectiveness

Meningococcal Polysaccharide Vaccine (Menomune) Uses: Immunize against *N. meningitidis* (meningococcus)*; recommended in some com lement deficiency, asplenia, lab workers w/ exposure; college students by some rofessional groups **Action:** Live vaccine, active immunization **Dose:** *Adults & eds.* >2 y: 0.5 mL SQ; ⊘ inject intradermally or IV; epinephrine (1:1000) must be vailable for anaphylactic/allergic Rxns **Caution:** [C, ?/–] **Contra:** Thimerosal sen itivity **Supplied:** Inj **SE:** Local inj site Rxns, HA **Notes:** Active against meningo occal serotypes A, C, Y, and W-135 but not group B **Interactions:** ↓ Effects w/ mmunoglobulin if admin. w/in 1 mo **NIPE:** Pain & inflammation at inj site

Meperidine (Demerol) [C–II] Uses: *Moderate to severe pain* **Action:** Narcotic analgesic **Dose:** *Adults.* 50–150 mg PO or IM q3–4h PRN. *Peds.*1–1.5 /kg/dose PO or IM q3–4h PRN, up to 100 mg/dose; ↓ in elderly and renal im airment **Caution:** [C/D (prolonged use or high doses at term, +] **Contra:** Recent r concomitant MAOIs, renal failure **Supplied:** Tabs 50, 100 mg; syrup 50 mg/mL; nj 10, 25, 50, 75, 100 mg/mL **SE:** Resp depression, Szs, sedation, constipation **Notes:** Analgesic effects potentiated w/ use of hydroxyzine; 75 mg IM = 10 mg of norphine IM; reduces Sz threshold **Interactions:** ↑ Effects w/ antihistamines, bar iturates, cimetidine, MAOIs, neuroleptics, selegiline, TCAs, St. John's wort, tOH; ↑ effects of INH; ↓ effects w/ phenytoin **Labs:** ↑ Serum amylase, lipase

Meprobamate (Equinil, Miltown) [C–IV] Uses: *Short-term relief f anxiety* **Action:** Mild tranquilizer; antianxiety **Dose:** *Adults.* 400 mg PO id–qid up to 2400 mg/d; SR 400–800 mg PO bid. *Peds. 6–12 y:* 100–200 mg bid–tid; SR 200 mg bid; ↓ in renal/liver insufficiency **Caution:** [D, +/–] **Contr** Narrow-angle glaucoma, porphyria, PRG **Supplied:** Tabs 200, 400, 600 mg; S caps 200, 400 mg **SE:** May cause drowsiness, syncope, tachycardia, edema **Inte actions:** ↑ Effects w/ antihistamines, barbiturates, CNS depressants, narcotic EtOH

Mercaptopurine [6-MP] (Purinethol) Uses: *Acute leukemias 2nd-line Rx of CML and NHL, maint ALL in children, immunosuppressant for a toimmune Dzs (Crohn's Dz) **Action:** Antimetabolite; mimics hypoxanthine **Dos** 80–100 mg/m²/d or 2.5–5 mg/kg/d; maint 1.5–2.5 mg/kg/d; concurrent allopurine therapy requires a 67–75% dose reduction of 6-MP because of interference w/ me tabolism by xanthine oxidase; ↓ in renal, hepatic insufficiency **Caution:** [D, **Contra:** Severe hepatic Dz, bone marrow suppression, PRG **Supplied:** Tabs 50 m **SE:** Mild hematologic toxicity; uncommon GI toxicity, except mucositis, stomat tis, and diarrhea; rash, fever, eosinophilia, jaundice, and hepatitis **Notes:** Us proper procedures for handling; take on empty stomach; ensure adequate hydratic **Interactions:** ↑ Effects w/ allopurinol; ↑ risk of bone marrow suppression v trimethoprim-sulfamethoxazole; ↓ effects of warfarin **Labs:** False ↑ serum glu cose, uric acid **NIPE:** ↑ Fluid intake to 2–3 L/d; may take 4+ wk for improvemen

Meropenem (Merrem) Uses: *Intraabdominal infections, bacteri meningitis* **Action:** Carbapenem; inhibits cell wall synthesis, a β-lactam. *Spe trum:* Excellent gram(+) except MRSA and *E. faecium;* excellent gram(–) includ ing extended-spectrum β-lactamase producers; good anaerobic **Dose:** *Adults.* IV q8h. *Peds.* 20–40 mg/kg IV q 8h; ↓ in renal insufficiency **Caution:** [B, ?] **Con tra:** β-Lactam sensitivity **Supplied:** Inj 1 g/30 mL, 500 mg/20 mL **SE:** Less Sz po tential than imipenem; diarrhea, thrombocytopenia **Notes:** Overuse can ↑ bacteria resistance **Interactions:** ↑ Effects w/ probenecid **Labs:** ↑ LFTs, BUN, creatinin eosinophils ↓ Hmg, Hct, WBCs **NIPE:** Monitor for superinfection

Mesalamine (Rowasa, Asacol, Pentasa) Uses: *Mild to modera distal ulcerative colitis, proctosigmoiditis, or proctitis* **Action:** Unknown; ma topically inhibit prostaglandins **Dose:** *Retention enema:* qd hs or insert 1 supp bi *PO:* 800–1000 mg PO 3–4×/d; ↓ initial dose in elderly **Caution:** [B, M] **Contra** Salicylate sensitivity **Supplied:** Tabs 400 mg; caps 250 mg; supp 500 mg; recta susp 4 g/60 mL **SE:** HA, malaise, abdominal pain, flatulence, rash, pancreatiti pericarditis **Notes:** May discolor urine yellow-brown **Interactions:** ↓ Effect c digoxin **Labs:** ↑ LFTs, amylase, lipase

Mesna (Mesnex) Uses: *↓ Ifosfamide- and cyclophosphamide-induced h morrhagic cystitis* **Action:** Antidote **Dose:** 20% of the ifosfamide dose (±) or cy clophosphamide dose IV 15 min prior to and 4 and 8 h after chemotherap **Caution:** [B; ?/–] **Contra:** Thiol sensitivity **Supplied:** Inj 100 mg/mL; tablets 40 mg **SE:** Hypotension, allergic Rxns, HA, GI upset, taste perversion **Notes:** Hydra tion helps ↓ hemorrhagic cystitis **Interactions:** ↓ Effects of warfarin **Labs:** False urine ketones

Mesoridazine (Serentil) WARNING: Can prolong QT interval in a dose-related fashion; torsades de points reported Uses: *Schizophrenia,* acute and chronic alcoholism, chronic brain syndrome Action: Phenothiazine antipsychotic Dose: Initial, 25–50 mg PO or IV tid; ↑ to 300–400 mg/d max Caution: [C, ?/–] Contra: Phenothiazine sensitivity, coadministration w/ drugs that cause QT_c prolongation, CNS depression Supplied: Tabs 10, 25, 50, 100 mg; PO conc 25 mg/mL; inj 25 mg/mL SE: Low incidence of EPS; hypotension, xerostomia, constipation, skin discoloration, tachycardia, lowered Sz threshold, blood dyscrasias, pigmentary retinopathy at high doses Interactions: ↑ Effects w/ antimalarials, BBs, chloroquine, TCAs, EtOH; ↑ effects of antidepressants, nitrates, antihypertensives; ↑ QT interval w/ amiodarone, azole antifungals, disopyramide, fluoxetine, macrolides, paroxetine, procainamide, quinidine, quinolones, TCAs, verapamil; ↓ effects w/ attapulgite, barbiturates, caffeine, tobacco; ↓ effects of barbiturates, guanethidine, guanadrel, levodopa, Li, sympathomimetics Labs: False + PRG test; ↑ serum glucose, cholesterol; ↓ uric acid NIPE: Photosensitivity—use sunscreen

Metaproterenol (Alupent, Metaprel) Uses: *Asthma and reversible bronchospasm* Action: Sympathomimetic bronchodilator Dose: *Adults.* Inhal: 2–3 inhal q3–4h, 12 inhal max/24 h; wait 2 min between inhal. *PO:* 20 mg q6–8h. *Peds.* Inhal: 0.5 mg/kg/dose, 15 mg/dose max inhaled q4–6h by neb or 1–2 puffs q4–6h. *PO:* 0.3–0.5 mg/kg/dose q6–8h Caution: [C, ?/–] Contra: Tachycardia, other arrhythmias Supplied: Aerosol 0.65 mg/inhal; soln for inhal 0.4, 0.6, 5%; tabs 10, 20 mg; syrup 10 mg/5 mL SE: Fewer β_1 effects than isoproterenol and longer acting; nervousness, tremor, tachycardia, HTN Interactions: ↑ Effects w/ sympathomimetic drugs, xanthines; ↑ risk of arrhythmias w/ cardiac glycosides, halothane, levodopa, theophylline, thyroid hormones; ↑ HTN w/ MAOIs; ↓ effects w/ BBs Labs: ↑ Serum K^+ NIPE: Separate additional aerosol use by 5 min

Metaxalone (Skelaxin) Uses: *Painful musculoskeletal conditions* Action: Centrally acting skeletal muscle relaxant Dose: 800 mg PO 3–4×/d Caution: [C, ?/–] Contra: Severe hepatic/renal impairment; caution in anemia Supplied: Tabs 400 mg SE: N/V, HA, drowsiness, hepatitis Interactions: ↑ Sedating effects w/ CNS depressants, EtOH Labs: False + urine glucose using Benedict's test

Metformin (Glucophage, Glucophage XR) WARNING: Associated w/ lactic acidosis Uses: *Type 2 DM* Action: ↓ Hepatic glucose production and intestinal absorption of glucose; improves insulin sensitivity Dose: *Adults.* Initial dose 500 mg PO bid; may ↑ 2550 mg/d max (administer w/ AM and PM meals); can convert total daily dose to qd dose of XR formulation). *Peds.* 10–16 y: 500 mg PO bid, ↑ by 500 mg weekly up to 2000 mg/d in ÷ doses; ⊘ use XR formulation in peds Caution: [B, +/–] Contra: ⊘ use if SCr >1.4 in females or >1.5 in males; contra in hypoxemic conditions, including acute CHF/sepsis; ⊘ EtOH; hold dose before and 48 h after ionic contrast Supplied: Tabs 500, 850, 1000 mg; XR tabs 500 mg SE: Anorexia, N/V, rash, lactic acidosis (rare, but serious) Interactions: ↑

Effects w/ amiloride, cimetidine, digoxin, furosemide, MAOIs, morphine, procainamide, quinidine, quinine, ranitidine, triamterene, trimethoprim, vancomycin ↓ effects w/ corticosteroids, CCBs, diuretics, estrogens, INH, oral contraceptives phenothiazines, phenytoin, sympathomimetics, thyroid drugs, tobacco **NIPE:** Take w/ food; ⊘ dehydration, EtOH

Methadone (Dolophine) [C-II]
Uses: *Severe pain; detoxification and maint of narcotic addiction* **Action:** Narcotic analgesic **Dose:** *Adults.* 2.5–10 m IM q3–8h or 5–15 mg PO q8h; titrate as needed *Peds.* 0.7 mg/kg/24 h PO or IM q8h; ↑ slowly to ⊘ resp depression; ↓ in renal Dz **Caution:** [B/D (prolonged use or high doses at term), + (w/ doses ≥ 20 mg/24 h)], severe liver Dz **Supplied:** Tabs 5, 10, 40 mg; PO soln 5, 10 mg/5 mL; PO conc 10 mg/mL; inj 10 mg/mL **SE:** Resp depression, sedation, constipation, urinary retention, ventricular arrhythmia **Notes:** Equianalgesic w/ parenteral morphine; longer half-life; prolongs QT interval **Interactions:** ↑ Effects w/ cimetidine, CNS depressants, EtOH; ↑ effects of anticoagulants, EtOH, antihistamines, barbiturates, glutethimide, methocarbamol; ↓ effects w/ carbamazepine, nelfinavir, phenobarbital, phenytoin, primidone, rifampin, ritonavir **Labs:** ↑ Serum amylase, lipase

Methenamine (Hiprex, Urex, others)
Uses: *Suppression or elimination of bacteriuria associated w/ chronic/ recurrent UTI* **Action:** Converted t formaldehyde and ammonia in acidic urine; nonspecific bactericidal action **Dose:** *Adults.* Hippurate: 1 g bid. *Mandelate:* 1 g qid pc and hs *Peds 6–12 y.* Hippurate 25–50 mg/kg/d ÷ bid. *Mandelate:* 50–75 mg/kg/d ÷ qid (take w/ food and ascorbi acid; adequate hydration) **Caution:** [C, +] **Contra:** Renal insufficiency, severe hepatic Dz, and severe dehydration; allergy to sulfonamides **Supplied:** *Methenamine hippurate* (Hiprex, Urex): 1-g tabs. *Methenamine mandelate:* 500-mg, 1-g EC tab **SE:** Rash, GI upset, dysuria, ↑ LFTs **Interactions:** ↓ Effects w/ acetazolamide antacids **Labs:** ↑ Serum catecholamines, urine glucose, urobilinogen; ↓ urine estriol, estrogens **NIPE:** Fluids to 2–3 L/d; take w/ food

Methimazole (Tapazole)
Uses: *Hyperthyroidism, thyrotoxicosis,* an prep for thyroid surgery or radiation **Action:** Blocks the formation of T_3 and T **Dose:** *Adults.* Initial: 15–60 mg/d PO ÷ tid. *Maint:* 5–15 mg PO qd. *Peds.* Initia 0.4–0.7 mg/kg/24 h PO ÷ tid. *Maint:* ⅓–⅔ of the initial dose PO qd; take w/ foo **Caution:** [D, +/–] **Contra:** Breast-feeding **Supplied:** Tabs 5, 10 mg **SE:** GI upset dizziness, blood dyscrasias **Notes:** Follow clinically and w/ TFT **Interactions:** ↑ Effects of digitalis glycosides, metroprolol, propranolol; ↓ effects of anticoagulants, theophylline; ↓ effects w/ amiodarone **Labs:** ↑ LFTs, PT **NIPE:** Take w food

Methocarbamol (Robaxin)
Uses: *Relief of discomfort associated w painful musculoskeletal conditions* **Action:** Centrally acting skeletal muscle re laxant **Dose:** *Adults.* 1.5 g PO qid for 2–3 d, then 1-g PO qid maint therapy; IV form rarely indicated. *Peds.* 15 mg/kg/dose, may repeat PRN (recommended fo tetanus only) **Caution:** [C, +] **Contra:** Myasthenia gravis, renal impairment; cau

ion in Sz disorders **Supplied:** Tabs 325, 500, 750 mg; inj 100 mg/mL **SE:** Can discolor urine; drowsiness, GI upset **Interactions:** ↑ Effects w/ CNS depressant, EtOH **Labs:** ↑ Urine 5-HIAA, urine vanillylmandelic acid **NIPE:** Monitor for blurred vision, nystagmus, diplopia

Methotrexate (Folex, Rheumatrex) **Uses:** *ALL and AML (including leukemic meningitis), trophoblastic tumors (chorioepithelioma, choriocarcinoma, chorioadenoma destruens, hydatidiform mole), breast CA, Burkitt's lymphoma, mycosis fungoides, osteosarcoma, head and neck CA, Hodgkin's and NHL, lung CA; psoriasis; and RA* **Action:** Inhibits dihydrofolate reductase-mediated gen. of tetrahydrofolate **Dose:** *CA:* Varies per protocol. *RA:* 7.5 mg/wk PO as a single dose or 2.5 mg q12h PO for 3 doses/wk; "high-dose" Rx requires leucovorin rescue to limit hematologic and mucosal toxicity; ↓ in renal/hepatic impairment **Caution:** [D, –] **Contra:** Severe renal/hepatic impairment, PRG/lactation **Supplied:** Tabs 2.5, 5, 7.5, 10, 15 mg; inj 2.5, 25 mg/mL; preservative-free inj 25 mg/mL **SE:** Myelosuppression, N/V/D, anorexia, mucositis, hepatotoxicity (transient and reversible; may progress to atrophy, necrosis, fibrosis, cirrhosis), rashes, dizziness, malaise, blurred vision, alopecia, photosensitivity, renal failure, pneumonitis, and, rarely, pulmonary fibrosis; chemical arachnoiditis and HA w/ IT delivery **Notes:** Monitor blood counts, LFTs, renal Fxn tests, CXR, and MTX levels **Interactions:** ↑ Effects w/ chloramphenicol, cyclosporine, etretinate, NSAIDs, phenylbutazone, phenytoin, penicillin, probenecid, salicylates, sulfonamides, sulfonylureas, EtOH; ↑ effects of cyclosporine, tetracycline, theophylline; ↓ effects w/ antimalarials, aminoglycosides, binding resins, cholestyramine, folic acid; ↓ effects of digoxin **Labs:** ↑ AST, ALT, alkaline phosphatase, bilirubin, cholesterol **NIPE:** ↑ Risk of photosensitivity—use sunscreen, ↑ fluids 2–3 L/d

Methyldopa (Aldomet) **Uses:** *HTN* **Action:** Centrally acting antihypertensive **Dose:** *Adults.* 250–500 mg PO bid–tid (max 2–3 g/d) or 250 mg–1 g IV q6–8h. *Peds.* 10 mg/kg/24 h PO in 2–3 ÷ doses (max 40 mg/kg/24 h ÷ q6–12h) or 5–10 mg/kg/dose IV q6–8h to total dose of 20–40 mg/kg/24 h;↓ dose in renal insufficiency and in elderly **Caution:** [B (PO), C (IV), +] **Contra:** Liver Dz; MAOIs **Supplied:** Tabs 125, 250, 500 mg; PO susp 50 mg/mL; inj 50 mg/mL **SE:** Can discolor urine; initial transient sedation or drowsiness frequent; edema, hemolytic anemia; hepatic disorders **Interactions:** ↑ Effects w/ anesthetics, diuretics, levodopa, Li, methotrimeprazine, thioxanthenes, vasodilators, verapamil; ↑ effects of haloperidol, Li, tolbutamide; ↓ effects w/ amphetamines, Fe, phenothiazines, TCAs; ↓ effects of ephedrine **Labs:** Interference w/ SCr, glucose, AST, catecholamines; urine catecholamines, uric acid; false ↓ serum cholesterol, triglycerides **NIPE:** After 1–2 mo tolerance may develop

Methylergonovine (Methergine) **Uses:** *Postpartum bleeding (uterine subinvolution)* **Action:** Ergotamine derivative **Dose:** 0.2 mg IM after delivery of placenta, may repeat at 2–4-h intervals or 0.2–0.4 mg PO q6–12h for 2–7 d **Caution:** [C, ?] **Contra:** HTN, PRG **Supplied:** Injectable forms; tabs 0.2 mg **SE:**

IV doses should be given over a period of >1 min w/ frequent BP monitoring HTN, N/V **Interactions:** ↑ Vasoconstriction w/ ergot alkaloids, sympathomime ics, tobacco **NIPE:** ⊘ Smoking

Methylprednisolone (Solu-Medrol)   [See Steroids, Table 4, page 27 **Interactions:** ↑ Effects w/ cyclosporine, clarithromycin, erythromycin, estrogen ketoconazole, oral contraceptives, troleandomycin, grapefruit juice; ↑ effects c cyclosporine; ↓ effects w/ aminoglutethimide, barbiturates, carbamazepine, choles tyramine, colestipol, INH, phenytoin, phenobarbital, rifampin; ↓ effects of antico agulants, hypoglycemics, INH, salicylates, vaccines **Labs:** ↓ Skin test Rxns; fals ↑ serum cortisol, digoxin, theophylline, & urine glucose **NIPE:** ⊘ DC abruptly, ⊘ infections or vaccines

Metoclopramide (Reglan, Clopra, Octamide)   **Uses:** *Relief o diabetic gastroparesis, symptomatic GERD; chemotherapy-induced N/V, facilitat small-bowel intubation and radiologic evaluation of the upper GI tract,* stimulat gut in prolonged postop ileus **Action:** Stimulates motility of the upper GI trac blocks dopamine in the chemoreceptor trigger zone **Dose:** *Adults.* Diabetic gastro paresis: 10 mg PO 30 min ac & hs for 2–8 wk PRN, or same dose given IV for 1 d, then switch to PO. *Reflux:* 10–15 mg PO 30 min ac and hs. *Antiemetic:* 1– mg/kg/dose IV 30 min before chemotherapy, then q2h for 2 doses, then q3h for doses. *Peds.* Reflux: 0.1 mg/kg/dose PO qid. *Antiemetic:* 1–2 mg/kg/dose IV as fc adults **Caution:** [B, –] Concomitant drugs w/ extrapyramidal ADRs **Contra:** S disorders, GI obstruction **Supplied:** Tabs 5, 10 mg; syrup 5 mg/5 mL; soln 1 mg/mL; inj 5 mg/mL **SE:** Dystonic Rxns common w/ high doses, treat w/ I diphenhydramine; restlessness, drowsiness, diarrhea **Interactions:** ↑ Risk of sero tonin syndrome w/ sertraline, venlafaxine; ↑ effects of acetaminophen, ASA, CN depressants, cyclosporine, levodopa, Li, succinylcholine, tetracyclines, EtOH; effects w/ anticholinergics, narcotics; ↓ effects of cimetidine, digoxin **Labs:** Serum ALT, AST, amylase **NIPE:** Monitor for extrapyramidal effects

Metolazone (Mykrox, Zaroxolyn)   **Uses:** *Mild/moderate essentia HTN and edema of renal Dz or cardiac failure* **Action:** Thiazide-like diuretic; in hibits Na reabsorption in the distal tubules **Dose:** *HTN:* 2.5–5 mg PO. *Edema* 5–20 mg/d PO. *Peds.* 0.2–0.4 mg/kg/d PO ÷ q12h–qd **Caution:** [D, +] **Contra** Thiazide or sulfonamide sensitivity, anuria **Supplied:** *Tabs:* Mykrox (rapid acting 0.5 mg, Zaroxolyn 2.5, 5, 10 mg **SE:** Monitor fluid and electrolyte status durin Rx; dizziness, hypotension, tachycardia, CP, photosensitivity; Mykrox and Zarox olyn not bioequivalent **Interactions:** ↑ Effects w/ antihypertensives, barbiturates narcotics, nitrates, EtOH, food; ↑ effects of digoxin, Li; ↑ hyperglycemia w/ BB diazoxide; ↑ hypokalemia w/ amphotericin B, corticosteroids, mezlocillir piperacillin, ticarcillin; ↓ effects w/ cholestyramine, colestipol, hypoglycemics, ir sulin, NSAIDs, salicylates; ↓ effects of methenamine **Labs:** ↑ Serum and urin glucose, serum cholesterol, triglycerides, uric acid **NIPE:** ↑ Risk of photosensitiv ity—use sunscreen; ↑ risk of gout; monitor electrolytes

Metoprolol (Lopressor, Toprol XL) **WARNING:** ⊘ acutely stop therapy as marked worsening of angina can result **Uses:** *HTN, angina, AMI, and CHF* **Action:** β-Adrenergic receptor blocker **Dose:** *Angina:* 50–100 mg PO bid. *HTN:* 100–450 mg/d PO. *AMI:* 5 mg IV ×3 doses, then 50 mg PO q6h ×48 h, then 100 mg PO bid. *CHF:* 12–25 mg/d PO ×2 wk, ↑ at 2-wk intervals to 200 mg/max, use low dose in Pts w/ greatest severity; ↓ in hepatic failure **Caution:** [C, +] Uncompensated CHF, bradycardia, heart block **Contra:** Arrhythmia w/tachycardia **Supplied:** Tabs 50, 100 mg; ER tabs 50, 100, 200 mg; inj 1 mg/mL **SE:** Drowsiness, insomnia, erectile dysfunction, bradycardia, bronchospasm **Interactions:** ↑ Effects w/ cimetidine, dihydropyridines, diltiazem, fluoxetine, hydralazine, methimazole, oral contraceptives, propylthiouracil, quinidine, quinolones; ↑ effects of hydralazine; ↑ bradycardia w/ digoxin, dipyridamole, verapamil; ↓ effects w/ barbiturates, NSAIDs, rifampin; ↓ effects of isoproterenol, theophylline **Labs:** ↑ BUN, SCr, LFTs, uric acid **NIPE:** Take w/ food, ⊘ DC abruptly—withdraw over 2 wk

Metronidazole (Flagyl, MetroGel) **Uses:** *Bone/joint, endocarditis, intraabdominal, meningitis, and skin infections; amebiasis; trichomoniasis; bacterial vaginosis* **Action:** Interferes w/ DNA synthesis. *Spectrum:* Excellent coverage for anaerobic infections including *C. difficile,* also *H. pylori* in combination therapy **Dose:** *Adults.* Anaerobic infections: 500 mg IV q6–8h. *Amebic dysentery:* 750 mg/d PO for 5–10 d. *Trichomoniasis:* 250 mg PO tid for 7 d or 2 g PO ×1. *C. difficile infection:* 500 mg PO or IV q8h for 7–10 d (PO preferred; IV only if Pt NPO). *Vaginosis:* 1 applicatorful intravaginally bid or 500 mg PO bid for 7 d. *Acne rosacea/skin:* Apply bid. *Peds.* Anaerobic infections: 15 mg/kg/24 h PO or IV ÷ q6h. *Amebic dysentery:* 35–50 mg/kg/24 h PO in 3 ÷ doses for 5–10 d; ↓ in hepatic failure **Caution:** [B, M] ⊘ EtOH **Contra:** 1st tri of PRG **Supplied:** Tabs 250, 500 mg; XR tabs 750 mg; caps 375 mg; topical lotion and gel 0.75%; gel, vaginal 0.75% (5 g/applicator 37.5 mg in 70-g tube), cream 1% **SE:** May cause disulfiram-like Rxn; dizziness, HA, GI upset, anorexia, urine discoloration **Notes:** For Trichomoniasis, Rx Pt's partner; no aerobic bacteria activity; used in combination in serious mixed infections **Interactions:** ↑ Effects w/ cimetidine; ↑ effects of carbamazepine, fluorouracil, Li, warfarin; ↓ effects w/ barbiturates, cholestyramine, colestipol, phenytoin **Labs:** May cause ↓/zero values for LFTs, triglycerides, glucose **NIPE:** Take w/ food, possible metallic taste

Mexiletine (Mexitil) **Uses:** *Suppression of symptomatic ventricular arrhythmias*; diabetic neuropathy **Action:** Class IB antiarrhythmic **Dose:** *Adults.* 200–300 mg PO q8h; 1200 mg/d max. *Peds.* 2.5–5 mg/kg PO q 8h; drug interactions w/ hepatic enzyme inducers and suppressors requiring dosage changes (administer w/ food or antacids) **Caution:** [C, +] May worsen severe arrhythmias **Contra:** Cardiogenic shock or 2nd-/3rd-degree AV block w/o pacemaker **Supplied:** Caps 150, 200, 250 mg **SE:** Monitor LFTs; lightheadedness, dizziness, anxiety, incoordination, GI upset, ataxia, hepatic damage, blood dyscrasias **Interactions:** ↑ Effects w/ fluvoxamine, quinidine, caffeine; ↑ effects of theophylline; ↓ effects w/ atropine, hydantoins, phenytoin, phenobarbital, rifampin, tobacco **Labs:** ↑ LFTs, + ANA

Mezlocillin (Mezlin) **Uses:** *Infections caused by susceptible gram(–) bacteria involving the skin, bone, resp tract, urinary tract, abdomen, and septicemia* **Action:** Bactericidal; inhibits cell wall synthesis. *Spectrum:* Gram(–) *Klebsiella, Proteus, E. coli, Enterobacter, P. aeruginosa,* and *Serratia* **Dose:** *Adults.* 3 g IV q4–6h. *Peds.* 200–300 mg/kg/d ÷ q4–6h; ↓ in renal/hepatic insufficiency **Caution:** [B, M] **Contra:** Penicillin sensitivity **Supplied:** Inj **SE:** GI upset, agranulocytosis, thrombocytopenia **Notes:** Often used w/ aminoglycoside **Interactions:** ↑ Effect w/ probenecid; ↑ effects of MRX **Labs:** ↑ LFTs, BUN, SCr; ↓ serum K⁺

Miconazole (Monistat, others) **Uses:** *Candidal infections, dermatomycoses (various tinea forms)* **Action:** Fungicide; alters permeability of the fungal cell membrane **Dose:** Apply to area bid for 2–4 wk. *Intravaginally:* applicatorful or supp hs for 3 (4% or 200 mg) or 7 d (2% or 100 mg) **Caution:** [C ?] Azole sensitivity **Supplied:** Topical cream 2%; lotion 2%; powder 2%; spray 2%; vaginal supp 100, 200 mg; vaginal cream 2%, 4% [OTC] **SE:** Vaginal burning may potentiate warfarin **Notes:** Antagonistic to amphotericin B in vivo **Interactions:** ↑ Effects of anticoagulants, cisapride, loratadine, phenytoin, quinidine; ↓ effects w/ amphotericin B; ↓ effects of amphotericin B **Labs:** ↑ Protein

Midazolam (Versed) [C-IV] **Uses:** *Preoperative sedation, conscious sedation for short procedures and mechanically ventilated Pts, induction of general anesthesia* **Action:** Short-acting benzodiazepine **Dose:** *Adults.* 1–5 mg IV or IM titrate to effect. *Peds.* Preop: 0.25–1 mg/kg, 20 mg max PO. *Conscious sedation.* 0.08 mg/kg IM × 1. *General anesthesia:* 0.15 mg/kg IV, then 0.05 mg/kg/dose q2min for 1–3 doses PRN to induce anesthesia (↓ in elderly, w/ use of narcotics or CNS depressants) **Caution:** [D, +/–] CYP3A4 substrate, several drug interactions **Contra:** Narrow-angle glaucoma; use of amprenavir, nelfinavir, ritonavir **Supplied:** Inj 1, 5 mg/mL; syrup 2 mg/mL **SE:** Monitor for resp depression; hypotension in conscious sedation, nausea **Notes:** Reversal w/ flumazenil **Interactions:** ↑ Effects w/ azole antifungals, antihistamines, cimetidine, CCBs, CNS depressants, erythromycin, INH, phenytoin, protease inhibitors, grapefruit juice, EtOH; ↓ effects w/ rifampin, tobacco; ↓ effects of levodopa

Mifepristone [RU 486] (Mifeprex) **WARNING:** Pt counseling and information required **Uses:** *Termination of intrauterine pregnancies of <49 d* **Action:** Antiprogestin; ↑ prostaglandins, resulting in uterine contraction **Dose:** Administered w/ 3 office visits: day 1, three 200-mg tablets PO; day 3 if no abortion, two 200-mg misoprostol PO; on or about day 14, verify termination of PRG **Caution:** [X, –] **Contra:** Anticoagulation therapy, bleeding disorders **Supplied:** Tabs 200 mg **SE:** Abdominal pain and 1–2 wk of uterine bleeding **Notes:** Must be administered under physician's supervision **Interactions:** ↑ Effects w/ azole antifungals, erythromycin, grapefruit juice; ↓ effects w/ carbamazepine, dexamethasone, phenytoin, phenobarbital, rifampin, St. John's wort

Miglitol (Glyset) Uses: *Type 2 DM* Action: α-Glucosidase inhibitor; delays digestion of ingested carbohydrates Dose: Initial 25 mg PO tid; maint 50–100 mg tid (w/ 1st bite of each meal) Caution: [B, –] Contra: Obstructive or inflammatory GI disorders; ⊘ if SCr >2 Supplied: Tabs 25, 50, 100 mg SE: Used alone or in combination w/ sulfonylureas; flatulence, diarrhea, abdominal pain Interactions: ↑ Effects w/ celery, coriander, juniper berries, ginseng, garlic; ↓ effects w/ INH, niacin; ↓ effects of digoxin, propranolol, ranitidine

Milrinone (Primacor) Uses: *CHF* Action: + Inotrope and vasodilator; little chronotropic activity Dose: 50 μg/kg, then 0.375–0.75 μg/kg/min inf; ↓ dose in renal impairment Caution: [C, ?] Contra: Hypersensitivity to drug or amrinone Supplied: Inj 1 μg/mL SE: Arrhythmias, hypotension, HA Notes: Carefully monitor fluid/electrolyte status and BP/HR Interactions: ↑ Hypotension w/ disopyramide

Mineral Oil Uses: *Constipation* Action: Emollient laxative Dose: *Adults.* 5–45 mL PO PRN. *Peds.* >6 y: 5–20 mL PO bid Caution: [C, ?] N/V, difficulty swallowing, bedridden Pts Contra: Appendicitis, diverticulitis, ulcerative colitis Supplied: Liq [OTC] SE: Lipid pneumonia, anal incontinence, ↓ vitamin absorption Interactions: ↑ Effects w/ stool softeners; ↓ effects of cardiac glycosides, oral contraceptives, sulfonamides, warfarin

Minoxidil (Loniten, Rogaine) Uses: *Severe HTN; male and female pattern baldness* Action: Peripheral vasodilator; stimulates vertex hair growth Dose: *Adults.* PO: 2.5–10 mg PO bid–qid *Topical:* Apply bid to affected area. *Peds.* 0.2–1 mg/kg/24 h ÷ PO q12–24h; ↓ PO dose in elderly Caution: [C, +] Contra: Pheochromocytoma, hypersensitivity to components Supplied: Tabs 2.5, 5, 10 mg; topical soln (Rogaine) 2% SE: Pericardial effusion and volume overload may occur w/ PO use; hypertrichosis after chronic use; edema, ECG changes, weight gain Interactions: ↑ Hypotension w/ guanethidine Labs: ↑ Alkaline phosphatase, BUN, creatinine; ↓ Hmg, Hct

Mirtazapine (Remeron) WARNING: Closely monitor for worsening depression or emergence of suicidality, particularly in pediatric Pts Uses: *Depression* Action: Tetracyclic antidepressant Dose: 15 mg PO hs, up to 45 mg/d hs Caution: [C, ?] Contra: MAOIs w/in 14 d Supplied: Tabs 15, 30, 45 mg SE: Somnolence, ↑ cholesterol, constipation, xerostomia, weight gain, agranulocytosis Notes: ⊘ ↑ Dose at intervals of less than 1–2 wk Interactions: ↑ Effects w/ CNS depressants, fluvoxamine; ↑ risk of HTN crisis w/ MAOIs Labs: ↑ ALT, cholesterol, triglycerides

Misoprostol (Cytotec) Uses: *Prevention of NSAID-induced gastric ulcers*; induction of labor, incomplete and therapeutic abortion Action: Prostaglandin w/ both antisecretory and mucosal protective properties Dose: *Ulcer prevention:* 200 μg PO qid w/ meals; in females, start on 2nd or 3rd day of next normal menstrual period; 25–50 μg for induction of labor (term); 400 μg on day 3 of mifepristone for PRG termination (take w/ food) Caution: [X, –] Contra: PRG, component hypersensitivity **Supplied:** Tabs 100, 200 µg **SE:** Can cause miscarriage w/ potentially dangerous bleeding; HA, GI Sxs common (diarrhea, abdominal pain, constipation) **Interactions:** ↑ HA & GI symptoms w/ phenylbutazone

Mitomycin (Mutamycin) **Uses:** *Stomach, pancreas,* breast, colon CA, squamous cell carcinoma of the anus; non-small-cell lung, head, and neck, cervical, and breast CA; bladder CA (intravesically) **Action:** Alkylating agent; may also generate oxygen free radicals, induces DNA strand breaks **Dose:** 20 mg/m q6–8wk or 10 mg/m² in combination w/ other myelosuppressive drugs; bladder CA 20–40 mg in 40 mL NS via a urethral catheter once/wk for 8 wk, followed by monthly Rxs for 1 y; ↓ dose in renal/hepatic impairment **Caution:** [D, –] **Contra:** Thrombocytopenia, leukopenia, coagulation disorders, SCr > 1.7 mg/dL **Supplied:** Inj **SE:** Myelosuppression (may persist up to 3–8 wk after dose and may be cumulative minimized by a lifetime dose <50–60 mg/m²), N/V, anorexia, stomatitis, and renal toxicity; microangiopathic hemolytic anemia (similar to hemolytic–uremic syndrome) w/ progressive renal failure; venoocclusive Dz of the liver, interstitial pneumonia, alopecia (rare); extravasation Rxns can be severe **Interactions:** ↑ Bronchospasm w/ vinca alkaloids; ↑ bone marrow suppression w/ antineoplastics

Mitotane (Lysodren) **Uses:** *Palliative Rx of inoperable adrenocortical carcinoma* **Action:** Unclear; induces mitochondrial injury in adrenocortical cells **Dose:** 8–10 g/d in 3–4 ÷ doses (begin at 2 g/d w/ glucocorticoid replacement); ↓ in hepatic insufficiency; adequate hydration necessary **Caution:** [C, ?] **Supplied:** Tabs 500 mg **SE:** Anorexia, N/V/D; acute adrenal insufficiency may be precipitated by physical stresses (shock, trauma, infection); Rx w/ steroids; allergic Rxns (rare); visual disturbances, hemorrhagic cystitis, albuminuria, hematuria, HTN or hypotension, minor aches, fever **Interactions:** ↑ Effects of CNS depressants EtOH; ↓ effects of corticosteroids, phenytoin, phenobarbital, warfarin **Labs:** ↓ Protein-bound I **NIPE:** Full effects may take 2–3 mo

Mitoxantrone (Novantrone) **Uses:** *AML (w/ cytarabine), ALL, CML, CAP, MS,* breast CA, and NHL **Action:** DNA-intercalating agent; inhibitor of DNA topoisomerase II **Dose:** Per specific protocols; ↓ dose in hepatic failure leukopenia, thrombocytopenia; maintain hydration **Caution:** [D, –] **Contra:** PRG **Supplied:** Inj 2 mg/mL **SE:** Myelosuppression, N/V, stomatitis, alopecia (infrequent), cardiotoxicity, urine discoloration **Interactions:** ↑ Bone marrow suppression w/ antineoplastics; ↓ effects of live virus vaccines **Labs:** ↑ AST, ALT, uric acid **NIPE:** ↑ fluids to 2–3 L/d, ⊘ vaccines, infection

Modafinil (Provigil) **Uses:** *Improve wakefulness in Pts w/ excessive daytime sleepiness associated w/ narcolepsy* **Action:** Possible mechanisms include altered dopamine and norepinephrine release; ↓ GABA-mediated neurotransmission **Dose:** 200 mg PO q AM **Caution:** [C, ?/–] ↑ effects of warfarin, diazepam phenytoin; ↓ effects of oral contraceptives, cyclosporine, theophylline **Contra:** Component hypersensitivity **Supplied:** Tablets 100 mg, 200 mg **SE:** HA, N, D, paresthesias, rhinitis, agitation **Notes:** Consider lower doses in elderly Pts, reduce dose by 50% in Pts w/ hepatic impairment; use w/ caution in Pts w/ CV Dz **Interactions:** ↑ Effects of CNS stimulants, diazepam, phenytoin, propranolol, TCAs, warfarin; ↓ effect of cyclosporine, oral contraceptives, theophylline **NIPE:** Take w/o regard to food, monitor BP, use barrier contraception

Moexipril (Univasc) **Uses:** *HTN, post-MI,* DN **Action:** ACEI **Dose:** 7.5–30 mg in 1–2 ÷ doses 1 h ac **Caution:** [C (1st tri, D 2nd and 3rd tri), ?] **Contra:** ACEI sensitivity **Supplied:** Tabs 7.5, 15 mg; ↓ dose in renal impairment **SE:** Hypotension, edema, angioedema, HA, dizziness, cough **Interactions:** ↑ Effects with diuretics, antihypertensives, EtOH, probenecid, garlic; ↑ effects of insulin, Li; ↑ risk of hyperkalemia with K suppl, K-sparing diuretics; ↓ effects with antacids, ASA, NSAIDS, ephedra, yohimbe, ginseng **Labs:** ↑ BUN, creatinine, K+, ALT, AST, serum alkaline phosphatase; ↓ serum cholesterol; false + test for urine acetone **NIPE:** May alter sense of taste, may cause cough, ⊘ salt substitutes, ⊘ PRG, use barrier contraception.

Molindone (Moban) **Uses:** *Psychotic disorders* **Action:** Piperazine phenothiazine **Dose:** *Adults.* 50–75 mg/d, ↑ to 225 mg/d if necessary. *Peds* 3–5 y: 1–2.5 mg/d in 4 ÷ doses. *5–12 y:* 0.5–1.0 mg/kg/d in 4 ÷ doses **Caution:** [C, ?] Narrow-angle glaucoma **Contra:** Drug or EtOH-induced CNS depression **Supplied:** Tabs 5, 10, 25, 50, 100 mg; conc 20 mg/mL **SE:** Hypotension, tachycardia, arrhythmias, EPS, Szs, constipation, xerostomia, blurred vision **Interactions:** ↑ Effects w/ antihypertensives; ↑ hyperkalemia w/ K-sparing diuretics, K suppls, salt substitutes, trimethoprim; ↑ effects of insulin, Li; ↓ effects w/ ASA, NSAIDs **Labs:** ↑ Serum K+, BUN, creatinine **NIPE:** Take w/o food, monitor for persistent cough

Montelukast (Singulair) **Uses:** *Prophylaxis and Rx of chronic asthma, seasonal allergic rhinitis* **Action:** Leukotriene receptor antagonist **Dose:** *Asthma: Adults & Peds.* > 15y: 10 mg/d PO taken in PM. *Peds. 2–5 y:* 4 mg/d PO taken in PM. *6–14 y:* 5 mg/d PO in PM. *Rhinitis: Adults & Peds.* > 15y: 10 mg qd **Peds:** *2–5 y:* 4 mg qd. *6–14 y:* 5 mg qd **Caution:** [B, M] **Contra:** Component hypersensitivity **Supplied:** Tabs 10 mg; chew tabs 4, 5 mg **SE:** HA, dizziness, fatigue, rash, GI upset, Churg–Strauss syndrome **Notes:** Not for acute asthma attacks **Interactions:** ↑ ↓ Effects w/ phenobarbital, rifampin **Labs:** ↑ AST, ALT

Morphine (Avinza XR, Duramorph, MS Contin, Kadian SR, Oramorph SR, Roxanol) [C-II] **Uses:** *Relief of severe pain* **Action:** Narcotic analgesic **Dose:** *Adults.* PO: 5–30 mg q4h PRN; SR tabs 30–60 mg q8–12h (⊘ chew/crush). IV/IM: 2.5–15 mg q2–6h; supp 10–30 mg q4h. *Peds.* 0.1–0.2 mg/kg/dose IM/IV q2–4h PRN to a max of 15 mg/dose **Caution:** [B (D if prolonged use or high doses at term), +/–] **Contra:** Severe edema, resp depression, GI obstruction **Supplied:** Immediate-release tabs 10, 14, 20 mg; MS Contin CR tabs 15, 30, 60, 100, 200 mg; Oramorph SR CR tabs 15, 30, 60, 100 mg; Kadian SR caps 20, 30 50, 60, 100 mg; Avinza XR caps 30, 60, 90, 120 mg; soln 10, 20, 100 mg; supp 5, 10, 20 mg; inj 2, 4, 5, 8, 10, 15 mg/mL; Duramorph preservative-free inj 0.5, 1 mg/mL; suppository 5, 10, 20, 30 mg **SE:** Narcotic SE (resp depression, sedation, constipation, N/V, pruritus) **Notes:** May require scheduled dosing to relieve severe chronic pain; MS Contin commonly used SR form (Ⓢ crush) **Interactions:** ↑ Effects w/ cimetidine, CNS depressants, dextroamphetamine, TCAs, EtOH, kava kava, valerian, St. John's wort; ↑ effects of warfarin; ↑ risk of HTN crisis w/ MAOIs; ↓ effects w/ opioids, phenothiazines **Labs:** ↑ Serum amylase, lipase

Moxifloxacin (Avelox) **Uses:** *Acute sinusitis, acute bronchitis, skin/soft tissue infections, conjunctivitis, and community-acquired pneumonia* **Action:** Quinolone; inhibits DNA gyrase. *Spectrum:* Excellent gram(+) coverage except MRSA and *E. faecium;* good gram(−) coverage except *P. aeruginosa, S. maltophilia,* and *Acinetobacter* sp; good anaerobic coverage **Dose:** 400 mg/d PO (Ⓢ cation products, antacids) /IV qd. *Ophth:* 1 gt tid ×7d **Caution:** [C, ?/−] Quinolone sensitivity; interactions w/ Mg-, Ca-, Al-, and Fe-containing products and class IA and III antiarrhythmic agents **Contra:** Quinolone or component sensitivity **Supplied:** Tabs 400 mg, inj, ophth 0.5% **SE:** Dizziness, nausea, QT prolongation, Szs, photosensitivity, tendon rupture **Notes:** Take 4 h before or 8 h after antacids **Interactions:** ↑ Effects w/ probenecid; ↑ effects of diazepam, theophylline, caffeine, metoprolol, propranolol, phenytoin, warfarin; ↓ effects w/ antacids, didanosine, Fe salts, Mg, sucralfate, NaHCO₃, zinc **Labs:** ↑ LFTs, BUN, SCr, amylase, PT, triglycerides, cholesterol; ↓ Hmg, Hct **NIPE:** Ⓢ Give to children <18 y; ↑ fluids to 2–3 L/d

Mupirocin (Bactroban) **Uses:** *Impetigo; eradication of MRSA in nasal carriers* **Action:** Inhibits bacterial protein synthesis **Dose:** *Topical:* Apply small amount to affected area. *Nasal:* Apply bid in nostrils **Caution:** [B, ?] **Contra:** Ⓢ Use concurrently w/ other nasal products **Supplied:** Oint 2%; cream 2% **SE:** Local irritation, rash **Interactions:** ↓ Bacterial action w/ chloramphenicol **NIPE:** Ⓢ Use w/ other nasal drugs

Muromonab-CD3 (Orthoclone OKT3) **WARNING:** Can cause anaphylaxis; monitor fluid status **Uses:** *Acute rejection following organ transplantation* **Action:** Blocks T-cell Fxn **Dose:** *Adults.* 5 mg/d IV for 10–14 d. *Peds.* 0.1 mg/kg/d for 10–14 d **Caution:** [C, ?/−] Murine sensitivity, fluid overload **Contra:** HF/fluid overload, Hx of Szs, PRG, uncontrolled HTN **Supplied:** Inj 5 mg/5 mL **SE:** Murine antibody; fever and chills after the 1st dose (premedicate w/ steroid/APAP/antihistamine); monitor closely for anaphylaxis or pulmonary edema **Notes:** Use 0.22- micron filter for administration **Interactions:** ↑ Effects w/ immunosuppressives; ↑ effects of live virus vaccines; ↑ risk of CNS effects & encephalopathy w/ indomethacin **Labs:** ↑ AST, ALT **NIPE:** Ⓢ Immunizations, exposure to infection

Mycophenolate Mofetil (CellCept) **WARNING:** ↑ Risk of infections, possible development of lymphoma **Uses:** *Prevent organ rejection after transplant* **Action:** Inhibits immunologically mediated inflammatory responses **Dose:** *Adults.*

1 g PO bid; *Peds.* BSA 1.2–1.5 m²: 750 mg PO bid; *BSA >1.5 m²:* 1 g PO bid; may taper up to 600 mg/m² PO bid; used w/ steroids and cyclosporine; ↓ in renal insufficiency or neutropenia. *IV:* Infuse over at least 2 hr. *PO:* Take on empty stomach, ⊘ open capsules **Caution:** [C, ?/–] **Contra:** Component hypersensitivity; IV use in polysorbate 80 allergy **Supplied:** Caps 250, 500 mg; inj 500 mg **SE:** N/V/D, pain, fever, HA, infection, HTN, anemia, leukopenia, edema **Interactions:** ↑ Effects w/ acyclovir, ganciclovir, probenecid; ↓ effects of acyclovir, ganciclovir; ↓ effects w/ antacids, cholestyramine, cyclosporine, Fe, food; ↓ effects of oral contraceptives, phenytoin, theophylline **Labs:** ↑ LFTs **NIPE:** Use barrier contraception during and 6 wk after drug therapy, ⊘ exposure to infection; take w/o food

Nabumetone (Relafen) Uses: *Arthritis and pain* Action: NSAID; inhibits prostaglandins **Dose:** 1000–2000 mg/d ÷ qd–bid w/ food **Caution:** [C (D 3rd tri), +] **Contra:** Peptic ulcer, NSAID sensitivity, severe hepatic Dz **Supplied:** Tabs 500, 750 mg **SE:** Dizziness, rash, GI upset, edema, peptic ulcer **Interactions:** ↑ Effects w/ aminoglycosides; ↓ effects of anticoagulants, hypoglycemics, Li, MRX, thrombolytics; ↑ GI effects w/ ASA, corticosteroids, K suppls, NSAIDs, EtOH; ↓ effects of antihypertensives, diuretics **Labs:** ↑ LFTs, BUN, SCr; ↓ serum glucose, Hmg, Hct, plts **NIPE:** Photosensitivity—use sunscreen

Nadolol (Corgard) Uses: *HTN and angina* Action: Competitively blocks β-adrenergic receptors, β₁, β₂ **Dose:** 40–80 mg/d; ↑ to 240 mg/d (angina) or 320 mg/d (HTN) may be needed; ↓ in renal insufficiency and elderly **Caution:** [C (1st tri); D if 2nd or 3rd tri), +] **Contra:** Uncompensated CHF, shock, heart block, asthma **Supplied:** Tabs 20, 40, 80, 120, 160 mg **SE:** Nightmares, paresthesias, hypotension, bradycardia, fatigue **Interactions:** ↑ Effects w/ antihypertensives, diuretics, nitrates, EtOH; ↑ effects of aminophylline, lidocaine; ↑ risk of HTN w/ clonidine, ephedrine, epinephrine, MAOIs, phenylephrine, pseudoephedrine; ↑ bradycardia w/ digitalis glycosides, ephedrine, epinephrine, phenylephrine, pseudoephedrine; ↓ effects w/ ampicillin, antacids, clonidine, NSAIDs, thyroid meds; ↑ effects of glucagon, theophylline **Labs:** ↑ K⁺, cholesterol, triglycerides, BUN, uric acid **NIPE:** May ↑ cold sensitivity; ⊘ DC abruptly

Nafcillin (Nallpen) Uses: *Infections caused by susceptible strains of Staphylococcus and Streptococcus* Action: Bactericidal; inhibits cell wall synthesis. *Spectrum:* Good gram(+) **Dose:** *Adults.* 1–2 g IV q4–6h. *Peds.* 50–200 mg/kg/d ÷ q4–6h **Caution:** [B, ?] Penicillin allergy **Supplied:** Inj **SE:** Interstitial nephritis, diarrhea, fever, nausea **Notes:** No adjustments for renal Fxn **Interactions:** ↑ Effects of MRX; ↓ effects w/ chloramphenicol, macrolides, tetracyclines; ↓ effects of cyclosporine, oral contraceptives, tacrolimus, warfarin **Labs:** ↑ Serum protein **NIPE:** Aminoglycosides not compatible, risk of drug inactivation w/ fruit juice/carbonated drinks; monitor for superinfection

Naftifine (Naftin) Uses: *Tinea pedis, cruris, and corporis* Action: Antifungal antibiotic **Dose:** Apply bid **Caution:** [B, ?] **Contra:** Component sensitivity **Supplied:** 1% cream; gel **SE:** Local irritation

Nalbuphine (Nubain) Uses: *Moderate to severe pain; preop and obstetrical analgesia* Action: Narcotic agonist–antagonist; inhibits ascending pain pathways Dose: *Adults.* 10–20 mg IM or IV q4–6h PRN; max of 160 mg/d; single max dose, 20 mg. *Peds.*0.2 mg/kg IV or IM to a max dose of 20 mg; ↓ in hepatic insufficiency Caution: [B (D if prolonged or high doses at term), ?] Contra: Sulfite sensitivity Supplied: Inj 10, 20 mg/mL SE: Causes CNS depression and drowsiness; caution in Pts receiving opiatesInteractions: ↑ CNS depression w/ cimetidine, CNS depressants; EtOH ↑ effects of digitoxin, phenytoin, rifampin Labs: ↑ Serum amylase, lipase

Naloxone (Narcan) Uses: *Opioid addiction (diagnosis) and OD* Action: Competitive narcotic antagonist Dose: *Adults.* 0.4–2.0 mg IV, IM, or SQ q5min; max total dose, 10 mg. *Peds.*0.01–1 mg/kg/dose IV, IM, or SQ; repeat IV q3min × 3 doses PRN Caution: [B, ?] May precipitate acute withdrawal in addicts Supplied: Inj 0.4, 1.0 mg/mL; neonatal inj 0.02 mg/mL SE: Hypotension, tachycardia, irritability, GI upset, pulmonary edema Notes: If no response after 10 mg, suspect nonnarcotic cause Interactions: ↓ Effects of opioids

Naltrexone (ReVia) Uses: *EtOH and narcotic addiction* Action: Competitively binds to opioid receptors Dose: 50 mg/d PO; ⊘ give until opioid-free for 7–10 d Caution: [C, M] Contra: Acute hepatitis, liver failure; opioid use Supplied: Tabs 50 mg SE: May cause hepatotoxicity; insomnia, GI upset, joint pain, HA, fatigue Interactions: ↑ Lethargy & somnolence w/ thioridazine; ↓ effects of opioids

Naphazoline and Antazoline (Albalon-A Ophthalmic, others), Naphazoline and Pheniramine Acetate (Naphcon A) Uses: *Relieve ocular redness and itching caused by allergy* Action: Vasoconstrictor and antihistamine Dose: 1–2 gtt up to 4×/d Caution: [C, +] Contra: Glaucoma, children <6 y, and w/ contact lenses Supplied: Soln 15 mL SE: CV stimulation, dizziness, local irritation Interactions: ↑ Risk of HTN crisis w/ MAOIs, TCAs

Naproxen (Aleve, Naprosyn, Anaprox) Uses: *Arthritis and pain* Action: NSAID; inhibits prostaglandins Dose: *Adults & Peds.* >12 y: 200–500 mg bid–tid to a max of 1500 mg/d; ↓ dose in hepatic impairment Caution: [B (D 3rd tri), +] Contra: NSAID sensitivity, peptic ulcer Supplied: Tabs 200, 250, 375, 500 mg; delayed-release (EC) tabs 375, 500 mg; susp 125 mg/5 mL SE: Dizziness, pruritus, GI upset, peptic ulcer, edema Interactions: ↑ Effects w/ aminoglycosides; ↑ effects of anticoagulants, hypoglycemics, Li, MRX, thrombolytics; ↑ GI effects w/ ASA, corticosteroids, K suppls, NSAIDs, EtOH; ↓ effects of antihypertensives, diuretics Labs: ↑ Urine 5-HIAA NIPE: Take w/ food

Naratriptan (Amerge) Uses: *Acute migraine attacks* Action: Serotonin 5-HT$_1$ receptor antagonist Dose: 1–2.5 mg PO once; repeat PRN in 4 h; ↓ dose in mild renal/hepatic insufficiency, take w/ fluids Caution: [C, M] Contra: Severe renal/hepatic impairment, ⊘ in angina, ischemic heart Dz, uncontrolled

HTN, cerebrovascular syndromes, and ergot use **Supplied:** Tabs 1, 2.5 mg **SE:** Dizziness, sedation, GI upset, paresthesias, ECG changes, coronary vasospasm, arrhythmias **Interactions:** ↑ Effects w/ MAOIs, SSRIs; ↑ effects of ergot drugs; ↓ effects w/ nicotine

Nateglinide (Starlix) **Uses:** * Type 2 DM* **Action:** ↑ pancreatic release of insulin **Dose:** 120 mg PO tid 1–30 min pc; ↓ to 60 mg tid if near target HbA$_{1c}$ (take 1 – 30 min ac) **Caution:** [C, –]. Caution w/ drugs metabolized by CYP2C9/3A4 **Contra:** Diabetic ketoacidosis, type 1 DM **Supplied:** Tabs 60, 120 mg **SE:** Hypoglycemia, URI; salicylates, nonselective BBs may enhance hypoglycemia **Interactions:** ↑ Effects w/ nonselective BBs, MAOIs, NSAIDs, salicylates, ↓ effects w/ corticosteroids, niacin, sympathomimetics, thiazide diuretics, thyroid meds **Labs:** ↑ Uric acid

Nedocromil (Tilade) **Uses:** *Mild–moderate asthma* **Action:** Antiinflammatory agent **Dose:** *Inhal:* 2 inhal 4×/d **Caution:** [B, ?/–] **Contra:** Component hypersensitivity **Supplied:** Met-dose inhaler **SE:** Chest pain, dizziness, dysphonia, rash, GI upset, infection **Notes:** Not for acute asthma attacks **NIPE:** May take 2–4 wk for full therapeutic effect

Nefazodone (Serzone) **WARNING:** Fatal hepatitis and liver failure possible, DC if LFT >3× ULN, ⊘ re-treat; closely monitor for worsening depression or emergence of suicidality, particularly in pediatric Pts **Uses:** *Depression* **Action:** Inhibits neuronal uptake of serotonin and norepinephrine **Dose:** Initially 100 mg PO bid; usual 300–600 mg/d in 2 ÷ doses **Caution:** [C, ?] **Contra:** MAOIs, pimozide, cisapride, carbamazepine **Supplied:** Tabs 100, 150, 200, 250 mg **SE:** Postural hypotension and allergic Rxns; HA, drowsiness, xerostomia, constipation, GI upset, liver failure **Notes:** Monitor LFTs, HR/BP **Interactions:** ↑ Effects w/ benzodiazepines, buspirone; ↑ effects of alprazolam, buspirone, carbamazepine, cyclosporine, digoxin, triazolam; ↑ risk of QT prolongation w/ astemizole, cisapride, pimozide; ↑ risk of serious and/or fatal Rxn w/ MAOIs; ↓ effects of propranolol **Labs:** ↑ LFTs, cholesterol; ↓ Hct **NIPE:** Take w/o food; may take 2–4 wk for full therapeutic effects

Nelfinavir (Viracept) **Uses:** *HIV infection* **Action:** Protease inhibitor; results in formation of immature, noninfectious virion **Dose:** *Adults.* 750 mg PO tid or 1250 mg PO bid. *Peds.* 20–30 mg/kg PO tid; take w/ food **Caution:** [B, ?] Many significant drug interactions **Contra:** Phenylketonuria, triazolam/midazolam use or any other drug highly dependent on CYP3A4 **Supplied:** Tabs 250 mg; PO powder **SE:** Food ↑ absorption; interacts w/ St. John's wort; dyslipidemia, lipodystrophy, diarrhea, rash **Interactions:** ↑ Effects w/ erythromycin, ketoconazole, indinavir, ritonavir; ↑ effects of barbiturates, carbamazepine, cisapride, ergot alkaloids, erythromycin, lovastatin, midazolam, phenytoin, saquinavir, simvastatin, triazolam; ↓ effects w/ barbiturates, carbamazepine, phenytoin, rifabutin, rifampin; ↓ effects of oral contraceptives **Labs:** ↑ LFTs **NIPE:** Take w/ food; use barrier contraception

Neomycin, Bacitracin, & Polymyxin B (Neosporin Ointment) (See Bacitracin, Neomycin, and Polymyxin B Topical)

Neomycin, Colistin, and Hydrocortisone (Cortisporin-TC Otic Drops); Neomycin, Colistin, Hydrocortisone, & Thonzonium (Cortisporin-TC Otic Suspension) Uses: *External otitis,* infections of mastoid/fenestration cavities **Action:** Antibiotic w/antiinflammatory **Dose: Adults.** 4–5 gtt in ear(s) tid–qid. **Peds.** 3–4 gtt in ear(s) tid–qid **Caution:** [C, ?] **Supplied:** Otic gtt and susp **SE:** Local irritation

Neomycin & Dexamethasone (AK-Neo-Dex Ophthalmic, NeoDecadron Ophthalmic) Uses: *Steroid-responsive inflammatory conditions of the cornea, conjunctiva, lid, and anterior segment* **Action:** Antibiotic w/ antiinflammatory corticosteroid **Dose:** 1–2 gtt in eye(s) q3–4h or thin coat tid–qid until response, then ↓ to qd **Caution:** [C, ?] **Supplied:** Cream neomycin 0.5%/dexamethasone 0.1%; oint neomycin 0.35%/dexamethasone 0.05%; soln neomycin 0.35%/dexamethasone 0.1% **SE:** local irritation **Notes:** Use under supervision of ophthalmologist

Neomycin & Polymyxin B (Neosporin Cream) [OTC] Uses: *Infection in minor cuts, scrapes, and burns* **Action:** Bactericidal **Dose:** Apply bid–qid **Caution:** [C, ?] **Contra:** component hypersensitivity **Supplied:** Cream neomycin 3.5 mg/polymyxin B 10,000 Units/g **SE:** Local irritation **Notes:** Different from Neosporin oint

Neomycin, Polymyxin B, & Dexamethasone (Maxitrol) Uses: *Steroid-responsive ocular conditions w/ bacterial infection* **Action:** Antibiotic w/ antiinflammatory corticosteroid **Dose:** 1–2 gtt in eye(s) q4–6h; apply oint in eye(s) 3–4×/d **Caution:** [C, ?] **Supplied:** Oint neomycin sulfate 3.5 mg/polymyxin B sulfate 10,000 Units/dexamethasone 0.1%/g; susp identical/5 mL **SE:** Local irritation **Notes:** Use under supervision of ophthalmologist

Neomycin-Polymyxin Bladder Irrigant [Neosporin GU Irrigant] Uses: *Continuous irrigant for prophylaxis against bacteriuria and gram(−) bacteremia associated w/ indwelling catheter use* **Action:** Bactericide **Dose:** 1 mL irrigant in 1 L of 0.9% NaCl; cont bladder irrigation w/ 1 L of soln/24 h **Caution:** [D] **Contra:** Component hypersensitivity **Supplied:** Soln neomycin sulfate 40 mg and polymyxin B sulfate 200,000 Units/mL; amp 1, 20 mL **SE:** Neomycin-induced ototoxicity or nephrotoxicity (rare) **Notes:** Potential for bacterial or fungal superinfection; not for inj

Neomycin, Polymyxin, & Hydrocortisone (Cortisporin Ophthalmic and Otic) Uses: *Ocular and otic bacterial infections* **Action:** Antibiotic and antiinflammatory **Dose:** *Otic:* 3–4 gtt in the ear(s) 3–4×/d. *Ophth:* Apply a thin layer to the eye(s) or 1 gtt 1–4×/d **Caution:** [C, ?] **Supplied:** Otic susp; ophth soln; ophth oint **SE:** Local irritation

Neomycin, Polymyxin B, & Prednisolone (Poly-Pred Ophthalmic) Uses: *Steroid-responsive ocular conditions w/ bacterial infection*

Action: Antibiotic and antiinflammatory **Dose:** 1–2 gtt in eye(s) q4–6h; apply oint in eye(s) 3–4×/d **Caution:** [C, ?] **Supplied:** Susp neomycin 0.35%/polymyxin B 10,000 Units/prednisolone 0.5%/mL **SE:** Irritation **Notes:** Use under supervision of ophthalmologist

Neomycin Sulfate (Myciguent) [OTC]
Uses: *Hepatic coma and preoperative bowel prep* **Action:** Aminoglycoside, poorly absorbed PO; suppresses GI bacterial flora **Dose:** *Adults.* 3–12 g/24 h PO in 3–4 ÷ doses. *Peds.* 50–100 mg/kg/24 h PO in 3–4 ÷ doses **Caution:** [C, ?/–] Renal failure, neuromuscular disorders, hearing impairment **Contra:** Intestinal obstruction **Supplied:** Tabs 500 mg; PO soln 125 mg/5 mL **SE:** Hearing loss w/ long-term use; rash, N/V **Notes:** ⊘ use parenterally due to ↑ toxicity; part of the Condon bowel prep

Nesiritide (Natrecor)
Uses: *Acutely decompensated CHF* **Action:** Human B-type natriuretic peptide **Dose:** 2 µg/kg IV bolus, then 0.01 µg/kg/min IV **Caution:** [C, ?/–] In Pts whom vasodilators are not appropriate **Contra:** SBP <90, cardiogenic shock **Supplied:** Vials 1.5 mg **SE:** Hypotension, HA, GI upset, arrhythmias, ↑ Cr **Notes:** Requires continuous BP monitoring **Interactions:** ↑ Hypotension w/ ACEIs, nitrates **Labs:** ↑ Creatinine

Nevirapine (Viramune)
WARNING: Reports of fatal hepatotoxicity even after short-term use; severe life-threatening skin Rxns (Stevens–Johnson, toxic epidermal necrolysis, and hypersensitivity Rxns); monitor closely during 1st 8 wk of Rx **Uses:** *HIV infection* **Action:** Nonnucleoside RT inhibitor **Dose:** *Adults.* Initial 200 mg/d × 14 d, then 200 mg bid. *Peds.* <8 y: 4 mg/kg/d × 14 d, then 7 mg/kg bid. >8 y: 4 mg/kg/d × 14 d, then 4 mg/kg bid **Caution:** [C, +/–] OCP **Supplied:** Tabs 200 mg; susp 50 mg/5 mL **SE:** Life-threatening rash; HA, fever, diarrhea, neutropenia, hepatitis **Notes:** Give w/out regard to food **Interactions:** ↑ Effects w/ clarithromycin, erythromycin; ↓ effects w/ rifabutin, rifampin, St. John's wort; ↓ effects of clarithromycin, indinavir, ketoconazole, methadone, oral contraceptives, protease inhibitors, warfarin **NIPE:** Use barrier contraception

Niacin (Niaspan)
Uses: *Adjunctive in significant hyperlipidemia* **Action:** Inhibits lipolysis; ↓ esterification of triglycerides; ↑ lipoprotein lipase activity **Dose:** 1–6 g ÷ doses tid; 9 g/d max **Caution:** [A (C if doses >RDA), +] **Contra:** Liver Dz, peptic ulcer, arterial hemorrhage **Supplied:** SR caps 125, 250, 300, 400, 500 mg; tabs 25, 50, 100, 250, 500 mg; SR tabs 150, 250, 500, 750 mg; elixir 50 mg/5 mL **SE:** Upper body and facial flushing and warmth following dose; may cause GI upset; HA, flatulence, paresthesias, liver damage, may exacerbate peptic ulcer, gout, or glucose control in DM. **Notes:** Administer w/ food; flushing may be ↓ by taking an ASA or NSAID 30–60 min prior to dose **Interactions:** ↑ Effects of antihypertensives, anticoagulants; ↓ effects of hypoglycemics, probenecid, sulfinpyrazone **Labs:** False ↑ urinary catecholamines, false + urine glucose, ↑ LFTs, uric acid **NIPE:** EtOH & hot beverages ↑ flushing

Nicardipine (Cardene)
Uses: *Chronic stable angina and HTN*; prophylaxis of migraine **Action:** CCB **Dose:** *Adults.* PO: 20–40 mg PO tid. *SR:* 30–60 mg

PO bid. *IV:* 5 mg/h IV cont inf; ↑ by 2.5 mg/h q15min to max 15 mg/h. **Peds.** PO: 20–30 mg PO q 8h. *IV:* 0.5 – 5 μg/kg/min; ↓ in renal/hepatic impairment **Caution:** [C, ?/–] Heart block, CAD **Contra:** Cardiogenic shock **Supplied:** Caps 20, 30 mg; SR caps 30, 45, 60 mg; inj 2.5 mg/mL **SE:** Flushing, tachycardia, hypotension, edema, HA **Notes:** *PO-to-IV conversion:* 20 mg tid = 0.5 mg/h, 30 mg tid = 1.2 mg/h, 40 mg tid = 2.2 mg/h; take w/ food (not high fat) **Interactions:** ↑ Effects w/ azole antifungals, cimetidine, ranitidine, grapefruit juice; ↑ effects of cyclosporine, carbamazepine, prazosin, quinidine, tacrolimus; ↑ hypotension w/ antihypertensives, fentanyl, nitrates, quinidine, EtOH; ↑ dysrhythmias w/ digoxin, disopyramide, phenytoin; ↓ effects w/ NSAIDs, rifampin **Labs:** ↑ LFTs **NIPE:** ↑ Risk of photosensitivity—use sunscreen

Nicotine Gum (Nicorette) [OTC]
Uses: *Aid to smoking cessation for the relief of nicotine withdrawal* **Action:** Systemic delivery of nicotine **Dose:** Chew 9–12 pieces/d PRN; max 30 pieces/d **Caution:** [C, ?] **Contra:** Life-threatening arrhythmias, unstable angina **Supplied:** 2 mg, 4 mg/piece; mint, orange, original flavors **SE:** Tachycardia, HA, GI upset, hiccups **Notes:** Must stop smoking and perform behavior modification for max effect **Interactions:** ↑ Effects w/ cimetidine; ↑ effects of catecholamines, cortisol; ↑ hemodynamic & A-V blocking effects of adenosine; ↓ effects w/ coffee, cola **NIPE:** Chew 30 min for full dose of nicotine; ↓ absorption w/ coffee, soda, juices, wine w/in 15 min

Nicotine Nasal Spray (Nicotrol NS)
Uses: *Aid to smoking cessation for the relief of nicotine withdrawal* **Action:** Systemic delivery of nicotine **Dose:** 0.5 mg/actuation; 1–2 sprays/h, 10 sprays/h max **Caution:** [D, M] **Contra:** Life-threatening arrhythmias, unstable angina **Supplied:** Nasal inhaler 10 mg/mL **SE:** Local irritation, tachycardia, HA, taste perversion **Notes:** Must stop smoking and perform behavior modification for max effect **Interactions:** ↑ Effects w/ cimetidine, blue cohash; ↑ effects of catecholamines, cortisol; ↑ hemodynamic & A-V blocking effects of adenosine **NIPE:** ⊘ in Pts w/ chronic nasal disorders or severe reactive airway Dz; ↑ incidence of cough

Nicotine Transdermal (Habitrol, Nicoderm CQ [OTC], Nicotrol [OTC])
Uses: *Aid to smoking cessation for the relief of nicotine withdrawal* **Action:** Systemic delivery of nicotine **Dose:** Individualized; 1 patch (14–22 mg/d), and taper over 6 wk **Caution:** [D, M] **Contra:** Life-threatening arrhythmias, unstable angina **Supplied:** Habitrol and Nicoderm CQ 7, 14, 21 mg of nicotine/24 h; Nicotrol 5, 10, 15 mg/24 h **SE:** Insomnia, pruritus, erythema, local site Rxn, tachycardia **Notes:** Nicotrol worn for 16 h to mimic smoking patterns; others worn for 24 h; must stop smoking and perform behavior modification for max effect **Interactions:** ↑ Effects w/ cimetidine, blue cohash; ↑ effects of catecholamines, cortisol; ↑ hemodynamic & A-V blocking effects of adenosine; ↑ HTN w/ bupropion **NIPE:** Change application site daily

Nifedipine (Procardia, Procardia XL, Adalat, Adalat CC)
Uses: *Vasospastic or chronic stable angina and HTN*; tocolytic **Action:** CCB

Dose: Adults. SR tabs 30–90 mg/d. *Tocolysis:* 10–20 mg PO q4–6h. *Peds.*0.6–0.9 mg/kg/24 h ÷ tid–qid **Caution:** [C, +] Heart block, aortic stenosis **Contra:** Immediate-release prep for urgent or emergent HTN; acute MI **Supplied:** Caps 10, 20 mg; SR tabs 30, 60, 90 mg **SE:** HA common on initial Rx; reflex tachycardia may occur w/ regular release dosage forms; peripheral edema, hypotension, flushing, dizziness **Notes:** Adalat CC and Procardia XL not interchangeable; SL administration is neither safe nor effective and should be abandoned **Interactions:** ↑ Effects w/ antihypertensives, azole antifungals, cimetidine, cisapride, CCBs, diltiazem, famotidine, nitrates, quinidine, ranitidine, EtOH, grapefruit juice; ↑ effects of digitalis glycosides, phenytoin, vincristine; ↓ effects w/ barbiturates, nafcillin, NSAIDs, phenobarbital, rifampin, St. John's wort, tobacco; ↓ effects of quinidine **Labs:** ↑ LFTs **NIPE:** Take w/o regard to food; ↑ risk of photosensitivity—use sunscreen

Nilutamide (Nilandron) WARNING: Interstitial pneumonitis possible; most cases in 1st 3 mo; follow CXR before Rx **Uses:** *Combination w/ surgical castration for metastatic CAP* **Action:** Nonsteroidal antiandrogen **Dose:** 300 mg/d in ÷ doses for 30 d, then 150 mg/d **Caution:** [N/A] **Contra:** Severe hepatic impairment or resp insufficiency **Supplied:** Tabs 150 mg **SE:** Hot flashes, loss of libido, impotence, N/V/D, gynecomastia, hepatic dysfunction (follow LFTs), interstitial pneumonitis **Notes:** May cause a severe Rxn when taken w/ EtOH **Interactions:** ↑ Effects of phenytoin, theophylline, warfarin **Labs:** ↑ LFTs **NIPE:** Take w/o regard to food; visual adaptation may be delayed

Nimodipine (Nimotop) Uses: *Prevent vasospasm following subarachnoid hemorrhage* **Action:** CCB **Dose:** 60 mg PO q4h for 21 d; ↓ dose in hepatic failure **Caution:** [C, ?] **Contra:** Component hypersensitivity **Supplied:** Caps 30 mg **SE:** Hypotension, HA, constipation **Notes:** Caps may be administered via NG tube if caps cannot be swallowed whole **Interactions:** ↑ Effects w/ antihypertensives, cimetidine, nitrates, omeprazole, protease inhibitors, quinidine, valproic acid, EtOH, grapefruit juice; ↑ effects of phenytoin **Labs:** ↑ LFTs **NIPE:** ↑ Risk of photosensitivity—use sunscreen

Nisoldipine (Sular) Uses: *HTN* **Action:** CCB **Dose:** 10–60 mg/d PO; ⊘ take w/ grapefruit juice or high-fat meal; ↓ starting doses in elderly or hepatic impairment **Caution:** [C, ?] **Supplied:** ER tabs 10, 20, 30, 40 mg **SE:** Edema, HA, flushing **Interactions:** ↑ Effects w/ antihypertensives, azole antifungals, cimetidine, famotidine, nitrates, ranitidine, EtOH, high-fat foods; ↑ effects of tacrolimus; ↓ effects w/ NSAIDs, phenytoin, rifampin **Labs:** ↑ Serum creatine kinase, BUN, creatinine

Nitazoxanide (Alinia) Uses: * *Cryptosporidium-* or *Giardia*-induced diarrhea in Pts 1–11 y* **Action:** Antiprotozoal. *Spectrum: Cryptosporidium* or *Giardia* **Dose: Peds.** 12–47 mo: 5 mL (100 mg) PO q 12h × 3 d. *4–11 y:* 10 mL (200 mg) PO q 12h × 3 d; take w/ food **Caution:** [B, ?] **Contra:** **Supplied:** 100 mg/5 mL PO susp **SE:** Abdominal pain **Notes:** Susp contains sucrose; likely to interact w/highly protein-bound drugs

Nitrofurantoin (Macrodantin, Furadantin, Macrobid)
WARNING: Pulmonary Rxns possible **Uses:** *Prevention and Rx UTI* **Action:** Bacteriostatic; interferes w/ carbohydrate metabolism. *Spectrum:* Susceptible gram(−) and some gram(+) bacteria; *Pseudomonas, Serratia,* and most sp. *Proteus* generally resistant **Dose:** *Adults.* Suppression: 50–100 mg/d PO. *Rx:* 50–100 mg PO qid. *Peds.*4–7 mg/kg/24 h in 4 ÷ doses; take w/ food, milk, or antacid **Caution:** [B, +] ⊘ if CrCl <50 mL/min, PRG at term **Contra:** Renal failure, infants < 1 mo **Supplied:** Caps and tabs 50, 100 mg; SR caps 100 mg; susp 25 mg/5 mL **SE:** GI side effects common; dyspnea and a variety of acute and chronic pulmonary Rxns, peripheral neuropathy **Notes:** Macrocrystals (Macrodantin) cause less nausea than other forms of the drug **Interactions:** ↑ Effects w/ anticholinergics, probenecid, sulfinpyrazone; ↓ effects w/ antacids, quinolones **Labs:** False + urine glucose; false ↑ serum bilirubin, creatinine **NIPE:** Take w/ food; may discolor urine

Nitroglycerin (Nitrostat, Nitrolingual, Nitro-Bid Ointment, Nitro-Bid IV, Nitrodisc, Transderm-Nitro, others) **Uses:** *Angina pectoris, acute and prophylactic therapy, CHF, BP control* **Action:** Relaxation of vascular smooth muscle, dilates coronary arteries **Dose:** *Adults.* SL: 1 tab q5min SL PRN for 3 doses. *Translingual:* 1–2 met-doses sprayed onto PO mucosa q3–5min, max 3 doses. *PO:* 2.5–9 mg tid. *IV:* 5–20 µg/min, titrated to effect. *Topical:* Apply ½ in. of oint to the chest wall tid, wipe off at night. *TD:* 0.2–0.4 mg/h/patch qd. *Peds.* 1 µg/kg/min IV, titrated to effect. **Caution:** [B, ?] Restrictive cardiomyopathy **Contra:** *IV:* Pericardial tamponade, constrictive pericarditis. *PO:* Concurrent use w/ sildenafil, tadalafil, vardenfil, head trauma, closed-angle glaucoma **Supplied:** SL tabs 0.3, 0.4, 0.6 mg; translingual spray 0.4 mg/dose; SR caps 2.5, 6.5, 9, 13 mg; SR tabs 2.6, 6.5, 9.0 mg; inj 0.5, 5, 10 mg/mL; oint 2%; TD patches 0.1, 0.2, 0.4, 0.6 mg/h; buccal CR 2, 3 mg **SE:** HA, hypotension, light-headedness, GI upset **Notes:** Tolerance to nitrates develops w/ chronic use after 1–2 wk; minimize by providing nitrate-free period each day, using shorter-acting nitrates tid, and removing long-acting patches and oint before hs to prevent development of tolerance **Interactions:** ↑ Hypotensive effects w/ antihypertensives, phenothiazines, sildenafil, EtOH; ↓ effects w/ ergot alkaloids; ↓ effects of SL tabs & spray w/ antihistamines, phenothiazines, TCAs **Labs:** False ↑ cholesterol, triglycerides **NIPE:** Replace SL tabs q6 mo & keep in original container

Nitroprusside (Nipride, Nitropress) **Uses:** *Hypertensive crisis, CHF, controlled hypotension periop (↓ bleeding),* aortic dissection, pulmonary edema **Action:** ↓ Systemic vascular resistance **Adult & Peds** 0.5–10 µg/kg/min IV inf, titrate to effect; usual dose 3 µg/kg/min **Caution:** [C, ?] ↓ cerebral perfusion **Contra:** High output failure, compensatory HTN **Supplied:** Inj 25 mg/mL **SE:** Excessive hypotensive effects, palpitations, HA **Notes:** Thiocyanate (metabolite), excreted by the kidney; thiocyanate toxicity at levels of 5–10 mg/dL, more likely when used for > 2–3 d; to treat aortic dissection, use BB concomitantly **Interactions:** ↑ Effects w/ antihypertensives, anesthetics, guanabenz, guanfacine, sildenafil; ↓ effects w/ estrogens, sympathomimetics **NIPE:** Discard colored soln other than light brown

Nizatidine (Axid)   **Uses:** *Duodenal ulcers, GERD, heartburn* **Action:** H$_2$-receptor antagonist **Dose:** *Adults.* Active ulcer: 150 mg PO bid or 300 mg PO hs; maint 150 mg PO hs. *GERD:* 300 mg PO bid; maint PO bid. *Heartburn:* 75 mg PO bid. *Peds.* GERD: 10 mg/kg PO bid in ÷ doses, 150 mg bid max ↓ dose in renal impairment **Caution:** [B, +] **Contra:** H$_2$ receptor antagonist sensitivity **Supplied:** Caps 75, 150, 300 mg **SE:** Dizziness, HA, constipation, diarrhea **Interactions:** ↑ Effects of glipizide, glyburide, nifedipine, nitrendipine, nisoldipine, salicylates, tolbutamide; ↓ effects w/ antacids, tomato/mixed veg juice; ↓ effects of azole antifungals, delavirdine, didanosine **Labs:** False + urobilinogen **NIPE:** Smoking ↑ gastric acid secretion

Norepinephrine (Levophed)   **Uses:** *Acute hypotension, cardiac arrest (adjunct)* **Action:** Peripheral vasoconstrictor acts on arterial/venous beds **Dose:** *Adults.* 8–12 µg/min IV, titrate. *Peds.* 0.05–0.1 mg/kg/min IV, titrate **Caution:** [C, ?] **Contra:** Hypotension due to hypovolemia **Supplied:** Inj 1 mg/mL **SE:** Bradycardia, arrhythmia **Notes:** Correct volume depletion as much as possible before vasopressors; interaction w/ TCAs leads to severe HTN; infuse into large vein to avoid extravasation; phentolamine 5–10 mg/10 mL NS injected locally for extravasation **Interactions:** ↑ HTN w/ antihistamines, BBs, ergot alkaloids, guanethidine, MAOIs, methyldopa, oxytocic meds, TCAs; ↑ risk of arrhythmias w/ cyclopropane, halothane

Norethindrone Acetate/Ethinyl Estradiol (FemHRT)   **WARNING:** Estrogens and progestins should not be used for the prevention of CV Dz; the WHI study reported ↑ risks of MI, breast CA, and DVT in postmenopausal women during 5 y of Rx w/ estrogens combined w/ medroxyprogesterone acetate relative to placebo **Uses:** *Rx of moderate to severe vasomotor Sxs associated w/ menopause; prevention of osteoporosis.* **Action:** Hormone replacement **Dose:** 1 tablet qd **Caution:** [X, –] **Contra:** PRG; Hx breast cancer; estrogen-dependent neoplasia; abnormal genital bleeding; Hx DVT, PE, or related disorders; recent (w/in past year) arterial thromboembolic Dz (CVA, MI) **Supplied:** 1 mg norethindrone/5 µg ethinyl estradiol tablets **SE:** thrombosis, dizziness, HA, libido changes **Notes:** Use in women w/ intact uterus **Interactions:** ↑ Effects of caffeine; ↓ effects with barbiturates, carbamazepine, fosphenytoin, phenytoin, rifampin **Labs:** Effects hepatic Fxn tests and endocrine Fxn tests **NIPE:** ⊘ PRG, cigarette smoking

Norfloxacin (Noroxin)   **Uses:** *Complicated and uncomplicated UTI due to gram(–) bacteria, prostatitis, gonorrhea,* and infectious diarrhea **Action:** Quinolone, inhibits DNA gyrase. *Spectrum:* Susceptible *E. faecalis, E. coli, K. pneumoniae, P. mirabilis, P. aeruginosa, S. epidermidis, S. saprophyticus* **Dose:** 400 mg PO bid. *Gonorrhea:* 800 mg single dose. *Prostatitis:* 400 mg PO bid **Caution:** [C, –] Tendinitis/tendon rupture, quinolone sensitivity, dose ↓ in renal impairment **Contra:** Hx of hypersensitivity or tendinitis w/ fluoroquinolones **Supplied:**

Tabs 400 mg **SE:** Photosensitivity, HA, GI **Notes:** Drug interactions w/ antacids, theophylline, and caffeine; good conc in the kidney and urine, poor blood levels; ⊘ use for urosepsis **Interactions:** ↑ Effects w/ probenecid; ↑ effects of diazepam, theophylline, caffeine, metoprolol, propranolol, phenytoin, warfarin; ↓ effects w/ antacids, didanosine, Fe salts, Mg, sucralfate, NaHCO₃, zinc; ↓ effects w/ food; **Labs:** ↑ LFTs, BUN, SCr **NIPE:** ⊘ Give to children <18 y; ↑ fluids to 2–3 L/d; may cause photosensitivity—use sunscreen

Norgestrel (Ovrette) **Uses:** *Contraceptive* **Action:** Prevent follicular maturation and ovulation **Dose:** 1 tab/d; begin day 1 of menses **Caution:** [X, ?] **Contra:** Thromboembolic disorders, breast CA, PRG, severe hepatic Dz **Supplied:** Tabs 0.075 mg **SE:** Edema, breakthrough bleeding, thromboembolism **Notes:** Progestin-only products have higher risk of failure in prevention of PRG **Interactions:** ↓ Effects w/ barbiturates, carbamazepine, hydantoins, griseofulvin, penicillins, rifampin, tetracyclines, St. John's wort **NIPE:** Photosensitivity—use sunscreen; DC drug if suspect PRG—use barrier contraception until confirmed

Nortriptyline (Aventyl, Pamelor) **Uses:** *Endogenous depression* **Action:** TCA; ↑ the synaptic CNS concs of serotonin and/or norepinephrine **Dose:** *Adults.* 25 mg PO tid–qid; doses >150 mg/d ⊘. *Elderly.* 10–25 mg hs. *Peds.* 6–7 y: 10 mg/d. *8–11 y:* 10–20 mg/d. *>11 y:* 25–35 mg/d. ↓ Dose w/ hepatic insufficiency **Caution:** [D, +/–] Narrow-angle glaucoma, CV Dz **Contra:** TCA hypersensitivity, use w/ MAOI **Supplied:** Caps 10, 25, 50, 75 mg; soln 10 mg/5 mL **SE:** Anticholinergic side effects (blurred vision, urinary retention, xerostomia) **Notes:** Max effect seen after 2 wk **Interactions:** ↑ Effects w/ antihistamines, CNS depressants, cimetidine, fluoxetine, oral contraceptives, phenothiazines, quinidine, EtOH; ↑ effects of anticoagulants; ↑ risk of HTN w/ clonidine, levodopa, sympathomimetics; ↓ effects w/ barbiturates, carbamazepine, rifampin **Labs:** ↑ Serum bilirubin, alkaline phosphatase **NIPE:** Concurrent use w/ MAOIs have resulted in HTN, Szs, death; ↑ risk of photosensitivity—use sunscreen

Nystatin (Mycostatin) **Uses:** *Mucocutaneous Candida infections (oral, skin, vaginal)* **Action:** Alters membrane permeability. *Spectrum:* Susceptible *Candida* sp **Dose:** *Adults and children.* PO: 400,000–600,000 Units PO "swish and swallow" qid. *Vaginal:* 1 tab vaginally hs for 2 wk. *Topical:* Apply bid–tid to affected area. *Peds.* Infants: 200,000 Units PO q6h. **Caution:** [B (C PO), +] **Supplied:** PO susp 100,000 Units/mL; PO tabs 500,000 Units; troches 200,000 Units; vaginal tabs 100,000 U; topical cream and oint 100,000 Units/g **SE:** GI upset, Stevens–Johnson syndrome **Notes:** Not absorbed PO; not effective for systemic infections **NIPE:** Store susp up to 10 d in refrigerator

Octreotide (Sandostatin, Sandostatin LAR) **Uses:** *Suppresses/ inhibits severe diarrhea associated w/ carcinoid and neuroendocrine GI tumors (eg, VIPoma, ZE syndrome)*; bleeding esophageal varices **Action:** Long-acting peptide; mimics natural hormone somatostatin **Dose:** *Adults.* 100–600 μg/d SQ/IV in 2–4 ÷ doses; start 50 μg qd–bid. *Sandostatin LAR (depot):* 10–30 mg IM

¼wk *Peds.*1–10 μg/kg/24 h SQ in 2–4 ÷ doses. **Caution:** [B, +] Hepatic/renal impairment **Supplied:** Inj 0.05, 0.1, 0.2, 0.5, 1 mg/mL; 10, 20, 30 mg/5 mL depot **SE:** N/V, abdominal discomfort, flushing, edema, fatigue, cholelithiasis, hyper-/hypoglycemia, hepatitis **Interactions:** ↓ Effects of cyclosporine **Labs:** Small ↑ LFTs, ↓ serum thyroxine **NIPE:** May alter effects of hypoglycemics

Ofloxacin (Floxin, Ocuflox Ophthalmic) Uses: *Lower resp tract, skin and skin structure, and UTI, prostatitis, uncomplicated gonorrhea, and *Chlamydia* infections; topical for bacterial conjunctivitis; otitis externa; if perforated ear drum >12 y* **Action:** Bactericide; inhibits DNA gyrase. *Spectrum: S. pneumoniae, S. aureus, S. pyogenes, H. influenzae, P. mirabilis, N. gonorrhoeae, C. trachomatis, E. coli* **Dose:** *PO:* **Adults.** 200–400 mg PO bid or IV q12h. *Ophth:* **Adults & Peds.** >1 y: 1–2 gtt in eye(s) q2–4h for 2 d, then qid for 5 more d. *Otic:* **Adults & Peds.** >12 y: 10 gtt in ear(s) bid for 10 d. *Peds.* 1–12 y: 5 gtt in ear(s) bid for 10 d. ↓ in renal impairment; take on empty stomach **Caution:** [C, –] Interactions w/ antacids, sucralfate, and Al-, Ca-, Mg-, Fe-, or Zn-containing products (↓ absorption) **Contra:** Quinolone hypersensitivity **Supplied:** Tabs 200, 300, 400 mg; inj 20, 40 mg/mL; ophth and otic 0.3% **SE:** N/V/D, photosensitivity, insomnia, and HA **Notes:** Ophth form can be used in ears **Interactions:** ↑ Effects w/ cimetidine, probenecid, St. John's wort; ↑ effects of cyclosporine, procainamide, theophylline, warfarin, caffeine; ↓ effects w/ antacids, antineoplastics, Ca, didanosine, Fe, NaHCO₃, sucralfate, zinc **NIPE:** Take w/o food; use sunscreen; ↑ fluids to 2–3 L/d

Olanzapine (Zyprexa, Zyprexa Zydis) Uses: *Bipolar mania, schizophrenia,* psychotic disorders **Action:** Dopamine and serotonin antagonist **Dose:** 5–10 mg/d, ↑ weekly PRN to 20 mg/d max **Caution:** [C, –] **Supplied:** Tabs 2.5, 5, 7.5, 10, 15, 20 mg; PO disintegrating tabs 5, 10, 15, 20 mg **SE:** HA, somnolence, orthostatic hypotension, tachycardia, dystonia, xerostomia, constipation **Notes:** Takes weeks to titrate to therapeutic dose; cigarette smoking ↓ levels **Interactions:** ↑ Effects w/ fluvoxamine, probenecid; ↑ sedation w/ CNS depressants, EtOH; ↑ Szs w/ anticholinergics, CNS depressants; ↑ hypotension w/ antihypertensives, diazepam; ↓ effects w/ activated charcoal, carbamazepine, omeprazole, rifampin, St. John's wort, tobacco; ↓ effects of dopamine agonists, levodopa **Labs:** ↑ LFTs **NIPE:** ↑ Risk of tardive dyskinesia, photosensitivity—use sunscreen, body temp impairment

Olopatadine (Patanol) Uses: *Allergic conjunctivitis* **Action:** H₁-receptor antagonist **Dose:** 1–2 gtt in eye(s) bid q6–8h **Caution:** [C, ?] **Supplied:** Soln 0.1% 5 mL **SE:** Local irritation, HA, rhinitis **Notes:** ⊘ instill if wearing contact lenses

Olsalazine (Dipentum) Uses: *Maint of remission of ulcerative colitis* **Action:** Topical antiinflammatory activity **Dose:** 500 mg PO bid; take w/ food **Caution:** [C, M] Salicylate sensitivity **Supplied:** Caps 250 mg **SE:** Diarrhea, HA, blood dyscrasias, hepatitis **Labs:** ↑ LFTs

Omalizumab (Xolair) Uses: *Moderate to severe asthma in Pts, ≥12 y w/ reactivity to an allergen and whose Sxs are inadequately controlled w/ inhaled steroids* **Action:** Anti-IgE antibody **Dose:** 150–375 mg SQ q2–4wk (dose/frequency determined by total serum IgE level and body weight—see package labeling) **Caution:** [B,?/–] **Contra:** Hx of component hypersensitivity **Supplied:** 150 mg in single-use 5-mL vial **SE:** Site Rxn, sinusitis, HA, anaphylaxis reported w/in 2 h of administration in 3 Pts **Notes:** Continue other asthma medications as indicated **Interactions:** No drug interaction studies done **NIPE:** ⊘ DC abruptly; not for acute bronchospasm; admin w/in 8 h of reconstitution and store in refrigerator

Omeprazole (Prilosec) **Uses:** *Duodenal and gastric ulcers, ZE syndrome, GERD,* and *H. pylori* infections **Action:** Proton pump inhibitor **Dose:** 20–40 mg PO qd–bid **Caution:** [C, –] **Supplied:** Caps 10, 20, 40 mg **SE:** HA, diarrhea **Notes:** Combination (ie, antibiotic) therapy necessary for *H. pylori* infection **Interactions:** ↑ Effects of carbamazepine, diazepam, digoxin, glipizide, glyburide, nifedipine, nimodipine, nisoldipine, nitrendipine, phenytoin, tolbutamide, warfarin; ↓ effects w/ sucralfate; ↓ effects of ampicillin, cefpodoxime, cefuroxime, enoxacin, cyanocobalamin, ketoconazole **Labs:** ↑ LFTs; **NIPE:** Take w/o food

Ondansetron (Zofran) **Uses:** *Prevent chemo-associated and postop N/V* **Action:** Serotonin receptor antagonist **Dose:** *Chemo: Adults & Peds.* 0.15 mg/kg/dose IV prior to chemo, then 4 and 8 h after 1st dose or 4–8 mg PO tid; give 1st dose 30 min prior to chemo. For chemo, administer on a schedule, not PRN. *Postop: Adults.* 4 mg IV immediately before induction of anesthesia or postop. *Peds.* <40 kg: 0.1 mg/kg. *>40 kg:* 4 mg IV ↓ dose w/ hepatic impairment **Caution:** [B, +/–] **Supplied:** Tabs 4, 8 mg; inj 2 mg/mL **SE:** Diarrhea, HA, constipation, dizziness **Interactions:** ↓ Effects w/ rifampin; **Labs:** ↑ Fibrinogen, AST, ALT, serum bilirubin, ↓ Hmg, serum albumin, transferrin, gamma globulin **NIPE:** Food ↑ absorption

Oprelvekin (Neumega) **Uses:** *Prevent severe thrombocytopenia due to chemo* **Action:** Promotes proliferation and maturation of megakaryocytes (interleukin-11) **Dose:** *Adults.* 50 μg/kg/d SQ for 10–21 d. *Peds.* >12 y: 75–100 μg/kg/d SQ for 10–21 d. <12 y: Use only in clinical trials. **Caution:** [C, ?/–] **Supplied:** 5 mg powder for inj **SE:** Tachycardia, palpitations, arrhythmias, edema, HA, dizziness, insomnia, fatigue, fever, nausea, anemia, dyspnea **Interactions:** None noted **Labs:** ↓ Hmg, albumin **NIPE:** Monitor for peripheral edema; use med w/in 3 h of reconstitution

Oral Contraceptives, Biphasic, Monophasic, Triphasic, Progestin Only (see Table 7, page 276) **Uses:** *Birth control and regulation of anovulatory bleeding* **Action:** *Birth control:* Suppresses LH surge, prevents ovulation; progestins thicken cervical mucus; inhibits fallopian tubule cilia, ↓ endometrial thickness to ↓ chances of fertilization. *Anovulatory bleeding:* Cyclic hormones mimic body's natural cycle and help regulate endometrial lining, resulting in regular bleeding q28d; may also reduce uterine bleeding and dysmenorrhea **Dose:** 28-d cycle pills taken qd; 21-d cycle pills taken qd, no pills taken during the last 7 d of the cycle (during menses) **Caution:** [X, +] Migraine, HTN, DM, sickle cell Dz, gallbladder Dz **Contra:** Undiagnosed abnormal vaginal bleeding, PRG, estrogen-dependent malignancy, hypercoagulation disorders, liver Dz, hemiplegic migraine, and smokers >35 y **Supplied:** 28-d cycle pills (21 hormonally active pills + 7 placebo/Fe suppl); 21-d cycle pills (21 hormonally active pills) **SE:** Intramenstrual bleeding, oligomenorrhea, amenorrhea, ↑ appetite/weight gain, loss of libido, fatigue, depression, mood swings, mastalgia, HA, melasma, ↑ vaginal discharge, acne/greasy skin, corneal edema, nausea **Notes:** Taken correctly, 99.9% effective for preventing PRG; not protective against STDs; encourage additional barrier contraceptive; long term, can ↓ risk of ectopic PRG, benign breast Dz, ovarian and uterine CA. *Rx for menstrual cycle control:* Start w/ a monophasic pill; pill must be taken for 3 mo before switching to another brand; if abnormal bleeding continues, change to pill w/ higher estrogen dose. *Rx for birth control:* Choose pill w/ most beneficial side effect profile for particular Pt; side effects numerous and due to Sxs of estrogen excess or progesterone deficiency; each pill's side effect profile is unique (found in package insert); tailor Rx to specific Pt

Orlistat (Xenical) Uses: *Manage obesity in Pts w/ BMI ≥ 30 kg/m² or ≥ 27 kg/m² in presence of other risk factors; type 2 DM, dyslipidemia* **Action:** Reversible inhibitor of gastric and pancreatic lipases. **Dose:** 120 mg PO tid w/ a fat-containing meal **Caution:** [B, ?] May ↓ cyclosporine levels and ↓ daily dose requirements for warfarin **Contra:** Cholestasis, chronic malabsorption **Supplied:** Capsules 120 mg **SE:** Abdominal pain/discomfort, fatty/oily stools, fecal urgency **Notes:** ⊘ Administer if meal contains no fat; GI effects ↑ w/ higher-fat meals; suppl w/ fat-soluble vitamins **Interactions:** ↑ Effects of pravastatin; ↓ effects of cyclosporine, fat-soluble vitamins **Labs:** Monitor warfarin, ↓ serum glucose, total cholesterol, LDL **NIPE:** ⊘ Administer if meal contains no fat; GI effects ↑ w/ higher-fat meals; supplement w/ fat-soluble vitamins

Orphenadrine (Norflex) Uses: *Muscle spasms* **Action:** Central atropine-like effects cause indirect skeletal muscle relaxation, euphoria, and analgesia **Dose:** 100 mg PO bid, 60 mg IM/IV q12h **Caution:** [C, +] **Contra:** Glaucoma, GI obstruction, cardiospasm, MyG **Supplied:** Tabs 100 mg; SR tabs 100 mg; inj 30 mg/mL **SE:** Drowsiness, dizziness, blurred vision, flushing, tachycardia, constipation **Interactions:** ↑ CNS depression w/ anxiolytics, butorphanol, hypnotics, MAOIs, nalbuphine, opioids, pentazocine, phenothiazines, tramadol, TCAs, kava kava, valerian, EtOH; ↑ effects w/ anticholinergics **NIPE:** Impaired body temp regulation

Oseltamivir (Tamiflu) Uses: *Prevention and Rx influenza A and B* **Action:** Inhibits viral neuraminidase **Dose:** *Adults.* 75 mg PO bid for 5 d. *Peds.* PO bid dosing: <15 kg: 30 mg. *16–23 kg:* 45 mg. *24–40 kg:* 60 mg; >40 kg: As adults; ↓ dose in renal impairment **Caution:** [C, ?/–] **Contra:** Component hypersensitivity **Supplied:** Caps 75 mg, powder 12 mg/mL **SE:** N/V, insomnia **Notes:** Initiate w/in 48 h of Sx onset or exposure **Interaction:** ↑ Effects w/ probenecid **NIPE:** Take w/o regard to food

Oxacillin (Bactocill, Prostaphlin) Uses: *Infections caused by susceptible strains of *S. aureus* and *Streptococcus** Action: Bactericidal; inhibits cell wall synthesis. *Spectrum:* Excellent gram(+), poor gram(–) Dose: *Adults.* 250–500 mg (1 g severe) IM/IV q4–6h. *Peds.* 150–200 mg/kg/d IV ÷ q4–6h; ↓ dose in significant renal Dz Caution: [B, M] Contra: Penicillin sensitivity Supplied: Inj; caps 250, 500 mg; soln 250 mg/5 mL SE: GI upset, interstitial nephritis, blood dyscrasias Interactions: ↑ Effects w/ disulfiram, probenecid; ↑ effects of anticoagulants, MRX; ↓ effects w/ chloramphenicol, tetracyclines, carbonated drinks, fruit juice, food; ↓ effects of oral contraceptives Labs: False + urine and serum protein NIPE: Take w/o food

Oxaprozin (Daypro) Uses: *Arthritis and pain* Action: NSAID; inhibits prostaglandins synthesis Dose: 600–1200 mg/d; ↓ dose in renal/hepatic impairment Caution: [C (D in 3rd tri or near term), ?] ASA/NSAID sensitivity, peptic ulcer, bleeding disorders Supplied: Caps 600 mg SE: CNS inhibition, sleep disturbance, rash, GI upset, peptic ulcer, edema, renal failure Interactions: ↑ Effects of aminoglycosides, anticoagulants, ASA, diuretics, Li, MRX, ↓ effects of antihypertensives NIPE: ↑ Risk of photosensitivity—use sunscreen; take w/ food

Oxazepam (Serax) [C-IV] Uses: *Anxiety, acute EtOH withdrawal,* anxiety w/ depressive Sxs Action: Benzodiazepine Dose: *Adults.* 10–15 mg PO tid–qid; severe anxiety and EtOH withdrawal may require up to 30 mg qid. *Peds.* 1 mg/kg/d in ÷ doses Caution: [D, ?] Supplied: Caps 10, 15, 30 mg; tabs 15 mg SE: Sedation, ataxia, dizziness, rash, blood dyscrasias, dependence Notes: ⊘ Abrupt discontinuation; metabolite of diazepam (Valium) Interactions: ↑ CNS effects w/ anticonvulsants, antidepressants, antihistamines, barbiturates, MAOIs, opioids, phenothiazines, kava kava, lemon balm, sassafras, valerian, EtOH; ↑ effects w/ cimetidine; ↓ effects w/ oral contraceptives, phenytoin, theophylline, tobacco; ↓ effects of levodopa Labs: False ↑ serum glucose NIPE: ⊘ DC abruptly

Oxcarbazepine (Trileptal) Uses: *Partial Szs,* bipolar disorders Action: Blocks voltage-sensitive Na⁺ channels, stabilization of hyperexcited neural membranes Dose: *Adults.* 300 mg PO bid, ↑ weekly to target maint 1200–2400 mg/d. *Peds.* 8–10 mg/kg bid, 500 mg/d max, ↑ weekly to target maint dose; ↓ in renal insufficiency Caution: [C, –] Cross-sensitivity to carbamazepine Contra: Sensitivity to components Supplied: Tabs 150, 300, 600 mg SE: Hyponatremia, HA, dizziness, fatigue, somnolence, GI upset, diplopia, mental conc difficulties Notes: ⊘ Abruptly DC, check Na⁺ if fatigue reported Interactions: ↑ Effects w/ benzodiazepines, EtOH; ↑ effects of phenobarbital, phenytoin; ↓ effects w/ barbiturates, carbamazepine, phenobarbital, valproic acid, verapamil; ↓ effects of CCBs, oral contraceptives Labs: ↓ Thyroid levels, serum Na NIPE: Take w/o regard to food; use barrier contraception

Oxiconazole (Oxistat) Uses: *Tinea pedis, tinea cruris, and tinea corporis* Action: Antifungal antibiotic *Spectrum:* Most strains of *Epidermophyton floccosum, Trichophyton mentagrophytes, Trichophyton rubrum, Malassezia furfur*

Dose: Apply bid **Caution:** [B, M] **Contra:** Component hypersensitivity **Supplied:** Cream 1%; lotion **SE:** Local irritation

Oxybutynin (Ditropan, Ditropan XL) **Uses:** *Symptomatic relief of urgency, nocturia, and incontinence associated w/ neurogenic or reflex neurogenic bladder* **Action:** Direct smooth muscle antispasmodic; ↑ bladder capacity **Dose:** **Adults & Peds.** > 5 y: 5 mg PO tid–qid; XL 5 mg PO qd; ↑ to 30 mg/d PO (5 and 10 mg). **Peds.** 1–5 y: 0.2 mg/kg/dose bid–qid (syrup 5 mg/5 mL); ↓ dose in elderly; periodic drug holidays recommended **Caution:** [B, ? (use w/ caution)] **Contra:** Glaucoma, MyG, GI or GU obstruction, ulcerative colitis, megacolon **Supplied:** Tabs 5 mg; XL tabs 5, 10, 15 mg; syrup 5 mg/5 mL **SE:** Anticholinergic side effects; drowsiness, xerostomia, constipation, tachycardia**Interactions:** ↑ Effects w/ CNS depressants, EtOH; ↑ effects of atenolol, digoxin, nitrofurantoin; ↑ anticholinergic effects w/ antihistamines, anticholinergics; ↓ effects of haloperidol, levodopa **NIPE:** ↓ Temp regulation; ↑ photosensitivity—use sunscreen

Oxybutynin Transdermal System (Oxytrol) **Uses:** *Rx of overactive bladder* **Action:** Direct smooth muscle antispasmodic; ↑ bladder capacity **Dose:** One 3.9 mg/d system apply 2×/wk to abdomen, hip, or buttock **Caution:** [B, ?/–] **Contra:** Urinary or gastric retention, uncontrolled narrow-angle glaucoma **Supplied:** 3.9 mg/d transdermal system **SE:** Anticholinergic effects, itching/redness at application site **Notes:** ⊘ Reapplication to the same site w/in 7 d **Interactions:** ↑ Effects w/ anticholinergics **NIPE:** Metabolized by the cytochrome P450 CYP3A4 enzyme system

Oxycodone [Dihydrohydroxycodeinone] (OxyContin, OxyIR, Roxicodone) [C-II] **WARNING:** Swallow whole, ⊘ crush; high abuse potential **Uses:** *Moderate/severe pain, usually in combination w/ nonnarcotic analgesics* **Action:** Narcotic analgesic **Dose:** **Adults.** 5 mg PO q6h PRN. **Peds.** 6–12 y: 1.25 mg PO q6h PRN. >12 y: 2.5 mg q6h PRN. ↓ In severe liver Dz **Caution:** [B (D if prolonged use or near term), M] **Contra:** Hypersensitivity, resp depression **Supplied:** Immediate-release caps (OxyIR) 5 mg; tabs (Percolone) 5 mg; CR (OxyContin) 10, 20, 40, 80 mg; liq 5 mg/5 mL; soln conc 20 mg/mL **SE:** Hypotension, sedation, dizziness, GI upset, constipation, risk of abuse **Notes:** OxyContin used for chronic CA pain; may be sought after as drug of abuse **Interactions:** ↑ CNS & resp. depression w/ amitriptyline, barbiturates, cimetidine, clomipramine, MAOIs, nortriptyline, protease inhibitors, TCAs **Labs:** False ↑ serum amylase, lipase **NIPE:** Take w/ food

Oxycodone & Acetaminophen (Percocet, Tylox) [C-II] **Uses:** *Moderate to severe pain* **Action:** Narcotic analgesic **Dose:** **Adults.** 1–2 tabs/caps PO q4–6h PRN (acetaminophen max dose 4 g/d). **Peds** Oxycodone 0.05–0.15 mg/kg/dose q 4–6h PRN, up to 5 mg/dose **Caution:** [B (D if prolonged use or near term), M] **Contra:** Hypersensitivity, resp depression **Supplied:** Percocet tabs, mg oxycodone/mg APAP: 2.5/325, 5/325, 7.5/325, 10/325, 7.5/500, 10/650; Tylox caps 5 mg oxycodone, 500 mg APAP; soln 5 mg oxycodone and 325 mg APAP/5 mL **SE:** Hypotension, sedation, dizziness, GI upset, constipation **Interactions:** CNS & resp depression w/ amitriptylline, barbiturates, cimetidine, clomipramine MAOIs, nortriptylline, protease inhibitors, TCAs **Labs:** False ↑ serum amylase, li pase **NIPE:** Take w/ food

Oxycodone & Aspirin (Percodan, Percodan-Demi) [C-I
Uses: *Moderate–moderately severe pain* **Action:** Narcotic analgesic w/ NSAID **Dose:** *Adults.* 1–2 tabs/caps PO q4–6h PRN. *Peds.*Oxycodone 0.05–0.1 mg/kg/dose q 4–6h PRN, up to 5 mg/dose; ↓ dose in severe hepatic failure **Caution:** [B (D if prolonged use or near term), M] Peptic ulcer **Contra:** Componen hypersensitivity **Supplied:** Percodan 4.5 mg oxycodone hydrochloride, 0.38 mg oxycodone terephthalate, 325 mg ASA; Percodan-Demi 2.25 mg oxycodone hy drochloride, 0.19 mg oxycodone terephthalate, 325 mg ASA **SE:** Sedation, dizzi ness, GI upset, constipation **Interactions:** ↑ CNS & resp. depression w amitriptylline, barbiturates, cimetidine, clomipramine, MAOIs, nortriptylline, pro tease inhibitors, TCAs; ↑ effects of anticoagulants **Labs:** False ↑ serum amylase lipase **NIPE:** Take w/ food

Oxymorphone (Numorphan) [C-II] **Uses:** *Moderate to severe pain sedative* **Action:** Narcotic analgesic **Dose:** 0.5 mg IM, SQ, IV initially, 1–1.5 m q4–6h PRN. *PR:* 5 mg q4–6h PRN **Caution:** [B, ?] **Contra:** ↑ ICP, severe resp de pression **Supplied:** Inj 1, 1.5 mg/mL; supp 5 mg **SE:** Hypotension, sedation, GI upset, constipation, histamine release **Notes:** Chemically related to hydromor phone **Interactions:** ↑ Effects w/ CNS depressants, cimetidine, neuroleptics EtOH; ↓ effects w/ phenothiazines **Labs:** False ↑ amylase, lipase

Oxytocin (Pitocin) **Uses:** *Induction of labor and control of postpartum he morrhage*; promote milk letdown in lactating women **Action:** Stimulate muscula contractions of the uterus and milk flow during nursing **Dose:** 0.001–0.00 Units/min IV inf; titrate 0.02 Units/min max. *Breast-feeding:* 1 spray in both nos trils 2–3 min before feeding **Caution:** [Uncategorized, no anomalies expected, +/– **Contra:** Where vaginal delivery is not favorable, fetal distress **Supplied:** Inj 1 Units/mL; nasal soln 40 Units/mL **SE:** Uterine rupture and fetal death; arrhyth mias, anaphylaxis, water intoxication **Notes:** Monitor vital signs; nasal form fo breast-feeding only **Interactions:** ↑ Pressor effects w/ sympathomimetics

Paclitaxel (Taxol) **Uses:** *Ovarian and breast CA* **Action:** Mitotic spindl poison promotes microtubule assembly and stabilization against depolymerizatio **Dose:** See specific protocols; use glass or polyolefin containers using polyethyl ene-lined nitroglycerin tubing sets; PVC inf sets result in leaching of plasticizer; ↓ dose in hepatic failure; maintain hydration **Caution:** [D, –] **Contra:** Neutropeni <1500 WBC/mm³; solid tumors **Supplied:** Inj 6 mg/mL **SE:** Myelosuppressio peripheral neuropathy, transient ileus, myalgia, bradycardia, hypotension, mucosi tis, N/V/D, fever, rash, HA, and phlebitis; hematologic toxicity schedule-depen dent; leukopenia dose-limiting by 24-h inf; neurotoxicity dose-limiting by shor (1–3 h) inf **Notes:** Hypersensitivity Rxns (dyspnea, hypotension, urticaria, rash usually w/in 10 min of starting inf; minimize w/corticosteroid, antihistamine (H_1-and H_2-antagonist) pretreatment. **Interactions:** ↑ Effects w/ BBs, cyclosporine, dexamethasone, diazepam, digoxin, etoposide, ketoconazole, midazolam, quinidine, teniposide, troleandomycin, verapamil, vincristine; ↑ risk of bleeding w/ anticoagulants, plt inhibitors, thrombolytics; ↑ myelosuppression when cisplatin is admin before paclitaxel; ↓ effects w/ carbamazepine, phenobarbital; ↓ effects of ve virus vaccines **Labs:** ↑ ALT, AST, serum bilirubin, alkaline phosphatase **NIPE:** Ⓢ PRG, breast-feeding, live virus vaccines; use barrier contraception

Palivizumab (Synagis) Uses: *Prevent RSV infection* Action: Monoclonal antibody Dose: *Peds.* 15 mg/kg IM monthly, typically Nov–Apr Caution: [C, ?] Caution in renal or hepatic dysfunction Contra: Hypersensitivity Supplied: Vials 50, 100 mg SE: URI, rhinitis, cough, ↑ LFT, local irritation NIPE: Use drug w/in 6 h after reconstitution; Ⓢ inj in gluteal site; for prophylaxis

Palonosetron (Aloxi) WARNING: May prolong QT_c interval Uses: *Prevention of acute and delayed N/V w/ moderately and highly emetogenic cancer chemo* Action: 5HT3 serotonin receptor antagonist Dose: 0.25 mg IV 30 min prior to chemo; Ⓢ repeat w/in 7 d Caution: [B, ?] Contra: Component hypersensitivity Supplied: 0.25 mg/5 mL vial SE: HA, constipation, dizziness, abdominal pain, anxiety Interactions: Potential for drug interactions low

Pamidronate (Aredia) Uses: *Hypercalcemia of malignancy and Paget's Dz; palliation of symptomatic bone mets* Action: Inhibits normal and abnormal bone resorption Dose: *Hypercalcemia:* 60 mg IV over 4 h or 90 mg IV over 24 h. *Paget's:* 30 mg/d IV slow inf for 3 d Caution: [C, ?/–] Contra: PRG Supplied: Powder for inj 30, 60, 90 mg SE: Fever, tissue irritation at inj site, uveitis, fluid overload, HTN, abdominal pain, N/V, constipation, UTI, bone pain, hypokalemia, hypocalcemia, hypomagnesemia, hypophosphatemia Interactions: ↓ Serum Ca levels w/ foscarnet; ↓ effects w/ Ca, vitamin D NIPE: Ⓢ Ingest food w/ Ca or vitamins w/ minerals before or 2–3 h after admin of drug

Pancrelipase (Pancrease, Cotazym, Creon, Ultrase) Uses: *Exocrine pancreatic secretion deficiency (CF, chronic pancreatitis, other pancreatic insufficiency) and for steatorrhea of malabsorption syndrome* Action: Pancreatic enzyme suppl Dose: 1–3 caps (tabs) w/meals and snacks; dosage ↑ to 8 caps (tabs); Ⓢ crush or chew EC products; dosage is dependent on digestive requirements of Pt; Ⓢ antacids Caution: [C, ?/–] Contra: Hypersensitivity to pork products Supplied: Caps, tabs SE: N/V, abdominal cramps Notes: Each Pt should receive individualized enzymatic therapy Interactions: ↓ Effects w/ antacids w/ Ca or Mg; ↓ effects of Fe Labs: ↑ Serum and urine uric acid NIPE: Take w/ food; stress adherence to diet (usually low-fat, high-protein, high-calorie)

Pancuronium (Pavulon) Uses: *Paralysis of Pts on mechanical ventilation* Action: Nondepolarizing neuromuscular blocker Dose: *Adults.* 2–4 mg IV q2–4h PRN. *Peds.* 0.02–0.1 mg/kg/dose q2–4h PRN; ↓ dose for renal/hepatic impairment; intubate Pt and keep on controlled ventilation; use adequate sedation or analgesia **Caution:** [C, ?/–] **Contra:** Component or bromide sensitivity **Supplied** Inj 1, 2 mg/mL **SE:** Tachycardia, HTN, pruritus, other histamine Rxns **Interactions:** ↑ Effects w/ aminoglycosides, bacitracin, clindamycin, enflurane, K-depleting diuretics, isoflurane, lidocaine, Li, metocurine, quinine, sodium colistimethate, succinylcholine, tetracycline, trimethaphan, tubocurarine, verapamil; ↓ effects w/ carbamazepine, phenytoin, theophylline

Pantoprazole (Protonix) **Uses:** *GERD, erosive gastritis,* ZE syndrome, PUD **Action:** Proton pump inhibitor **Dose:** 40 mg/d PO; ⊘ crush or chew tabs; 40 mg IV/d (not >3 mg/min and use Protonix filter) **Caution:** [B, ?/–] **Supplied:** Tabs 40 mg; inj **SE:** Chest pain, anxiety, GI upset, ↑ levels on LFTs

Paregoric [Camphorated Tincture of Opium] [C-III] **Uses:** *Diarrhea,* pain, and neonatal opiate withdrawal syndrome **Action:** Narcotic **Dose:** *Adults.* 5–10 mL PO qd–qid PRN. *Peds.* 0.25–0.5 mL/kg qd–qid. *Neonatal withdrawal syndrome:* 3–6 gtt PO q3–6 h PRN to relieve Sxs for 3–5 d, then taper over 2–4 wk **Caution:** [B (D if prolonged use or high dose near term, +] **Contra:** Tincture (children); convulsive disorder **Supplied:** Liq 2 mg morphine = 20 m opium/5 mL **SE:** Hypotension, sedation, constipation **Notes:** Contains anhydrous morphine from opium; short-term use only **Interactions:** ↓ Effects of ampicillin esters, azole antifungals, Fe salts **Labs:** ↑ LFTs, SCr **NIPE:** Take w/o regard to food

Paroxetine (Paxil, Paxil CR) **WARNING:** Closely monitor for worsening depression or emergence of suicidality, particularly in pediatric Pts **Uses:** *Depression, OCD, panic disorder, social anxiety disorder,* PMDD **Action:** SSRI **Dose:** 10–60 mg PO single daily dose in AM; CR 25 mg/d PO; ↑ 12.5 mg/wk max range 26–62.5 mg/d) **Caution:** [B, ?/] **Contra:** MAOI **Supplied:** Tabs 10, 20, 30 40 mg; susp 10 mg/5 mL; CR 12.5, 25 mg **SE:** Sexual dysfunction, HA, somnolence, dizziness, GI upset, diarrhea, xerostomia, tachycardia **Interactions:** ↑ Effects w/ cimetidine; ↑ effects of BBs, dexfenfluramine, dextromethorphan fenfluramine, haloperidol, MAOIs, theophylline, thioridazine, TCAs, warfarin, S John's wort, EtOH; ↓ effects w/ cyproheptadine, phenobarbital, phenytoin; ↓ effects of digoxin, phenytoin **Labs:** ↑ LFTs **NIPE:** Take w/o regard to food, ma take up to 4 wk for full effect

Pegfilgrastim (Neulasta) **Uses:** *↓ Frequency of infection in Pts w nonmyeloid malignancies receiving myelosuppressive anticancer drugs that caus febrile neutropenia* **Action:** Colony-stimulating factor **Dose:** *Adults.* 6 mg SQ 1/chemo cycle. *Peds.* 100 μg/kg SQ × 1/chemo cycle **Caution:** [C, M] in sickle cel **Contra:** Hypersensitivity to drugs used to treat *E. coli* or to filgrastim **Supplied** *Syringes:* 6 mg/0.6 mL **SE:** HA, fever, weakness, fatigue, dizziness, insomnia edema, N/V/D, stomatitis, anorexia, constipation, taste perversion, dyspepsia, ab dominal pain, granulocytopenia, neutropenic fever, ↑ LFT, uric acid, arthralgia myalgia, bone pain, ARDS, alopecia, splenic rupture, aggravation of sickle cell D **Notes:** Never give between 14 d before and 24 h after dose of cytotoxic chemo **In**

ractions: ↑ Effects w/ Li **Labs:** ↑ Alkaline phosphatase, LDH, uric acid **NIPE:** Exposure to infection

eg Interferon Alfa-2a (Pegasys) **Uses:** *Chronic hepatitis C w/ mpensated liver Dz* **Action:** Biologic response modifier **Dose:** 180 μg (1 mL) Q qwk × 48 wk; ↓ in renal impairment **Caution:** [C, ?/–] **Contra:** Autoimmune patitis, decompensated liver Dz **Supplied:** 180 μg/mL inj **SE:** Depression, in- mnia, suicidal behavior, GI upset, neutropenia and thrombocytopenia, alopecia, uritus **Notes:** May aggravate neuropsychiatric, autoimmune, ischemic, and infec- ous disorders **NIPE:** ⊘ Exposure to infection, use barrier contraception

eg Interferon Alfa-2b (PEG-Intron) **Uses:** *Rx hepatitis C* **Ac- on:** Immune modulation **Dose:** 1 μg/kg/wk SQ; 1.5 μg/kg/wk combined w/rib- virin **Caution:** [C, ?/–] w/psychiatric Hx **Contra:** Autoimmune hepatitis, ecompensated liver Dz, hemoglobinopathy **Supplied:** Vials 50, 80, 120, 150 g/0.5 mL **SE:** Depression, insomnia, suicidal behavior, GI upset, neutropenia and rombocytopenia, alopecia, pruritus **Notes:** ↓ Flu-like Sxs by giving hs or /APAP; follow CBC and plts **Interactions:** ↑ Myelosuppression w/ antineoplas- cs; ↑ effects of doxorubicin, theophylline; ↑ neurotoxicity w/ vinblastine **Labs:** ↑ LT, ↓ neutrophils, plts **NIPE:** Maintain hydration; use barrier contraception

emetrexed (Alimta) **Uses:** *W/ cisplatin in nonresectable esothelioma* **Action:** Antifolate antineoplastic **Dose:** 500 mg/m² IV over 10 min ay 1 of each 21-d cycle; 30 min after, 75 mg/m² cisplatin IV over 2 h; ↓ dose ased on hematologic or neural toxicity **Caution:** [D, –] Renal/hepatic/BM impair- ent **Contra:** Component sensitivity **Supplied:** 500-mg vial **SE:** Neutropenia, eukopenia, thrombocytopenia, N/V/D, anorexia, stomatitis, renal failure, neuropa- y, fever, fatigue, mood changes, dyspnea, anaphylactic Rxns **Notes:** ⊘ NSAIDs, llow CBC and plts

emirolast (Alamast) **Uses:** *Allergic conjunctivitis* **Action:** Mast cell tabilizer **Dose:** 1–2 gtt in each eye qid **Caution:** [C, ?/–] **Supplied:** 1 mg/mL SE: A, rhinitis, cold/flu symptoms, local irritation **Notes:** Wait 10 min before insert- g contact lenes

enbutolol (Levatol) **Uses:** *HTN* **Action:** β-Adrenergic receptor locker, β₁, β₂ **Dose:** 20–40 mg/d; ↓ in hepatic insufficiency **Caution:** [C (1st tri; of 2nd/3rd tri), M] **Contra:** Asthma, cardiogenic shock, cardiac failure, heart lock, bradycardia **Supplied:** Tabs 20 mg **SE:** Flushing, hypotension, fatigue, hy- erglycemia, GI upset, sexual dysfunction, bronchospasm **Interactions:** ↑ Effects / CCBs, fluoroquinolones; ↑ bradycardia w/ adenosine, amiodarone, digitalis, ipyridamole, epinephrine, neuroleptics, phenylephrine, physostigmine, tacrine; ↑ ffects of lidocaine, verapamil; ↓ effects w/ antacids, NSAIDs; ↓ effects of insulin, ypoglycemics, theophylline **Labs:** ↑ Serum glucose, BUN, K⁺, lipoprotein, riglycerides, uric acid **NIPE:** ↑ Cold sensitivity

enciclovir (Denavir) **Uses:** *Herpes simplex (herpes labialis/cold sores)* **Action:** Competitive inhibitor of DNA polymerase **Dose:** Apply at 1st sign of lesions, then q2h for 4 d **Caution:** [B, ?/–] **Contra:** Hypersensitivity **Supplie** Cream 1% [OTC] **SE:** Erythema, HA **Notes:** ⊘ apply to mucous membranes

Penicillin G, Aqueous (Potassium or Sodium) (Pfizerpe **Pentids)** **Uses:** *Bacteremia, endocarditis, pericarditis, resp tract infectio meningitis, neurosyphilis, skin/skin structure infections* **Action:** Bactericide: i hibits cell wall synthesis. *Spectrum:* Most gram(+) (not staphylococci, strep cocci, *N. meningitidis*, syphilis, clostridia, and anaerobes (not *Bacteroides*) **Dos** **Adults.** 400,000–800,000 Units PO qid; IV doses vary depending on indicatio range 0.6–24 MU/d in ÷ doses q4h. **Peds.** Newborns <1 wk: 25,000–50,0 Units/kg/dose IV q12h. **Infants 1 wk–<1 mo:** 25,000–50,000 Units/kg/dose IV q8 **Children:** 100,000–300,000 Units/kg/24h IV ÷ q4h; ↓ in renal impairment **Ca** **tion:** [B, M] **Contra:** Hypersensitivity **Supplied:** Tabs 200,000, 250,000, 400,0 800,000 Units; susp 200,000, 400,000 Units/5 mL; powder for inj **SE:** Hypersens tivity Rxns; interstitial nephritis, diarrhea, Szs **Notes:** Contains 1.7 mEq of K⁺/M **Interactions:** ↑ Effects w/ probenecid; ↑ effects of MRX; ↑ risk of bleeding anticoagulants; ↓ effects w/ chloramphenicol, macrolides, tetracyclines; ↓ effec of oral contraceptives **Labs:** ↑ LFTs, ↓ serum albumin, folate **NIPE:** Monitor f superinfection; use barrier contraception

Penicillin G Benzathine (Bicillin) **Uses:** *Single-dose regimen f* streptococcal pharyngitis, rheumatic fever, glomerulonephritis prophylaxis, ar syphilis* **Action:** Bactericide; inhibits cell wall synthesis. *Spectrum:* See Penicill G **Dose:** **Adults.** 1.2–2.4 MU deep IM inj q2–4wk. **Peds.** 50,000 Units/kg/dose, 2 MU/dose max; deep IM inj q2–4 wk **Caution:** [B, M] **Contra:** Hypersensitivi **Supplied:** Inj 300,000, 600,000 Units/mL; Bicillin L-A contains the benzathi salt only; Bicillin C-R contains a combination of benzathine and procaine (300,0 Units procaine w/ 300,000 Units benzathine/mL or 900,000 Units benzathine w 300,000 Units procaine/2 mL) **SE:** Pain at inj site, acute interstitial nephritis, an phylaxis **Notes:** Sustained action w/detectable levels up to 4 wk; drug of choice f Rx of noncongenital syphilis **Interactions:** See Penicillin G

Penicillin G Procaine (Wycillin, others) **Uses:** *Resp tract infe* tions, scarlet fever, skin and soft tissue infections, syphilis* **Action:** Bactericid inhibits cell wall synthesis. *Spectrum:* Penicillin G-sensitive organisms that respond to low, persistent serum levels **Dose:** **Adults.** 0.6–4.8 MU/d in ÷ dose q12–24h; give probenecid at least 30 min prior to penicillin to prolong actio **Peds.** 25,000–50,000 Units/kg/24h IM ÷ qd–bid **Caution:** [B, M] **Contra:** Hyperse sitivity **Supplied:** Inj 300,000, 500,000, 600,000 Units/mL **SE:** Pain at inj site, i terstitial nephritis, anaphylaxis **Notes:** Long-acting parenteral penicillin; bloc levels up to 15 h **Interactions:** See Penicillin G, Aqueous

Penicillin V (Pen-Vee K, Veetids, others) **Uses:** Susceptible strep tococci infections, otitis media, URIs, skin/soft tissue infections (penicillin-sens tive staph) **Action:** Bactericidal; inhibits cell wall synthesis. *Spectrum:* Mos gram(+), including streptococci **Dose:** **Adults.** 250–500 mg PO q6h, q8h, q12

Peds. 25–50 mg/kg/25h PO in 4 doses; ↓ in renal Dz; take on empty stomach **Caution:** [B, M] **Contra:** Hypersensitivity **Supplied:** Tabs 125, 250, 500 mg; susp 125, 250 mg/5 mL **SE:** GI upset, interstitial nephritis, anaphylaxis, convulsions **Notes:** Well-tolerated PO penicillin; 250 mg = 400,000 Units of penicillin G **Interactions:** See Penicillin G, Aqueous

Pentamidine (Pentam 300, NebuPent) Uses: *Rx and prevention of PCP* **Action:** Inhibits DNA, RNA, phospholipid, and protein synthesis **Dose:** *Rx: Adults & Peds.* 4 mg/kg/24 h IV qd for 14–21 d. *Prevention: Adults & Peds.* >5 y: 300 mg once q4wk, administered via Respirgard II neb; IV requires ↓ dose in renal impairment **Caution:** [C, ?] **Contra:** Component hypersensitivity **Supplied:** Inj 300 mg/vial; aerosol 300 mg **SE:** Associated w/ pancreatic islet cell necrosis leading to hyperglycemia; CP, fatigue, dizziness, rash, GI upset, pancreatitis, renal impairment, blood dyscrasias **Notes:** Follow CBC (leukopenia and thrombocytopenia); monitor glucose and pancreatic Fxn monthly for the 1st 3 mo; monitor for hypotension following IV administration **Interactions:** ↑ Nephrotoxic effects w/ aminoglycosides, amphotericin B, capreomycin, cidofovir, cisplatin, cyclosporine, colistin, ganciclovir, methoxyflurane, polymyxin B, vancomycin; ↑ bone marrow suppression w/ antineoplastics, radiation therapy **Labs:** ↑ LFTs, serum K⁺ **NIPE:** Reconstitute w/ sterile H_2O only, inhalation may cause metallic taste; ↑ fluids to 2–3 L/d

Pentazocine (Talwin) [C-IV] Uses: *Moderate to severe pain* **Action:** Partial narcotic agonist–antagonist **Dose:** *Adults.* 30 mg IM or IV; 50–100 mg PO q3–4h PRN. *Peds.* 5–8 y: 15 mg IM q4h PRN. *8–14 y:* 30 mg IM q4h PRN; ↓ dose in renal/hepatic impairment **Caution:** [C (1st tri, D if prolonged use or high doses near term), +/–] **Contra:** Hypersensitivity **Supplied:** Tabs 50 mg (+ naloxone 0.5 mg); inj 30 mg/mL **SE:** Associated w/ considerable dysphoria; drowsiness, GI upset, xerostomia, Szs **SE:** 30–60 mg IM equianalgesic to 10 mg of morphine IM **Interactions:** ↑ CNS depression w/ antihistamines, barbiturates, hypnotics, phenothiazines, EtOH; ↑ effects w/ cimetidine; ↑ effects of digitoxin, phenytoin, rifampin; ↓ effects of opioids **Labs:** ↑ Serum amylase, lipase **NIPE:** May cause withdrawal in Pts using opioids

Pentobarbital (Nembutal, others) [C-II] Uses: *Insomnia, convulsions,* and induced coma following severe head injury **Action:** Barbiturate **Dose:** *Adults.* Sedative: 20–40 mg PO or PR q6–12h. *Hypnotic:* 100–200 mg PO or PR hs PRN. *Induced coma:* Load 5–10 mg/kg IV, then maint 1–3 mg/kg IV cont inf to keep the serum level between 20 and 50 mg/mL. *Peds.* Hypnotic: 2–6 mg/kg/dose PO hs PRN. *Induced coma:* See adult dosage **Caution:** [D, +/–] Significant hepatic impairment **Contra:** Hypersensitivity **Supplied:** Caps 50, 100 mg; elixir 18.2 mg/5 mL (= 20 mg pentobarbital); supp 30, 60, 120, 200 mg; inj 50 mg/mL **SE:** Can cause resp depression, hypotension when used aggressively IV for cerebral edema; bradycardia, hypotension, sedation, lethargy, hangover, rash, Stevens–Johnson syndrome, blood dyscrasias, resp depression **Notes:** Tolerance to sedative–hypnotic effect acquired w/in 1–2 wk **Interactions:** ↑ Effects w/ chloramphenicol, MAOIs, narcotic analgesics, kava kava, valerian, EtOH; ↓ effects of BBs, CCBs, corticosteroids, cyclosporine, digitoxin, disopyramide, doxycycline, estrogen, griseofulvin, neuroleptics, oral anticoagulants, oral contraceptives, propafenone, quinidine, tacrolimus, theophylline, TCAs **Labs:** ↑ Ammonia; ↓ bilirubin

Pentosan Polysulfate Sodium (Elmiron) **Uses:** *Relief of pain/discomfort associated w/ interstitial cystitis* **Action:** Acts as buffer on bladder wall **Dose:** 100 mg PO tid on empty stomach w/ water 1 h ac or 2 h pc **Caution:** [B, ?/–] **Contra:** Hypersensitivity **Supplied:** Caps 100 mg **SE:** Alopecia, N/D, HA, ↑ LFTs, anticoagulant effects, thrombocytopenia **Notes:** Reassess Pts after 3 mo **Interactions:** Risk of ↑ anticoagulation w/ anticoagulants, ASA, thrombolytics

Pentoxifylline (Trental) **Uses:** *Symptomatic management of peripheral vascular Dz* **Action:** Lowers blood cell viscosity by restoring erythrocyte flexibility **Dose:** *Adults.* 400 mg PO tid pc; treat for at least 8 wk to see full effect; ↓ to bid if GI or CNS effects occur **Caution:** [C, +/–] **Contra:** Cerebral or retinal hemorrhage **Supplied:** Tabs 400 mg **SE:** Dizziness, HA, GI upset **Interactions:** ↑ Effects w/ cimetidine, fluoroquinolones, H$_2$ antagonists, warfarin; ↑ effects of antihypertensives, theophylline **Labs:** ↓ Serum Ca^{2+}, Mg^{2+} **NIPE:** Take w/ food

Pergolide (Permax) **Uses:** *Parkinson's Dz* **Action:** Centrally active dopamine receptor agonist **Dose:** Initially, 0.05 mg PO qhs, titrated q2–3d to desired effect; usual maint 2–3 mg/d in ÷ doses **Caution:** [B, ?/–] **Contra:** Ergot sensitivity **Supplied:** Tabs 0.05, 0.25, 1.0 mg **SE:** Dizziness, somnolence, confusion, nausea, constipation, dyskinesia, rhinitis, MI **Notes:** May cause hypotension during initiation of therapy **Interactions:** ↑ Risk of dyskinesia w/ levodopa; ↑ hypotension w/ antihypertensives; ↓ effects w/ antipsychotics, butyrophenones, haloperidol, metoclopramide, phenothiazines, thioxanthenes **Labs:** ↓ Prolactin **NIPE:** Take w/ food

Perindopril Erbumine (Aceon) **Uses:** *HTN,* CHF, DN, post-MI **Action:** ACEI **Dose:** 4–8 mg/d; ⊘ taking w/ food; ↓ in elderly/renal impairment **Caution:** [C (1st tri, D 2nd and 3rd tri), ?/–] ACE-inhibitor-induced angioedema, **Contra:** Bilateral renal artery stenosis, primary hyperaldosteronism **Supplied:** Tabs 2, 4, 8 mg **SE:** HA, hypotension, dizziness, GI upset, cough **Notes:** Can use w/ diuretics **Interactions:** ↑ Effects w/ antihypertensives, diuretics; ↑ effects of cyclosporine, insulin, Li, sulfonylureas, tacrolimus; ↓ effects w/ NSAIDs **Labs:** ↑ Serum K$^+$, LFTs, uric acid, cholesterol, creatinine **NIPE:** ↓ Effects if taken w/ food; risk of persistent cough

Permethrin (Nix, Elimite) **Uses:** *Eradication of lice and scabies* **Action:** Pediculicide **Dose:** Adults & Peds. Saturate hair and scalp; allow 10 min before rinsing **Caution:** [B, ?/–] **Contra:** Hypersensitivity **Supplied:** Topical liq 1%; cream 5% **SE:** Local irritation **Notes:** Disinfect clothing, bedding, combs/brushes **NIPE:** Drug remains on hair up to 2 wk, reapply in 1 wk if live lice

Perphenazine (Trilafon) Uses: *Psychotic disorders, severe nausea,* intractable hiccups **Action:** Phenothiazine; blocks brain dopaminergic receptors **Dose:** *Antipsychotic:* 4–16 mg PO tid; max 64 mg/d. *Hiccups:* 5 mg IM q6h PRN or 1 mg IV at intervals not <1–2 mg/min, 5 mg max. **Peds.** 1–6 y: 4–6 mg/d PO in ÷ doses. *6–12 y:* 6 mg/d PO in ÷ doses. *>12 y:* 4–16 mg PO 2–4 ×/d; ↓ in hepatic insufficiency **Caution:** [C, ?/–] Narrow-angle glaucoma, severe hyper-/hypotension **Contra:** Phenothiazine sensitivity, bone marrow depression, severe liver or cardiac Dz **Supplied:** Tabs 2, 4, 8, 16 mg; PO conc 16 mg/5 mL; inj 5 mg/mL **SE:** Hypotension, tachycardia, bradycardia, EPS, drowsiness, Szs, photosensitivity, skin discoloration, blood dyscrasias, constipation **Interactions:** ↑ Effects w/ antidepressants; ↑ effects of anticholinergics, antidepressants, propranolol, phenytoin; ↓ CNS effects w/ CNS depressants, EtOH; ↓ effects w/ antacids, Li, phenobarbital, caffeine, tobacco; ↓ effects of levodopa, Li **Labs:** ↑ Serum cholesterol, glucose, ↓ uric acid, false + urine PRG test **NIPE:** Take oral dose w/ food; risk of photosensitivity—use sunscreen

Phenazopyridine (Pyridium, others) Uses: *Lower urinary tract irritation* **Action:** Local anesthetic on urinary tract mucosa **Dose:** *Adults.* 100–200 mg PO tid. **Peds.** 6–12 y: 12 mg/kg/24 h PO in 3 ÷ doses; ↓ in renal insufficiency **Caution:** [B, ?] Hepatic Dz **Contra:** Renal failure **Supplied:** Tabs 100, 200 mg **SE:** GI disturbances; causes red-orange urine color, which can stain clothing; HA, dizziness, acute renal failure, methemoglobinemia **Labs:** Interferes w/ urinary tests for glucose, ketones, bilirubin, protein, steroids **NIPE:** Urine may turn red; take pc

Phenelzine (Nardil) Uses: *Depression* **Action:** MAOI **Dose:** 15 mg tid. *Elderly:* 15–60 mg/d in ÷ doses **Caution:** [C, –] Interactions w/ SSRI, ergots, triptans **Contra:** CHF, Hx liver Dz **Supplied:** Tabs 15 mg **SE:** May cause postural hypotension; edema, dizziness, sedation, rash, sexual dysfunction, xerostomia, constipation, urinary retention **Notes:** May take 2–4 wk to see effect; ⊘ tyramine-containing foods **Interactions:** ↑ HTN Rxn w/ amphetamines, fluoxetine, levodopa, metaraminol, phenylephrine, phenylpropanolamine, pseudoephedrine, reserpine, sertraline, tyramine, EtOH, foods w/ tyramine, caffeine, tryptophan; ↑ effects of barbiturates, narcotics, sedatives, sumatriptan, TCAs, ephedra, ginseng **Labs:** ↓ Glucose, false + ↑ in bilirubin & uric acid

Phenobarbital [C-IV] Uses: *Sz disorders,* insomnia, and anxiety **Action:** Barbiturate **Dose:** *Adults.* Sedative–hypnotic: 30–120 mg/d PO or IM PRN. *Anticonvulsant:* Load 10–12 mg/kg in 3 ÷ doses, then 1–3 mg/kg/24 h PO, IM, or IV. **Peds.** Sedative–hypnotic: 2–3 mg/kg/24 h PO or IM hs PRN. *Anticonvulsant:* Load 15–20 mg/kg ÷ in 2 equal doses 4 h apart, then 3–5 mg/kg/24h PO ÷ in 2–3 doses. **Caution:** [D, M] **Contra:** Porphyria, liver dysfunction **Supplied:** Tabs 8, 15, 16, 30, 32, 60, 65, 100 mg; elixir 15, 20 mg/5 mL; inj 30, 60, 65, 130 mg/mL **SE:** Bradycardia, hypotension, hangover, Stevens–Johnson syndrome, blood dyscrasias, resp depression **Notes:** Tolerance develops to sedation; paradoxic hyperactivity seen in pediatric Pts; long half-life allows single daily dosing (see Table

2, page 265) **Interactions:** ↑ CNS depression w/ CNS depressants, anesthetics, antianxiety meds, antihistamines, narcotic analgesics, EtOH, Indian snakeroot, kava kava; ↑ effects w/ chloramphenicol, MAOIs, procarbazine, valproic acid; ↓ effects w/ rifampin; ↓ effects of anticoagulants, BBs, carbamazepine, clozapine, corticosteroids, doxorubicin, doxycycline, estrogens, felodipine, griseofulvin, haloperidol, methadone, metronidazole, oral contraceptives, phenothiazines, quinidine, TCAs, theophylline, verapamil **Labs:** ↑ LFTs, creatinine, ↑ or ↓ bilirubin **NIPE:** May take 2–3 wk for full effects, ⊘ DC abruptly

Phenylephrine (Neo-Synephrine)

Uses: *Vascular failure in shock, hypersensitivity, or drug-induced hypotension; nasal congestion; mydriatic* **Action:** α-Adrenergic agonist **Dose:** *Adults.* Mild/moderate hypotension: 2–5 mg IM or SQ elevates BP for 2 h; 0.1–0.5 mg IV elevates BP for 15 min. *Severe hypotension/shock:* Cont inf at 100–180 mg/min; after BP stabilized, maint rate of 40–60 mg/min. *Nasal congestion:* 1–2 sprays/nostril PRN. *Ophth:* 1 gtt 15–30 min before exam. *Peds.* Hypotension: 5–20 μg/kg/dose IV q10–15 min or 0.1–0.5 mg/kg/min IV inf, titrate to effect. *Nasal congestion:* 1 spray/nostril q3–4h PRN **Caution:** [C, +/–] HTN, acute pancreatitis, hepatitis, coronary Dz, narrow-angle glaucoma, hyperthyroidism **Contra:** Bradycardia, arrhythmias **Supplied:** Inj 10 mg/mL; nasal soln 0.125, 0.16, 0.25, 0.5, 1%; ophth soln 0.12, 2.5, 10% **SE:** Arrhythmias, HTN, peripheral vasoconstriction activity potentiated by oxytocin, MAOIs, and TCAs; HA, weakness, necrosis, ↓ renal perfusion **Notes:** Promptly restore blood volume if loss has occurred; use large veins for inf to avoid extravasation; phentolamine 10 mg in 10–15 mL of NS for local inj as antidote for extravasation **Interactions:** ↑ HTN w/ BBs, MAOIs; ↑ pressor response w/ guanethidine, methyldopa, reserpine, TCAs

Phenytoin (Dilantin)

Uses: *Sz disorders* **Action:** Inhibits Sz spread in the motor cortex **Dose:** *Load: Adults & Peds.* 15–20 mg/kg IV, max inf rate 25 mg/min or PO in 400-mg doses at 4-h intervals. *Maint: Adults.* Initially, 200 mg PO or IV bid or 300 mg hs; then follow serum levels. *Peds.* 4–7 mg/kg/24h PO or IV ÷ qd–bid; ⊘ PO susp if possible due to erratic absorption **Caution:** [D, +] **Contra:** Heart block, sinus bradycardia **Supplied:** Caps 30, 100 mg; chew tabs 50 mg; PO susp 30, 125 mg/5 mL; inj 50 mg/mL **SE:** Nystagmus and ataxia early signs of toxicity; gum hyperplasia w/ long-term use. *IV:* Hypotension, bradycardia, arrhythmias, phlebitis; peripheral neuropathy, rash, blood dyscrasias, Stevens–Johnson syndrome **Notes:** Follow levels (see Table 2, page 265); phenytoin is bound to albumin, and levels reflect bound and free phenytoin; in the presence of ↓ albumin and azotemia, low phenytoin levels may be therapeutic (normal free levels); changes in dosage (↑ or ↓) should not be carried out at intervals shorter than 7–10 d **Interactions:** ↑ Effects w/ amiodarone, allopurinol, chloramphenicol, disulfiram, INH, omeprazole, sulfonamides, quinolones, trimethoprim; ↑ effects of Li; ↓ effects w/ cimetidine, cisplatin, diazoxide, folate, pyridoxine, rifampin; ↓ effects of zole antifungals, benzodiazepines, carbamazepine, corticosteroids, cyclosporine, igitalis glycosides, doxycycline, furosemide, levodopa, oral contraceptives, quinine, tacrolimus, theophylline, thyroid meds, valproic acid **Labs:** ↑ Serum cholesterol, glucose, alkaline phosphatase **NIPE:** Take w/ food; may alter urine color; use arrier contraception; ⊘ DC abruptly

Physostigmine (Antilirium) **Uses:** *Antidote for TCA, atropine, and copolamine OD; glaucoma* **Action:** Reversible cholinesterase inhibitor **Dose: Adults.** 2 mg IV or IM q 20 min. **Peds.** 0.01–0.03 mg/kg/dose IV q15–30 min up to total of 2 mg if needed **Caution:** [C, ?] **Contra:** GI or GU obstruction, CV Dz **Supplied:** Inj 1 mg/mL; ophth oint 0.25% **SE:** Rapid IV admin associated w/ convulsions; cholinergic side effects; asystole sweating, salivation, lacrimation, GI upset, changes in heart rate **Notes:** Excessive readministration of physostigmine an result in cholinergic crisis; cholinergic crisis reversed w/ atropine **Interactions:** ↑ Resp depression w/ succinylcholine, ↑ effects w/ cholinergics, jaborandi ree, pill-bearing spurge **Labs:** ↑ ALT, AST, serum amylase

Phytonadione [Vitamin K] (AquaMEPHYTON, others) **Uses:** *Coagulation disorders caused by faulty formation of factors II, VII, IX, and X*; hyperalimentation* **Action:** Cofactor for the production of factors II, VII, IX, and X **Dose: Adults and Children.** Anticoagulant-induced prothrombin deficiency: 1–10 mg PO or IV slowly. *Hyperalimentation:* 10 mg IM or IV qwk. **Infants.** 0.5–1 mg/dose IM, SQ, or PO **Caution:** [C, +] **Contra:** Hypersensitivity **Supplied:** Tabs 5 mg; inj 2, 10 mg/mL **SE:** Anaphylaxis can result from IV dosage; administer IV slowly; GI upset (PO), inj site Rxns **Notes:** W/ parenteral Rx, the 1st change in prothrombin usually seen in 12–24 h **Interactions:** ↓ Effects w/ antibiotics, cholestyramine, colestipol, salicylates, sucralfate; ↓ effects of oral anticoagulants **Labs:** Falsely ↑ urine steroids

Pimecrolimus (Elidel) **Uses:** *Atopic dermatitis* **Action:** T-lymphocyte inhibition **Dose:** Apply bid for at least 1 wk following resolution **Caution:** [C, ?/–] Caution w/ local infection, lymphadenopathy **Contra:** Hypersensitivity **Supplied:** Ointment 0.03%, 0.1%; 30-g, 60-g tubes **SE:** Phototoxicity, local irritation/burning, flu-like Sxs **Notes:** apply to dry skin only; wash hands after use

Pindolol (Visken) **Uses:** *HTN* **Action:** β-Adrenergic receptor blocker, β_1, β_2, ISA **Dose:** 5–10 mg bid, 60 mg/d max; ↓ in hepatic/renal failure **Caution:** [B (1st tri; D if 2nd or 3rd tri), +/–] **Contra:** Uncompensated CHF, cardiogenic shock, bradycardia, heart block, asthma, COPD **Supplied:** Tabs 5, 10 mg **SE:** Insomnia, dizziness, fatigue, edema, GI upset, dyspnea; fluid retention may exacerbate CHF **Interactions:** ↑ Effects w/ amiodarone, antihypertensives, diuretics; ↓ effects w/ NSAIDs; ↓ effect of hypoglycemics **Labs:** ↑ LFTs, uric acid **NIPE:** ⊘ DC abruptly; ↑ cold sensitivity

Pioglitazone (Actos) **Uses:** *Type 2 DM* **Action:** ↑ Insulin sensitivity **Dose:** 15–45 mg/d **Caution:** [C, –] **Contra:** Hepatic impairment **Supplied:** Tabs

15, 30, 45 mg **SE:** Weight gain, URI, HA, hypoglycemia, edema **Interactions:** ↑ Effects w/ ketoconazole; ↓ effects of oral contraceptives **Labs:** ↑ LFTs, ↓ Hmg, Hct **NIPE:** Take w/o regard to food; use barrier contraception

Piperacillin (Pipracil) **Uses:** *Infections of skin, bone, resp tract, urinary tract, and abdomen, and septicemia* **Action:** 4th-gen PCN; bactericidal; inhibits cell wall synthesis. *Spectrum:* Primarily gram(+) better *Enterococcus, H. influenza,* not staph; gram(–) *E. coli, Proteus, Shigella, Pseudomonas,* not β-lactamase-producing **Dose:** *Adults.* 3 g IV q4–6h. *Peds.* 200–300 mg/kg/d IV ÷ q4–6h; ↓ dose in renal failure **Caution:** [B, M] Penicillin sensitivity **Supplied:** Inj **SE:** ↓ Plt aggregation, interstitial nephritis, renal failure, anaphylaxis, hemolytic anemia **Notes:** Often used in combination w/ aminoglycoside **Interactions:** ↑ Effects w/ probenecid; ↑ effects of anticoagulants, MRX; ↓ effects w/ macrolides, tetracyclines; ↓ effects of oral contraceptives **Labs:** ↑ LFTs, BUN, creatinine, + direct Coombs' test, ↓ K⁺ **NIPE:** Inactivation of aminoglycosides if drugs given together—admin at least 1 h apart

Piperacillin–Tazobactam (Zosyn) **Uses:** *Infections involving skin, bone, resp tract, urinary tract, and abdomen, and septicemia* **Action:** PCN plus β-lactamase inhibitor; bactericidal; inhibits cell wall synthesis. *Spectrum:* Good gram(+), excellent gram(–); covers β-lactamase producers **Dose:** *Adults.* 3.375–4.5 g IV q6h; ↓ dose in renal failure **Caution:** [B, M] Penicillin or β-lactam sensitivity **Supplied:** Inj **SE:** Diarrhea, HA, insomnia, GI upset, serum sickness-like Rxn, pseudomembranous colitis **Notes:** Often used in combination w/ aminoglycoside. See Piperacillin Interactions; **Additional Labs:** ↓ Hmg, Hct, protein, albumin

Pirbuterol (Maxair) **Uses:** *Prevention and Rx of reversible bronchospasm* **Action:** β₂-Adrenergic agonist **Dose:** 2 inhal q4–6h; max 12 inhal/d **Caution:** [C, ?/–] **Supplied:** Aerosol 0.2 mg/actuation; Autohaler dry powder 0.2 mg/actuation **SE:** Nervousness, restlessness, trembling, HA, taste changes, tachycardia **Interactions:** ↑ Effects w/ epinephrine, sympathomimetics; ↑ vascular effects w/ MAOIs, TCAs; ↓ effects w/ BBs **NIPE:** Rinse mouth after use; shake well before use

Piroxicam (Feldene) **Uses:** *Arthritis and pain* **Action:** NSAID; inhibits prostaglandins **Dose:** 10–20 mg/d **Caution:** [B (1st tri; D if 3rd tri or near term), +] GI bleeding **Contra:** ASA or NSAID sensitivity **Supplied:** Caps 10, 20 mg **SE:** Dizziness, rash, GI upset, edema, acute renal failure, peptic ulcer **Interactions:** ↑ Effects w/ probenecid; ↑ effects of aminoglycosides, anticoagulants, hypoglycemics, Li, MRX; ↑ risk of bleeding w/ ASA, corticosteroids, NSAIDs, feverfew, garlic, ginger, ginkgo biloba, EtOH; ↓ effect w/ ASA, antacids, cholestyramine; ↓ effect of BBs, diuretics **Labs:** ↑ BUN, LFTs, serum Cl, serum Na, PT **NIPE:** Take w/ food, full effect after 2 wk admin, ↑ risk of photosensitivity—use sunscreen

Plasma Protein Fraction (Plasmanate, others) **Uses:** *Shock and hypotension* **Action:** Plasma volume expander **Dose:** Initial, 250–500 mL IV (not >10 mL/min); subsequent inf depends on clinical response. *Peds.* 10–15

mL/kg/dose IV; subsequent inf depends on clinical response **Caution:** [C, +] **Contra:** Renal insufficiency, CHF **Supplied:** Inj 5% **SE:** Hypotension associated w/ rapid inf; hypocoagulability, metabolic acidosis, PE **Notes:** 130–160 mEq Na/L; not substitute for RBC

Pneumococcal 7-Valent Conjugate Vaccine (Prevnar) Uses: *Immunization against pneumococcal infections in infants and children* **Action:** Active immunization **Dose:** 0.5 mL IM/dose; series of 3 doses; 1st dose at 2 mo of age w/ subsequent doses q2mo **Caution:** [C, +] Thrombocytopenia **Contra:** Diphtheria toxoid sensitivity, febrile illness **Supplied:** Inj **SE:** Local Rxns, arthralgia, fever, myalgia

Pneumococcal Vaccine, Polyvalent (Pneumovax-23) Uses: *Immunization against pneumococcal infections in Pts predisposed or at high risk (all people ≥65 y of age)* **Action:** Active immunization **Dose:** 0.5 mL IM. **Caution:** [C, ?] **Contra:** ⊘ vaccinate during immunosuppressive therapy **Supplied:** Inj 25 mg each of polysaccharide isolates per 0.5-mL dose **SE:** Fever, inj site Rxn, hemolytic anemia, thrombocytopenia, anaphylaxis **Interactions:** ↓ Effects w/ corticosteroids, immunosuppressants

Podophyllin (Podocon-25, Condylox Gel 0.5%, Condylox) Uses: *Topical therapy of benign growths (genital and perianal warts [condylomata acuminata],* papillomas, fibromas) **Action:** Direct antimitotic effect; exact mechanism unknown **Dose:** *Condylox gel and Condylox:* Apply 3 consecutive d/wk for 4 wk. *Podocon-25:* Use sparingly on the lesion, leave on for 1–4 h, then thoroughly wash off **Caution:** [C, ?] Immunosuppression **Contra:** DM, bleeding lesions **Supplied:** Podocon-25 (w/benzoin) 15-mL bottles; Condylox gel 0.5% 3.5 g clear gel; Condylox soln 0.5% 3.5 g clear **SE:** Local Rxns, significant absorption; anemias, tachycardia, paresthesias, GI upset, renal/hepatic damage **Notes:** Podocon-25 applied only by the clinician; ⊘ dispense

Polyethylene Glycol [PEG]—Electrolyte Solution (GoLYTELY, CoLyte) Uses: *Bowel prep prior to examination or surgery* **Action:** Osmotic cathartic **Dose:** *Adults.* Following 3–4-h fast, drink 240 mL of soln q10min until 4 L consumed. *Peds.* 25–40 mL/kg/h for 4–10 h **Caution:** [C, ?] **Contra:** GI obstruction, bowel perforation, megacolon, ulcerative colitis **Supplied:** Powder for reconstitution to 4 L **SE:** Cramping or nausea, bloating **Notes:** 1st BM should occur in approximately 1 h

Polyethylene Glycol [PEG] 3350 (MiraLax) Uses: *Occasional constipation* **Action:** Osmotic laxative **Dose:** 17 g powder (1 heaping tablespoon) in 8 oz (1 cup) of water and drink; max 14 d **Caution:** [C, ?] R/o bowel obstruction before use **Contra:** GI obstruction, allergy to PEG **Supplied:** Powder for reconstitution; bottle cap holds 17 g **SE:** Upset stomach, bloating, cramping, gas, severe diarrhea, hives **Notes:** Can add to water, juice, soda, coffee, or tea

Polymyxin B & Hydrocortisone (Otobiotic Otic) Uses: *Superficial bacterial infections of external ear canal* **Action:** Antibiotic antiinflammatory combination **Dose:** 4 gtt in ear(s) tid–qid **Caution:** [B, ?] **Supplied:** Soln polymyxin B 10,000 Units/hydrocortisone 0.5%/mL **SE:** Local irritation **Notes:** Useful in neomycin allergy

Potassium Citrate (Urocit-K) **Uses:** *Alkalinize urine, prevention of urinary stones (uric acid, Ca stones if hypocitraturic)* **Action:** Urinary alkalinizer **Dose:** 10–20 mEq PO tid w/ meals, max 100 mEq/d **Caution:** [A, +] **Contra:** Severe renal impairment, dehydration, hyperkalemia, peptic ulcer; use of K-sparing diuretics or salt substitutes **Supplied:** 540-, 1080-mg tabs **SE:** GI upset, hypocalcemia, hyperkalemia, metabolic alkalosis **Notes:** Tabs 540 mg = 5 mEq, 1080 mg = 10 mEq **Interactions:** ↑ Risk of hyperkalemia w/ ACEIs, K-sparing diuretics

Potassium Citrate & Citric Acid (Polycitra-K) **Uses:** *Alkalinize urine, prevent urinary stones (uric acid, Ca stones if hypocitraturic)* **Action:** Urinary alkalinizer **Dose:** 10–20 mEq PO tid w/ meals, max 100 mEq/d **Caution:** [A, +] **Contra:** Severe renal impairment, dehydration, hyperkalemia, peptic ulcer; use of K-sparing diuretics or salt substitutes **Supplied:** Soln 10 mEq/5 mL; powder 30 mEq/packet **SE:** GI upset, hypocalcemia, hyperkalemia, metabolic alkalosis **Interactions:** ↑ Risk of hyperkalemia w/ ACEIs, K-sparing diuretics

Potassium Iodide [Lugol's Solution] (SSKI, Thyro-Block) **Uses:** *Thyroid storm,* reduction of vascularity before thyroid surgery, block thyroid uptake of radioactive isotopes of I, thin bronchial secretions **Action:** I suppl **Dose:** *Adults & Peds.* >2 y: Preop thyroidectomy: 50–250 mg PO tid (2–6 gtt strong I soln); administer 10 d preop. *Peds.* 1 y: Thyroid crisis: 300 mg (6 gtt SSKI q8h). *Peds.* <1 y: ½ adult dose **Caution:** [D, +] Hyperkalemia, tuberculosis, PE, bronchitis, renal impairment **Contra:** I sensitivity **Supplied:** Tabs 130 mg; soln (SSKI) 1 g/mL; Lugol's soln, strong I 100 mg/mL; syrup 325 mg/5 mL **SE:** Fever, HA, urticaria, angioedema, goiter, GI upset, eosinophilia **Interactions:** ↑ Risk of hypothyroidism w/ antithyroid drugs and Li; ↑ risk of hyperkalemia w/ ACEIs, K-sparing diuretics, K suppls **Labs:** May alter TFTs **NIPE:** Take pc w/ food or milk

Potassium Supplements (Kaon, Kaochlor, K-Lor, Slow-K, Micro-K, Klorvess, others) **Uses:** *Prevention or Rx of hypokalemia* (eg, diuretic use) **Action:** K suppl **Dose:** *Adults.* 20–100 mEq/d PO ÷ qd–bid; IV 10–20 mEq/h, max 40 mEq/h and 150 mEq/d (monitor K⁺ levels frequently w/high-dose IV). *Peds.* Calculate K deficit; 1–3 mEq/kg/d PO ÷ qd–qid; IV max dose 0.5–1 mEq/kg/h **Caution:** [A, +] Renal insufficiency, use w/inSAIDs and ACEIs **Contra:** Hyperkalemia **Supplied:** PO forms (see Table 8, page 280); injectable forms **SE:** Can cause GI irritation; bradycardia, hyperkalemia, heart block **Notes:** Mix powder and liquid w/ beverage (unsalted tomato juice, etc); follow serum K⁺; Cl⁻ salt recommended in coexisting alkalosis; for coexisting acidosis use acetate, bicarbonate, citrate, or gluconate salt **Interactions:** ↑ Effects w/ ACEI, K-sparing diuretics, salt substitutes **NIPE:** Take w/ food

Pramipexole (Mirapex) **Uses:** *Parkinson's Dz* **Action:** Dopamine agonist **Dose:** 1.5–4.5 mg/d, initial 0.375 mg/d in 3 ÷ doses; titrate slowly **Caution:**

C, ?/–] **Contra:** Component hypersensitivity **Supplied:** Tabs 0.125, 0.25, 1, 1.5 ng **SE:** Postural hypotension, asthenia, somnolence, abnormal dreams, GI upset, PS **Interactions:** ↑ Effects w/ cimetidine, diltiazem, quinidine, quinine, ranitine, triamterene, verapamil; ↑ effects of levodopa; ↑ CNS depression w/ CNS deressants, EtOH; ↓ effects w/ antipsychotics, butyrophenones, metoclopramide, henothiazines, thioxanthenes **NIPE:** May take w/ food; ⊘ DC abruptly

Pramoxine (Anusol Ointment, Proctofoam-NS, others) Uses: *Relief of pain and itching from hemorrhoids and anorectal surgery*; topical or burns and dermatosis **Action:** Topical anesthetic **Dose:** Apply cream, oint, gel, r spray freely to anal area q3h **Caution:** [C, ?] **Supplied:** [OTC] All 1%; foam Proctofoam-NS), cream, oint, lotion, gel, pads, spray **SE:** Contact dermatitis NIPE: ⊘ Use on large areas

Pramoxine + Hydrocortisone (Enzone, Proctofoam-HC) Uses: *Relief of pain and itching from hemorrhoids* **Action:** Topical anesthetic, ntiinflammatory **Dose:** Apply freely to anal area tid–qid **Caution:** [C, ?/–] **Supplied:** Cream pramoxine 1% acetate 0.5/1%; foam pramoxine 1% hydrocortisone % ; lotion pramoxine 1% hydrocortisone 0.25/1/2.5%, pramoxine 2.5% and hylrocortisone 1% **SE:** Contact dermatitis **NIPE:** ⊘ Use on large areas

Pravastatin (Pravachol) Uses: ↓ Cholesterol **Action:** HMG-CoA reducase inhibitor **Dose:** 10–40 mg PO hs; ↓ dose in significant renal/hepatic insuffiiency **Caution:** [X, –] **Contra:** Liver Dz or persistent LFT ↑ **Supplied:** Tabs 10, 20, 40 mg **SE:** Use caution w/ concurrent gemfibrozil; HA, GI upset, hepatitis, myopathy, renal failure **Interactions:** ↑ Risk of myopathy & rhabdomyolysis w/ clarthromycin, clofibrate, cyclosporine, danazol, erythromycin, fluoxetine, gemfibrozil, niacin, nefazodone, troleandomycin; ↑ effects w/ azole antifungals, cimetidine, grapefruit juice; ↓ effects w/ cholestyramine, isradipine **Labs:** ↑ LFTs **NIPE:** ⊘ PRG, breast-feeding; take w/o regard to food; full effect may take up to 4 wks; ↑ risk of photosensitivity—use sunscreen

Prazosin (Minipress) Uses: *HTN* **Action:** Peripherally acting α-adrenergic blocker **Dose:** *Adults.* 1 mg PO tid; can ↑ to max daily dose of up to 20 mg/d. *Peds.* 5–25 μg/kg/dose q6h, up to 25 μg/kg/dose **Caution:** [C, ?] **Contra:** Component hypersensitivity **Supplied:** Caps 1, 2, 5 mg **SE:** Dizziness, edema, palpitaions, fatigue, GI upset **Notes:** Can cause orthostatic hypotension, take the 1st dose hs; tolerance develops to this effect; tachyphylaxis may result **Interactions:** ↑ Hypotension w/ antihypertensives, diuretics, nitrates, EtOH; ↓ effects w/ NSAIDs, butcher's broom **Labs:** ↑ Serum Na levels, vanillylmandelic acid level; alters test for pheochromocytoma **NIPE:** ⊘ DC abruptly

Prednisolone [See Table 4, page 271] **Interactions:** ↑ Effects w/ clarithromycin, erythromycin, estrogen, ketoconazole, oral contraceptives, troleandomycin; ↓ effects w/ antacids, aminoglutethimide, barbiturates, cholestyramine, colestipol, phenytoin, rifampin; ↓ effects of anticoagulants, hypoglycemics, INH, salicylates, vaccine toxoids **Labs:** False – skin allergy tests; false ↑ cortisol, digoxin, theophylline **NIPE:** ⊘ Use live virus vaccines, ⊘ DC abruptly; take w/ food.

Prednisone [See Table 4, page 271] **Interactions:** ↑ Effects w/ clarithromycin, cyclosporine, erythromycin, estrogen, ketoconazole, oral contraceptives, troleandomycin; ↓ effects w/ antacids, aminoglutethimide, barbiturates, carbamazepine, cholestyramine, colestipol, phenytoin, rifampin; ↓ effects of anticoagulants, hypoglycemics, INH, salicylates, vaccine toxoids **Labs:** False − skin allergy tests, false ↑ cortisol, digoxin, theophylline **NIPE:** Take w/ food; ⊘ use live virus vaccine, ⊘ DC abruptly, infection may be masked

Probenecid (Benemid, others) **Uses:** *Prevent gout and hyperuricemia; prolongs serum levels of penicillins or cephalosporins* **Action:** Renal tubular blocking agent **Dose:** *Adults.* Gout: 250 mg bid for 1 wk, then 0.5 g PO bid; can ↑ by 500 mg/mo up to 2–3 g/d. *Antibiotic effect:* 1–2 g PO 30 min before antibiotic dose. *Peds.* >2y: 25 mg/kg, then 40 mg/kg/d PO ÷ qid **Caution:** [B, ?] **Contra:** High-dose ASA, moderate–severe renal impairment, age <2 y **Supplied:** Tabs 500 mg **SE:** HA, GI upset, rash, pruritus, dizziness, blood dyscrasias **Notes:** ⊘ Use during acute gout attack **Interactions:** ↑ Effects of acyclovir, allopurinol; ↑ effects of benzodiazepines, cephalosporins, ciprofloxacin, clofibrate, dapsone, dyphylline, MRX, NSAIDs, olanzapine, rifampin, sulfonamides, sulfonylureas zidovudine; ↓ effects w/ niacin, EtOH; ↓ effects of penicillamine **Labs:** False + urine glucose; false ↑ level of theophylline **NIPE:** Take w/ food, ↑ fluids to 2–3 L/d; ⊘ ASA, NSAIDs, salicylates

Procainamide (Pronestyl, Procan) **Uses:** *Supraventricular and ventricular arrhythmias* **Action:** Class 1A antiarrhythmic; depresses the excitability of cardiac muscle to electrical stimulation and slows conduction in the atrium, bundle of His, ventricle **Dose:** *Adults.* Recurrent VF/VT: 20 mg/min IV (max total 17 mg/kg). *Maint:* 1–4 mg/min. *Stable wide-complex tachycardia of unknown origin, AF w/ rapid rate in WPW:* 20 mg/min IV until arrhythmia suppression, hypotension, QRS widens >50%, then 1–4 mg/min. *Chronic dosing:* 50 mg/kg/d PO in ÷ doses q4–6h. *Peds.* Chronic maint: 15–50 mg/kg/24 h PO ÷ q3–6h; ↓ in renal/hepatic impairment **Caution:** [C, +] **Contra:** Complete heart block, 2nd- or 3rd-degree heart block w/o pacemaker, torsades de pointes, SLE **Supplied:** Tabs and caps 250, 375, 500 mg; SR tabs 250, 500, 750, 1000 mg; inj 100, 500 mg/mL **SE:** Can cause hypotension and a lupus-like syndrome; GI upset, taste perversion, arrhythmias, tachycardia, heart block, angioneuropathic edema **Notes:** Follow levels (see Table 2, page 265) **Interactions:** ↑ Effects w/ acetazolamide, amiodarone, cimetidine, ranitidine, trimethoprim; ↑ effects of anticholinergics, antihypertensives; ↓ effects w/ procaine, EtOH **Labs:** ↑ LFTs, + Coombs' test **NIPE:** Take w/ food if GI upset, ⊘ crush SR tab

Procarbazine (Matulane) **WARNING:** Highly toxic; handle w/ care **Uses:** *Hodgkin's Dz,* NHL, brain tumors **Action:** Alkylating agent; inhibits DNA and RNA synthesis **Dose:** Refer to specific protocol **Caution:** [D, ?] W/

EtOH ingestion **Contra:** Inadequate bone marrow reserve **Supplied:** Caps 50 mg **SE:** Myelosuppression, hemolytic Rxns (w/ G6PD deficiency), N/V/D; disulfiram-like Rxn; cutaneous Rxns; constitutional Sxs, myalgia, and arthralgia; CNS effects, azoospermia, and cessation of menses **Interactions:** ↑ CNS depression w/ antihistamines, antihypertensives, barbiturates, CNS depressants, narcotics, phenothiazines; ↑ effects of hypoglycemics; ↑ risk of HTN w/ guanethidine, levodopa, MAOIs, methyldopa, sympathomimetics, TCAs, tyramine-containing foods; ↓ effects of digoxin **NIPE:** Disulfiram-like Rxn w/ EtOH; ↑ fluids to 2–3 L/d; ↑ risk of photosensitivity—use sunscreen; ⊘ exposure to infection

Prochlorperazine (Compazine) **Uses:** *N/V, agitation, and psychotic disorders* **Action:** Phenothiazine; blocks postsynaptic dopaminergic CNS receptors **Dose:** *Adults.* Antiemetic: 5–10 mg PO tid–qid or 25 mg PR bid or 5–10 mg deep IM q4–6h. *Antipsychotic:* 10–20 mg IM acutely or 5–10 mg PO tid–qid for maint; ↑ doses may be required for antipsychotic effect. *Peds.* 0.1–0.15 mg/kg/dose IM q4–6h or 0.4 mg/kg/24 h PO ÷ tid–qid **Caution:** [C, +/–] Narrow-angle glaucoma, severe liver/cardiac Dz **Contra:** Phenothiazine sensitivity, bone marrow suppression **Supplied:** Tabs 5, 10, 25 mg; SR caps 10, 15, 30 mg; syrup 5 mg/5 mL; supp 2.5, 5, 25 mg; inj 5 mg/mL **SE:** EPS common; treat w/ diphenhydramine **Interactions:** ↑ Effects w/ chloroquine, indomethacin, narcotics, procarbazine, SSRIs, pyrimethamine; ↑ effects of antidepressants, BBs, EtOH; ↓ effects w/ antacids, anticholinergics, barbiturates, tobacco; ↓ effects of guanethidine, levodopa, Li **Labs:** False + urine bilirubin, amylase, phenylketonuria, ↑ serum prolactin **NIPE:** ⊘ DC abruptly; ↑ risk of photosensitivity—use sunscreen; urine may turn pink/red

Promethazine (Phenergan) **Uses:** *N/V, motion sickness* **Action:** Phenothiazine; blocks postsynaptic mesolimbic dopaminergic receptors in the brain **Dose:** *Adults.* 12.5–50 mg PO, PR, or IM bid–qid PRN. *Peds.* 0.1–0.5 mg/kg/dose PO or IM q2–6h PRN **Caution:** [C, +/–] **Contra:** Component hypersensitivity, narrow-angle glaucoma **Supplied:** Tabs 12.5, 25, 50 mg; syrup 6.25 mg/5 mL, 25 mg/5 mL; supp 12.5, 25, 50 mg; inj 25, 50 mg/mL **SE:** Drowsiness, tardive dyskinesia, EPS, lowered Sz threshold, hypotension, GI upset, blood dyscrasias, photosensitivity **Interactions:** ↑ Effects w/ CNS depressants, MAOIs, EtOH; ↑ effects of antihypertensives; ↓ effects w/ anticholinergics, barbiturates, tobacco; ↓ effect of levodopa **NIPE:** Effects skin allergy tests; use sunscreen for photosensitivity

Propafenone (Rythmol) **Uses:** *Life-threatening ventricular arrhythmias and AF* **Action:** Class IC antiarrhythmic; blocks the fast inward Na current in heart muscle and Purkinje fibers, and slows the rate of ↑ of phase 0 of the action potential **Dose:** *Adults.* 150–300 mg PO q8h. *Peds.* 8–10 mg/kg/d ÷ in 3–4 doses; may ↑ 2 mg/kg/d, to max of 20 mg/kg/d **Caution:** [C, ?] Amprenavir or ritonavir use **Contra:** Uncontrolled CHF, bronchospasm, cardiogenic shock, conduction disorders **Supplied:** Tabs 150, 225, 300 mg **SE:** Dizziness, unusual taste, 1st-degree heart block, arrhythmias, prolongation of QRS and QT intervals; fatigue, GI upset, blood dyscrasias **Interactions:** ↑ Effects w/ cimetidine, quinidine; ↑ effects of anticoagulants, BBs, digitalis glycosides, theophylline; ↓ effects w/ rifampin, phenobarbital, rifabutin **Labs:** ↑ ANA titers **NIPE:** Take w/o regard to food

Propantheline (Pro-Banthine) Uses: *PUD,* symptomatic Rx of small intestine hypermotility, spastic colon, ureteral spasm, bladder spasm, pylorospasm **Action:** Antimuscarinic agent **Dose: Adults.** 15 mg PO ac and 30 mg PO hs; ↓ dose in elderly. **Peds.** 2–3 mg/kg/24h PO ÷ tid–qid **Caution:** [C, ?] **Contra:** Narrow-angle glaucoma, ulcerative colitis, toxic megacolon, GI or GU obstruction **Supplied:** Tabs 7.5, 15 mg **SE:** Anticholinergic side effects (xerostomia and blurred vision common) **Interactions:** ↑ Anticholinergic effects w/ antihistamines, antidepressants, atropine, haloperidol, phenothiazines, quinidine, TCAs; ↑ effects of atenolol, digoxin; ↓ effects w/ antacids **NIPE:** May cause heat intolerance, ↑ risk of photosensitivity—use sunscreen

Propofol (Diprivan) Uses: *Induction or maint of anesthesia; continuous sedation in intubated Pts* **Action:** Sedative–hypnotic; mechanism unknown **Dose: Adults.** Anesthesia: 2–2.5 mg/kg induction, then 0.1–0.2 mg/kg/min inf. *ICU sedation:* 5–50 µg/kg/min cont inf; ↓ dose in elderly, debilitated, or ASA II or IV Pts. **Peds. Anesthesia.** 2.5–3.5 mg/kg induction; then 125–300 µg/kg/min **Caution:** [B, +] **Contra:** When general anesthesia is contraindicated **Supplied:** Inj 10 mg/mL **SE:** May ↑ triglycerides w/ extended dosing; hypotension, pain at inj site, apnea, anaphylaxis **Notes:** 1 mL of propofol contains 0.1 g fat **Interactions:** ↑ Effects w/ antihistamines, opioids, hypnotics, EtOH **Labs:** ↓ Serum cortisol levels

Propoxyphene (Darvon); Propoxyphene & Acetaminophen (Darvocet); & Propoxyphene & Aspirin (Darvon Compound-65, Darvon-N + Aspirin) [C-IV] Uses: *Mild–moderate pain* **Action:** Narcotic analgesic **Dose:** 1–2 PO q4h PRN; ↓ in hepatic impairment, elderly **Caution:** [C (D if prolonged use), M] Hepatic impairment (APAP), peptic ulcer (ASA); severe renal impairment **Contra:** Hypersensitivity **Supplied:** *Darvon:* Propoxyphene HCl caps 65 mg. *Darvon-N:* Propoxyphene napsylate 100-mg tabs. *Darvocet-N:* Propoxyphene napsylate 50 mg/APAP 325 mg. *Darvocet-N 100:* Propoxyphene napsylate 100 mg/APAP 650 mg. *Darvon Compound-65:* Propoxyphene HCl caps 65-mg/ASA 389 mg/caffeine 32 mg. *Darvon-N w/ ASA:* Propoxyphene napsylate 100 mg/ASA 325 mg **SE:** OD can be lethal; hypotension, dizziness, sedation, GI upset, ↑ levels on LFTs **Interactions:** ↑ CNS depression w/ antidepressants, antihistamines, barbiturates, glutethimide, methocarbamol, protease inhibitors, EtOH, St. John's wort; ↑ effects of BBs, carbamazepine, MAOIs, phenobarbital, TCAs, warfarin; ↓ effects w/ tobacco **Labs:** ↑ LFTs, serum amylase, lipase **NIPE:** Take w/ food if GI upset

Propranolol (Inderal) Uses:* HTN, angina, MI, hyperthyroidism, essential tremor, hypertropic subaortic stenosis, pheochromocytoma; prevents migraines and atrial arrhythmias* **Action:** β-Adrenergic receptor blocker, β₁, β₂; only BB to block conversion of T_4 to T_3 **Dose:** *Adults.* Angina: 80–320 mg/d PO ÷ bid–qid or 80–160 mg/d SR. *Arrhythmia:* 10–80 mg PO tid–qid or 1 mg IV slowly, repeat q5min up to 5 mg. *HTN:* 40 mg PO bid or 60–80 mg/d SR, ↑ weekly to max 640 mg/d. *Hypertrophic subaortic stenosis:* 20–40 mg PO tid–qid. *MI:* 180–240 mg PO ÷ tid–qid. *Migraine prophylaxis:* 80 mg/d ÷ qid–tid, ↑ weekly to max 160–240 mg/d ÷ tid–qid; wean off if no response in 6 wk. *Pheochromocytoma:* 30–60 mg/d ÷ tid–qid. *Thyrotoxicosis:* 1–3 mg IV single dose; 10–40 mg PO q6h. *Tremor:* 40 mg PO bid, ↑ as needed to max 320 mg/d. **Peds.** Arrhythmia: 0.5–1.0 mg/kg/d ÷ tid–qid, ↑ as needed q3–7d to max 60 mg/d; 0.01–0.1 mg/kg IV over 10 min, max dose 1 mg. *HTN:* 0.5–1.0 mg/kg ÷ bid, ↑ as needed q3–7d to 2 mg/kg/d max; ↓ dose in renal impairment **Caution:** [C (1st tri, D if 2nd or 3rd tri), +] **Contra:** Uncompensated CHF, cardiogenic shock, bradycardia, heart block, PE, severe resp Dz **Supplied:** Tabs 10, 20, 40, 60, 80 mg; SR caps 60, 80, 120, 160 mg; oral soln 4, 8, 80 mg/mL; inj 1 mg/mL **SE:** Bradycardia, hypotension, fatigue, GI upset, erectile dysfunction, hypoglycemia **Interactions:** ↑ Effects w/ antihypertensives, cimetidine, fluvoxamine, flecainide, hydralazine, methimazole, neuroleptics, nitrates, propylthiouracil, quinidine, quinolones, theophylline, EtOH; ↑ effects of digitalis, glycosides, hypoglycemics, hydralazine, lidocaine, neuroleptics, rizatriptan; ↓ effects w/ NSAIDs, phenobarbital, phenytoin, rifampin, tobacco **Labs:** ↑ LFTs, BUN, K+, serum lipoprotein, triglycerides, uric acid; ↑ or ↓ serum glucose **NIPE:** ⊘ DC abruptly; ↑ cold sensitivity

Propylthiouracil [PTU] **Uses:** *Hyperthyroidism* **Action:** Inhibits production of T_3 and T_4 and conversion of T_4 to T_3 **Dose:** *Adults.* Initial: 100 mg PO q8h (may need up to 1200 mg/d); after Pt euthyroid, taper dose by ½ q4–6wk to maint, 50–150 mg/24 h; can usually be DC in 2–3 y; ↓ dose in elderly **Peds.** Initial: 5–7 mg/kg/24 h PO ÷ q8h. *Maint:* ⅓–⅔ of initial dose **Caution:** [D, –] **Contra:** Hypersensitivity **Supplied:** Tabs 50 mg **SE:** Monitor Pt clinically; monitor TFT, fever, rash, leukopenia, dizziness, GI upset, taste perversion, SLE-like syndrome **Interactions:** ↑ Effects w/ iodinated glycerol, Li, KI, NaI **Labs:** ↑ LFTs, PT; ↑ effects of anticoagulants **NIPE:** Take w/ food for GI upset; omit dietary sources of I; full effects take 6–12 wk

Protamine (generic) **Uses:** *Reversal of heparin effect* **Action:** Neutralizes heparin by forming a stable complex **Dose:** Based on amount of heparin reversal desired; give IV slowly; 1 mg reverses approximately 100 Units of heparin given in the preceding 3–4 h, 50 mg max dose **Caution:** [C, ?] **Contra:** Hypersensitivity **Supplied:** Inj 10 mg/mL **SE:** Follow coagulation studies; may have anticoagulant effect if given w/out heparin; hypotension, bradycardia, dyspnea, hemorrhage

Pseudoephedrine (Sudafed, Novafed, Afrinol, others) **Uses:** *Decongestant* **Action:** Stimulates α-adrenergic receptors, resulting in vasoconstriction **Dose:** Adults. 30–60 mg PO q6–8h; SR caps 120 mg PO q12h. *Peds.*4 mg/kg/24 h PO ÷ qid; ↓ dose in renal insufficiency **Caution:** [C, +] **Contra:**

Poorly controlled HTN or CAD Dz and in MAOIs **Supplied:** Tabs 30, 60 mg; caps 60 mg; SR tabs 120, 240 mg; SR caps 120 mg; liq 7.5 mg/0.8 mL, 15, 30 mg/5 mL **SE:** HTN, insomnia, tachycardia, arrhythmias, nervousness, tremor **Notes:** Ingredient in many cough and cold preps **Interactions:** ↑ Risk of HTN crisis w/ MAOIs; ↑ effects w/ BBs, sympathomimetics; ↓ effects w/ TCAs; ↓ effect of methyldopa, reserpine

Psyllium (Metamucil, Serutan, Effer-Syllium) **Uses:** *Constipation and diverticular Dz of the colon* **Action:** Bulk laxative **Dose:** 1 tsp (7 g) in a glass of water qd–tid **Caution:** [B, ?] Psyllium in effervescent (Effer-Syllium) form usually contains K⁺; use caution in Pts w/ renal failure; phenylketonuria (in products w/ aspartame) **Contra:** ⊘ use if suspected bowel obstruction **Supplied:** Granules 4, 25 g/tsp; powder 3.5 g/packet **SE:** Diarrhea, abdominal cramps, bowel obstruction, constipation, bronchospasm **Interactions:** ↓ Effects of digitalis glycosides, K-sparing diuretics, nitrofurantoin, salicylates, tetracyclines, warfarin **NIPE:** Psyllium dust inhalation may cause wheezing, runny nose, watery eyes

Pyrazinamide (generic) **Uses:** *Active TB in combination w/ other agents* **Action:** Bacteriostatic; mechanism unknown **Dose:** **Adults.** 15–30 mg/kg/24 h PO ÷ tid–qid; max 2 g/d. **Peds.** 15–30 mg/kg/d PO ÷ qd–bid; dosage regimen differs for directly observed therapy; ↓ dose for renal/hepatic impairment **Caution:** [C, +/−] **Contra:** Severe hepatic damage, acute gout **Supplied:** Tabs 500 mg **SE:** Hepatotoxicity, malaise, GI upset, arthralgia, myalgia, gout, photosensitivity **Notes:** Use in combination w/ other anti-TB drugs; consult *MMWR* for the latest TB recommendations; dosage regimen differs for directly observed therapy **Interactions:** ↓ Effects of cyclosporine, tacrolimus **Labs:** False + urine ketones **NIPE:** ↑ Risk of photosensitivity—use sunscreen; ↑ fluids to 2 L/d

Pyridoxine [Vitamin B₆] **Uses:** *Rx and prevention of vitamin B₆ deficiency* **Action:** Suppl of vitamin B₆ **Dose:** **Adults.** Deficiency: 10–20 mg/d PO. *Drug-induced neuritis:* 100–200 mg/d; 25–100 mg/d prophylaxis. **Peds.** 5–25 mg/d × 3 wk **Caution:** [A (C if doses exceed RDA), +] **Contra:** Component hypersensitivity **Supplied:** Tabs 25, 50, 100 mg; inj 100 mg/mL **SE:** Allergic Rxns, HA, nausea **Interactions:** ↑ Pyridoxine needs w/ chloramphenicol, cycloserine, hydralazine, immunosuppressant drugs, INH, oral contraceptives, penicillamine, high-protein diet; ↓ effects of levodopa, phenobarbital, phenytoin **Labs:** False ↑ urobilinogen **NIPE:** Lactation suppressed w/ pyridoxine

Quazepam (Doral) [C-IV] **Uses:** *Insomnia* **Action:** Benzodiazepine **Dose:** 7.5–15 mg PO hs PRN; ↓ dose in the elderly, hepatic failure **Caution:** [X, ?/−] Narrow-angle glaucoma **Contra:** PRG, sleep apnea **Supplied:** Tabs 7.5, 15 mg **SE:** Sedation, hangover, somnolence, resp depression **Notes:** ⊘ DC abruptly **Interactions:** ↑ Effects w/ azole antifungals, cimetidine, digoxin, disulfiram, INH, levodopa, macrolides, neuroleptics, phenytoin, quinolones, SSRIs, verapamil, grapefruit juice, EtOH; ↓ effects w/ carbamazepine, rifampin, rifabutin, tobacco **NIPE:** ⊘ Breastfeed, PRG, DC abruptly; use barrier contraception

Quetiapine (Seroquel)
Uses: *Acute exacerbations of schizophrenia* **Action:** Serotonin and dopamine antagonism **Dose:** 150–750 mg/d; initiate at 25–100 mg bid–tid; slowly ↑ dose; ↓ dose for hepatic and geriatric Pts **Caution:** [C, –] **Contra:** Component hypersensitivity **Supplied:** Tabs 25, 100, 200 mg **SE:** Multiple reports of confusion w/ nefazodone; HA, somnolence, weight gain, orthostatic hypotension, dizziness, cataracts, neuroleptic malignant syndrome, tardive dyskinesia, QT prolongation **Interactions:** ↑ Effects w/ azole antifungals, cimetidine, macrolides, EtOH; ↑ effects of antihypertensives, lorazepam; ↓ effects w/ barbiturates, carbamazepine, glucocorticoids, phenytoin, rifampin, thioridazine; ↓ effects of dopamine antagonists, levodopa **Labs:** ↑ LFTs, cholesterol, triglycerides **NIPE:** ↑ risk of cataract formation, tardive dyskinesia; take w/o regard to food; ↓ body temp regulation

Quinapril (Accupril)
WARNING: ACEIs used during the 2nd and 3rd tri of PRG can cause injury and even death to the developing fetus **Uses:** *HTN, CHF, DN, post-MI* **Action:** ACEI **Dose:** 10–80 mg PO qd single dose; ↓ in renal impairment **Caution:** [D, +] **Contra:** ACEI sensitivity or angioedema **Supplied:** Tabs 5, 10, 20, 40 mg **SE:** Dizziness, HA, hypotension, ↓ renal Fxn, angioedema, taste perversion, cough **Interactions:** ↑ Effects w/ diuretics, antihypertensives; ↑ effects of insulin, Li; ↓ effects w/ ASA, NSAIDs; ↓ effects of quinolones, tetracyclines **Labs:** ↑ BUN, SCr **NIPE:** ↓ Absorption w/ high-fat foods; ↑ risk of cough

Quinidine (Quinidex, Quinaglute)
Uses: *Prevention of tachydysrhythmias, malaria* **Action:** Class 1A antiarrhythmic; ↑ the refractory period in atrial and ventricular muscle, in SA and AV conduction systems, and the Purkinje fibers **Dose:** *Adults.* Conversion of AF or flutter: Use after digitalization, 200 mg q2–3h for 8 doses; then ↑ daily dose to a max of 3–4 g or until normal rhythm. *Peds.* 15–60 mg/kg/24 h PO in 4–5 ÷ doses; ↓ dose in renal impairment **Caution:** [C, +] Ritonavir use **Contra:** Digitalis toxicity and AV block; conduction disorders **Supplied:** *Sulfate:* Tabs 200, 300 mg; SR tabs 300 mg. *Gluconate:* SR tabs 324 mg; inj 80 mg/mL **SE:** Extreme hypotension may be seen w/ IV administration; syncope, QT prolongation, GI upset, arrhythmias, fatigue, cinchonism (tinnitus, hearing loss, delirium, visual changes), fever, hemolytic anemia, thrombocytopenia, rash **Notes:** Follow serum levels (see Table 2, page 265); sulfate salt is 83% quinidine; gluconate salt is 62% quinidine; must use in combination w/ drug that slows AV conduction (eg, digoxin, diltiazem, BB) **Interactions:** ↑ Effects w/ acetazolamide, antacids, amiodarone, azole antifungals, cimetidine, K, macrolides, NaHCO₃, thiazide diuretics, lily-of-the-valley, pheasant's eye herb, scopolia root, squill; ↑ effects of anticoagulants, dextromethorphan, digitalis glycosides, disopyramide, haloperidol, metoprolol, nifedipine, procainamide, propafenone, propranolol, TCAs, verapamil; ↓ effects w/ barbiturates, disopyramide, nifedipine, phenobarbital, phenytoin, rifampin, sucralfate **NIPE:** Take w/ food, ↑ risk of photosensitivity—use sunscreen

Quinupristin–Dalfopristin (Synercid)
Uses: *Infections caused by vancomycin-resistant E. faecium and other gram(+) organisms* **Action:** Inhibits

both the early and late phases of protein synthesis at the ribosomes. *Spectrum:* Susceptible infections due to vancomycin-resistant *Enterococcus faecium,* methicillin-susceptible *Staphylococcus aureus,* and *Streptococcus pyogenes; not* active against *Enterococcus faecalis* **Dose:** *Adults & Peds* 7.5 mg/kg IV q8–12h (use central line if possible); not compatible w/ NS or heparin; flush IV lines w/ dextrose; ↓ in hepatic failure **Caution:** [B, M] **Contra:** Hypersensitivity **Supplied:** Inj 500 mg (150 mg quinupristin/350 mg dalfopristin) **SE:** Hyperbilirubinemia, inf site Rxns and pain, arthralgia, myalgia **Notes:** Multiple drug interactions **Interactions:** ↑ Effects of CCBs, carbamazepine, cyclosporine, diazepam, disopyramide, docetaxel, lovastatin, methylprednisolone, midazolam, paclitaxel, protease inhibitors, quinidine, tacrolimus, vinblastine **Labs:** ↑ LFTs, BUN, creatinine, Hct; ↑ or ↓ serum glucose, K⁺

Rabeprazole (Aciphex)
Uses: *PUD, GERD, ZE* **Action:** Proton pump inhibitor **Dose:** 20 mg/d; may be ↑ to 60 mg/d; ∅ crush tabs **Caution:** [B, ?/–] **Supplied:** Tabs 60 mg **SE:** HA, fatigue, GI upset **Interactions:** ↑ Effects of cyclosporine, digoxin; ↓ effects of ketoconazole **Labs:** ↑ LFTs, TSH **NIPE:** Take w/o regard to food; ↑ risk of photosensitivity—use sunscreen

Raloxifene (Evista)
Uses: *Prevention of osteoporosis* **Action:** Partial antagonist of estrogen that behaves like estrogen **Dose:** 60 mg/d **Caution:** **Contra:** Thromboembolism, PRG **Supplied:** Tabs 60 mg **SE:** Chest pain, insomnia, rash, hot flashes, GI upset **Interactions:** ↓ Effects w/ ampicillin, cholestyramine **NIPE:** ∅ PRG, breast-feeding; take w/o regard to food; ↑ risk of venous thromboembolic effects

Ramipril (Altace)
WARNING: ACEIs used during the 2nd and 3rd tri of PRG can cause injury and even death to the developing fetus **Uses:** *HTN, CHF, DN, post-MI* **Action:** ACEI **Dose:** 2.5–20 mg/d PO ÷ qd–bid; ↓ in renal failure **Caution:** [D, +] **Contra:** ACE-inhibitor-induced angioedema **Supplied:** Caps 1.25, 2.5, 5, 10 mg **SE:** Cough, HA, dizziness, hypotension, renal impairment, angioedema **Notes:** May use in combination w/ diuretics **Interactions:** ↑ Effects w/ α-adrenergic blockers, loop diuretics; ↑ effects of insulin, Li; ↑ risk of hyperkalemia w/ K⁺, K-sparing diuretics, K salt substitutes, trimethoprim; ↓ effects w/ ASA, NSAIDs, food; **Labs:** ↑ BUN, creatinine, K⁺, ↓ Hmg, Hct, cholesterol **NIPE:** ↑ Risk of photosensitivity—use sunscreen; ↓ risk of cough esp w/ capsaicin; take w/o food

Ranitidine Hydrochloride (Zantac)
Uses: *Duodenal ulcer, active benign ulcers, hypersecretory conditions, and GERD* **Action:** H₂-receptor antagonist **Dose:** *Adults.* Ulcer: 150 mg PO bid, 300 mg PO hs, or 50 mg IV q6–8h; or 400 mg IV/d cont inf, then maint of 150 mg PO hs. *Hypersecretion:* 150 mg PO bid, up to 600 mg/d. *GERD:* 300 mg PO bid; maint 300 mg PO hs. *Peds.*0.75–1.5 mg/kg/dose IV q6–8h or 1.25–2.5 mg/kg/dose PO q12h; ↓ dose in renal failure **Caution:** [B, +] **Contra:** Component hypersensitivity **Supplied:** Tabs 75, 150, 300 mg; syrup 15 mg/mL; inj 25 mg/mL **SE:** Dizziness, sedation, rash, GI upset **Notes:**

PO and parenteral doses differ **Interactions:** ↑ Effects of glipizide, glyburide, lido-caine, nifedipine, nitrendipine, nisoldipine, procainamide, TCAs, theophylline, tolbutamide, warfarin; ↓ effects w/ antacids, tobacco; ↓ effects of cefuroxime, cef-podoxime, diazepam, enoxacin, ketoconazole, itraconazole, oxaprozin **Labs:** ↑ SCr, LFTs, false + urine protein **NIPE:** ASA, NSAIDs, EtOH, caffeine ↑ stomach acid production

Rasburicase (Elitek) Uses: *Elevated plasma uric acid due to tumor lysis (peds)* **Action:** Catalyzes uric acid **Dose:** *Peds.* 0.15 or 0.20 mg/kg IV over 30 min, qd × 5 **Caution:** [C, ?/–] Falsely ↓ uric acid values **Contra:** Anaphylaxis, screen for G6PD deficiency to ⊘ hemolysis, methemoglobinemia **Supplied:** 1.5 mg inj **SE:** Fever, neutropenia, GI upset, HA, rash

Repaglinide (Prandin) Uses: *Type 2 DM* **Action:** Stimulates insulin release from pancreas **Dose:** 0.5–4 mg ac, start 1–2 mg, ↑ to 16 mg/d max; take pc **Caution:** [C, ?/–] **Contra:** DKA, type 1 DM **Supplied:** Tabs 0.5, 1, 2 mg **SE:** HA, hyper-/hypoglycemia, GI upset **Interactions:** ↑ Effects w/ ASA, BBs, chloram-phenicol, erythromycin, ketoconazole, miconazole, MAOIs, NSAIDs, probenecid, sulfa drugs, warfarin, celery, coriander, dandelion root, fenugreek, garlic, ginseng, juniper berries; ↓ effects w/ barbiturates, carbamazepine, CCBs, corticosteroids, diuretics, estrogens, INH, oral contraceptives, phenytoin, phenothiazines, rifampin, sympathomimetics, thiazide diuretics, thyroid drugs **NIPE:** Take 15 min before meal; skip drug if meal skipped

Reteplase (Retavase) Uses: *Post-AMI* **Action:** Thrombolytic agent **Dose:** 10 Units IV over 2 min, 2nd dose in 30 min 10 Units IV over 2 min **Cau-tion:** [C, ?/–] **Contra:** Internal bleeding, spinal surgery or trauma, Hx CNS vascu-lar malformations, uncontrolled hypotension, sensitivity to thrombolytics **Supplied:** Inj 10.8 Units/2 mL **SE:** Bleeding, allergic Rxns **Interactions:** ↑ Risk of bleeding w/ ASA, abciximab, dipyridamole, heparin, NSAIDs, oral anticoagu-lants, vitamin K antagonists **Labs:** ↓ Fibrinogen, plasminogen **NIPE:** Monitor ECG during Rx for ↑ risk of reperfusion arrhythmias

Ribavirin (Virazole) Uses: *RSV infection in infants and hepatitis C (in combination w/ interferon alfa-2b)* **Action:** Unknown **Dose:** *RSV:* 6 g in 300 mL sterile water inhaled over 12–18 h. *Hep C:* 600 mg PO bid in combination w/ inter-feron alfa-2b (see Rebetron) **Caution:** [X, ?] **Contra:** PRG, autoimmune hepatitis, CrCl <50 mL/min **Supplied:** Powder for aerosol 6 g; caps 200 mg **SE:** May accu-mulate on soft contact lenses; fatigue, HA, GI upset, anemia, myalgia, alopecia, bronchospasm **Notes:** Aerosolized by a SPAG; monitor Hbg/Hct frequently; PRG test monthly **Interactions:** ↓ Effects w/ Al, Mg, simethicone; ↓ effect of zidovu-dine **Labs:** ↑ Bilirubin, uric acid, ↓ Hmg **NIPE:** ⊘ PRG, breast-feeding; ↑ risk of photosensitivity—use sunscreen; take w/o regard to food

Rifabutin (Mycobutin) Uses: *Prevention of MAC infection in AIDS Pts w/ a CD4 count <100* **Action:** Inhibits DNA-dependent RNA polymerase activity **Dose:** *Adults.* 150–300 mg/d PO. *Peds.* 1 y: 15–25 mg/kg/d PO. *2–10 y:* 4.4–18.8

mg/kg/d PO. *14–16 y:* 2.8–5.4 mg/kg/d PO **Caution:** [B; ?/–] WBC <1000/mm³ or plts <50,000/mm³; ritonavir **Contra:** Hypersensitivity **Supplied:** Caps 150 mg **SE:** Discolored urine, rash, neutropenia, leukopenia, myalgia, ↑ LFTs **Notes:** Adverse effects/drug interactions similar to rifampin **Interactions:** ↑ Effects w/ ritonavir; ↓ effects of anticoagulants, anticonvulsants, barbiturates, benzodiazepines, BBs, clofibrate, corticosteroids, cyclosporine, dapsone, delavirdine, digoxin, eprosartan, fluconazole, hypoglycemics, ketoconazole, nifedipine, oral contraceptives, propafenone, protease inhibitors, quinidine, tacrolimus, theophylline **Labs:** ↑ ALT, AST, alkaline phosphatase **NIPE:** Urine and body fluids may turn reddish brown in color, discoloration of soft contact lenses, use barrier contraception, take w/o food

Rifampin (Rifadin) **Uses:** *TB and Rx and prophylaxis of *N. meningitidis, H. influenzae,* or *S. aureus* carriers* **Action:** Inhibits DNA-dependent RNA polymerase activity **Dose:** *Adults.* N. meningitidis and H. influenzae carrier: 600 mg/d PO for 4 d. *TB:* 600 mg PO or IV qd or 2 ×/wk w/ combination therapy regimen. *Peds.* 10–20 mg/kg/dose PO or IV qd–bid; ↓ dose in hepatic failure **Caution:** [C, +] Amprenavir, multiple drug interactions **Contra:** Hypersensitivity, presence of active meningitidis infection **Supplied:** Caps 150, 300 mg; inj 600 mg **SE:** Orange-red discoloration of bodily fluids, ↑ LFTs, flushing, HA **Notes:** Never use as single agent for active TB; multiple drug interactions **Interactions:** ↓ Effects w/ aminosalicylic acid; ↓ effects of acetaminophen, aminophylline, amiodarone, anticoagulants, barbiturates, BBs, CCBs, chloramphenicol, clofibrate, delavirdine, digoxin, disopyramide, doxycycline, enalapril, estrogens, haloperidol, hypoglycemics, hydantoins, methadone, morphine, nifedipine, ondansetron, oral contraceptives, phenytoin, protease inhibitors, quinidine, repaglinide, sertraline, sulfapyridine, sulfones, tacrolimus, theophylline, thyroid drugs, tocainide, TCAs, theophylline, verapamil, zidovudine, zolpidem **Labs:** ↑ LFTs, uric acid; affects serum folate and vit B₁₂ levels **NIPE:** Use barrier contraception, take w/o food, reddish brown color in urine and body fluids, stains soft contact lenses

Rifapentine (Priftin) **Uses:** *Pulmonary TB* **Action:** Inhibits DNA-dependent RNA polymerase. *Spectrum: M. tuberculosis* **Dose:** *Intensive phase:* 600 mg PO 2×/wk for 2 mo; separate doses by 3 or more days. *Continuation phase:* 600 mg/wk for 4 mo; should be part of 3–4 drug regimen **Caution:** [C, red/orange breast milk] ↓ efficacy of protease inhibitors, antiepileptics, BBs, CCBs **Contra:** Hypersensitivity to rifamycins **Supplied:** 150-mg tabs **SE:** Neutropenia, hyperuricemia, HTN, HA, dizziness, rash, GI upset, blood dyscrasias, ↑ LFTs, hematuria, discolored secretions **Notes:** Monitor LFTs for liver dysfunction

Rimantadine (Flumadine) **Uses:** *Prophylaxis and Rx of influenza A viral infections* **Action:** Antiviral agent **Dose:** *Adults & Peds.* >9 y: 100 mg PO bid. *Peds.* 1–9 y: 5 mg/kg/d PO, 150 mg/d max; use qd in severe renal/hepatic impairment & elderly; initiate w/in 48 h of Sx onset **Caution:** [C, –] W/ cimetidine

Contra: Component and amantadine hypersensitivity **Supplied:** Tabs 100 mg; syrup 50 mg/5 mL **SE:** Orthostatic hypotension, edema, dizziness, GI upset, lowered Sz threshold **Notes:** ⊘ in PRG or breast-feeding **Interactions:** ↑ Effects w/ cimetidine; ↓ effects w/ acetaminophen, ASA

Rimexolone (Vexol Ophthalmic) **Uses:** *Postop inflammation and uveitis* **Action:** Steroid **Dose:** *Adults & Peds.* >2 y: Uveitis: 1–2 gtt/h daytime and q2h at night, taper to 1 gt q4h. *Postop:* 1–2 gtt qid ≤ 2 wk **Caution:** [C, ?/–] Ocular infections **Supplied:** Susp 1%; **SE:** Blurred vision, local irritation **Notes:** Taper dose to zero **NIPE:** Shake well, ⊘ touch eye w/ dropper

Risedronate (Actonel) **Uses:** *Paget's Dz; treat/prevent glucocorticoid-induced osteoporosis or postmenopausal osteoporosis* **Action:** Bisphosphonate; inhibits osteoclast-mediated bone resorption **Dose:** *Paget's:* 30 mg/d for 2 mo. *Osteoporosis Rx/prevention:* 5 mg qd or 35 mg qwk; take 30 min before 1st food/drink of the day; maintain upright position for at least 30 min after **Caution:** [C, ?/–] Ca suppls & antacids ↓ absorption **Contra:** Hypersensitivity, hypocalcemia, esophageal abnormalities, unable to stand/sit for 30 min, ⊘ in CrCl < 30 mL/min **Supplied:** Tabs 5, 30, 35 mg **SE:** HA, diarrhea, abdominal pain, arthralgia; flu-like Sxs, rash, esophagitis, bone pain **Notes:** Monitor LFT, Ca^{2+}, PO^{3+}, K^+ **Interactions:** ↓ Effects w/ antacids, Ca^{2+}, food **Labs:** Interference w/ bone-imaging agents **NIPE:** EtOH intake and cigarette smoking promote osteoporosis

Risperidone (Risperdal) **Uses:** *Psychotic disorders (schizophrenia),* *dementia of the elderly, bipolar disorder, mania, Tourette's disorder, autism* **Action:** Benzisoxazole antipsychotic agent **Dose:** *Adults.* 0.5–6 mg PO bid. *Peds/Adolescents.* 0.25 mg PO bid, titrate up q5–7d; ↓ starting dose in elderly, renal/hepatic impairment **Caution:** [C, –], ↑ hypotension w/ antihypertensives, clozapine **Contra:** Component hypersensitivity **Supplied:** Tabs 0.25, 0.5, 1, 2, 3, 4 mg; soln 1 mg/mL **SE:** Orthostatic hypotension, EPS w/ higher doses, tachycardia, arrhythmias, sedation, dystonias, neuroleptic malignant syndrome, sexual dysfunction, constipation, xerostomia, blood dyscrasias, cholestatic jaundice, weight gain **Notes:** Several weeks to see effect **Interactions:** ↑ Effects w/ clozapine, CNS depressants, EtOH; ↑ effects of antihypertensives; ↓ effects w/ carbamazepine; ↓ effects of levodopa **Labs:** ↑ LFTs, serum prolactin **NIPE:** ↑ Risk photosensitivity—use sunscreen, extrapyramidal effects; may alter body temp regulation

Ritonavir (Norvir) **Uses:** *HIV* **Actions:** Protease inhibitor; inhibits maturation of immature noninfectious virions to mature infectious virus **Dose:** *Adults.* Start at 300 mg PO bid and titrate over 1 wk to 600 mg PO bid (titration ↓ GI SE). *Peds.* ≥2 y: 250 mg/m^2 titrate to 400 mg bid (dose adjustments required w/ amprenavir, indinavir, nelfinavir, and saquinavir; take w/ food) **Caution:** [B, +] W/ ergotamine, amiodarone, bepridil, flecainide, propafenone, quinidine, pimozide, midazolam, triazolam **Contra:** Concurrent ergotamine, amiodarone, bepridil, flecainide, propafenone, quinidine, pimozide, midazolam, triazolam, St. John's wort **Supplied:** Caps 100 mg; soln 80 mg/mL **SE:** ↑ triglycerides, ↑ LFTs, N/V/D/C, abdominal pain, taste perversion, anemia, weakness, HA, fever, malaise, rash, paresthesias **Notes:** Store in refrigerator **Interactions:** ↑ Effects w/ erythromycin, interleukins, grapefruit juice, food; ↑ effects of amiodarone, astemizole, atorvastatin, barbiturates, bepridil, bupropion, cerivastatin, cisapride, clorazepate, clozapine, clarithromycin, despiramine, diazepam, encainide, ergot alkaloids, estazolam, flecainide, flurazepam, indinavir, ketoconazole, lovastatin, meperidine, midazolam, nelfinavir, phenytoin, pimozide, piroxicam, propafenone, propoxyphene, quinidine, rifabutin, saquinavir, sildenafil, simvastatin, SSRIs, TCAs, terfenadine, triazolam, troleandomycin, zolpidem; ↓ effects w/ barbiturates, carbamazepine, phenytoin, rifabutin, rifampin, St. John's wort, tobacco; ↓ effects of didanosine, hypnotics, methadone, oral contraceptives, sedatives, theophylline, warfarin **Labs:** ↑ Serum glucose, LFTs, triglycerides, uric acid **NIPE:** Food ↑ absorption; use barrier contraception; disulfiram-like Rxn w/ disulfiram, metronidazole

Rivastigmine (Exelon) **Uses:** *Mild–moderate dementia associated w/ Alzheimer's Dz* **Action:** Enhances cholinergic activity **Dose:** 1.5 mg bid; ↑ to 6 mg bid, w/ ↑ at 2-wk intervals (take w/ food) **Caution:** [B, ?] BBs, CCBs, smoking, neuromuscular blockade, digoxin **Contra:** Hypersensitivity to rivastigmine or carbamates **Supplied:** Caps 1.5, 3, 4.5, 6 mg; soln 2 mg/mL **SE:** Dose-related GI effects, N/V/D; dizziness, insomnia, fatigue, tremor, diaphoresis, HA **Notes:** Swallow capsules whole, ⊘ break, chew, or crush; ⊘ concurrent EtOH use **Interactions:** ↑ Risk of GI bleed w/ NSAIDs; ↓ effects w/ nicotine; ↓ effects of anticholinergics **NIPE:** Take w/ food

Rizatriptan (Maxalt) (See Table 11, page 283)

Rocuronium (Zemuron) **Uses:** *Skeletal muscle relaxation during rapid-sequence intubation, surgery, or mechanical ventilation* **Action:** Nondepolarizing neuromuscular blockade **Dose:** *Rapid sequence intubation:* 0.6–1.2 mg/kg IV. *Continuous inf:* 4–16 µg/kg/min IV; ↓ in hepatic impairment **Caution:** [C, ?] Aminoglycosides, vancomycin, tetracycline, polymyxins enhance blockade **Contra:** Component or pancuronium hypersensitivity **Supplied:** 10 mg/mL 5,10 mL vials **SE:** BP changes, tachycardia **Notes:** N/A **Interactions:** ↑ Effects w/ MAOIs, propranolol; ↑ vasospastic Rxn w/ ergot-containing drugs; ↑ risk of hyperreflexia, incoordination, weakness w/ SSRIs **NIPE:** Food delays drug action; ⊘ take >30 mg/24 h

Rofecoxib (Vioxx) **Uses:** *Osteoarthritis, RA, acute pain, and primary dysmenorrhea* **Action:** NSAID; COX-2 inhibitor (withdrawn in 2004 by manufacturer due to indications of ↑ cardiac risk w/ long-term use)

Ropinirole (Requip) **Uses:** *Rx of Parkinson's Dz* **Action:** Dopamine agonist **Dose:** Initial 0.25 mg PO tid, w/ weekly ↑ 0.25 mg per dose, to 3 mg **Caution:** [C, ?/–] Severe CV, renal, or hepatic impairment **Contra:** Component hypersensitivity **Supplied:** Tabs 0.25, 0.5, 1, 2, 5 mg **SE:** Syncope, postural hypotension, N/V, HA, somnolence, hallucinations, dyskinesias **Notes:** DC requires a 7-d taper **Interactions:** ↑ Risk of bleeding w/ ASA, NSAIDs, feverfew, garlic, ginger, horse chestnut, red clover, EtOH, tobacco; ↑ effects of amitriptyline, Li, MRX, theophylline, warfarin; ↑ risk of photosensitivity w/ dong quai—use sunscreen, St. John's wort; ↓ effects w/ antacids, rifampin; ↓ effects of ACEIs, diuretics **Labs:** ↑ ALT, AST **NIPE:** Take w/ food

Rosiglitazone (Avandia) **Uses:** Type 2 DM **Action:** ↑ Insulin sensitivity **Dose:** 4–8 mg/d PO or in 2 ÷ doses (w/out regard to meals) **Caution:** [C, –] Not for DKA **Contra:** Active liver Dz, use w/ caution in ESRD (renal elimination) **Supplied:** Tabs 2, 4, 8 mg **SE:** Weight gain, hyperlipidemia, HA, edema, fluid retention, exacerbate CHF, hyper-/hypoglycemia, hepatic damage **Notes:** Take w/ or w/o meals **Interactions:** ↑ Risk of hypoglycemia w/ insulin, ketoconazole, oral hypoglycemics, fenugreek, garlic, ginseng, glucomannan; ↓ effects of oral contraceptives **Labs:** ↑ ALT, total cholesterol, LDL, HDL, ↓ Hmg, Hct **NIPE:** Use barrier contraception

Rosuvastatin (Crestor) **Uses:** *Rx primary hypercholesterolemia and mixed dyslipidemia* **Action:** HMG-CoA reductase inhibitor **Dose:** 5–40 mg PO daily; max 5 mg/d w/ cyclosporine, 10 mg/d w/ gemfibrozil or CrCl < 30 mL/min (Ⓢ Al-/Mg-based antacids for 2 h after) **Caution:** [X,?/–] **Contra:** Active liver Dz or unexplained ↑ LFT **Supplied:** Tabs 5, 10, 20, 40 mg **SE:** Myalgia, constipation, asthenia, abdominal pain, nausea, myopathy, rarely rhabdomyolysis **Notes:** May ↑ warfarin effect; monitor LFTs baseline, 12 wk, then q6mo **Interactions:** ↑ Effects of warfarin; ↑ risk of myopathy w/ cyclosporine, fibrates, niacin, statins **Labs:** ↑ ALT, AST, CK; + urine protein, Hmg; **NIPE:** Ⓢ PRG or breast-feeding

Salmeterol (Serevent) **Uses:** *Asthma, exercise-induced asthma, COPD* **Action:** Sympathomimetic bronchodilator, β₂-agonist **Dose:** *Adults & Peds.* ≥12 y: 1 diskus-dose inhaled bid **Caution:** [C, ?/–] **Contra:** Acute asthma; w/in 14 d of MAOI **Supplied:** Dry powder discus **SE:** HA, pharyngitis, tachycardia, arrhythmias, nervousness, GI upset, tremors **Notes:** Not for acute attacks; should also prescribe short-acting β-agonist **Interactions:** ↑ Effects w/ MAOIs, TCAs; ↓ effects w/ BBs **Labs:** ↓ serum K⁺ **NIPE:** Shake canister before use, inhale q12h, not for acute exacerbations

Saquinavir (Fortovase) **Uses:** *HIV infection* **Action:** HIV protease inhibitor **Dose:** 1200 mg PO tid w/in 2 h pc (dose adjust w/ ritonavir, delavirdine, lopinavir, and nelfinavir) **Caution:** [B, +] W/ rifampin, ketoconazole, statins, sildenafil **Contra:** Hypersensitivity, sun exposure w/o sunscreen/clothing, triazolam, midazolam, ergots **Supplied:** Caps 200 mg **SE:** Dyslipidemia, lipodystrophy, rash, hyperglycemia, GI upset, weakness, hepatic dysfunction **Notes:** Take 2h after meal, Ⓢ direct sunlight **Interactions:** ↑ Effects w/ clarithromycin, delavirdine, erythromycin, indinavir, ketoconazole, nelfinavir, ritonavir, grapefruit juice, food; ↑ effects of astemizole, cisapride, clarithromycin, ergot alkaloids, erythromycin, lovastatin, midazolam, phenytoin, sildenafil, simvastatin, terfenadine, triazolam; ↓ effects w/ barbiturates, carbamazepine, dexamethasone, efavirenz, phenytoin, rifabutin, rifampin, St. John's wort; ↓ effects of oral contraceptives **Labs:** ↑ LFTs, ↓

eutrophils **NIPE:** Use barrier contraception; ↑ risk of photosensitivity—use sunscreen

Sargramostim [GM-CSF] (Prokine, Leukine) Uses: *Myeloid recovery following BMT or chemo* **Action:** Activates mature granulocytes and macrophages **Dose:** *Adults & Peds.* 250 μg/m²/d IV for 21 d (BMT) **Caution:** [C, /–] Li, corticosteroids **Contra:** >10% blasts, hypersensitivity to yeast, concurrent chemo/RT **Supplied:** Inj 250, 500 μg **SE:** Bone pain, fever, hypotension, tachycardia, flushing, GI upset, myalgia **Notes:** Rotate inj sites; use APAP PRN for pain **Interactions:** ↑ Effects w/ corticosteroids, Li **Labs:** ↑ Serum glucose, BUN, creatinine, LFTs; ↓ albumin, Ca²⁺ **NIPE:** ⊘ Exposure to infection

Scopolamine, Scopolamine Transdermal (Scopace, Transderm-Scop) Uses: *Prevent N/V associated w/ motion sickness, anesthesia, and opiates; mydriatic,* cyclplegic, Rx iridiocyclitis **Action:** Anticholinergic, antiemetic **Dose:** 1 patch behind ear q3d; apply > 4 h before exposure: 0.4–0.8 PO, repeat PRN q4–6h; ↓ in elderly **Caution:** [C, +] APAP, levodopa, ketoconazole, digitalis, KCl **Contra:** Narrow-angle glaucoma, GI or GU obstruction, thyrotoxicosis, paralytic ileus **Supplied:** Patch 1.5 mg, tabs 0.4 mg, ophthal 0.25% **SE:** Xerostomia, drowsiness, blurred vision, tachycardia, constipation **Notes:** ⊘ Blink excessively after admin eye drops, wait 5 min to use other eye drops; activity w/ patch requires several hours **Interactions:** ↑ Effects w/ antihistamines, amantadine, antidepressants, disopyramide, opioids, procainamide, quinidine, TCAs, EtOH; ↓ effects of acetaminophen, digoxin, ketoconazole, levodopa, K⁺, phenothiazines, riboflavin **NIPE:** ⊘ DC abruptly; wash hands after applying patch; may cause heat intolerance

Secobarbital (Seconal) [C-II] Uses: *Insomnia,* preanesthetic agent **Action:** Rapid-acting barbiturate **Dose:** *Adults.* 100–200 mg, 100–300 mg preop. *Peds.* 2–6 mg/kg/dose, 100 mg/max; ↓ in elderly **Caution:** [D, +] CYP2C9, 3A3/4, 3A5–7 inducer; ↑ tox w/ other CNS depressants **Contra:** Porphyria, PRG **Supplied:** Caps 100 mg **SE:** Tolerance in 1–2 wk; resp depression, CNS depression, porphyria, photosensitivity **Interactions:** ↑ Effects w/ MAOIs, valproic acid, EtOH, kava kava, valerian; ↑ effects of meperidine; ↓ effects of anticoagulants, BBs, CCBs, CNS depressants, chloramphenicol, corticosteroids, cyclosporine, digitoxin, disopyramide, doxycycline, estrogen, griseofulvin, methadone, neuroleptics, oral contraceptives, propafenone, quinidine, tacrolimus, theophylline **NIPE:** ⊘ PRG, breast-feeding; use barrier contraception

Selegiline (Eldepryl) Uses: *Parkinson's Dz* **Action:** MAOI **Dose:** 5 mg PO bid; ↓ in elderly **Caution:** [C, ?] Meperidine, SSRI, TCAs **Contra:** Concurrent meperidine **Supplied:** Tabs/caps 5 mg **SE:** Nausea, dizziness, orthostatic hypotension, arrhythmias, tachycardia, edema, confusion, xerostomia **Notes:** ↓ carbidopa/levodopa if used in combo **Interactions:** ↑ Risk of serotonin syndrome w/ dextroamphetamine, dextromethorphan, fenfluramine, meperidine, methylphenidate, sibutramine, venlafaxine; ↑ risk of hypertension w/ dextroamphetamine, levodopa, methylphenidate, SSRIs, tyramine containing foods, EtOH, ephedra, ginseng, ma-huang, St. John's wort **Labs:** False ↑ uric acid, urine protein; false + urine ketones, urine glucose

Selenium Sulfide (Exsel Shampoo, Selsun Blue Shampoo, Selsun Shampoo) Uses: *Scalp seborrheic dermatitis,* itching and flaking of the scalp due to *dandruff*; tinea versicolor **Action:** Antiseborrheic **Dose:** *Dandruff, seborrhea:* Massage 5–10 mL into wet scalp, leave on 2–3 min, rinse, and repeat; use 2×/wk, then once q1–4wk PRN. *Tinea versicolor:* Apply 2.5% qd for 7 d on area and lather w/ small amounts of water; leave on skin for 10 min, then rinse **Caution:** [C, ?] **Contra:** Open wounds **Supplied:** Shampoo [OTC] 1, 2.5% **SE:** Dry or oily scalp, lethargy, hair discoloration, local irritation **Notes:** ⊘ Use more than 2×/wk **NIPE:** ⊘ Use on excoriated skin; may cause reversible hair loss; rinse thoroughly after use

Sertaconazole (Ertaczo) Uses: *Topical Rx interdigital tinea pedis* **Action:** Imidazole antifungal. *Spectrum: Trichophyton rubrum, T. mentagrophytes, Epidermophyton floccosum* **Dose:** *Adults & Peds.* > 12: Apply between toes and immediate surrounding healthy skin bid × 4 wk **Caution:** [C, ?] **Contra:** Component allergy **Supplied:** 2% cream **SE:** Contact dermatitis, dry/burning skin, tenderness **Notes:** Use in immunocompetent Pts

Sertraline (Zoloft) WARNING: Closely monitor Pts for worsening depression or emergence of suicidality, particularly in pediatric Pts Uses: *Depression, panic disorders, obsessive–compulsive disorder (OCD), posttraumatic stress disorders (PTSD),* social anxiety disorder, eating disorders, premenstrual disorders **Action:** Inhibits neuronal uptake of serotonin **Dose:** *Adults.* Depression: 50–200 mg PO qd. *PTSD:* 25 mg PO qd ×1 wk, then 50 mg PO qd, max 200 mg/d. *Peds.*6–12 y: 25 mg PO qd. *13–17 y:* 50 mg PO qd **Caution:** [C, ?/–] W/ haloperidol (serotonin syndrome), sumatriptan, linezolid, hepatic impairment **Contra:** MAOI use w/in 14 d; concomitant pimozide **Supplied:** Tabs 25, 50, 100 mg **SE:** Can activate manic/hypomanic state; weight loss; insomnia, somnolence, fatigue, tremor, xerostomia, nausea, dyspepsia, diarrhea, ejaculatory dysfunction, ↓ libido, hepatotoxicity **Interactions:** ↑ Effects w/ cimetidine, MAOIs, tryptophan, St. John's wort; ↑ effects of clozapine, diazepam, hydantoins, sumatriptan, tolbutamide, TCAs, warfarin, EtOH; ↓ effects w/ carbamazepine, rifampin **Labs:** ↑ LFTs, triglycerides, ↓ uric acid

Sevelamer (Renagel) Uses: Reduce serum phosphorus in ESRD **Action:** Binds intestinal phosphate **Dose:** 2–4 capsules PO tid w/ meals; adjust based on serum phosphorus **Caution:** [C, ?] **Contra:** Bowel obstruction **Supplied:** Capsules 403 mg **SE:** BP changes, N/V/D, dyspepsia, thrombosis **Notes:** ⊘ Open or chew capsules; may ↓ fat-soluble vitamin absorption; 800 mg sevelamer = 667 mg Ca acetate **Interactions:** ↓ Effects of antiarrhythmics, anticonvulsants when given w/ sevelamer **Labs:** Monitor serum bicarbonate, Ca, Cl, P **NIPE:** Must be admin with meals, take daily multivitamin, take 1 h before or 3 h after other meds

Sibutramine (Meridia) [C-IV] Uses: *Obesity* Action: Blocks uptake of norepinephrine, serotonin, and dopamine Dose: 10 mg/d PO, may ↓ to 5 mg after 4 wk Caution: [C, –] SSRIs, Li, dextromethorphan, opioids Contra: MAOI w/in 14 d, uncontrolled HTN, arrhythmias Supplied: Caps 5, 10, 15 mg SE: HA, insomnia, xerostomia, constipation, rhinitis, tachycardia, HTN Notes: Use w/ low-calorie diet, monitor BP and HR Interactions: ↑ Risk of serotonin syndrome w/ dextromethorphan, ergots, fentanyl, Li, meperidine, MAOIs, naratriptan, penta-zocine, rizatriptan, sumatriptan, SSRIs, tromethorphan, tryptophan, zolmitriptan, St. John's wort; ↑ effects w/ cimetidine, erythromycin, ketoconazole; ↑ CNS de-pression w/ EtOH NIPE: ⊘ EtOH; take early in the day to avoid insomnia

Sildenafil (Viagra) Uses: *Erectile dysfunction* Action: Smooth muscle relaxation and ↑ inflow of blood to the corpus cavernosum; inhibits phosphodi-esterase type 5 responsible for cGMP breakdown; ↑ cGMP activity Dose: 25–100 mg PO 1 h before sexual activity, max once daily; ↓ if >65 y; ⊘ fatty foods w/ dose Caution: [B, ?] Potent CYP3A4 inhibitors (eg, protease inhibitors) Contra: W/ nitrates; retinitis pigmentosa; hepatic/severe renal impairment Supplied: Tabs 25, 50, 100 mg SE: HA; flushing; dizziness; blue haze visual disturbance (usually reversible) Notes: Cardiac events in absence of nitrates debatable Interactions: ↑ Effects w/ amlodipine, cimetidine, erythromycin, indinavir, itraconazole, ketocona-zole, nelfinavir, protease inhibitors, ritonavir, saquinavir, grapefruit juice; ↑ risk of hypotension w/ antihypertensives, nitrates; ↓ effects w/ rifampin NIPE: High-fat food delays absorption; ↑ risk of cardiac arrest if used w/ nitrates

Silver Nitrate (Dey-Drop, others) Uses: *Removal of granulation tis-sue and warts; prophylaxis in burns* Action: Caustic antiseptic and astringent Dose: Adults & Peds Apply to moist surface 2–3×/wk for several weeks or until ef-fect Caution: [C, ?] Contra: ⊘ use on broken skin Supplied: Topical impregnated applicator sticks, oint 10%, soln 10, 25, 50%; ophth 1% amp SE: May stain tissue black, usually resolves; local irritation, methemoglobinemia Notes: DC if redness or irritation develop; no longer used in US for newborn prevention of gonococo-cal conjunctivitis

Silver Sulfadiazine (Silvadene) Uses: *Prevention & Rx of infection in 2nd- and 3rd-degree burns* Action: Bactericidal Dose: Adults & Peds. Asepti-cally cover the affected area w/ ¹⁄₁₆-in. coating bid Caution: [B unless near term, ?/–] Contra: Infants < 2 mo, PRG near term Supplied: Cream 1% SE: Itching, rash, skin discoloration, blood dyscrasias, hepatitis, allergy Notes: Systemic ab-sorption w/ extensive application

Simethicone (Mylicon) Uses: Flatulence Action: Defoaming action Dose: Adults & Peds. 40–125 mg PO pc and hs PRN Caution: [C, ?] Contra: In-testinal perforation or obstruction Supplied: [OTC] Tabs 80, 125 mg; caps 125 mg; gtt 40 mg/0.6 mL SE: Diarrhea, nausea Notes: Available in combination products OTC Interactions: ↓ Effects of topical proteolytic enzymes

Simvastatin (Zocor) Uses: ↓ Cholesterol Action: HMG-CoA reductase inhibitor Dose: 5–80 mg PO; w/ meals; ↓ in renal insufficiency Caution: [X, –] ⊘ concurrent use of gemfibrozil Contra: PRG, liver Dz Supplied: Tabs 5, 10, 20, 40 mg SE: HA, GI upset, myalgia, myopathy manifested as muscle pain, tenderness or weakness w/ creatine kinase 10× ULN, hepatitis Notes: follow LFTs Interactions: ↑ Effects w/ amprenavir, azole antifungals, cyclosporine, danazol, diltiazem, gemfibrozil, indinavir, macrolides, nefazodone, nelfinavir, ritonavir, saquinavir, verapamil, grapefruit juice; ↑ effects of digoxin, warfarin; ↓ effects w/ cholestyramine, colestipol, fluvastatin, isradipine Labs: ↑ LFTs NIPE: Take w/ food and in the evening; ⊘ PRG, breast-feeding

Sirolimus [Rapamycin] (Rapamune) WARNING: Can cause immunosuppression and infections Uses: Prophylaxis of organ rejection Action: Inhibits T-lymphocyte activation Dose: *Adults.* >40 kg: 6 mg PO on day 1, then 2 mg/d PO. *Adults.* <40 kg: Peds. ≥13 y: 3 mg/m² load, then 1 mg/m²/d (in water or orange juice); ⊘ drink grapefruit juice while on sirolimus); take 4 h after cyclosporine; ↓ in hepatic impairment Caution: [C, ?/–] Grapefruit juice, ketoconazole Contra: Component hypersensitivity Supplied: Soln 1 mg/mL, tab 1 mg SE: HTN, edema, CP, fever, HA, insomnia, acne, rash, ↑ cholesterol, GI upset, ↑ or ↓ K⁺, infections, blood dyscrasias, arthralgia, tachycardia, renal impairment, hepatic artery thrombosis, graft loss and death in de novo liver transplant Notes: Routine levels not needed except in liver failure (trough 9–17 ng/mL) Interactions: ↑ Effects w/ azole antifungals, cimetidine, cyclosporine, diltiazem, macrolides, nicardipine, protease inhibitors, verapamil, grapefruit juice; ↓ effects w/ carbamazepine, phenobarbital, phenytoin, rifabutin, rifapentine, rifampin; ↓ effects of live virus vaccines Labs: ↑ LFTs, BUN, creatinine, cholesterol, triglycerides NIPE: Take w/o regard to food; ⊘ PRG while taking drug and for 12 wk after drug DC

Smallpox Vaccine (Dryvax) Uses: Immunization against smallpox (variola virus) Action: Active immunization (live attenuated vaccinia virus) Dose: *Adults (routine nonemergency)* or all ages (emergency): 2–3 punctures w/ bifurcated needle dipped in vaccine into deltoid, posterior triceps muscle; check site for Rxn in 6–8 d; if major Rxn, site scabs, and heals, leaving scar; if mild/equivocal Rxn, repeat using 15 punctures Caution: [X, N/A] Contra: *Nonemergency use:* Febrile illness, immunosuppression, Hx eczema and their household contacts. *Emergency:* No absolute contraindications Supplied: Vial for reconstitution: 100 million pock-forming Units/mL SE: Malaise, fever, regional lymphadenopathy, encephalopathy, rashes, spread of inoculation to other sites administered; Stevens–Johnson syndrome, eczema vaccinatum w/severe disability

Sodium Bicarbonate [NaHCO₃] Uses: *Alkalinization of urine,* RTA, *metabolic acidosis,* hyperkalemia, TCA OD* Action: Alkalinizing agent Dose: *Adults.* Cardiac arrest: Initiate ventilation, 1 mEq/kg/dose IV; can repeat 0.5 mEq/kg in 10 min once or based on acid–base status. *Metabolic acidosis:* 2–5 mEq/kg IV over 8 h and PRN based on acid–base status. *Alkalinize urine:* 4 g (48 mEq) PO, then 1–2 g q4h; adjust based on urine pH; 2 amp/1 L D$_5$W at 100–250 mL/h V, monitor urine pH and serum bicarbonate. *Chronic renal failure:* 1–3 mEq/kg/d. *Distal RTA:* 1 mEq/kg/d PO. *Peds.* >1 y: Cardiac arrest: See Adult dosage. *Peds.* <1 y: ECC: Initiate ventilation, 1:1 dilution 1 mEq/mL dosed 1 mEq/kg IV; can repeat w/ 0.5 mEq/kg in 10 min ×1 or based on acid–base status. *Chronic renal failure:* See Adult dosage. *Distal RTA:* 2–3 mEq/kg/d PO. *Proximal RTA:* 5–10 mEq/kg/d; titrate based on serum bicarbonate. *Urine alkalinization:* 84–840 mg/kg/d (1–10 mEq/kg/d) in ÷ doses; adjust based on urine pH **Caution:** [C, ?] **Contra:** Alkalosis, hypernatremia, severe pulmonary edema, hypocalcemia **Supplied:** Powder, tabs; 300 mg = 3.6 mEq; 325 mg = 3.8 mEq; 520 mg = 6.3 mEq; 600 mg = 7.3 mEq; 650 mg = 7.6 mEq; inj 1 mEq/1 mL vial or amp **SE:** Belching, edema, flatulence, hypernatremia, metabolic alkalosis **Notes:** 1 g neutralizes 12 mEq of acid; 50 mEq bicarb = 50 mEq Na; can make 3 amps in 1 L D$_5$W to = D$_5$NS w/ 150 mEq bicarb **Interactions:** ↑ Effects of anorexiants; amphetamines, ephedrine, flecainide, mecamylamine, pseudoephedrine, quinidine, sympathomimetics; ↓ effects of BBs, cefpodoxime, cefuroxime, ketoconazole, Li, MRX, quinolones, salicylates, sulfonylureas, tetracyclines **Labs:** False + urinary protein **NIPE:** ⊘ Take w/in 2 h of other drugs; ↑ risk of milk-alkali syndrome w/ long-term use or when taken w/ milk

Sodium Citrate (Bicitra) **Uses:** Alkalinize urine; dissolve uric acid and cysteine stones **Action:** Urinary alkalinizer **Dose:** *Adults.* 2–6 tsp (10–30 mL) diluted in 1–3 oz water pc and hs. *Peds.* 1–3 tsp (5–15 mL) diluted in 1–3 oz water pc and hs; best pc **Caution:** [C, +] **Contra:** Al-based antacids; severe renal impairment or Na-restricted diets **Supplied:** 15- or 30-mL unit dose: 16 (473 mL) or 4 (118 mL) fl oz **SE:** Tetany, metabolic alkalosis, hyperkalemia, GI upset; ⊘ use of multiple 50-mL amps; can cause hypernatremia/hyperosmolality **Notes:** 1 mL = 1 mEq Na and 1 mEq bicarb **Interactions:** ↑ Effects of amphetamines, ephedrine, flecainide, pseudoephedrine, quinidine; ↓ effects of barbiturates, chlorpropamide, Li, salicylates **NIPE:** Dilute w/ water; take pc to ⊘ laxative effect

Sodium Oxybate (Xyrem) [C-III] **Uses:** *Narcolepsy-associated cataplexy* **Action:** Inhibitory neurotransmitter **Dose:** *Adults & Peds.* ≥ 16 y: 2.25 g PO qhs, second dose 2.5–4 h later; may ↑ 9 g/d max **Caution:** [B, ?/–] **Contra:** Succinic semialdehyde dehydrogenase deficiency; potentiates EtOH **Supplied:** 500 mg/mL 180-mL PO soln **SE:** Confusion, depression, diminished level of consciousness, incontinence, significant vomiting, resp depression, psychiatric Sxs **Notes:** May lead to dependence; synonym for γ-hydroxybutyrate (GHB), abused recreationally and as a "date rape drug"; controlled distribution requires prescriber and Pt registration; must be administered when Pt in bed **Interactions:** ↑ Risk of CNS depression w/ sedatives, hypnotics, EtOH **NIPE:** Dilute w/ 2 oz water, ⊘ eat w/in 2 h of taking this drug

Sodium Phosphate (Visicol) Uses: Bowel evacuation prior to colonoscopy **Action:** Hyperosmotic laxative **Dose:** 3 tabs w/ at least 8 oz clear liquid every 15 min (20 tabs total the night before procedure; 3–5 h before colonoscopy, repeat the process) **Caution:** [C, ?] Renal impairment, electrolyte disturbances **Contra:** Megacolon, bowel obstruction, CHF, ascites, unstable angina, gastric retention, bowel perforation, colitis, hypomotility. **Supplied:** Tablets 2 g **SE:** QT prolongation, diarrhea, hypernatremia, flatulence, cramps **Interactions:** May bind with Al- & Mg-containing antacids and sucralfate; ↑ risk of hypoglycemia with bisphosphonates; ↓ absorption of other meds **Labs:** Monitor electrolytes; **NIPE:** Drink clear liq 12 h before start of this med; ⊘ take w/ drugs that prolong QT interval, ⊘ take other laxatives

Sodium Polystyrene Sulfonate (Kayexalate) Uses: *Hyperkalemia* **Action:** Na^+/K^+ ion-exchange resin **Dose:** *Adults.* 15–60 g PO or 30–60 g PR q6h based on serum K^+. *Peds.* 1 g/kg/dose PO or PR q6h based on serum K^+ (given w/agent, eg, sorbitol, to promote movement through the bowel) **Caution:** [C, M] **Contra:** Hypernatremia **Supplied:** Powder; susp 15 g/60 mL sorbitol **SE:** Can cause hypernatremia, hypokalemia, Na retention, GI upset, fecal impaction; enema acts more quickly than PO form; PO route is most effective **Interactions:** ↑ Risk of systemic alkalosis w/ Ca- or Mg-containing antacids **NIPE:** Mix w/ chilled fluid other than orange juice

Sorbitol (generic) Uses: *Constipation* **Action:** Laxative **Dose:** 30–60 mL of a 20–70% soln PRN **Caution:** [B, +] **Contra:** Anuria **Supplied:** Liq 70% soln **SE:** Edema, electrolyte losses, lactic acidosis, GI upset, xerostomia **Notes:** May be vehicle for many liquid formulations (eg, zinc, Kayexalate) **NIPE:** ⊘ Use unless soln clear

Sotalol (Betapace) **WARNING:** Monitor Pts for 1st 3 d of therapy to reduce risks of induced arrhythmia **Uses:** *Ventricular arrhythmias, AF* **Action:** β-Adrenergic-blocking agent **Dose:** *Adults.* 80 mg PO bid; may be ↑ to 240–320 mg/d. *Peds.* Neonates: 9 mg/m² tid. *1–19 mo:* 20 mg/m² tid. *20–23 mo:* 29.1 mg/m² tid. ≥ *2 y:* 30 mg/m² tid; ↓ in renal failure **Caution:** [B (1st tri) (D if 2nd or 3rd tri), +] **Contra:** Asthma, bradycardia, prolonged QT interval, 2nd- or 3rd-degree heart block w/o pacemaker, cardiogenic shock, uncontrolled CHF, CrCl <40 mL/min **Supplied:** Tabs 80, 120, 160, 240 mg **SE:** Bradycardia, CP, palpitations, fatigue, dizziness, weakness, dyspnea **Notes:** Betapace should not be substituted for Betapace AF because of significant differences in labeling **Interactions:** ↑ Effects w/ ASA, antihypertensives, nitrates, oral contraceptives, fluoxetine, prazosin, sulfinpyrazone, verapamil, EtOH; ↑ risk of prolonged QT interval w/ amiodarone, amitriptyline, bepridil, disopyramide, erythromycin, gatifloxacin, haloperidol, imipramine, moxifloxacin, quinidine, pimozide, procainamide, sparfloxacin, thioridazine; ↑ effects of lidocaine; ↓ effects w/ antacids, clonidine, NSAIDs, thyroid drugs; ↓ effects of hypoglycemics, terbutaline, theophylline **Labs:** ↑ BUN, serum glucose, lipoprotein, triglycerides, K⁺, uric acid **NIPE:** May ↑ sensitivity to cold; DC MAOIs 14 d before drug; take w/o food

Sotalol (Betapace AF)
WARNING: To minimize risk of induced arrhythmia, Pts initiated/reinitiated on Betapace AF should be placed for a minimum of 3 d (on their maint dose) in a facility that can provide cardiac resuscitation, continuous ECG monitoring, and calculations of CrCl; Betapace should not be substituted for Betapace AF because of differences in labeling **Uses:** *Maintain sinus rhythm for symptomatic A fib/flutter* **Action:** β-Adrenergic-blocking agent **Dose:** *Adults.* Initial CrCl >60 mL/min: 80 mg PO q12h. *CrCl 40–60 mL/min:* 80 mg PO q2h; ↑ to 120 mg during hospitalization; monitor QT interval 2–4 h after each dose, w/ dose reduction or discontinuation if QT interval >500 ms. *Peds.*Neonates: 9 mg/m² tid. *1–19 mo:* 20 mg/m² tid. *20–23 mo:* 29.1 mg/m² tid. *≥ 2 y:* 30 mg/m² tid; all dosage ranges may be doubled as max daily dose; allow ≥ 36 h between dosage titrations **Caution:** [B (1st tri; D if 2nd or 3rd tri), +] **Contra:** Asthma, bradycardia, prolonged QT interval, 2nd- or 3rd-degree heart block w/o pacemaker, cardiogenic shock, uncontrolled CHF, CrCl <40 mL/min; caution if converting from previous antiarrhythmic therapy **Supplied:** Tabs 80, 120, 160 mg **SE:** Bradycardia, CP, palpitations, fatigue, dizziness, weakness, dyspnea **Notes:** Routinely evaluate renal Fxn and QT interval

Sparfloxacin (Zagam)
Uses: *Community-acquired pneumonia, acute exacerbations of chronic bronchitis* **Action:** Quinolone antibiotic; inhibits DNA gyrase **Dose:** 400 mg PO day 1, then 200 mg q24h × 10 d; ↓ in renal impairment **Caution:** [C, ?/–] W/ theophylline, caffeine, sucralfate, warfarin, and antacids **Contra:** QT prolongation; w/ drugs that prolong QT interval **Supplied:** Tabs 200 mg **SE:** ↑ overall phototoxicity (even from daylight through windows); restlessness, N/V/D, rash, ruptured tendons, ↑ LFTs, sleep disorders, confusion, convulsions **Notes:** Protect from sunlight up to 5 d after last dose **Interactions:** ↑ Effects w/ cimetidine, probenecid; ↑ effects of cyclosporine, diazepam, metroprolol, theophylline, warfarin, caffeine; ↑ risk of prolonged QT interval w/ amiodarone, bepridil, disopyramide, erythromycin, pentamidine, phenothiazines, procainamide, propranolol, quinidine, sotalol, TCAs; ↓ effects w/ antacids, antineoplastics, didanosine, sucralfate **NIPE:** ↑ Risk of tendon rupture & photosensitivity—use sunscreen; take w/o regard to food; ↑ fluids to 2–3 L/d

Spironolactone (Aldactone)
Uses: *Hyperaldosteronism, ascites from CHF or cirrhosis* **Action:** Aldosterone antagonist; K-sparing diuretic **Dose:** *Adults.* 25–100 mg PO qid; CHF (NYHA class III–IV) 25–50 mg/d. *Peds.* 1–3.3 mg/kg/24 h PO ÷ bid-qid. *Neonates.* 0.5–1 mg/kg/dose q8h; w/food **Caution:** [D, +] **Contra:** Hyperkalemia, renal failure, anuria **Supplied:** Tabs 25, 50, 100 mg **SE:** Hyperkalemia and gynecomastia, arrhythmia, sexual dysfunction, confusion, dizziness **Interactions:** ↑ Risk of hyperkalemia w/ ACEIs, K suppls, K-sparing diuretics, ↑ K diet; ↑ effects of Li; ↓ effects w/ salicylates; ↓ effects of anticoagulants

Labs: False ↑ of corticosteroids, digoxin **NIPE:** Take w/ food; ↑ risk of gynecomastia; maximum effects of drug may take 2–3 wk

Stavudine (Zerit) **WARNING:** Lactic acidosis and severe hepatomegaly w/ steatosis and pancreatitis reported **Uses:** *Advanced HIV* **Action:** Reverse transcriptase inhibitor **Dose:** *Adults.* *>60 kg:* 40 mg bid. *<60 kg:* 30 mg bid. *Peds.* Birth–13 d: 0.5 mg/kg q12h. *>14 d and <30 kg:* 1 mg/kg q12h. *≥30 kg:* Adult dose; ↓ in renal failure **Caution:** [C, +] **Contra:** Hypersensitivity **Supplied:** Caps 15, 20, 30, 40 mg; soln 1 mg/mL **SE:** Peripheral neuropathy, HA, chills, fever, malaise, rash, GI upset, anemias, lactic acidosis, ↑ levels on LFTs, pancreatitis **Notes:** Take w/ plenty of water **Interactions:** ↑ Risk of pancreatitis w/ didanosine; ↑ effects w/ probenecid; ↑ effects w/ zidovudine **Labs:** ↑ LFTs **NIPE:** Take w/o regard to food

Steroids, Systemic (See also Table 4, page 271) The following relates only to the commonly used systemic glucocorticoids **Uses:** *Endocrine disorders* (adrenal insufficiency), *rheumatoid disorders, collagen–vascular Dzs, dermatologic Dzs, allergic states, cerebral edema,* nephritis, nephrotic syndrome, immunosuppression for transplantation, hypercalcemia, malignancies (breast, lymphomas), preoperatively (in any Pt who has been on steroids in the previous year, known hypoadrenalism, preop for adrenalectomy), inj into joints/tissue **Action:** Glucocorticoid **Dose:** Varies w/ use and institutional protocols. *Adrenal insufficiency, acute: Adults.* Hydrocortisone: 100 mg IV; then 300 mg/d ÷ q6h; convert to 50 mg PO q8h ×6 doses, taper to 30–50 mg/d ÷ bid. *Peds.* Hydrocortisone: 1–2 mg/kg IV, then 150–250 mg/d ÷ tid. *Adrenal insufficiency, chronic (physiologic replacement):* May need mineralocorticoid suppl such as fludrocortisone acetate. *Adults.* Hydrocortisone: 20 mg PO qAM, 10 mg PO qPM; cortisone 0.5–0.75 mg/kg/d ÷ bid; cortisone 0.25–0.35 mg/kg/d IM; dexamethasone 0.03–0.15 mg/kg/d or 0.6–0.75 mg/m²/d ÷ q6–12h PO, IM, IV. *Peds.* Hydrocortisone 0.5–0.75 mg/kg/d PO tid; hydrocortisone succinate 0.25–0.35 mg/kg/d IM. *Asthma, acute: Adults.* Methylprednisolone: 60 mg PO/IV q6h or dexamethasone 12 mg IV q6h. *Peds.* Prednisolone: 1–2 mg/kg/d or prednisone 1–2 mg/kg/d ÷ qd–bid for up to 5 d; methylprednisolone 2–4 mg/kg/d IV ÷ tid; dexamethasone 0.1–0.3 mg/kg/d divided q6h. *Congenital adrenal hyperplasia: Peds.* Hydrocortisone: Initial dosage 30–36 mg/m²/d PO ÷ ⅓ dose ×AM, ⅔ dose qPM *Maint:* 20–25 mg/m²/d ÷ bid. *Extubation/airway edema: Adults.* Dexamethasone: 0.5–1 mg/kg IM/IV ÷ q6h (start 24 h prior to extubation; continue × 4 more doses). *Peds.* Dexamethasone: 0.1–0.3 mg/kg/d ÷ q6h × 3–5 d (start 48–72h before extubation) *Immunosuppressive/antiinflammatory: Adults & Older Peds.* Hydrocortisone: 15–240 mg PO, IM, IV q12h *Methylprednisolone:* 4–48 mg/d PO, taper to lowest effective dose *Methylprednisolone Na succinate:* 10–80 mg/d IM. *Adults.* Prednisone or prednisolone: 5–60 mg/d PO ÷ qd–qid. *Infants & Younger Children.* Hydrocortisone: 2.5–10 mg/kg/d PO ÷ q6–8h; 1–5 mg/kg/d IM/IV ÷ bid. *Nephrotic syndrome: Peds.* Prednisolone or prednisone: 2 mg/kg/d PO tid–qid until urine is protein-free for 5 d, use up to 28 d; for persistent proteinuria, 4 mg/kg/dose PO qod max 120 mg/d for an additional 28 d; maint 2 mg/kg/dose qod for 28 d; taper over 4–6 wk (max 80 mg/d). *Septic shock* (controversial): *Adults.* Hydrocortisone: 500 mg–1 g IM/IV q2–6h. *Peds.* Hydrocortisone: 50 mg/kg IM/IV, repeat q4–24 h PRN. *Status asthmaticus:* *Adults & Peds* Hydrocortisone: 1–2 mg/kg/dose IV q6h; then ↓ by 0.5–1 mg/kg q6h. *Rheumatic Dz: Adults. Intraarticular:* Hydrocortisone acetate 25–37.5 mg large joint, 10–25 mg small joint; methylprednisolone acetate 20–80 mg large joint, 4–10 mg small joint. *Intrabursal:* Hydrocortisone acetate 25–37.5 mg. *Intraganglial:* Hydrocortisone acetate 25–37.5 mg. *Tendon sheath:* Hydrocortisone acetate 5–12.5 mg. *Perioperative steroid coverage:* Hydrocortisone 100 mg IV night before surgery, 1 h preop, intraop, and 4, 8, and 12 h postop; postop d #1 100 mg IV q6h; postop d #2 100 mg IV q8h; postop d #3 100 mg IV q12h; postop d #4 50 mg IV q12h; postop d #5 25 mg IV q12h; resume prior PO dosing if chronic use or DC if only perioperative coverage required. *Cerebral edema:* Dexamethasone 10 mg IV; then 4 mg IV q4–6h   **Caution:** [C, ?/–] **Contra:** Active varicella infection, serious infection except TB, fungal infections **Supplied: See Table 4, page 271 SE:** All can cause ↑ appetite, hyperglycemia, hypokalemia, osteoporosis, nervousness, insomnia, "steroid psychosis," adrenal suppression **Notes:** Hydrocortisone succinate administered systemically, acetate form intraarticular; **NIPE:** Never abruptly DC steroids, especially in chronic Rx; taper dose

Streptokinase (Streptase, Kabikinase) Uses: *Coronary artery thrombosis, acute massive PE, DVT, and some occluded vascular grafts* Action:
Activates plasminogen to plasmin that degrades fibrin **Dose: Adults.** PE: Load 250,000 Units peripheral IV over 30 min, then 100,000 Units/h IV for 24–72 h. *Coronary artery thrombosis:* 1.5 M Units IV over 60 min. *DVT or arterial embolism:* Load as w/ PE, then 100,000 Units/h for 72 h. **Peds.** 3500–4000 Units/kg IV over 30 min, followed by 1000–1500 Units/kg/h. *Occluded catheter* (controversial): 10,000–25,000 Units in NS to final volume of catheter (leave in place for 1h, aspirate and flush catheter w/ NS) **Caution:** [C, +] **Contra:** Streptococcal infection or streptokinase use in last 6 mo, active bleeding, CVA, TIA, spinal surgery, or trauma in last month, vascular anomalies, severe hepatic or renal Dz, endocarditis, pericarditis, severe uncontrolled HTN **Supplied:** Powder for inj 250,000, 600,000, 750,000, 1,500,000 Units **SE:** Bleeding, hypotension, fever, bruising, rash, GI upset, hemorrhage, anaphylaxis **Notes:** If maint inf inadequate to maintain thrombin clotting time 2–5× control, refer to the package insert for adjustments; antibodies remain 3–6 mo following dose **Interactions:** ↑ Risk of bleeding w/ anticoagulants, ASA, heparin, indomethacin, NSAIDs, dong quai, feverfew, garlic, ginger, horse chestnut, red clover; ↓ effects w/ aminocaproic acid **Labs:** ↑ PT, PTT

Streptomycin Uses: *TB,* streptococcal or enterococcal endocarditis **Action:** Aminoglycoside; interferes w/ protein synthesis **Dose: Adults.** Endocarditis: 1 g q12h 1–2 wk, then 500 mg q12h 1–4 wk; *TB:* 15 mg/kg/d (up to 1 g), directly observed therapy (DOT) 2×wk 20–30 mg/kg/dose (max 1.5gm), DOT 3×wk 25–30

mg/kg/dose (max 1g). **Peds.** 15 mg/kg/d; DOT 2×wk 20–40 mg/kg/dose (max 1 g); DOT 3×wk 25–30 mg/kg/dose (max 1 g); ↓ in renal failure, either IM or IV over 30–60 min **Caution:** [D, +] **Contra:** PRG **Supplied:** Inj 400 mg/mL (1-g vial) **SE:** ↑ incidence of vestibular and auditory toxicity, neurotoxicity, nephrotoxicity **Notes:** Monitor levels peak 20–30 μg/mL, trough < 5 μg/mL; toxic peak > 50, trough > 10 **Interactions:** ↑ Risk of nephrotoxicity w/ amphotericin B, cephalosporins, cisplatin, methoxyflurane, polymyxin B, vancomycin; ↑ risk of ototoxicity w/ carboplatin, furosemide, mannitol, urea; ↑ effects of anticoagulants **Labs:** False + urine glucose, false ↑ urine protein **NIPE:** ↑ fluid intake

Streptozocin (Zanosar) **Uses:** *Pancreatic islet cell tumors* and carcinoid tumors **Action:** DNA–DNA (interstrand) cross-linking; DNA, RNA, and protein synthesis inhibitor **Dose:** Refer to specific protocol; ↓ in renal failure **Caution:** [D, ?/–] **Contra:** Caution in renal failure, PRG **Supplied:** Inj 1 g **SE:** N/V, duodenal ulcers; myelosuppression rare (20%) and mild; nephrotoxicity (proteinuria and azotemia often heralded by hypophosphatemia) dose-limiting; hypo-/hyperglycemia may occur; phlebitis and pain at inj site of inj **Notes:** Monitor renal Fxn **Interactions:** ↑ Risk of nephrotoxicity w/ aminoglycosides, amphotericin B, cisplatin, vancomycin; ↑ effects of doxorubicin; ↓ effects w/ phenytoin **NIPE:** ⊘ PRG, breast-feeding; ↑ fluid intake to 2–3 L/d

Succimer (Chemet) **Uses:** *Lead poisoning (lead levels > 45 μg/mL)* **Action:** Heavy-metal chelating agent **Dose:** *Adults & Peds.* 10 mg/kg/dose q8h × 5 d, then 10 mg/kg/dose q12h for 14 d; ↓ in renal impairment **Caution:** [C, ?] **Contra:** Hypersensitivity **Supplied:** Caps 100 mg **SE:** Rash, fever, GI upset, hemorrhoids, metallic taste, drowsiness, ↑ LFTs **Notes:** Monitor lead levels, maintain adequate hydration, may open capsules **Labs:** False + urinary ketones, false ↑ serum CPK, false ↓ uric acid **NIPE:** ⊘ Take w/ other chelating agents; ↑ fluid intake to 2–3 L/d

Succinylcholine (Anectine, Quelicin, Sucostrin) **Uses:** *Adjunct to general anesthesia to facilitate ET intubation and to induce skeletal muscle relaxation during surgery or mechanically supported ventilation* **Action:** Depolarizing neuromuscular blocking agent **Dose:** *Adults.* 1–1.5 mg/kg IV over 10–30 s, followed by 0.04–0.07 mg/kg PRN or 10–100mcg/kg/min inf. *Peds.* 1–2 mg/kg/dose IV, followed by 0.3–0.6 mg/kg/dose q5min or use of CI ⊘; ↓ in severe liver Dz **Caution:** [C, M] **Contra:** At risk for malignant hyperthermia; myopathy; recent major burn, multiple trauma, extensive skeletal muscle denervation **Supplied:** Inj 20, 50, 100 mg/mL; powder for inj 500 mg, 1 g/vial **SE:** May precipitate malignant hyperthermia, resp depression, or prolonged apnea; multiple drugs potentiate succinylcholine; observe for CV effects (arrhythmias, hypotension, brady/tachycardia); ↑ intraocular pressure, postoperative stiffness, salivation, myoglobinuria **Notes:** May be given IVP or inf or IM in the deltoid **Interactions:** ↑ Effects w/ amphotericin B, aprotinin, BBs, clindamycin, lidocaine, Li, metoclopramide, oral contraceptives, oxytocin, phenothiazines, procainamide, procaine, quinidine, quinine, trimethaphan; ↓ effect w/ diazepam **Labs:** ↑ Serum K⁺

Sucralfate (Carafate) Uses: *Duodenal ulcers,* gastric ulcers, stomatitis, GERD, preventing stress ulcers, esophagitis **Action:** Forms ulcer-adherent complex that protects against acid, pepsin, and bile acid **Dose:** *Adults.* 1 g PO qid, 1 h ac and hs. **Peds.** 40–80 mg/kg/d ÷ q6h; continue 4–8 wk unless healing demonstrated by x-ray or endoscopy; separate from other drugs by 2 h; take on empty stomach ac **Caution:** [B, +] **Contra:** Component hypersensitivity **Supplied:** Tabs 1 g; susp 1 g/10 mL SE: Constipation frequent; diarrhea, dizziness, xerostomia **Notes:** Al may accumulate in renal failure **Interactions:** ↓ Effects of cimetidine, digoxin, levothyroxine, phenytoin, quinolones, quinidine, ranitidine, tetracyclines, theophylline, warfarin **NIPE:** Take w/o food

Sulfacetamide (Bleph-10, Cetamide, Sodium Sulamyd) Uses: *Conjunctival infections* **Action:** Sulfonamide antibiotic **Dose:** 10% oint apply qid and hs; soln for keratitis apply q2–3h based on severity **Caution:** [C, M] **Contra:** Sulfonamide sensitivity; age <2 mo **Supplied:** Oint 10%; soln 10, 15, 30% SE: Irritation, burning, blurred vision, brow ache, Stevens–Johnson syndrome, photosensitivity **Interactions:** ↓ Effects w/ tetracyclines **NIPE:** Not compatible w/ Ag-containing preps; purulent exudate inactivates drug; ↑ risk of photosensitivity—use sunscreen

Sulfacetamide & Prednisolone (Blephamide, others) Uses: *Steroid-responsive inflammatory ocular conditions w/ infection or a risk of infection* **Action:** Antibiotic and antiinflammatory **Dose:** *Adults and Peds.* >2 y: Apply oint to lower conjunctival sac qd–qid; soln 1–3 gtt 2–3 h while awake **Caution:** [C, ?/–] Sulfonamide sensitivity; age <2 mo **Supplied:** Oint sulfacetamide 10%/prednisolone 0.5%, sulfacetamide 10%/prednisolone 0.2%, sulfacetamide 10%/prednisolone 0.25%; susp sulfacetamide 10%/prednisolone 0.25%, sulfacetamide 10%/prednisolone 0.5%, sulfacetamide 10%/prednisolone 0.2% SE: Irritation, burning, blurred vision, brow ache, Stevens–Johnson syndrome, photosensitivity **Notes:** Ophth susp can be used as an otic agent **Interactions:** ↓ Effects w/ tetracyclines **NIPE:** Not compatible w/ Ag-containing preps; purulent exudate inactivates drug; ↑ risk of sensitivity to light; ⊘ DC abruptly

Sulfasalazine (Azulfidine, Azulfidine EN) Uses: *Ulcerative colitis, RA, juvenile RA,* active Crohn's, ankylosing spondylitis, psoriasis **Action:** Sulfonamide; actions unclear **Dose:** *Adults.* Initially, 1 g PO tid–qid; ↑ to a max of 8 g/d in 3–4 ÷ doses; maint 500 mg PO qid. **Peds.** Initially, 40–60 mg/kg/24 h PO + q4–6h; maint, 20–30 mg/kg/24 h PO ÷ q6h. RA >6 y: 30–50 mg/kg/d in 2 doses, start w/ ¼–⅓ described maint dose, ↑ weekly until dose reached at 1 mo, 2 g/d max; ↓ in renal failure **Caution:** [B (D if near term), M] **Contra:** Sulfonamide or salicylate sensitivity, porphyria, GI or GU obstruction; ⊘ in hepatic impairment **Supplied:** Tabs 500 mg; EC tabs 500 mg; PO susp 250 mg/5 mL SE: Can cause severe GI upset; discolors urine; dizziness, HA, photosensitivity, oligospermia, anemias, Stevens–Johnson syndrome **Notes:** May cause yellow-orange skin discoloration or stain contact lenses; ⊘ long sunlight exposure **Interactions:** ↑ Effects of anticoag-lants, hypoglycemics, MRX, phenytoin, zidovudine; ↓ effects w/ antibiotics; ↓ effects of digoxin, folic acid, Fe, procaine, proparacaine, sulfonylureas, tetracaine **Labs:** False + urinary glucose; false ↑ serum conjugated bilirubin, creatinine; false ↓ serum unconjugated bilirubin, K⁺ **NIPE:** Take pc; ↑ fluids to 2–3 L/d; ↑ risk of photosensitivity—use sunscreen; skin & urine may become yellow-orange

Sulfinpyrazone (Anturane) **Uses:** *Acute and chronic gout* **Action:** Inhibits renal tubular absorption of uric acid **Dose:** 100–200 mg PO bid for 1 wk, ↑ PRN to maint of 200–400 mg bid; max 800 mg/d; take w/ food or antacids, plenty of fluids; ⊘ salicylates **Caution:** [C (D if near term), ?/–] **Contra:** ⊘ in renal impairment, ⊘ salicylates; peptic ulcer; blood dyscrasias, near term PRG, hypersensitivity **Supplied:** Tabs 100 mg; caps 200 mg **SE:** N/V, stomach pain, urolithiasis, leukopenia **Notes:** Take w/ plenty of water **Interactions:** ↑ Effects of anticoagulants, hypoglycemics, MRX; ↓ effects w/ ASA, cholestyramine, niacin, salicylates, EtOH; ↓ effects of acetaminophen, BBs, nitrofurantoin, theophylline, verapamil **Labs:** ↓ Serum uric acid **NIPE:** Take w/ food, ↑ fluids to 2–3 L/d

Sulindac (Clinoril) **Uses:** *Arthritis and pain* **Action:** NSAID; inhibits prostaglandins **Dose:** 150–200 mg bid w/ food **Caution:** [B (D if 3rd tri or near term), ?] **Contra:** NSAID or ASA sensitivity, ulcer, GI bleeding **Supplied:** Tabs 150, 200 mg **SE:** Dizziness, rash, GI upset, pruritus, edema, ↓ renal blood flow, renal failure (? fewer renal effects than other NSAIDs), peptic ulcer, GI bleeding **Interactions:** ↑ Effects w/ NSAIDs, probenecid; ↑ effects of aminoglycosides, anticoagulants, cyclosporine, digoxin, Li, MRX, K-sparing diuretics; ↑ risk of bleeding w/ ASA, NSAIDs, EtOH, dong quai, feverfew, garlic, ginger, horse chestnut, red clover; ↓ effects w/ antacids, ASA; ↓ effects of BBs, captopril, diuretics, hydralazine **Labs:** ↑ Serum Cl, Na, glucose, LFTs, PT **NIPE:** Take w/ food; ↑ risk of photosensitivity—use sunscreen; may take several weeks for full drug effect

Sumatriptan (Imitrex) **Uses:** Acute Rx of migraine attacks **Action:** Vascular serotonin receptor agonist **Dose:** *Adults.* SQ: 6 mg SQ as a single dose PRN; repeat PRN in 1 h to a max of 12 mg/24 h. *PO:* 25 mg, repeat in 2 h, PRN, 100 mg/d max PO dose; max 300 mg/d. *Nasal spray:* 1 spray into 1 nostril, may repeat in 2 h to a max of 40 mg/24 h. *Peds. Nasal spray: 6–9 y: 5–20 mg/d. 12–17 y: 5–20 mg, up to 40 mg/d* **Caution:** [C, M] **Contra:** Angina, ischemic heart Dz, uncontrolled HTN, ergot use, MAOI use w/in 14 d **Supplied:** Inj 6 mg/mL; orally disintegrating tabs 25, 50, 100 mg; nasal spray 5, 20 mg **SE:** Pain and bruising at the inj site; dizziness, hot flashes, paresthesias, CP, weakness, numbness, coronary vasospasm, HTN **Interactions:** ↑ Effects of weakness, incoordination and hyperreflexia w/ ergots, MAOIs, and SSRIs, horehound, St. John's wort **NIPE:** Admin drug as soon as possible after onset of migraine

Tacrine (Cognex) **Uses:** *Mild/moderate Alzheimer's dementia* **Action:** Cholinesterase inhibitor **Dose:** 10–40 mg PO qid to 160 mg/d; separate doses from food **Caution:** [C, ?] **Contra:** Previous tacrine-induced jaundice **Supplied:** Caps 10, 20, 30, 40 mg **SE:** ↑ LFT, HA, dizziness, GI upset, flushing, confusion, ataxia, myalgia, bradycardia **Notes:** Serum conc > 20 ng/mL assoc w/ more SE **Interactions:** ↑ Effects w/ cimetidine, quinolones, SSRIs, ↑ effects of BBs, cholinergics, cholinesterase inhibitors, succinylcholine, theophylline; ↓ effects w/ tobacco, food, ↓ effects of anticholinergics, levodopa **Labs:** ↑ ALT **NIPE:** If taken w/ food ↓ drug plasma levels by 30%; may take up to 6 wk for ALT elevations

Tacrolimus [FK 506] (Prograf, Protopic) **Uses:** Prophylaxis against organ rejection, eczema **Action:** Macrolide immunosuppressant **Dose:** *Adults. IV:* 0.05–0.1 mg/kg/d cont inf. *PO:* 0.15–0.3 mg/kg/d ÷ 2 doses. *Peds.* IV: 0.03–0.05 mg/kg/d as cont inf. *PO:* 0.15–0.2 mg/kg/d PO ÷ q 12 h. *Adults & Peds. Eczema:* Apply bid, continue 1 wk after clearing; ↓ in hepatic/renal impairment **Caution:** [C, –] ⊘ use w/ cyclosporine **Contra:** Component hypersensitivity **Supplied:** Caps 1, 5 mg; inj 5 mg/mL; oint 0.03, 0.1% **SE:** Neurotoxicity and nephrotoxicity, HTN, edema, HA, insomnia, fever, pruritus, hypo-/hyperkalemia, hyperglycemia, GI upset, anemia, leukocytosis, tremors, paresthesias, pleural effusion, Szs, lymphoma **Notes:** Monitor drug levels

Tadalafil (Cialis) **Uses:** Erectile dysfunction **Action:** Phosphodiesterase 5 inhibitor **Dose:** *Adults.* 10 mg PO before sexual activity w/o regard to meals (20 mg max); ↓ 5 mg (10 mg max) in renal and mild hepatic insufficiency **Caution:** [B, –] **Contra:** Nitrates, α-blockers (except tamsulosin), severe hepatic insufficiency **Supplied:** 5-, 10-, 20-mg tabs **SE:** HA, flushing, dyspepsia, rhinitis, back pain, myalgia **Notes:** Longest acting of class (36 h) **Interactions:** ↑ Effects w/ ketoconazole, ritonavir, and other cytochrome P450 CYP3A4 inhibitors; ↑ hypotension w/ antihypertensives, EtOH; ↓ effects w/ P450 CYP3A4 inducers such as rifampin, antacids **NIPE:** ↑ Risk of priapism; use barrier contraception to prevent STDs

Talc (Sterile Talc Powder) **Uses:** ↓ recurrence of malignant pleural effusions (pleurodesis) **Action:** Sclerosing agent **Dose:** Mix slurry: 50 mL NS w/5-g vial, mix, distribute 25 mL into two 60-mL syringes, volume to 50 mL/syringe w/ NS. Infuse each into chest tube, flush w/ 25 mL NS. Keep tube clamped and have Pt change positions q15min for 2 h, unclamp tube **Caution:** [X, –] **Contra:** Further surgery on site planned **Supplied:** 5 g powder **SE:** Pain, infection **Notes:** May add 10–20 mL 1% lidocaine/syringe; must have chest tube in place, monitor closely while tube clamped (tension pneumothorax), not antineoplastic

Tamoxifen (Nolvadex) **Uses:** *Breast CA (postmenopausal, estrogen receptor-+), reduction of breast CA in women at high-risk, metastatic male breast CA,* *mastalgia, pancreatic CA, gynecomastia, ovulation induction* **Action:** Nonsteroidal antiestrogen; mixed agonist–antagonist effect **Dose:** 20–40 mg/d (typically 10 mg bid or 20 mg/d) **Caution:** [D, –] **Contra:** Caution in leukopenia, thrombocytopenia, hyperlipidemia **Supplied:** Tabs 10, 20 mg **SE:** Uterine malignancy and thrombotic events noted in breast CA prevention trials; menopausal Sxs (hot flashes, N/V) in premenopausal Pts; vaginal bleeding and menstrual irregularities; skin rash, pruritus vulvae, dizziness, HA, peripheral edema; acute flare of bone metastasis pain and hypercalcemia; retinopathy reported (high dose) **Notes:** ↑ Risk of PRG in premenopausal women by inducing ovulation **Interactions:** ↑ Effects w/ bromocriptine, grapefruit juice; ↑ effects of warfarin, cyclosporine, warfarin; ↓ effects w/ antacids, aminoglutethimide, letrozole, medroxyprogesterone, rifamycins **Labs:** ↑ Ca²⁺, T₄, BUN, creatinine, LFTs **NIPE:** ⊘ PRG or breast-feeding; use barrier contraception; ↑ risk of photosensitivity—use sunscreen

Tamsulosin (Flomax) Uses: ***BPH*** **Action:** Antagonist of prostatic α-receptors **Dose:** 0.4 mg/d PO; ⊘ crush, chew, or open caps **Caution:** [B, ?] **Contra:** Female gender **Supplied:** Caps 0.4, 0.8 mg **SE:** HA, dizziness, syncope, somnolence, ↓ libido, GI upset, retrograde ejaculation, rhinitis, rash, angioedema **Notes:** Not for use as antihypertensive **Interactions:** ↑ Effects w/ cimetidine; ↑ hypotension w/ doxazosin, prazosin, terazosin **NIPE:** Ensure – test results for prostate CA before drug admin

Tazarotene (Tazorac) Uses: ***Facial acne vulgaris; stable plaque psoriasis up to 20% body surface area*** **Action:** Keratolytic **Dose:** *Adults & Peds.* >12 y: *Acne:* Cleanse face, dry, and apply thin film qd hs on acne lesions. *Psoriasis:* Apply hs **Caution:** [X, ?/–] **Contra:** Retinoid sensitivity **Supplied:** Gel 0.05, 0.1% **SE:** Burning, erythema, irritation, rash, photosensitivity, desquamation, bleeding, skin discoloration **Notes:** DC if excessive pruritus, burning, skin redness or peeling occur until Sxs resolve **Interactions:** ↑ Risk of photosensitivity w/ quinolones, phenothiazines, sulfonamides, tetracyclines, thiazide diuretics **NIPE:** ⊘ PRG or breast-feeding; use contraception; use sunscreen for ↑ photosensitivity risk

Tegaserod Maleate (Zelnorm) Uses: ***Short-term Rx of constipation-predominant IBS in women*** **Action:** 5HT4 serotonin agonist **Dose:** 6 mg PO bid pc for 4–6 wk; may continue for 2nd course **Caution:** [B, ?/–] **Contra:** Severe renal, moderate–severe hepatic impairment, Hx of bowel obstruction, gallbladder Dz, sphincter of Oddi dysfunction, abdominal adhesions **Supplied:** Tabs 2, 6 mg **SE:** ⊘ Administer if diarrhea present, as GI motility ↑; DC if abdominal pain worsens **Notes:** Maintain adequate hydration **NIPE:** Take ac

Telithromycin (Ketek) Uses: ***Exacerbation of chronic bacterial bronchitis, sinusitis, community-acquired pneumonia*** **Action:** Ketolide antibiotic, related to macrolides, blocks protein synthesis. *Spectrum:* Gram(+), gram(–) cocci (esp. *H. influenzae, S. pneumoniae, M. catarrhalis, Toxoplasma,* and anaerobic bacteria) **Dose:** *Bronchitis, sinusitis:* 800 mg PO daily × 5d. *Pneumonia:* 800 mg PO daily × 10 d **Caution:** [C, ?] CYP inducers (eg, rifampin, phenytoin, carbamazepine, phenobarbital) may ↓ telithromycin levels, use w/hepatically metabolized drugs **Contra:** W/ cisapride or pimozide, macrolide sensitivity **Supplied:** Tabs 400 mg **SE:** N/V/D, dizziness, prolonged QTc interval, ↑ LFTs **Notes:** Monitor for pseudomembranous colitis **Interactions:** ↑ QT interval & arrhythmias w/ antiarrhythmics, mesoridazine, quinolone antibiotics, thioridazine; ↑ effects of alprazolam, atorvastatin, benzodiazepines, CCBs, carbamazepine, cisapride, colchicine, cyclosporine, digoxin, ergot alkaloids, felodipine, lovastatin, mirtazapine, midazolam, nateglinide, nefazodone, pimozide, sildenafil, simvastatin, sirolimus, tacrolimus, tadalafil, triazolam, vardenafil, venlafaxine, verapamil; ↑ effects with azole antifungals, ciprofloxin, clarithromycin, diclofenac, doxycycline, erythromycin, imatinib, INH, nefazodone, nicardipine, propofol, protease inhibitors, quinidine, verapamil; ↓ effect with aminoglutethimide, carbamazepine, nafcillin, nevirapine, phenobarbital, phenytoin, rifampin, rifamycins **NIPE:** Take w/o regard to food; ⊘ chew or crush tablets.

Telmisartan (Micardis) Uses: *HTN, CHF,* DN **Action:** Angiotensin II receptor antagonist **Dose:** 40–80 mg/d **Caution:** [C (1st tri; D 2nd and 3rd tri), ?/–] **Contra:** Angiotensin II receptor antagonist sensitivity **Supplied:** Tabs 40, 80 mg **SE:** Edema, GI upset, HA, angioedema, renal impairment, orthostatic hypotension **Interactions:** ↑ Effects w/ EtOH; ↑ effects of digoxin; ↓ effects of warfarin **Labs:** ↑ Creatinine, ↓ Hmg **NIPE:** Take w/o regard to food; ⊘ PRG; use barrier contraception

Temazepam (Restoril) [C-IV] Uses: *Insomnia,* anxiety, depression, panic attacks **Action:** Benzodiazepine **Dose:** 15–30 mg PO hs PRN; ↓ dose in elderly **Caution:** [X, ?/–] Potentiates CNS depressive effects of opioids, barbs, EtOH, antihistamines, MAOIs, TCAs **Contra:** Narrow-angle glaucoma **Supplied:** Caps 7.5, 15, 30 mg **SE:** Confusion, dizziness, drowsiness, hangover **Notes:** Abrupt DC after >10 d use may cause withdrawal **Interactions:** ↑ Effects w/ cimetidine, disulfiram, kava kava, valerian; ↑ CNS depression w/ anticonvulsants, CNS depressants, EtOH; ↑ effects of haloperidol, phenytoin; ↓ effects w/ aminophylline, dyphylline, oral contraceptives, oxtriphylline, rifampin, theophylline, tobacco; ↓ effects of levodopa **NIPE:** ⊘ DC abruptly after prolonged use, use in PRG or breast-feeding

Tenecteplase (TNKase) Uses: *Restore perfusion and reduce mortality w/ AMI* **Action:** Thrombolytic; tPA **Dose:** 30–50 mg (see following table)

Tenecteplase Dosing

Weight (kg)	TNKase (mg)	TNKase[a] Volume (mL)
<60	30	6
≥60–70	35	7
≥70–80	40	8
≥80–90	45	9
≥90	50	10

[a]From one vial of reconstituted TNKase.

Caution: [C, ?], ↑ bleeding w/ concurrent NSAIDs, ticlodipine, clopidogrel, GPIIb/IIIa antagonists Contra: Bleeding, CVA, major surgery (intracranial, intraspinal) or trauma w/in 2 mo Supplied: Inj 50 mg, reconstitute w/ 10 mL sterile water SE: Bleeding, hypersensitivity Notes: ⊘ shake when reconstituting; do *not* se D₅W either in the IV line or to reconstitute Interactions: ↑ Risk of bleeding w/ nticoagulants, ASA, clopidogrel, dipyridamole, ticlopidine, vitamin K antagoists; ↓ effects w/ aminocaproic acid NIPE: Eval for S/Sxs bleeding

Fenofovir (Viread) Uses: *HIV infection* Action: Nucleotide RT inhibitor Dose: 300 mg PO qd w/ a meal Caution: [B, ?/–] Didanosine (separate dmin times), lopinavir, ritonavir Contra: CrCl <60 mL/min; caution w/ known isk factors for liver Dz Supplied: Tabs 300 mg SE: GI upset, metabolic syndrome, hepatotoxicity; separate didanosine doses by 2 h Notes: Take w/ fatty meal nteractions: ↑ Effects w/ acyclovir, cidofovir, ganciclovir, indinavir, lopinavir, ritonavir, valacyclovir, food; ↓ effects of didanosine, lamivudine, ritonavir Labs: ↑ LFTs, triglycerides, serum and urine glucose NIPE: Take w/ food, take 2 h before or 1 h after didanosine, lopinavir/ritonavir

Terazosin (Hytrin) Uses: *BPH and HTN* Action: α₁-Blocker (blood vessel and bladder neck/prostate) Dose: Initially, 1 mg PO hs; ↑ 20 mg/d max Caution: [C, ?] ↑ hypotension w/BB, CCB, ACEI Contra: α-Antagonist sensitivity Supplied: Tabs 1, 2, 5, 10 mg; caps 1, 2, 5, 10 mg SE: Hypotension and syncope following 1st dose; dizziness, weakness, nasal congestion, peripheral edema common; palpitations, GI upset Notes: Caution w/1st dose syncope; if for HTN, combine w/ thiazide diuretic Interactions: ↑ Effects w/ antihypertensives, diuretics; ↑ effects of finasteride; ↓ effects w/ NSAIDs, α-blockers, ephedra, garlic, ginseng, saw palmetto, yohimbe; ↓ effects of clonidine Labs: ↓ Albumin, Hmg, Hct, WBCs NIPE: Take w/o regard to food, ⊘ DC abruptly

Terbinafine (Lamisil) Uses: *Onychomycosis, athlete's foot, jock itch, ringworm,* cutaneous candidiasis, pityriasis versicolor Action: Inhibits squalene epoxidase resulting in fungal death Dose: *PO:* 250 mg/d PO for 6–12 wk. *Topical:* Apply to area; ↓ in renal/hepatic impairment Caution: [B, –] May ↑ effects of drug metab by CYP2D6 Contra: Liver Dz or kidney failure Supplied: Tabs 250 mg; cream 1% SE: HA, dizziness, rash, pruritus, alopecia, GI upset, taste perversion, neutropenia, retinal damage, Stevens–Johnson syndrome Notes: Effect may take months due to need for new nail growth; ⊘ use occlusive dressings Interactions: ↑ Effects w/ cimetidine; ↑ effects of dextromethorphan, theophylline, caffeine; ↓ effects w/ rifampin; ↓ effects of cyclosporine Labs: LFT abnormalities

Terbutaline (Brethine, Bricanyl) Uses: *Reversible bronchospasm (asthma, COPD); inhibition of labor (tocolytic)* Action: Sympathomimetic Dose: *Adults.* Bronchodilator: 2.5–5 mg PO qid or 0.25 mg SQ; may repeat in 15 min (max 0.5 mg in 4 h). *Met-dose inhaler:* 2 inhal q4–6h. *Premature labor:* Acutely 2.5–10 mg/min/IV, gradually ↑ as tolerated q10–20min; maint 2.5–5 mg PO q4–6h until term *Peds.* PO: 0.05–0.15 mg/kg/dose PO tid; max 5 mg/24h; ↓ in renal failure **Caution:** [B, +] ↑ toxicity w/MAOIs, TCAs; diabetes, HTN, hyperthyroidism **Contra:** Tachycardia, component hypersensitivity **Supplied:** Tabs 2.5, 5 mg; inj mg/mL; met-dose inhaler **SE:** HTN, hyperthyroidism; high doses may precipitat β₁-adrenergic effects; nervousness, trembling, tachycardia, HTN, dizziness **Notes** Caution w/ DM **Interactions:** ↑ Effects w/ MAOIs, TCAs; ↓ effects w/ BBs **Labs** ↑ LFTs, serum glucose **NIPE:** Take oral dose w/ food

Terconazole (Terazol 7) **Uses:** *Vaginal fungal infections* **Action:** Topi cal antifungal **Dose:** 1 applicatorful or 1 supp intravaginally hs for 3–7 d **Caution** [C, ?] **Contra:** Component hypersensitivity **Supplied:** Vaginal cream 0.4%, vagi nal supp 80 mg **SE:** Vulvar or vaginal burning **Notes:** Insert high into vagin **NIPE:** Insert cream or supp high into vagina, complete full course of Rx, ↻ inter course during drug Rx, ↑ risk of breakdown of latex condoms & diaphragms w drug

Teriparatide (Forteo) **Uses:** *Severe/refractory osteoporosis* **Action** PTH (recombinant) **Dose:** 20 μg SQ qd in thigh or abdomen **Caution:** [C, ?/– **Contra:** Osteosarcoma in animals; ⊘ administer if Paget's Dz, prior radiation bone mets, hypercalcemia; caution in urolithiasis **Supplied:** 3-mL prefilled devic (discard after 28 d) **SE:** Symptomatic orthostatic hypotension on administration N/D, ↑ Ca, leg cramps **Notes:** ⊘ for use > 2 y **Labs:** ↑ Serum Ca²⁺, uric acid, urin Ca²⁺ **NIPE:** ⊘ Take if Hx Paget's Dz, bone mets or malignancy, or Hx radiation therapy; take w/o regard to food; not used to prevent osteoporosis

Testosterone (AndroGel, Androderm, Striant, Testim, Testo derm) [CIII] **Uses:** *Male hypogonadism* **Action:** Testosterone replacement ↑ lean body mass and libido **Dose:** All daily dosing: *AndroGel:* 5g gel. *Andro derm:* two 2.5-mg or one 5-mg patch qd. *Striant:* 30-mg buccal tabs bid. *Testim* one 5-g gel tube. *Testoderm:* one 4- or 6-mg scrotal patch **Caution:** [N/A, N/A] **Supplied:** *AndroGel, Testim:* 5-g gel (50-mg test); *Androderm:* 2.5-, 5-mg patches *Striant:* 30-mg buccal tab; *Testoderm:* 4- or 6-mg scrotal patch **SE:** Site Rxns acne, edema, weight gain, gynecomastia, hypertension, ↑ in sleep apnea, prostate enlargement **Notes:** Injectable testosterone enanthate (Delatestryl; Testro-LA) and cypionate (Depo-Testosterone) require inj every 14-28 d w/ highly variable serum levels; PO agents methyltestosterone and oxandrolone associated w/ hepatitis and hepatic tumors; transdermal/mucosal forms preferred **Interactions:** ↑ Effects o anticoagulants, cyclosporine, insulin, hypoglycemics, oxyphenbutazone; ↑ effects with grapefruit juice; ↓ effects with St. John's wort **Labs:** ↑ AST, creatinine, Hgb Hct, LDL, serum alkaline phosphatase, bilirubin, Ca, K & Na; ↓ HDL, thyroid hor mones **NIPE:** Wear gloves if handling transdermal patches; topical drug may cause virilization in female partners. Apply Testoderm to dry shaved scrotal skin (⊘ use chemical depilatories), Androderm to nonscrotal skin, AndroGel to shoulder and upper arms, buccal system, on gum above incisors

Tetanus Immune Globulin **Uses:** *Passive immunization against tetanus* (suspected contaminated wound and unknown immunization status) **Ac**

ion: Passive immunization **Dose:** *Adults & Peds* 250–500 Units IM (higher doses f delayed therapy) **Caution:** [C, ?] **Contra:** Thimerosal sensitivity **Supplied:** Inj 250-unit vial or syringe **SE:** Pain, tenderness, erythema at inj site; fever, angioedema, muscle stiffness, anaphylaxis **Notes:** May begin active immunization series at different inj site if required **Interactions:** ↓ Immune response when admin w/ Td **NIPE:** Drug does not cause AIDs or hepatitis

Tetanus Toxoid **Uses:** *Tetanus prophylaxis* **Action:** Active immunization **Dose:** Based on previous immunization status **Caution:** [C, ?] **Contra:** Chloramphenicol use, neurologic Sxs w/ previous use, active infection (for routine primary immunization) **Supplied:** Inj tetanus toxoid, fluid, 4–5 Lf Units/0.5 mL; tetanus toxoid, adsorbed, 5, 10 Lf Units/0.5 mL **SE:** Local erythema, induration, sterile abscess; chills, fever, neurologic disturbances **Interactions:** Delay of active immunity if given w/ tetanus immune globulin; ↓ immune response if given to Pts taking corticosteroids or immunosuppressive drugs **NIPE:** Stress the need of timely completion of immunization series

Tetracycline (Achromycin V, Sumycin) **Uses:** *Broad-spectrum antibiotic* **Action:** Bacteriostatic; inhibits protein synthesis. *Spectrum:* Gram(+): *Staphylococcus, Streptococcus.* Gram(–): *H. pylori.* Atypicals: *Chlamydia, Rickettsia,* and *Mycoplasma* **Dose:** *Adults.* 250–500 mg PO bid–qid. *Peds.* >8 y: 25–50 mg/kg/24 h PO q6–12h; ↓ in renal/hepatic impairment **Caution:** [D, +] **Contra:** PRG, antacids, dairy products; children ≤8 y **Supplied:** Caps 100, 250, 500 mg; tabs 250, 500 mg; PO susp 250 mg/5 mL **SE:** Photosensitivity, GI upset, renal failure, pseudotumor cerebri, hepatic impairment **Notes:** Can stain tooth enamel and depress bone formation in children **Interactions:** ↑ Effects of anticoagulants, digoxin; ↓ effects w/ antacids, cimetidine, laxatives, penicillin, Fe suppl, dairy products; ↓ effects of oral contraceptives **Labs:** False – of urinary glucose, serum folate; false ↑ serum glucose; **NIPE:** ⊘ Take w/ dairy products, take w/o food; use barrier contraception

Thalidomide (Thalomid) **Uses:** *Erythema nodosum leprosum (ENL),* graft-versus-host Dz, aphthous ulceration in HIV-+ Pts **Action:** Inhibits neutrophil chemotaxis, ↓ monocyte phagocytosis **Dose:** *GVHD:* 100–1600 mg PO qd. *Stomatitis:* 200 mg bid for 5 d, then 200 mg qd for up to 8 wk. *ENL:* 100–300 mg PO qhs **Cautions:** [X, –] May ↑ HIV viral load; Hx Szs **Contra:** PRG; sexually active males not using latex condoms, or females not using 2 forms of contraception **SE:** Dizziness, drowsiness, rash, fever, orthostasis, Stevens–Johnson syndrome, peripheral neuropathy, Szs **Supplied:** 50-mg cap **Notes:** MD must register w/ STEPS risk management program; informed consent necessary; immediately DC if skin rash develops **Interactions:** ↑ Effects of barbiturates, CNS depressants, chlorpromazine, reserpine, ETOH; ↑ peripheral neuropathy with INH, Li, metronidazole, phenytoin **Labs:** Monitor LFTs, WBC, differential, PRG test before start of therapy & monthly during therapy **NIPE:** If also taking drugs that ↓ hormonal contraceptives (carbamazepine, griseofulvin, phenytoin, rifabutin, rifampin) use two other contraceptive methods; take 1 h pc—food will effect absorption; photosensitivity—use sunscreen; ⊘ PRG & breast-feeding

Theophylline (Theolair, Somophyllin, others) Uses: *Asthma, bronchospasm* Action: Relaxes smooth muscle of the bronchi and pulmonary blood vessels Dose: *Adults.* 900 mg PO ÷ q6h; SR products may be ÷ q8–12h (maint). *Peds.* 16–22 mg/kg/24 h PO ÷ q6h; SR products may be ÷ q8–12h (maint) ↓ dose in hepatic failure Caution: [C, +] Multiple interactions (eg, caffeine, smoking, carbamazepine, barbiturates, BBs, ciprofloxacin, E-mycin, INH, loop diuretics) Contra: Arrhythmia, hyperthyroidism, uncontrolled Szs Supplied: Elixir 80, 150 mg/15 mL; liq 80, 160 mg/15 mL; caps 100, 200, 250 mg; tabs 100, 125, 200, 225, 250, 300 mg; SR caps 50, 75, 100, 125, 200, 250, 260, 300 mg; SR tabs 100, 200, 250, 300, 400, 450, 500 mg SE: N/V, tachycardia, and Szs; nervousness, arrhythmias Notes: See drug levels in Table 2, page 265 Interactions: ↑ effects w/ allopurinol, BBs, CCBs, cimetidine, corticosteroids, macrolide antibiotics, oral contraceptives, quinolones, rifampin, tacrine, tetracyclines, verapamil, zileuton; ↑ effects of digitalis; ↓ effects w/ barbiturates, loop diuretics, thyroid hormones, tobacco, St John's wort; ↓ effects of benzodiazepines, Li, phenytoin Labs: False + ↑ uric acid, ↑ bilirubin, ESR NIPE: Use barrier contraception; take w/ food if GI upset; caffeine foods ↑ drug effects; smoking ↓ drug effects

Thiamine [Vitamin B₁] Uses: *Thiamine deficiency (beriberi), alcoholic neuritis, Wernicke's encephalopathy* Action: Dietary suppl Dose: *Adults.* Deficiency: 100 mg/d IM for 2 wk, then 5–10 mg/d PO for 1 mo. *Wernicke's encephalopathy:* 100 mg IV single dose, then 100 mg/d IM for 2 wk. *Peds.* 10–25 mg/d IM for 2 wk, then 5–10 mg/24 h PO for 1 mo Caution: [A (C if doses exceed RDA), +] Contra: Component hypersensitivity Supplied: Tabs 5, 10, 25, 50, 100, 500 mg; inj 100, 200 mg/mL SE: Angioedema, paresthesias, rash, anaphylaxis w/ rapid IV administration Notes: IV thiamine use associated w/ anaphylaxis Rxn; must give IV slowly Interactions: ↑ Effects of neuromuscular blocking drugs; Labs: False + uric acid; interference w/ theophylline levels

Thiethylperazine (Torecan) Uses: *N/V* Action: Antidopaminergic antiemetic Dose: 10 mg PO, PR, or IM qd–tid; ↓ in hepatic failure Caution: [X, ?] Contra: Phenothiazine and sulfite sensitivity, PRG Supplied: Tabs 10 mg; supp 10 mg; inj 5 mg/mL SE: EPS, xerostomia, drowsiness, orthostatic hypotension, tachycardia, confusion Interactions: ↑ Effects w/ atropine, CNS depressants, epinephrine, Li, MAOIs, TCAs, EtOH; ↑ effects of antihypertensives, phenytoin; ↓ effects of bromocriptine, cabergoline, levodopa Labs: ↑ Serum prolactin level, interferes w/ PRG test NIPE: May cause tardive dyskinesia; ↑ risk of photosensitivity—use sunscreen

6-Thioguanine [6-TG] (Tabloid) Uses: *AML, ALL, CML* Action: Purine-based antimetabolite (substitutes for natural purines interfering w/ nucleotide synthesis) Dose: 2–3 mg/kg/d; ↓ in severe renal/hepatic impairment Caution: [D, –] Contra: Resistance to mercaptopurine Supplied: Tabs 40 mg SE:

Myelosuppression (especially leukopenia and thrombocytopenia), N/V/D, anorexia, stomatitis, rash, hyperuricemia, rare hepatotoxicity **Interactions:** ↑ bleeding w/ anticoagulants, NSAIDs, salicylates, thrombolytics **Labs:** ↑ Serum and urine uric acid **NIPE:** Take w/o food; ↑ fluids to 2–3 L/d; ⊘ exposure to infection

Thioridazine (Mellaril) WARNING: Dose-related QT prolongation **Uses:** *Schizophrenia,* *psychosis* **Action:** Phenothiazine antipsychotic **Dose:** *Adults.* Initially, 50–100 mg PO tid; maint 200–800 mg/24 h PO in 2–4 ÷ doses. *Peds. >2 y:* 0.5–3 mg/kg/24 h PO in 2–3 ÷ doses **Caution:** [C, ?] Phenothiazines, QT_c-prolonging agents, AI **Contra:** Phenothiazine sensitivity **Supplied:** Tabs 10, 15, 25, 50, 100, 150, 200 mg; PO conc 30, 100 mg/mL; PO susp 25, 100 mg/5 mL **SE:** Low incidence of EPS; ventricular arrhythmias; hypotension, dizziness, drowsiness, neuroleptic malignant syndrome, Szs, skin discoloration, photosensitivity, constipation, sexual dysfunction, blood dyscrasias, pigmentary retinopathy, hepatic impairment **Notes:** ⊘ EtOH, dilute PO conc in 2–4 oz liquid **Interactions:** ↑ Effects w/ BBs; ↑ effects of anticholinergics, antihypertensives, antihistamines, CNS depressants, nitrates, EtOH; ↓ effects w/ barbiturates, Li, tobacco; ↓ effects of levodopa **Labs:** False + and − urine bilirubin and amylase; ↑ serum LFTs; **NIPE:** ↑ Risk of photosensitivity—use sunscreen, take w/ food; ⊘ DC abruptly; ↓ temp regulation; urine color change to reddish brown

Thiothixene (Navane) Uses: *Psychotic disorders* **Action:** Antipsychotic **Dose:** *Adults & Peds.* >12 y: Mild–moderate psychosis: 2 mg PO tid, up to 20–30 mg/d. *Severe psychosis:* 5 mg PO bid; ↑ to a max of 60 mg/24 h PRN. *IM use:* 16–20 mg/24 h ÷ bid–qid; max 30 mg/d. *Peds.* <12 y: 0.25 mg/kg/24 h PO ÷ q6–12h **Caution:** [C, ?] **Contra:** Phenothiazine sensitivity **Supplied:** Caps 1, 2, 5, 10, 20 mg; PO conc 5 mg/mL; inj 2, 5 mg/mL **SE:** Drowsiness, EPS most common; hypotension, dizziness, drowsiness, neuroleptic malignant syndrome, Szs, skin discoloration, photosensitivity, constipation, sexual dysfunction, blood dyscrasias, pigmentary retinopathy, hepatic impairment **Notes:** Dilute PO conc immediately before administration **Interactions:** ↑ Effects w/ BBs; ↑ effects of anticholinergics, antihistamines, BBs, CNS depressants, nitrates, EtOH; ↓ effects w/ barbiturates, Li, tobacco, caffeine; ↓ effects of levodopa **Labs:** ↑ Serum glucose, cholesterol; ↓ serum uric acid; false + urinary PRG test **NIPE:** ↑ risk of photosensitivity—use sunscreen; take w/ food; ⊘ DC abruptly; ↓ temp regulation; darkens urine color

Tiagabine (Gabitril) Uses: *Adjunctive therapy in Rx of partial Szs,* bipolar disorder **Action:** Inhibition of GABA **Dose:** *Adults and Peds.* ≥ 12 y: Initially 4 mg/d PO, ↑ by 4 mg during 2nd wk; ↑ PRN by 4–8 mg/d based on response, 56 mg/d max **Caution:** [C, M] **Contra:** Component hypersensitivity **Supplied:** Tabs 4, 12, 16, 20 mg **SE:** Dizziness, HA, somnolence, memory impairment, tremors **Notes:** Use gradual withdrawal; used in combination w/ other anticonvulsants **Interactions:** ↑ Effects w/ valproate; ↑ effects of CNS depressants,

EtOH; ↓ effects w/ barbiturates, carbamazepine, phenobarbital, phenytoin, primidone, rifampin, ginkgo biloba **NIPE:** Take w/ food; ⊘ DC abruptly

Ticarcillin (Ticar) Uses: Infections due to gram(–) bacteria (*Klebsiella, Proteus, E. coli, Enterobacter, P. aeruginosa*, and *Serratia*) involving the skin, bone resp tract, urinary tract, and abdomen, and septicemia **Action:** 4th-gen PCN, bactericidal; inhibits cell wall synthesis. *Spectrum:* Some gram(+), includes strep, fai enterococcus, not MRSA, gram(–), enhanced w/aminoglycoside use, good anaerobes (*Bactericides*) **Dose:** *Adults.* 3 g IV q4–6h. *Peds.* 200–300 mg/kg/d IV ÷ q4–6h; ↓ dose in renal failure **Caution:** [B, +] Penicillin sensitivity **Supplied:** In **SE:** Often used in combination w/ aminoglycosides; interstitial nephritis, anaphylaxis, bleeding, rash, hemolytic anemia **Notes:** Used w/ aminoglycosides **Interactions:** ↑ Effects w/ probenecid; ↑ effects of anticoagulants, MRX; ↓ effects w tetracyclines, ↓ effects of aminoglycosides **Labs:** False ↑ urine glucose, ↑ serum AST, ALT, alkaline phosphatase **NIPE:** Monitor for S/Sxs superinfection; frequen loose stools may be due to pseudomembranous colitis

Ticarcillin/Potassium Clavulanate (Timentin) Uses: *Infections involving the skin, bone, resp tract, urinary tract, and abdomen, and septicemia* **Action:** 4th-gen PCN bactericidal; inhibits cell wall synthesis; clavulanic acid blocks β-lactamase. *Spectrum:* Good gram(+) but not MRSA; good gram(–), and anaerobes **Dose:** *Adults.* 3.1 g IV q4–6h. *Peds.* 200–300 mg/kg/d IV ÷ q4–6h; ↓ dose in renal failure **Caution:** [B, +/–] Penicillin sensitivity **Supplied:** Inj **SE:** Hemolytic anemia **Notes:** Often used in combination w/ aminoglycosides; penetrates CNS w/ meningeal irritation; may cause false + proteinuria **Interactions:** ↑ Effects w/ probenecid; ↑ effects of anticoagulants, MRX; ↓ effects w/ tetracyclines, ↓ effects of aminoglycosides, oral contraceptives **Labs:** False ↑ urine glucose, false + urine proteins **NIPE:** Monitor for S/Sxs superinfection; frequent loose stools may be due to pseudomembranous colitis; use barrier contraception

Ticlopidine (Ticlid) **WARNING:** Neutropenia/agranulocytosis, TTP, and aplastic anemia reported **Uses:** *↓ Risk of thrombotic stroke,* protect grafts status post CABG, diabetic microangiopathy, ischemic heart Dz, DVT prophylaxis, graft prophylaxis after renal transplant **Action:** Plt aggregation inhibitor **Dose:** 250 mg PO bid w/ food **Caution:** [B, ?/–], ↑ toxicity of ASA, anticoagulation, NSAIDs, theophylline **Contra:** Bleeding, hepatic impairment, neutropenia, thrombocytopenia **Supplied:** Tabs 250 mg **SE:** Bleeding, GI upset, rash, ↑ on LFTs **Notes:** Follow CBC 1st 3 mo **Interactions:** ↑ Effects w/ anticoagulants, cimetidine, dong quai, evening primrose oil, feverfew, garlic, ginkgo biloba, ginseng, grapeseed extract, red clover; ↑ effects of ASA, carbamazepine, phenytoin, theophylline; ↓ effects w/ antacids; ↓ effects of cyclosporine, digoxin **Labs:** ↑ ALT, AST, serum alkaline phosphatase, cholesterol, triglycerides **NIPE:** Take w/ food

Timolol (Blocadren) **WARNING:** Exacerbation of ischemic heart Dz following abrupt withdrawal **Uses:** *HTN and MI* **Action:** β-adrenergic receptor blocker, β_1, β_2 **Dose:** *HTN:* 10–20 mg bid, up to 60 mg/d. *MI:* 10 mg bid **Caution:**

C (1st tri; D if 2nd or 3rd tri), +] **Contra:** Uncomplicated CHF, cardiogenic shock, bradycardia, heart block, COPD, asthma **Supplied:** Tabs 5, 10, 20 mg **SE:** Sexual dysfunction, arrhythmia, dizziness, fatigue, CHF **Interactions:** ↑ Effects w/ antihypertensives, ciprofloxacin, fentanyl, quinindine, ↑ bradycardia and myocardial depression w/ cardiac glycosides, diltiazem, tarcine, verapamil; ↑ effects of epinephrine, ergots, flecainide, lidocaine, nifedipine, phenothiazines, prazosin, verapamil; ↓ effects w/ barbiturates, cholestyramine, colestipol, NSAIDs, penicillin, rifampin, salicylates, sulfinpyrazone; ↓ effect of hypoglycemics, sulfonylureas, theophylline **Labs:** ↑ Serum glucose, BUN, K⁺, lipoprotein, triglycerides, uric acid **NIPE:** ⊘ DC abruptly; ↑ cold sensitivity,

Timolol, Ophthalmic (Timoptic) **Uses:** *Glaucoma* **Action:** BB **Dose:** 0.25% 1 gt bid; ↓ to qd when controlled; use 0.5% if needed; 1 gt/d gel **Caution:** C (1st tri; D 2nd or 3rd), ?/+] **Supplied:** Soln 0.25/0.5%; Timoptic XE (0.25, 0.5%) gel-forming soln **SE:** Local irritation. See Timolol **Additional NIPE:** Depress lacrimal sac 1 min after admin to lessen systemic absorption, admin other drops 10 min before gel

Tinzaparin (Innohep) **Uses:** *Rx of DVT w/ or w/out PE* **Action:** LMW heparin **Dose:** 175 Units/kg SQ qd at least 6 d until warfarin dose stabilized **Caution:** [B, ?] Pork hypersensitivity, active bleeding, mild–moderate renal dysfunction **Contra:** Hypersensitivity to sulfites, heparin, benzyl EtOH, HIT **Supplied:** 20,000 Units/mL **SE:** Bleeding, bruising, thrombocytopenia, pain at inj site, ↑ LFTs **Notes:** Anti-Xa levels monitoring tool; no effect on bleeding time, plt Fxn, PT, or aPTT **Interactions:** ↑ Bleeding w/ anticoagulants, cephalosporins, dextran, NSAIDs, penicillins, salicylates, thrombolytics **Labs:** ↑ ALT, AST **NIPE:** ⊘ Rub nj site, admin deep SQ inj, rotate abdominal inj sites

Tioconazole (Vagistat) **Uses:** *Vaginal fungal infections* **Action:** Topical antifungal **Dose:** 1 applicatorful intravaginally hs (single dose) **Caution:** [C, ?] **Contra:** Component hypersensitivity **Supplied:** Vaginal oint 6.5% **SE:** Local burning, itching, soreness, polyuria **Notes:** Insert high into vagina **Interactions:** Risk of inactivation of nonoxynol-9 spermacidal **NIPE:** Insert high into vaginal canal; may cause staining of clothing; refrain from intercourse during drug therapy; risk of latex breakdown of condoms and diaphragm

Tiotropium (Spiriva) **Uses:** Bronchospasm w/ COPD, bronchitis, and emphysema **Action:** Synthetic anticholinergic similar to atropine **Dose:** 1 cap/d inhaled using HandiHaler device, ⊘ use w/spacer **Caution:** [C, ?] BPH, narrow-angle glaucoma, MyG, renal impairment **Contra:** Acute bronchospasm **Supplied:** Caps 18 µg **SE:** URI, xerostomia **Notes:** Monitor FEV₁ or peak flow **Interactions:** ↑ Effects with other anticholinergic drugs **Labs:** Monitor peak flow & PFT **NIPE:** ⊘ For acute resp episode; take daily at same time each day

Tirofiban (Aggrastat) **Uses:** *ACS* **Action:** Glycoprotein IIB/IIIa inhibitor **Dose:** Initial 0.4 µg/kg/min for 30 min, followed by 0.1 µg/kg/min; use in combination w/ heparin; ↓ in renal insufficiency **Caution:** [B, ?/–] **Contra:** Bleed-

ing, intracranial neoplasm, vascular malformation, stroke/surgery/trauma w/in las
30 d, severe HTN **Supplied:** Inj 50, 250 µg/mL **SE:** Bleeding, bradycardia, coro
nary dissection, pelvic pain, rash **Interactions:** ↑ Bleeding risks w/ anticoagulants
antiplatlets, NSAIDs, salicylates, dong quai, feverfew, garlic, ginger, ginkgo, hors
chestnut; ↓ effects w/ levothyroxine, omeprazole **Labs:** ↓ Hmg, Hct, plts; **NIPE:**
⊘ Breast-feeding

Tobramycin (Nebcin) Uses: *Serious gram(–) infections* **Action:**
Aminoglycoside; inhibits protein synthesis. *Spectrum:* Gram(–) bacteria (includin
Pseudomonas) **Dose:** *Adults.* 1–2.5 mg/kg/dose IV q8–24h. *Peds.* 2.5 mg/kg/dos
IV q8h; ↓ w/ renal insufficiency **Caution:** [C, M] **Contra:** Aminoglycoside sensi
tivity **Supplied:** Inj 10, 40 mg/mL **SE:** Nephrotoxic and ototoxic **Notes:** Monitc
CrCl and serum concs for dosage adjustments (see Table 2, page 265) **Interac**
tions: ↑ Effects w/ carbenicillin, NSAIDs, ticarcillin; ↑ nephrotoxic, neurotoxic
and/or ototoxic effects w/ aminoglycosides, amphotericin B, cephalosporins, cis
platin, furosemide, mannitol, methoxyflurane, polymyxin B, urea, vancomyci
Labs: ↑ LFTs, BUN, creatinine, serum protein; ↓ serum K⁺, Na⁺, Ca²⁺, Mg²
NIPE: ↑ Fluids to 2–3 L/d; monitor for superinfection

Tobramycin Ophthalmic (AKTob, Tobrex) Uses: *Ocular bacteria
infections* **Action:** Aminoglycoside **Dose:** 1–2 gtt q4h; oint bid–tid; if severe, us
oint q3–4h, or 2 gtt q30–60min, then less frequently **Caution:** [C, M] **Contra**
Aminoglycoside sensitivity **Supplied:** Oint and soln tobramycin 0.3% **SE:** Ocula
irritation. See Tobramycin. **Additional NIPE:** Depress lacrimal sac for 1 min t
prevent systemic absorption; ↑ risk of blurred vision & burning

Tobramycin & Dexamethasone Ophthalmic (TobraDex
Uses: *Ocular bacterial infections associated w/ significant inflammation* **Action**
Antibiotic w/ antiinflammatory **Dose:** 0.3% oint apply q3–8h or soln 0.3% appl
1–2 gtt q1–4h **Caution:** [C, M] **Contra:** Aminoglycoside sensitivity **Supplied**
Oint and soln tobramycin 0.3% and dexamethasone 0.1% **SE:** Local irritation o
edema **Notes:** Use under ophthalmologist's direction. See Tobramycin. **Additiona**
NIPE: Eval intraocular pressure and lens if prolonged use

Tolazamide (Tolinase) Uses: *Type 2 DM* **Action:** Sulfonylurea; stimu
lates pancreatic insulin release; ↑ peripheral insulin sensitivity at peripheral sites;
hepatic glucose output **Dose:** 100–500 mg/d (no benefit >1 g/d) **Caution:** [C, +/–
Elderly, hepatic or renal impairment **Supplied:** Tabs 100, 250, 500 mg **Notes/SE**
HA, dizziness, GI upset, rash, hyperglycemia, photosensitivity, blood dyscrasia
Interactions: ↑ Effects w/ chloramphenicol, cimetidine, clofibrate, insulin
MAOIs, phenylbutazone, probenecid, salicylates, sulfonamides, garlic, ginseng; ↓
effects w/ diuretics **NIPE:** Risk of disulfiram-type Rxn w/ EtOH; take w/ food; us
sunscreen

Tolazoline (Priscoline) Uses: *Peripheral vasospastic disorders* **Action**
Competitively blocks α-adrenergic receptors **Dose:** *Adults.* 10–50 mg IM/IV/SC
qid. *Neonates.* 1–2 mg/kg IV over 10–15 min, then 1–2 mg/kg/h (adjust w/ ↓ rena

xn) **Caution:** [C, ?] **Contra:** CAD **Supplied:** Inj 25 mg/mL **SE:** Hypotension, peripheral vasodilation, tachycardia, arrhythmias, GI upset, blood dyscrasias, renal failure, GI bleeding **Interactions:** ↓ BP w/ epinephrine, norepinephrine, phenylephrine **NIPE:** Risk of disulfiram-type Rxn w/ EtOH

Tolbutamide (Orinase) Uses: *Type 2 DM* **Action:** Sulfonylurea; ↑ pancreatic insulin release; ↑ peripheral insulin sensitivity; ↓ hepatic glucose output **Dose:** 500–1000 mg bid; ↓ dose in hepatic failure **Caution:** [C, +] **Contra:** Sulfonylurea sensitivity **Supplied:** Tabs 500 mg **SE:** HA, dizziness, GI upset, rash, photosensitivity, blood dyscrasias, hypoglycemia **Interactions:** ↑ Effects w/ anticoagulants, antidepressants, chloramphenicol, insulin, H₂ antagonists, MAOIs, metformin, NSAIDs, phenylbutazone, probenecid, salicylates; ↓ effects w/ BBs, CCBs, cholestyramine, corticosteroids, hydantoins, INH, oral contraceptives, phenothiazines, phenytoin, rifampin, sympathomimetics, thiazides, thyroid drugs **NIPE:** Risk of disulfiram-type Rxn w/ EtOH; take w/ food; use barrier contraception; ↑ risk of photosensitivity—use sunscreen

Tolcapone (Tasmar) Uses: *Adjunct to carbidopa/levodopa in Parkinson's Dz* **Action:** Catechol-O-methyltransferase inhibitor slows metabolism of levodopa **Dose:** 100 mg PO tid w/ first daily levodopa/carbidopa dose, followed by doses 6 and 12 h later; ↓ in renal impairment **Caution:** [C, ?] **Contra:** Hepatic impairment; nonselective MAOI **Supplied:** Tablets 100 mg, 200 mg **SE:** Constipation, xerostomia, vivid dreams, hallucinations, anorexia, N/D, orthostasis, liver failure **Notes:** ⊘ Abruptly DC or ↓ dose; monitor LFTs **Interactions:** ↑ Effects of apomorphine, dobutamine, CNS depressants, desipramine, isoproterenol, levodopa, methyldopa, SSRIs, TCAs, warfarin, EtOH, gout kola, kava kava, St. John's wort, valerian; ↑ risk of hypertensive crisis with nonselective MAO inhibitors phenelzine, tranylcypromine) **Labs:** Monitor AST,ALT **NIPE:** May give w/o regard to food but food ↓ bioavailability of drug, may experience hallucinations

Tolmetin (Tolectin) Uses: *Arthritis and pain* **Action:** NSAID; inhibits prostaglandins **Dose:** 200–600 mg tid; 2000 mg/d max **Caution:** [C (D in 3rd tri or near term), +] **Contra:** NSAID or ASA sensitivity **Supplied:** Tabs 200, 600 mg; caps 400 mg **SE:** Dizziness, rash, GI upset, edema, GI bleeding, renal failure **Interactions:** ↑ Effect of aminoglycosides, anticoagulants, cyclosporine, digoxin, insulin, Li, MRX, K-sparing diuretics, sulfonylureas; ↑ effect w/ ASA, food; ↓ effect of furosemide, thiazides **Labs:** ↑ ALT, AST, serum K⁺, BUN, ↓ Hmg, Hct **NIPE:** Take w/ food if GI upset; ↑ risk of photosensitivity—use sunscreen

Tolnaftate (Tinactin) Uses: *Tinea pedis, tinea cruris, tinea corporis, tinea manus, tinea versicolor* **Action:** Topical antifungal **Dose:** Apply to area bid for 2–4 wk **Caution:** [C, ?] **Contra:** Nail and scalp infections **Supplied:** OTC 1% liq; gel; powder; cream; soln **SE:** Local irritation **Notes:** ⊘ Ocular contact, infection should improve in 7–10 d

Tolterodine (Detrol, Detrol LA) Uses: *Overactive bladder (frequency, urgency, incontinence)* **Action:** Anticholinergic **Dose:** Detrol 1–2 mg PO bid; Detrol LA 2–4 mg/d **Caution:** [C, ?/–] CYP2D6 & 3A3/4 inhibitor **Contra:** Urinary retention, gastric retention, or uncontrolled narrow-angle glaucoma **Supplied:** Tabs 1, 2 mg; Detrol LA tabs 2, 4 mg **SE:** Xerostomia, blurred vision **Interactions:** ↑ Effects w/ azole antifungals, macrolides, grapefruit juice, food; ↑ anticholinergic effects w/ amantadine, amoxapine, bupropion, clozapine, cyclobenzaprine, disopyramide, olanzapine, phenothiazines, TCAs **NIPE:** May cause blurred vision

Topiramate (Topamax) **Uses:** *Adjunctive Rx for complex partial Szs & tonic–clonic Szs,* bipolar disorder, neuropathic pain **Action:** Anticonvulsant **Dose:** *Adults.* Total dose 400 mg/d; see product information for 8-wk titration schedule. *Peds.* 2–16 y: Initially, 1–3 mg/kg/d PO qhs; titrate per product info to 5–9 mg/kg/d; ↓ in renal failure **Caution:** [C, ?/–] **Contra:** Component hypersensitivity **Supplied:** Tabs 25, 100, 200 mg; caps sprinkles 15, 25, 50 mg **SE:** May cause metabolic acidosis, kidney stones; fatigue, dizziness, psychomotor slowing, memory impairment, GI upset, tremor, nystagmus; acute secondary angle closure glaucoma requiring drug DC **Notes:** May be associated w/ weight loss; metabolic acidosis generally responsive to dose reduction or DC; DC requires taper **Interactions:** ↑ CNS effects w/ CNS depressants, EtOH; ↑ effects of phenytoin; ↓ effect w/ carbamazepine, phenytoin, valproate, ginkgo biloba; ↓ effects of digoxin, oral contraceptives **Labs:** ↑ LFTs **NIPE:** Take w/o regard to food; ⊘ DC abruptly; use barrier contraception; ↑ fluids to 2–3 L/d

Topotecan (Hycamtin) **WARNING:** Chemo precautions, bone marrow suppression possible **Uses:** *Ovarian CA (cisplatin-refractory), small-cell lung CA,* sarcoma, pediatric non-small-cell lung CA **Action:** Topoisomerase I inhibitor; interferes w/ DNA synthesis **Dose:** 1.5 mg/m^2/d as a 1-h IV inf for 5 consecutive days, repeated q3wk; ↓ in renal failure **Caution:** [D, –] **Contra:** PRG, breast-feeding **Supplied:** 4-mg vials **SE:** Myelosuppression, N/V/D, drug fever, skin rash **Interactions:** ↑ Myleosuppression w/ cisplatin, other neoplastic drugs, radiation therapy; ↑ in duration of neutropenia w/ filgrastim **Labs:** ↑ AST, ALT, bilirubin **NIPE:** Monitor CBC; ⊘ PRG, breast-feeding, immunizations; ⊘ exposure to infection; use barrier contraception

Torsemide (Demadex) **Uses:** *Edema, HTN, CHF, and hepatic cirrhosis* **Action:** Loop diuretic; inhibits reabsorption of Na$^+$ and Cl$^–$ in ascending loop of Henle and distal tubule **Dose:** 5–20 mg/d PO or IV **Caution:** [B, ?] **Contra:** Sulfonylurea sensitivity **Supplied:** Tabs 5, 10, 20, 100 mg; inj 10 mg/mL **SE:** Orthostatic hypotension, HA, dizziness, photosensitivity, electrolyte imbalance, blurred vision, renal impairment **Notes:** 20 mg torsemide = 40 mg furosemide **Interactions:** ↑ Risk of ototoxicity w/ aminoglycosides, cisplatin; ↑ effects w/ thiazides; ↑ effects of anticoagulants, antihypertensives, Li, salicylates; ↓ effects w/ barbiturates, carbamazepine, cholestyramine, NSAIDs, phenytoin, phenobarbital, probenicid, dandelion **NIPE:** Monitor electrolytes, BUN, creatinine, glucose, uric acid; take w/o regard to food; monitor for S/Sxs tinnitus

Tramadol (Ultram) Uses: *Moderate–severe pain* Action: Centrally acting analgesic Dose: *Adults.* 50–100 mg PO q4–6h PRN, not to exceed 400 mg/d. *Peds.* 0.5–1 mg/kg PO q 4–6h PRN Caution: [C, ?/–] Contra: Opioid dependency; MAOIs Supplied: Tabs 50 mg SE: Dizziness, HA, somnolence, GI upset, resp depression, anaphylaxis (sensitivity to codeine) Notes: ↓ Sz threshold, tolerance or dependence may develop Interactions: ↑ Effects w/ cimetidine, CNS depressants, MAOIs, phenothiazines, quinidine, TCAs, EtOH, St. John's wort; ↑ effects of digoxin, warfarin; ↓ effects w/ carbamazepine Labs: ↑ Creatinine, LFTs, Hmg NIPE: Take w/o regard to food

Tramadol/Acetaminophen (Ultracet) Uses: *Short-term Rx acute pain (<5 d)* Action: Centrally acting analgesic Dose: 2 tabs PO q4–6h PRN; 8 tabs/d max. *Elderly/renal impairment:* Lowest possible dose; 2 tabs q12h max if CrCl <30 Caution: [C, –] Szs, hepatic/renal impairment, r Hx addictive tendencies Contra: Acute intoxication Supplied: Tab 37.5 mg tramadol/325 mg APAP SE: SSRIs, TCAs, opioids, MAOIs ↑ risk of Szs; dizziness, somnolence, tremor, headache, N/V/D, constipation, xerostomia, liver toxicity, rash, pruritus, ↑ sweating, physical dependence Notes: ⊘ EtOH Interactions: ↑ effects w/ cimetidine, CNS depressants, MAOIs, phenothiazines, quinidine, TCAs, EtOH, St. John's wort; ↑ effects of digoxin, warfarin; ↓ effects w/ carbamazepine Labs: ↑ Creatinine, LFTs, ↓ Hmg NIPE: Take w/o regard to food; ⊘ take other acetaminophen-containing drugs

Trandolapril (Mavik) WARNING: Use in PRG in 2nd/3rd tri can result in fetal death Uses: *HTN,* CHF, LVD, post-AMI Action: ACEI Dose: *HTN:* 2–4 mg/d. *CHF/LVD:* 4 mg/d; ↓ in severe renal/hepatic impairment Caution: [D, +] ACEI sensitivity, angioedema w/ ACEIs Supplied: Tabs 1, 2, 4 mg SE: Hypotension, bradycardia, dizziness, hyperkalemia, GI upset, renal impairment, cough, angioedema Notes: Afro-Americans, minimal effective dose is 2 mg vs 1 mg in Caucasians Interactions: ↑ Effects w/ diuretics; ↑ effects of insulin, Li; ↓ effects w/ ASA, NSAIDs; NIPE: ⊘ if PRG or breast-feeding; ⊘ K-containing salt substitutes

Trastuzumab (Herceptin) Uses: *Metastatic breast cancer overexpress the HER2/neu protein* Action: Monoclonal antibody; binds human epidermal growth factor receptor 2 protein (HER2); mediates cellular cytotoxicity. Dose: Refer to specific protocol Caution: [B, ?] CV dysfunction, hypersensitivity/inf Rxns Contra: None known Supplied: Injectable SE: Anemia, cardiomyopathy, nephritic syndrome, pneumonitis Notes: Inf-related Rxns minimized w/ acetaminophen, diphenhydramine, and meperidine Interactions: ↑ Risk of cardiac dysfunction with anthracyclines, cyclophosphamide, doxorubicin, epirubicin; Labs: Monitor cardiac function; NIPE: ⊘ Use dextrose inf soln; ⊘ breast-feed for 6 mo following drug therapy

Trazodone (Desyrel) Uses: *Depression,* hypnotic, augment other antidepressants Action: Antidepressant; inhibits reuptake of serotonin and norepinephrine Dose: *Adults & Adolescents.* 50–150 mg PO qd–qid; max 600 mg/d. *Sleep:* 50

mg PO, qhs, PRN **Caution:** [C, ?/–] **Contra:** Component hypersensitivity **Supplied:** Tabs 50, 100, 150, 300 mg **SE:** Dizziness, HA, sedation, nausea, xerostomia, syncope, confusion, tremor, hepatitis, EPS **Notes:** May take 1–2 wk for symptomatic improvement **Interactions:** ↑ Effects w/ fluoxetine, phenothiazine; ↑ risk of serotonin syndrome w/ MAOIs, SSRIs, venlafaxine, St. John's wort; ↑ CNS depression w/ barbiturates, CNS depressants, opioids, sedatives, EtOH; ↑ hypotension w/ antihypertensive, neuroleptics; nitrates, EtOH; ↑ effects of clonidine, digoxin, phenytoin; ↓ effects w/ carbamazepine **NIPE:** Take w/ food; ↑ fluids to 2–3 L/d; ⊘ DC abruptly; ↑ risk of priapism

Treprostinil Sodium (Remodulin) Uses: *NYHA class II–IV pulmonary arterial hypertension* **Action:** Vasodilation, inhibition of plt aggregation **Dose:** 0.625–1.25 ng/kg/min cont inf **Caution:** [B, ?/–] **Contra:** Component hypersensitivity **Supplied:** 1, 2.5, 5, 10 mg/mL inj **SE:** Additive effects w/ anticoagulants, antihypertensives; inf site Rxns **Notes:** Initiate in monitored setting; ⊘ DC or reduce dose abruptly **Interactions:** ↑ Effects w/ antihypertensives; ↑ effects of anticoagulants **NIPE:** Teach care of inf site and pump; use barrier contraception; once med vial used discard after 14 d

Tretinoin, Topical [Retinoic Acid] (Retin-A, Avita, Renova) Uses: *Acne vulgaris, sun-damaged skin, wrinkles* (photoaging), some skin CA **Action:** Exfoliant retinoic acid derivative **Dose:** *Adults & Peds.* >12 y: Apply qd hs (if irritation develops, ↓ frequency). *Photoaging:* Start w/ 0.025%, ↑ to 0.1% over several months (apply only q3d if on neck area; dark skin may require bid application) **Caution:** [C, ?] **Contra:** Retinoid sensitivity **Supplied:** Cream 0.025, 0.05, 0.1%; gel 0.01, 0.025, 0.1%; microformulation gel 0.1%; liq 0.05% **SE:** ⊘ sunlight; edema; skin dryness, erythema, scaling, changes in pigmentation, stinging, photosensitivity **Interactions:** ↑ photosensitivity w/ quinolones, phenothiazines, sulfonamides, tetracyclines, thiazides, dong quai, St. John's wort; ↑ skin irritation w/ topical sulfur, resorcinol, benzoyl peroxide, salicylic acid; ↑ effects w/ vitamin A suppl and foods w/ excess vitamin A such as fish oils **NIPE:** ⊘ Apply to mucous membranes, wash skin and apply med after 30 min, wash hands after application; ⊘ breast-feeding, PRG use contraception; use sunscreen

Triamcinolone (Azmacort) Uses: *Chronic asthma* **Actions:** Topical steroid **Dose:** Two inhalations tid–qid or 4 inhal bid **Caution:** [C, ?] **SE:** Cough, oral candidiasis **Contra:** Component hypersensitivity **Supplied:** Inhaler 100 μg/met spray **Notes:** Instruct Pts to rinse their mouth after use; not for acute asthma **Interactions:** ↑ Effects w/ salmeterol, troleandomycin; ↓ effects with barbiturates, hydantoins, phenytoin, rifampin; ↓ effects of diuretics, insulin, oral hypoglycemics, K suppl, salicylates, somatrem, live virus vaccines **Labs:** ↑ serum glucose, lipids, amylase, sodium; ↓ skin test reaction, serum Ca, K⁺, thyroxine **NIPE:** Use bronchodilator several minutes before triamcinolone; allow 1 min between repeat inhalations

riamcinolone & Nystatin (Mycolog-II) Uses: *Cutaneous candidi-
sis* **Action:** Antifungal and antiinflammatory **Dose:** Apply lightly to area bid;
ax 25 mg/d **Caution:** [C, ?] **Contra:** Varicella; systemic fungal infections **Sup-
lied:** Cream and oint 15, 30, 60, 120 mg **SE:** Local irritation, hypertrichosis,
hanges in pigmentation **Notes:** For short-term use (<7 d) **Interactions:** ↓ Effects
/ barbiturates, phenytoin, rifampin; ↓ effects of salicylates, vaccines **NIPE:** ⊘
yes; ⊘ apply to open skin/wounds, eyes, mucous membranes

riamterene (Dyrenium) Uses: *Edema associated w/ CHF, cirrhosis*
ction: K-sparing diuretic **Dose:** *Adults.* 100–300 mg/24 h PO ÷ qd–bid. *Peds.*2–4
ng/kg/d in 1–2 ÷ doses; ↓ dose in renal/hepatic impairment **Caution:** [B (manu-
acturer; D expert opinion), ?/–] **Contra:** Hyperkalemia, renal impairment, DM;
aution w/ other K-sparing diuretics **Supplied:** Caps 50, 100 mg **SE:** Hyper-
alemia, blood dyscrasias, liver damage, and other Rxns **Interactions:** ↑ Risk of
yperkalemia w/ ACEIs, K suppls, K-sparing drugs, K-containing drugs, K salt
ubstitutes; ↑ effects w/ cimetidine, indomethacin; ↑ effects of amantadine, antihy-
ertensives, Li; ↓ effects of digitalis **Labs:** False ↑ serum digoxin **NIPE:** Take w/
ood, blue discoloration of urine, ↑ risk of photosensitivity—use sunscreen

riazolam (Halcion) [C-IV] Uses: *Short-term management of insom-
ia* **Action:** Benzodiazepine **Dose:** 0.125–0.25 mg/d PO hs PRN; ↓ dose in el-
erly **Caution:** [X, ?/–] **Contra:** Narrow-angle glaucoma; cirrhosis; concurrent
mprenavir, ritonavir, or nelfinavir **Supplied:** Tabs 0.125, 0.25 mg **SE:** Tachycar-
ia, CP, drowsiness, fatigue, memory impairment, GI upset **Notes:** Additive CNS
epression w/ EtOH and other CNS depressants **Interactions:** ↑ Effects w/ azole
ntifungals, cimetidine, clarithromycin, ciprofloxin, CNS depressants, disulfiram,
igoxin, erythromycin, fluvoxamine, INH, protease inhibitors, troleandomycin, ve-
apamil, EtOH, grapefruit juice, kava kava, valerian; ↓ effects of levodopa; ↓ ef-
ects w/ carbamazepine, phenytoin, rifampin, theophylline **NIPE:** ⊘ PRG or
reast-feeding; ⊘ DC abruptly after long-term use

riethanolamine (Cerumenex) [OTC] Uses: *Cerumen (ear wax) re-
noval* **Action:** Ceruminolytic agent **Dose:** Fill the ear canal and insert the cotton
lug; irrigate w/ water after 15 min; repeat PRN **Caution:** [C, ?] **Contra:** Perfo-
ated tympanic membrane, otitis media **Supplied:** Soln 6, 12 mL **SE:** Local der-
natitis, pain, erythema, pruritus **NIPE:** Warm soln to body temp before use for
etter effect

riethylenetriphosphamide (Thio-Tepa, Tespa, TSPA) Uses:
Hodgkin's and NHLs; leukemia; breast, ovarian, and bladder CAs (IV and in-
ravesical therapy), preparative regimens for allogeneic and ABMT in high doses
Action: Polyfunctional alkylating agent **Dose:** 0.5 mg/kg q1–4wk, 6 mg/m² IM or
V ×4 d q2–4wk, 15–35 mg/m² by cont IV infd over 48 h; 60 mg into the bladder
and retained 2 h q1–4wk; 900–125 mg/m² in ABMT regimens (highest dose w/o
ABMT is 180 mg/m²); 1–10 mg/m² (typically 15 mg) IT 1 or 2 ×/wk; 0.8 mg/kg in

1–2 L of soln may be instilled intraperitoneally; ↓ in renal failure **Caution:** [D, **Contra:** Component hypersensitivity **Supplied:** Inj 15 mg **SE:** Myelosuppressio N/V, dizziness, HA, allergy, paresthesias, alopecia

Trifluoperazine (Stelazine) **Uses:** *Psychotic disorders* **Action:** Ph nothiazine; blocks postsynaptic CNS dopaminergic receptors in the brain **Dose Adults.** 2–10 mg PO bid. **Peds.** 6–12 y: 1 mg PO qd–bid initially, gradually ↑ to mg/d; ↓ dose in elderly/debilitated Pts **Caution:** [C, ?/–] **Contra:** Hx bloc dyscrasias; phenothiazine sensitivity **Supplied:** Tabs 1, 2, 5, 10 mg; PO conc mg/mL; inj 2 mg/mL **SE:** Orthostatic hypotension, EPS, dizziness, neuroleptic ma lignant syndrome, skin discoloration, lowered Sz threshold, photosensitivity, bloc dyscrasias **Notes:** PO conc must be diluted to 60 mL or more prior to administra tion; requires several weeks for onset of effects

Trifluridine (Viroptic) **Uses:** *Herpes simplex keratitis and conjunctivitis **Action:** Antiviral **Dose:** 1 gt q2h (max 9 gtt/d); ↓ to 1 gt q4h after healing begin treat up to 14 d **Caution:** [C, M] **Contra:** Component hypersensitivity **Supplied** Soln 1% **SE:** Local burning, stinging **Interactions:** ↑ Hypotensive effects w/ ant hypertensives, nitrates, sulfadoxine-pyrimethamine, EtOH; ↑ effects of anticholiner gics; ↑ CNS depression w/ antihistamines, CNS depressants, narcotics, EtOH; effects w/ barbiturates, Li, caffeine, tobacco; ↓ effects of guanadrel, guanethidine levodopa **Labs:** ↑ LFTs, serum prolactin levels, ↓ Hmg, Hct, plts, false PRG test re sults + or – **NIPE:** Use sunscreen due to photosensitivity; affects body temperatu regulation; reddish brown urine color change; ⊘ DC abruptly after long-term use

Trihexyphenidyl (Artane) **Uses:** *Parkinson's Dz* **Action:** Blocks ex cess acetylcholine at cerebral synapses **Dose:** 2–5 mg PO qd–qid **Caution:** [C, + **Contra:** Narrow-angle glaucoma, GI obstruction, MyG, bladder obstructions **Sup plied:** Tabs 2, 5 mg; SR caps 5 mg; elixir 2 mg/5 mL **SE:** Dry skin, constipation xerostomia, photosensitivity, tachycardia, arrhythmias **Interactions:** ↑ Effects w MAOIs, phenothiazines, quinidine, TCAs; ↑ effects of amantadine, anticholiner gics, digoxin; ↓ effects w/ antacids, tacrine; ↓ effects of chlorpromazine, haloper dol, tacrine **Labs:** False ↑ T3, T4 **NIPE:** Take w/ food; monitor for urinar hesitancy or retention; ⊘ DC abruptly; ↑ risk of heat stroke

Trimethobenzamide (Tigan) **Uses:** *N/V* **Action:** Inhibits medullar chemoreceptor trigger zone **Dose:** **Adults.** 250 mg PO or 200 mg PR or IM tid–q PRN. **Peds.** 20 mg/kg/24 h PO or 15 mg/kg/24 h PR or IM in 3–4 ÷ doses **Caution** [C, ?] **Contra:** Benzocaine sensitivity **Supplied:** Caps 100, 250 mg; supp 100, 20 mg; inj 100 mg/mL **SE:** Drowsiness, hypotension, dizziness; hepatic impairmen blood dyscrasias, Szs, parkinsonian-like syndrome **Notes:** In the presence of vira infections, may mask emesis or mimic CNS effects of Reye's syndrome **Interac tions:** ↑ CNS depression w/ antidepressants, antihistamines, opioids, sedatives EtOH; ↑ risk of extrapyramidal effects

Trimethoprim (Trimpex, Proloprim) **Uses:** *UTI due to susceptibl gram(+) and gram(–) organisms;* suppression of UTI **Action:** Inhibits dihydrofo te reductase. *Spectrum:* Many gram(+) and (–) except *Bacteroides, Branhamella, rucella, Chlamydia, Clostridium, Mycobacterium, Mycoplasma, Nocardia, Neiseria, Pseudomonas,* and *Treponema* **Dose:** *Adults.* 100 mg/d PO bid or 200 mg/d O. **Peds.**4 mg/kg/d in 2 ÷ doses; ↓ in renal failure **Caution:** [C, +] **Contra:** legaloblastic anemia due to folate deficiency **Supplied:** Tabs 100, 200 mg; PO oln 50 mg/5 mL **SE:** Rash, pruritus, megaloblastic anemia, hepatic impairment, lood dyscrasias **Notes:** Take w/ plenty of water **Interactions:** ↑ Effects w/ dapone; ↑ effects of dapsone, phenytoin, procainamide; ↓ efficacy w/ rifampin **Labs:** LFTs, BUN, creatinine **NIPE:** ↑ Fluids to 2–3 L/d; ↑ risk of folic acid deficiency

rimethoprim (TMP)–Sulfamethoxazole (SMX) [Co-Trimoxa-zole] (Bactrim, Septra) **Uses:** *UTI Rx and prophylaxis, otitis media, siusitis, bronchitis* **Action:** SMX-inhibiting synthesis of dihydrofolic acid; MP-inhibiting dihydrofolate reductase to impair protein synthesis. *Spectrum:* Inludes *Shigella, P. jiroveci* (formerly *carinii*), and *Nocardia* infections, *Myoplasma, Enterobacter* sp, *Staphylococcus, Streptococcus,* and more **Dose:** **dults.** 1 DS tab PO bid or 5–20 mg/kg/24 h (based on TMP) IV in 3–4 ÷ doses. *P. roveci:* 15–20 mg/kg/d IV or PO (TMP) in 4 ÷ doses. *Nocardia:* 10–15 mg/kg/d V or PO (TMP) in 4 ÷ doses. *UTI prophylaxis:* 1 PO qd. **Peds.**8–10 mg/kg/24 h TMP) PO ÷ into 2 doses or 3–4 doses IV; ⊘ use in newborns; ↓ in renal failure; naintain hydration **Caution:** [B (D if near term), +] **Contra:** Sulfonamide sensiivity, porphyria, megaloblastic anemia w/ folate deficiency, significant hepatic imairment **Supplied:** Regular tabs 80 mg TMP/400 mg SMX; DS tabs 160 mg TMP/800 mg SMX; PO susp 40 mg TMP/200 mg SMX/5 mL; inj 80 mg TMP/ 400 mg SMX/5 mL **SE:** Allergic skin Rxns, photosensitivity, GI upset, Stevens–Johnson syndrome, blood dyscrasias, hepatitis **Notes:** Synergistic combiation, interacts w/ warfarin **Interactions:** ↑ Effect of dapsone, MRX, phenytoin, ulfonylureas, warfarin, zidovudine; ↓ effects w/ rifampin; ↓ effect of cyclosporine **Labs:** ↑ Serum bilirubin, alkaline phosphatase, creatinine **NIPE:** ↑ Risk of photosensitivity—use sunscreen; ↑ fluids to 2–3 L/d

Trimetrexate (Neutrexin) **WARNING:** Must be used w/ leucovorin to ⊘ toxicity **Uses:** *Moderate to severe PCP* **Action:** Inhibits dihydrofolate reducase **Dose:** 45 mg/m² IV q24h for 21 d; administer w/ leucovorin 20 mg/m² IV q6h or 24 d; ↓ in hepatic impairment **Caution:** [D, ?/–] **Contra:** MTX sensitivity **Supplied:** Inj **SE:** Sz, fever, rash, GI upset, anemias, ↑ LFTs, peripheral neuropahy, renal impairment **Notes:** Use cytotoxic cautions; inf over 60 min **Interactions:** ↑ Effects w/ azole antifungals, cimetidine, erythromycin; ↓ effects w/ rifabutin, riampin; ↓ effects of pneumococcal immunization **Labs:** ↑ LFTs, SCr **NIPE:** ⊘ PRG, breast-feeding use contraception; ⊘ exposure to infection

Triptorelin (Trelstar Depot, Trelstar LA) **Uses:** *Palliation of advanced CAP* **Action:** LHRH analogue; ↓ gonadotropin secretion when given continuously; transient surge in LH, FSH, testosterone, and estradiol after first dose; w/ chronic/continuous use (usually 2–4 wk), sustained ↓ LH and FSH w/ ↓ testicular and ovarian steroidogenesis similar to surgical castration **Dose:** 3.75 mg IM monthly or 11.25 mg IM q3mo **Caution:** [X, N/A] **Contra:** Not indicated in females **Supplied:** Inj depot 3.75 mg; LA 11.25 mg **SE:** Dizziness, emotional lability, fatigue, headache, insomnia HTN, diarrhea, vomiting, impotence, urinary retention, UTI, pruritus, anemia, inj site pain, musculoskeletal pain, allergic Rxns **Interactions:** ↑ Risk of severe hyperprolactinemia w/ antipsychotics, metoclopramide **Labs:** Suppression of pituitary-gonadal Fxn **NIPE:** ⊘ PRG or breast feeding; may cause hot flashes; initial ↑ bone pain

Trospium Chloride (Sanctura) **Uses:** Overactive bladder **Action:** Anticholinergic **Dose:** 20 mg PO bid; CrCl <30 mL/min, 20 mg qhs; >75 y ↓ dose; take 1 h ac or on empty stomach **Caution:** [C, ?] Hepatic impairment **Contra:** Urinary/gastric retention, narrow-angle glaucoma **Supplied:** 20-mg tabs **SE:** Xerostomia, constipation, HA **Notes:** Food impairs absorption **Interactions:** ↑ Effects may be seen when used with amiloride, digoxin, morphine, metformin, procainamide, quinidine, quinine, ranitidine, tenofovir, triamterene, trimethoprim, vancomycin; ↑ effects of these drugs may be seen amiloride, digoxin, morphine, metformin, procainamide, quinidine, quinine, ranitidine, tenofovir, triamterene, trimethoprim, vancomycin **NIPE:** Take w/o food 1 h ac

Trovafloxacin (Trovan) **WARNING:** Trovan has been associated w/ serious liver injury leading to need for liver transplantation and/or death. **Uses:** *Life-threatening infections* including pneumonia, complicated intraabdominal, gynecologic/pelvic, or skin infections **Action:** Fluoroquinolone antibiotic; inhibits DNA gyrase. *Spectrum:* Broad-spectrum gram(+) and gram(−), including anaerobes; TB typically resistant **Dose:** 200 mg/d; ↓ in hepatic impairment **Caution:** [C, −] Use w/ caution in children **Contra:** Hepatic impairment **Supplied:** Inj 5 mg/mL in 40 and 60 mL; tabs 100, 200 mg **SE:** Liver failure, dizziness, HA, nausea, rash **Notes:** Use restricted to hospitals; hepatotoxicity led to restricted availability **Interactions:** ↑ Risk of photosensitivity with dong quai, St John's wort; ↑ risk of tendon rupture if used with corticosteroids ↓ effects with antacids containing Al or Mg, Fe salts, Mg, sucralfate, vitamins/minerals containing Fe, zinc; IV morphine; dairy products **Labs:** Monitor LFTs **NIPE:** Admin antacids or IV morphine 2 h after trovafloxacin on empty stomach, take w/o regard to food and w/ 8 oz water, risk of photosensitivity–use sunscreen

Urokinase (Abbokinase) **Uses:** *PE, DVT, restore patency to IV catheters* **Action:** Converts plasminogen to plasmin that causes clot lysis **Dose:** *Adults & Peds* Systemic effect: 4400 Units/kg IV over 10 min, followed by 4400–6000 Units/kg/h for 12 h. *Restore catheter patency:* Inject 5000 Units into catheter and aspirate **Caution:** [B, +] **Contra:** ⊘ use w/in 10 d of surgery, delivery, or organ biopsy; bleeding, CVA, vascular malformation **Supplied:** Powder for inj 5000 Units/mL, 250,000-unit vial **SE:** Bleeding, hypotension, dyspnea, bronchospasm, anaphylaxis, cholesterol embolism **Interactions:** ↑ Risk of bleeding w/ anticoagulants, ASA, heparin, indomethacin, NSAIDs, phenylbutazone, feverfew, garlic, ginger, ginkgo biloba; ↓ effects w/ aminocaproic acid **Labs:** ↑ PT, PTT; ↓ fibrinogen, plasminogen

Valacyclovir (Valtrex) **Uses:** *Herpes zoster; genital herpes* **Action:** Prodrug of acyclovir; inhibits viral DNA replication. *Spectrum:* Herpes simplex I and II **Dose:** 1 g PO tid. *Genital herpes:* 500 mg bid × 7 d. *Herpes prophylaxis:* 500–1000 mg/d; ↓ in renal failure **Caution:** [B, +] **Supplied:** Caplets 500 mg **SE:** HA, GI upset, dizziness, pruritus, photophobia **Interactions:** ↑ Effects w/ cimetidine, probenecid **Labs:** ↑ LFTs, creatinine **NIPE:** Take w/o regard to food; ↑ fluids to 2–3 L/d; begin drug at first sign of S/Sxs

Valdecoxib (Bextra) (withdrawn in 2005 by manufacturer) **Uses:** *RA, osteoarthritis, primary dysmenorrhea* **Action:** COX-2 inhibition **Dose:** *Arthritis:* 10 mg PO qd. *Dysmenorrhea:* 20 mg PO bid, PRN **Caution:** [C, ?] Asthma, urticaria, allergic-type Rxns after ASA or NSAIDs, sulfonamide hypersensitivity **Supplied:** Tabs 10, 20 mg **SE:** ↑ LFT, GI ulceration or bleeding; dizziness, edema, HTN, HA, peptic ulcer, renal failure; serious hypersensitivity Rxns have occurred, including Stevens–Johnson syndrome **Interactions:** ↑ Effects w/ azole antifungals; ↑ effects of dextromethorphan, Li, warfarin; ↓ effects of ACEIs, diuretics **Labs:** ↑ LFTs, BUN, creatinine **NIPE:** Take w/ food if GI upset; ↑ fluids to 2–3 L/d

Valganciclovir (Valcyte) **Uses:** *CMV* **Action:** Ganciclovir prodrug; inhibits viral DNA synthesis **Dose:** Induction, 900 mg PO bid w/ food × 21 d, then 900 mg PO qd; ↓ in renal dysfunction **Caution:** [C, ?/–] Use w/ imipenem/cilastatin, nephrotoxic drugs **Contra:** Hypersensitivity to acyclovir, ganciclovir, valganciclovir; ANC < 500/mm²; plt < 25 K; Hgb < 8 g/dL **Supplied:** Tabs 450 mg **SE:** Bone marrow suppression **Notes:** Monitor CBC and Cr **Interactions:** ↑ Effects w/ cytotoxic drugs, immunosuppressive drugs, probenecid; ↑ risks of nephrotoxicity w/ amphotericin B, cyclosporine; ↑ effects w/ didanosine **Labs:** ↑ SCr **NIPE:** Take w/ food; ⊘ PRG, breast-feeding, EtOH, NSAIDs; use contraception for at least 3 mo after drug Rx

Valproic Acid (Depakene, Depakote) **Uses:** *Rx epilepsy, mania; prophylaxis of migraines,* Alzheimer's behavior disorder **Action:** Anticonvulsant; ↑ availability of GABA **Dose:** *Adults & Peds.* Szs: 30–60 mg/kg/24 h PO ÷ tid (after initiation of 10–15 mg/kg/24 h). *Mania:* 750 mg in 3 ÷ doses, ↑ 60 mg/kg/d max. *Migraines:* 250 mg bid, ↑ 1000 mg/d max; ↓ dose in hepatic impairment **Caution:** [D, +] **Contra:** Severe hepatic impairment **Supplied:** Caps 250 mg; syrup 250 mg/5 mL **SE:** somnolence, dizziness, GI upset, diplopia, ataxia, rash, thrombocytopenia, hepatitis, pancreatitis, prolonged bleeding times, alopecia, weight gain, hyperammonemic encephalopathy reported in Pts w/ urea cycle disorders **Notes:** Monitor LFTs and serum levels (see Table 2, page 265); phenobarbital and phenytoin may alter levels **Interactions:** ↑ Effects w/ clarithromycin, erythromycin, felbamate, INH, salicylates, troleandomycin; ↑ effects of anticoagulants, lamotrigine, nimodipine, phenobarbital, primidone, zidovudine; ↑ CNS depression w/ CNS depressants, haloperidol, loxapine, maprotiline, MAOIs, phenothiazines, thioxanthenes, TCAs, EtOH; ↓ effects w/ cholestyramine colestipol; ↓ effects of clozapine, rifampin **Labs:** ↑ LFTs; altered TFTs, false + urinary ketones **NIPE:** Take w/ food for GI upset; ∅ PRG, breast-feeding; DC abruptly

Valsartan (Diovan)
WARNING: Use during 2nd/3rd tri of PRG can cause fetal harm **Uses:** HTN, CHF, DN **Action:** Angiotensin II receptor antagonist **Dose:** 80–160 mg/d **Caution:** [C (1st tri); D 2nd and 3rd tri), ?/–] W/ K-sparing diuretics or K suppls **Contra:** Severe hepatic impairment, biliary cirrhosis, biliary obstruction, primary hyperaldosteronism, bilateral renal artery stenosis **Supplied:** Caps 80, 160 mg **SE:** Hypotension, dizziness **Interactions:** ↑ Effects w/ diuretics, Li; ↑ risk of hyperkalemia w/ K-sparing diuretics, K suppls, trimethoprim **Labs:** ↑ LFTs, K⁺, ↑ Hmg, Hct **NIPE:** Take w/o regard to food; ∅ PRG, breast-feeding use contraception

Vancomycin (Vancocin, Vancoled)
Uses: *Serious MRSA infections; enterococcal infections; PO Rx of C. difficile pseudomembranous colitis* **Action:** Inhibits cell wall synthesis. **Spectrum:** Gram(+) bacteria & some anaerobes (includes MRSA, *Staphylococcus* sp, *Enterococcus* sp, *Streptococcus* sp, *C. difficile*) **Dose:** *Adults.* 1 g IV q12h; for colitis 125–500 mg PO q6h. *Peds.*40–60 mg/kg/24 h IV in ÷ doses q6–12 h. *Neonates.* 10–15 mg/kg/dose q12h; (↓ in renal insufficiency **Caution:** [C, M] **Contra:** Component hypersensitivity; ∅ in Hx hearing loss **Supplied:** Caps 125, 250 mg; powder for PO soln; powder for inj 500 mg, 1000 mg, 10 g/vial **SE:** Ototoxic and nephrotoxic; GI upset (PO), neutropenia **Notes:** See drug levels (see Table 2, page 265); not absorbed PO, local effect in gut only; give IV dose slowly (over 1–3 h) to prevent "red-man syndrome" (a red flushing of the head, neck, and upper torso); IV product may be given PO for colitis **Interactions:** ↑ Ototoxicity and nephrotoxicity w/ ASA, aminoglycosides, cyclosporine, cisplatin, loop diuretics; ↓ effects of MRX **Labs:** ↑ BUN; **NIPE:** Take w/ food, ↑ fluid to 2–3 L/d

Vardenafil (Levitra)
WARNING: May prolong QT$_c$ interval **Uses:** *Erectile dysfunction* **Action:** Phosphodiesterase 5 inhibitor **Dose:** 10 mg PO 60 min before sexual activity; 2.5 mg if administered w/ CYP3A4 inhibitors; administer no more than once daily or in doses greater than 20 mg **Caution:** [B, –] W/ CV, hepatic, or renal Dz **Contra:** Nitrates **Supplied:** 2.5-mg, 5-mg, 10-mg, 20-mg tabs **SE:** Hypotension, headache, dyspepsia, priapism **Notes:** Concomitant α-blockers may cause hypotension **Interactions:** ↑ Effects w/ erythromycin, keotconazole, indinavir, ritonavir; ↑ effects of α-blockers, nitrates; ↓ effects of indinavir, ritonavir **NIPE:** Take w/o regard to food; ↑ risk of priapism

Varicella Virus Vaccine (Varivax)
Uses: *Prevention of varicella (chickenpox) infection* **Action:** Active immunization; live attenuated virus **Dose:** *Adults & Peds.* 0.5 mL SQ, repeat 4–8 wk **Caution:** [C, M] **Contra:** Immunocompromise; neomycin-anaphylactoid Rxn, blood dyscrasias; immunosuppressive drugs; ∅ PRG for 3 mo after **Supplied:** Powder for inj **SE:** May cause mild vari-

cella infection; fever, local Rxns, irritability, GI upset **Notes:** Recommended for all children and adults who have not had chickenpox **Interactions:** ↓ Effects w/ acyclovir, immunosuppressant drugs **NIPE:** ⊘ Aalicylates for 6 wk after immunization; ⊘ PRG for 3 mo after immunization

Vasopressin [Antidiuretic Hormone, ADH] (Pitressin) **Uses:** *DI; Rx postop abdominal distension*; adjunct Rx of GI bleeding & esophageal varices; pulseless VT & VF, adjunct systemic vasopressor (IV drip) **Action:** Posterior pituitary hormone, potent GI vasoconstrictor, potent peripheral vasoconstrictor **Dose:** *Adults & Peds* DI: 2.5–10 Units SQ or IM tid–qid or 1.5–5.0 Units IM q1–3d of the tannate. *GI hemorrhage:* 0.2–0.4 Units/min; ↓ dose in cirrhosis; caution in vascular Dz. *VT/VF:* 40 Units IVP × 1. *Vasopressor:* 0.01–0.1 Units/kg/min **Caution:** [B, +] **Contra:** Hypersensitivity **Supplied:** Inj 20 Units/mL **SE:** HTN, arrhythmias, fever, vertigo, GI upset, tremor **Notes:** Addition of vasopressor to concurrent norepinephrine or epinephrine infs **Interactions:** ↑ Vasopressor effects w/ guanethidine, neostigmine; ↑ antidiuretic effects w/ carbamazepine, chlorpropamide, clofibrate, phenformin urea, TCAs; ↓ antidiuretic effects w/ demeclocycline, epinephrine, heparin, Li, phenytoin, EtOH **Labs:** ↑ cortisol level **NIPE:** Take 1–2 glasses H$_2$O w/ drug

Vecuronium (Norcuron) **Uses:** *Skeletal muscle relaxation during surgery or mechanical ventilation* **Action:** Nondepolarizing neuromuscular blocker **Dose:** *Adults & Peds* 0.08–0.1 mg/kg IV bolus; maint 0.010–0.015 mg/kg after 25–40 min; additional doses q12–15min PRN; ↓ dose in severe renal/hepatic impairment **Caution:** [C, ?] Drug interactions causing ↑ effect of vecuronium (eg, aminoglycosides, tetracycline, succinylcholine) **Supplied:** Powder for inj 10 mg **SE:** Bradycardia, hypotension, itching, rash, tachycardia, CV collapse **Notes:** Fewer cardiac effects than w/ pancuronium **Interactions:** ↑ Neuromuscular blockade w/ aminoglycosides, BBs, CCBs, clindamycin, furosemide, lincomycin, quinidine, tetracyclines, thiazide diuretics, verapamil; ↑ resp depression w/ opioids; ↓ effects w/ phenytoin **NIPE:** Will not provide pain relief or sedation

Venlafaxine (Effexor) **WARNING:** Closely monitor for worsening depression or emergence of suicidality, particularly in pediatric Pts **Uses:** *Depression, generalized anxiety,* social anxiety disorder; obsessive–compulsive disorder, chronic fatigue syndrome, ADHD, autism **Action:** Potentiation of CNS neurotransmitter activity **Dose:** 75–375 mg/d ÷ into 2–3 equal doses; ↓ dose in renal/hepatic impairment **Caution:** [C, ?/–] **Contra:** MAOIs **Supplied:** Tabs 25, 37.5, 50, 75, 100 mg; ER caps 37.5, 75, 150 mg **SE:** HTN, ↑ mean HR, HA, somnolence, GI upset, sexual dysfunction; actuates mania or Szs **Notes:** ⊘ EtOH **Interactions:** ↑ Effects w/ cimetidine, desipramine, haloperidol, MAOIs; ↑ risk of serotonin syndrome w/ buspirone, Li, meperidine, sibutramine, sumatriptan, SSRIs, TCAs, trazodone, St. John's wort **Labs:** ↑ LFTs, creatinine **NIPE:** Take w/ food; ⊘ DC abruptly; DC MAOI 14 days before start of this drug; ↑ fluids to 2–3 L/d; may take 2–3 wk for full effects

Verapamil (Calan, Isoptin) Uses: *Angina, HTN, PSVT, AF, atrial flutter,* migraine prophylaxis, hypertrophic cardiomyopathy, bipolar Dz **Action:** CC▌ **Dose:** *Adults.* Arrhythmias: 2nd line for PSVT w/ narrow QRS complex and adequate BP 2.5–5 mg IV over 1–2 min; repeat 5–10 mg in 15–30 min PRN (30 m█ max). *Angina:* 80–120 mg PO tid, ↑ 480 mg/24 h max. *HTN:* 80–180 mg PO tid o▌ SR tabs 120–240 mg PO qd to 240 mg bid. *Peds* <1 y: 0.1–0.2 mg/kg IV over ▌ min (may repeat in 30 min). *1–16y:* 0.1–0.3 mg/kg IV over 2 min (may repeat i▌ 30 min); 5 mg max. *PO: 1–5 y:* 4–8 mg/kg/d in 3 ÷ doses. >5 y: 80 mg q6–8h; ↓ ▋ renal/hepatic impairment **Caution:** [C, +] Amiodarone/BBs/flecainide can caus▌ bradycardia; statins, midazolam, tacrolimus theophylline levels may be ↑ **Contra▌** Conduction disorders, cardiogenic shock; caution w/ elderly Pts **Supplied:** Tab▌ 40, 80, 120 mg; SR tabs 120, 180, 240 mg; SR caps 120, 180, 240, 360 mg; inj ▌ mg/2 mL **SE:** Gingival hyperplasia, constipation, hypotension, bronchospasm▌ heart rate or conduction disturbances **Interactions:** ↑ Effects w/ antihypertensives▌ nitrates, quinidine, EtOH, grapefruit juice; ↑ effects of buspirone, carbamazepine▌ cyclosporine, digoxin, prazosin, quinidine, theophylline, warfarin; ↓ effects w/ an▌ tineoplastics, barbiturates, NSAIDs, ↓ effects of Li, rifampin **Labs:** ↑ ALT, AST▌ alkaline phosphatase **NIPE:** Take w/ food; ↑ fluids and bulk foods to prevent con▌ stipation

Vinblastine (Velban, Velbe) **WARNING:** Chemotherapeutic agent▌ handle w/ caution **Uses:** *Hodgkin's and NHLs, mycosis fungoides, CAs (testis▌ renal cell, breast, non-small-cell lung, AIDS-related Kaposi's sarcoma,* choriocarcinoma), histiocytosis **Action:** Inhibits microtubule assembly **Dose:** 0.1–0.▌ mg/kg/wk (4–20 mg/m²); ↓ in hepatic failure **Caution:** [D, ?] **Contra:** Intrathecal▌ use **Supplied:** Inj 1 mg/mL **SE:** Myelosuppression (especially leukopenia), N/V▌ (rare), constipation, neurotoxicity (like vincristine but less frequent), alopecia▌ rash; myalgia tumor pain **Interactions:** ↑ Effects w/ erythromycin, itraconazole, ↓▌ effects w/ glutamic acid, tryptophan; ↓ effects of phenytoin **Labs:** ↑ Uric acid▌ **NIPE:** ↑ Fluids to 2–3 L/d; ⊘ PRG or breast-feeding; use contraception for at leas▌ 2 mo after drug; photosensitivity—use sunscreen; ⊘ admin immunizations

Vincristine (Oncovin, Vincasar PFS) **WARNING:** Chemotherapeu-▌ tic agent; handle w/ caution ***Fatal if administered intrathecally*** **Uses:**▌ *ALL, breast and small-cell lung carcinoma, sarcoma (eg, Ewing's, rhabdomyosarcoma), Wilms' tumor, Hodgkin's and NHLs, neuroblastoma, multiple myeloma*▌ **Action:** Promotes disassembly of mitotic spindle, causing metaphase arrest **Dose:**▌ 0.4–1.4 mg/m² (single doses 2 mg/max); ↓ dose in hepatic failure **Caution:** [D, ?]▌ **Contra:** Intrathecal use **Supplied:** Inj 1 mg/mL **SE:** Neurotoxicity commonly▌ dose limiting, jaw pain (trigeminal neuralgia), fever, fatigue, anorexia, constipation▌ and paralytic ileus, bladder atony; no significant myelosuppression w/ standard▌ doses; soft tissue necrosis possible w/ extravasation **Interactions:** ↑ Effects w/▌ CCBs; ↑ effects of MRX; ↑ risk of bronchospasm w/ mitomycin; ↓ effects of digoxin, phenytoin **NIPE:** ↑ Fluids to 2–3 L/d; reversible hair loss; ⊘ exposure to infection; ⊘ admin immunizations

Vinorelbine (Navelbine) **WARNING:** Chemotherapeutic agent; handle w/ caution **Uses:** *Breast and non-small-cell lung CA* (alone or w/ cisplatin) **Action:** Inhibits polymerization of microtubules, impairing mitotic spindle formation; semisynthetic vinca alkaloid **Dose:** 30 mg/m²/wk; ↓ dose in hepatic failure **Caution:** [D, ?] **Contra:** Intrathecal use **Supplied:** Inj 10 mg **SE:** Myelosuppression (especially leukopenia), mild GI effects, and infrequent neurotoxicity (6–29%); constipation and paresthesias (rare); tissue damage can result from extravasation **Interactions:** ↑ Risk of granulocytopenia w/ cisplatin, ↑ pulmonary effects w/ mitomycin, paclitaxel **Labs:** ↑ LFTs **NIPE:** ⊘ PRG or breast-feeding; use contraception; ⊘ infectious environment; ↑ fluids to 2–3 L/d

Vitamin B₁ See Thiamine

Vitamin B₆ See Pyridoxine

Vitamin B₁₂ See Cyanocobalamin

Vitamin K See Phytonadione

Voriconazole (VFEND) **Uses:** *Invasive aspergillosis, serious fungal infections* **Action:** Inhibits ergosterol synthesis. *Spectrum:* Several types of fungus including *Aspergillus, Scedosporium* sp, *Fusarium* sp **Dose:** *Adults and Peds.* ≥ 12 y: IV: 6 mg/kg q12h × 2, then 4 mg/kg bid; may ↓ to 3 mg/kg per dose. *PO: <40 kg:* 100 mg q12h, up to 150 mg; *>40 kg:* 200 mg q 12 h, up to 300 mg; ↓ dose in mild–moderate hepatic impairment; IV only one dose in renal impairment/ESRD **Caution:** [D, ?/–] **Contra:** Severe hepatic impairment **Supplied:** Tabs 50, 200 mg; 200-mg inj **SE:** Visual changes, fever, rash, GI upset, ↑ LFTs **Notes:** Must screen for multiple drug interactions (eg, ↑ dose when given w/ phenytoin); administer PO doses on empty stomach **Interactions:** ↑ Effects w/ delavirdine, efavirenz; ↑ effects of benzodiazepines, buspirone, CCBs, cisapride, cyclosporine, ergots, pimozide, quinidine, sirolimus, sulfonylureas, tacrolimus; ↓ effects w/ carbamazepine, mephobarbital, phenobarbital, rifampin, rifabutin **NIPE:** Take w/o food; ↑ risk of photosensitivity—use sunscreen; ⊘ PRG or breast-feeding

Warfarin (Coumadin) **Uses:** *Prophylaxis and Rx of PE and DVT, AF w/ embolization,* other postop indications **Action:** Inhibits vitamin K–dependent production of clotting factors in the order VII-IX-X-II **Dose:** *Adults.* Adjust to keep INR 2.0–3.0 for most; mechanical valves INR is 2.5–3.5. *ACCP guidelines:* 5 mg initially (unless rapid therapeutic INR needed), use 7.5–10 mg or if Pt elderly or has other bleeding risk factors ↓. *Alternative:* 10–15 mg PO, IM, or IV qd for 1–3 d; maint 2–10 mg/d PO, IV, or IM; follow daily INR initially to adjust dosage. *Peds.* 0.05–0.34 mg/kg/24 h PO, IM, or IV; follow PT/INR to adjust dosage; monitor vitamin K intake; ↓ in hepatic impairment or elderly **Caution:** [X, +] **Contra:** Severe hepatic or renal Dz, bleeding, peptic ulcer, PRG **Supplied:** Tabs 1, 2, 2.5, 3, 4, 5, 6, 7.5, 10 mg; inj **SE:** Bleeding caused by overanticoagulation (PT >3× control or INR >5.0–6.0) or injury and INR w/in therapeutic range; bleeding, alopecia, skin necrosis, purple toe syndrome **Notes:** INR preferred test; to rapidly correct overanticoagulation, use vitamin K, FFP or both; highly teratogenic; do *not* use in PRG. Caution Pt on taking warfarin w/ other meds, especially ASA. *Common warfarin interactions:* Potentiated by APAP, EtOH (w/ liver Dz), amiodarone, cimetidine, ciprofloxacin, co-trimoxazole, erythromycin, fluconazole, flu vaccine, INH, itraconazole, metronidazole, omeprazole, phenytoin, propranolol, quinidine, tetracycline. Inhibited by barbiturates, carbamazepine, chlordiazepoxide, cholestyramine, dicloxacillin, nafcillin, rifampin, sucralfate, high-vitamin K foods **Labs:** ↑ PTT; false ↓ serum theophylline levels **NIPE:** Reddish discoloration of urine; ⊘ PRG or breast-feeding; use barrier contraception; monitor for bleeding

Zafirlukast (Accolate) Uses: *Adjunctive Rx of asthma* **Action:** Selective and competitive inhibitor of leukotrienes **Dose:** *Adults and Peds.* ≥ 12 y:. 20 mg bid. *Peds.* 5–11 y: 10 mg PO bid (empty stomach) **Caution:** [B, –] Interacts w/ warfarin to ↑ INR **Contra:** Component hypersensitivity **Supplied:** Tabs 20 mg **SE:** Hepatic dysfunction, usually reversible on discontinuation; HA, dizziness, GI upset; Churg–Strauss syndrome **Notes:** Not for acute asthma, take on empty stomach **Interactions:** ↑ Effects w/ ASA; ↑ effects of CCBs, cyclosporine; ↑ risk of bleeding w/ warfarin; ↓ effects w/ erythromycin, theophylline, food **Labs:** ↑ ALT **NIPE:** Take w/o food; ⊘ use for acute asthma attack

Zalcitabine (Hivid) WARNING: Use w/ caution in Pts w/ neuropathy, pancreatitis, lactic acidosis, hepatitis Uses: *HIV* **Action:** Antiretroviral agent **Dose:** *Adults.* 0.75 mg PO tid. *Peds.* 0.015–0.04 mg/kg PO q 6h: ↓ dose in renal failure **Caution:** [C, +] **Contra:** Component hypersensitivity **Supplied:** Tabs 0.375, 0.75 mg **SE:** Peripheral neuropathy, pancreatitis, fever, malaise, anemia, hypo-/ hyperglycemia, hepatic impairment **Notes:** May be used in combination w/ zidovudine **Interactions:** ↑ Risk of peripheral neuropathy w/ amphotericin B, aminoglycosides, cisplatin, didanosine, disulfiram, foscarnet, INH, phenytoin, ribavirin, vincristine; ↑ effects w/ cimetidine, metoclopramide; probenecid; ↓ effects w/ antacids **Labs:** ↑ LFTs, lipase, triglycerides **NIPE:** Use barrier contraception; take w/o regard to food

Zaleplon (Sonata) Uses: *Insomnia* **Action:** A nonbenzodiazepine sedative–hypnotic, a pyrazolopyrimidine **Dose:** 5–20 mg hs PRN; ↓ dose in renal/hepatic insufficiency, elderly **Caution:** [C, ?/–] Caution in mental/psychological conditions **Contra:** Component hypersensitivity **Supplied:** Caps 5, 10 mg **SE:** HA, edema, amnesia, somnolence, photosensitivity **Notes:** Take immediately before desired onset **Interactions:** ↑ CNS depression w/ cimetidine, CNS depressants, imipramine, thioridazine, EtOH; ↓ effects w/ carbamazepine, phenobarbital, phenytoin, rifampin **NIPE:** Rapid effects of drug; take w/o food ⊘ DC abruptly

Zanamivir (Relenza) Uses: *Influenza A and B* **Action:** Inhibits viral neuraminidase **Dose:** *Adults & Peds.* >7 y: 2 inhal (10 mg) bid for 5 d; initiate w/in 48 h of Sxs **Caution:** [C, M] **Contra:** Pulmonary Dz **Supplied:** Powder for inhal 5

mg **SE:** Bronchospasm, HA, GI upset **Notes:** Uses a Diskhaler for administration **Labs:** ↑?LFTs, CPK **NIPE:** Does not reduce risk of transmitting virus

Zidovudine (Retrovir)
WARNING: Neutropenia, anemia, lactic acidosis, and hepatomegaly w/ steatosis **Uses:** *HIV infection, prevention of maternal transmission of HIV* **Action:** Inhibits RT **Dose:** *Adults.* 200 mg PO tid or 300 mg PO bid or 1–2 mg/kg/dose IV q4h. *PRG:* 100 mg PO 5×/d until the start of labor, then during labor 2 mg/kg over 1 h followed by 1 mg/kg/h until clamping of the umbilical cord. *Peds.* 160 mg/m²/dose q8h; ↓ dose in renal failure **Caution:** [C, ?/–] **Contra:** Life-threatening hypersensitivity **Supplied:** Caps 100 mg; tabs 300 mg; syrup 50 mg/5 mL; inj 10 mg/mL **SE:** Hematologic toxicity, HA, fever, rash, GI upset, malaise **Interactions:** ↑ Effects w/ fluconazole, phenytoin, probenecid, trimethoprim, valproic acid, vinblastine, vincristine; ↑ hematologic toxicity w/ adriamycin, dapsone, ganciclovir, interferon-α; ↓ effects w/ rifampin, ribavirin, stavudine **NIPE:** Take w/o food monitor for S/Sxs opportunistic infection; monitor for anemia

Zidovudine and Lamivudine (Combivir)
WARNING: Neutropenia, anemia, lactic acidosis, and hepatomegaly w/ steatosis **Uses:** *HIV infection* **Action:** Combination of RT inhibitors **Dose:** *Adults & Peds.* >12 y: 1 tab bid; ↓ in renal failure **Caution:** [C, ?/–] **Contra:** Component hypersensitivity **Supplied:** Caps zidovudine 300 mg/lamivudine 150 mg **SE:** Hematologic toxicity, HA, fever, rash, GI upset, malaise, pancreatitis **Interactions:** Combination product ↓ daily pill burden **Interactions:** ↑ Effects w/ fluconazole, phenytoin, probenecid, trimethoprim, valproic acid, vinblastine, vincristine; ↑ hematologic toxicity w/ adriamycin, dapsone, ganciclovir, interferon-α; ↓ effects w/ rifampin, ribavirin, stavudine **NIPE:** Take w/o food; monitor for S/Sxs opportunistic infection; monitor for anemia

Zileuton (Zyflo)
Uses: *Chronic Rx of asthma* **Action:** Inhibitor of 5-lipoxygenase **Dose:** *Adults and Peds.* ≥ 12 y: 600 mg PO qid **Caution:** [C, ?/–] **Contra:** Hepatic impairment **Supplied:** Tabs 600 mg **SE:** Hepatic damage, HA, GI upset, leukopenia **Notes:** Monitor LFTs every month × 3, then q2–3 mo; must take on a regular basis; not for acute asthma **Interactions:** ↑ Effects of propranolol, terfenadine, theophylline, warfarin **Labs:** ↑ LFTs, ↓ WBCs; **NIPE:** Take w/o regard to food

Ziprasidone (Geodon)
Uses: *Schizophrenia, acute agitation* **Action:** Atypical antipsychotic **Dose:** 20 mg PO bid w/ food, may ↑ in 2-d intervals up to 80 mg bid; agitation 10–20 mg IM PRN up to 40 mg/d; separate 10 mg doses by 2 h and 20 mg doses by 4h **Caution:** [C, –] W/ hypokalemia/hypomagnesemia **Contra:** QT prolongation, recent MI, uncompensated HF, meds that prolong QT interval **Supplied:** Caps 20, 40, 60, 80 mg; Inj 20 mg/mL **SE:** Bradycardia; rash, somnolence, resp disorder, EPS, weight gain, orthostatic hypotension **Notes:** Monitor electrolytes **Interactions:** ↑ Effects w/ ketoconazole; ↑ effects of antihypertensives; ↑ CNS depression w/ anxiolytics, sedatives, opioids, EtOH; TCAs, thioridazine, risk of prolonged QT w/ cisapride, chlorpromazine, clarithromycin,

diltiazem, erythromycin, levofloxacin, mefloquine, pentamidine, TCAs, thioridazine; ↓ effects w/ amphetamines, carbamazepine; ↓ effects of levodopa **Labs:** ↑ Prolactin, cholesterol, triglycerides **NIPE:** May take weeks before full effects, take w/ food, ↑ risk of tardive dyskinesia

Zoledronic Acid (Zometa) **Uses:** *Hypercalcemia of malignancy (HCM),* ↓ skeletal-related events in CAP, multiple myeloma, and metastatic bone lesions **Action:** Bisphosphonate; inhibits osteoclastic bone resorption **Dose:** *HCM:* 4 mg IV over at least 15 min; may re-treat in 7 d if adequate renal Fxn. *Bone lesions/myeloma:* 4 mg IV over at least 15 min, repeat q3–4wk PRN; prolonged w/ Cr ↑ **Caution:** [C, ?/–] Loop diuretics, aminoglycosides; ASA-sensitive asthmatics **Contra:** Bisphosphonate hypersensitivity **Supplied:** Vial 4 mg **SE:** Adverse effects ↑ w/ renal dysfunction; fever, flu-like syndrome, GI upset, insomnia, anemia; electrolyte abnormalities **Notes:** Requires vigorous prehydration; ⊘ exceed recommended doses/inf duration to minimize dose-related renal dysfunction; follow Cr **Interactions:** ↑ Risk of hypocalcemia w/ diuretics; ↑ risk of nephrotoxicity w/ aminoglycosides, thalidomide **NIPE:** ↑ Fluids to 2–3 L/d

Zolmitriptan (Zomig) **Uses:** *Acute Rx migraine* **Action:** Selective serotonin agonist; causes vasoconstriction **Dose:** Initial 2.5 mg PO, may repeat after 1 h to 10 mg max in 24 h **Caution:** [C, ?/–] **Contra:** Ischemic heart Dz, Prinzmetal's angina, uncontrolled HTN, accessory conduction pathway disorders, ergots, MAOIs **Supplied:** Tabs 2.5, 5 mg **SE:** Dizziness, hot flashes, paresthesias, chest tightness, myalgia, diaphoresis **Interactions:** ↑ Effects w/ cimetidine, MAOIs, oral contraceptives, propranolol; ↑ risk of prolonged vasospasms w/ ergots; ↑ risk of serotonin syndrome w/ sibutramine, SSRIs **NIPE:** Admin to relieve migraines; not for prophylaxis

Zolpidem (Ambien) [C-IV] **Uses:** *Short-term Rx of insomnia* **Action:** Hypnotic agent **Dose:** 5–10 mg PO hs PRN; ↓ in elderly, hepatic insufficiency **Caution:** [B, –] **Contra:** Breast-feeding **Supplied:** Tabs 5, 10 mg **SE:** HA, dizziness, drowsiness, nausea, myalgia **Notes:** May be habit-forming **Interactions:** ↑ CNS depression w/ CNS depressants, sertraline, EtOH ↑ effects of ketoconazole; ↓ effects of rifampin; **NIPE:** Take w/o food; ⊘ DC abruptly if long-term use; may develop tolerance to drug

Zonisamide (Zonegran) **Uses:** *Adjunct Rx complex partial Szs* **Action:** Anticonvulsant **Dose:** Initial 100 mg/d PO; may ↑ to 400 mg/d **Caution:** [C, –] ↑ toxicity w/ CYP3A4 inhibitor; ↓ levels w/ concurrent carbamazepine, phenytoin, phenobarbital, valproic acid **Contra:** Hypersensitivity to sulfonamides; oligohidrosis and hypothermia in peds **Supplied:** Caps 100 mg **SE:** Dizziness, drowsiness, confusion, ataxia, memory impairment, paresthesias, psychosis, nystagmus, diplopia, tremor; anemia, leukopenia; GI upset, nephrolithiasis, Stevens–Johnson syndrome; monitor for ↓ sweating and ↑ body temperature **Notes:** Swallow capsules whole **Interactions:** ↓ Effects w/ carbamazepine, phenobarbital, phenytoin, valproic acid **Labs:** ↑ serum alkaline phosphatase, ALT, AST, creatinine, BUN, ↓ glucose, Na **NIPE:** ⊘ DC

COMMONLY USED MEDICINAL HERBS

Arnica (*Arnica montana*) Uses: ↓ Swelling & inflammation from acne, blunt injury, bruises, rashes, sprains **Action:** Sesquiterpenoids have shown antibacterial, antiinflammatory, & analgesic properties; **Available forms:** Topical cream, spray, oint, tinc; for poultice dilute tinc 3–10 × w/ water & apply PRN **Contra:** Poisonous, ⊘ take internally; ⊘ if Pt allergic to arnica, chrysanthemums, marigold, sunflowers **Notes/SE:** Arrhythmias, abdominal pain, cardiac arrest, contact dermatitis, coma, death, hepatic failure, HTN, nervousness, restlessness **Interactions:** ↑ Risk of bleeding w/ ASA, heparin, warfarin, angelica, anise, asafetida, bogbean, boldo, capsicum, celery, chamomile, clove, danshen, fenugreek, feverfew, garlic, ginger, ginkgo, ginseng, horse chestnut, horseradish, licorice, meadowsweet, onion, papain, passion flower, poplar bark, prickly ash, quassia wood, red clover, turmeric, wild carrot, wild lettuce, willow; ↓ effects of antihypertensives **Labs:** None **NIPE:** ⊘ Apply to broken skin, ⊘ use in PRG & lactation, serious liver & kidney damage w/ internal use, ingestion of flowers & root can cause death, prolonged topical use ↑ risk of allergic reaction

Astragalus (*Astragalus membranaceus*) Uses: Rx of resp infections, enhancement of immune system, & heart failure **Action:** Root saponins ↑ diuresis, ↓ BP; antiinflammatory action related to the stimulation of macrophages, ↑ antibody formation & ↑ T-lymphocyte proliferation **Available forms:** Caps/tabs 1–4 g tid, PO; liq ext 4–8 mL/d (1:2 ratio) ÷ doses; dry ext 250 mg (1:8 ratio) tid, PO **Notes/SE:** Immunosuppression w/ doses > 28 g **Interactions:** ↑ Effect of acyclovir, anticoagulants, antihypertensives, antithrombotics, antiplts, interleukin-2, interferon; ↓ effect of cyclophosphamide **Labs:** ↑ PT, INR **NIPE:** Use cautiously in immunosuppressed Pts or those w/ autoimmune Dz

Butcher's Broom (*Ruscus aculeatus*) Uses: Rx of circulatory disorders such as PVD, varicose veins, & leg edema; hemorrhoids; diuretic; laxative; inflammation; arthritis **Action:** Vasoconstriction due to direct activation of the α-receptors of the smooth-muscle cells in vascular walls **Available forms:** Raw ext 7–11 mg once/d, PO; tea 1 tsp in 1 cup water; topical oint apply PRN **Notes/SE:** GI upset, N/V **Interactions:** ↑ Effects of anticoagulants, MAOIs; ↓ effects of antihypertensives **Labs:** None **NIPE:** Hypertensive crisis may occur if admin w/ MAOIs; ⊘ use in PRG & lactation

Black Cohosh (*Cimicifuga racemosa*) Uses: Antitussive; smooth muscle relaxant; management of menopausal symptoms esp hot flashes, sleep disturbance & anxiety, premenstrual syndrome, & dysmenorrhea. Antiinflammatory, peripheral vasodilation, & sedative effects **Action:** Estrogenic activity w/ some studies showing ↓ in LH; vasodilation activity causing ↑ blood flow & hypotensive effects; antimicrobial activity **Available forms:** Dried root/rhizome caps 40–200 mg ONCE/D; fluid ext (1:1) 2–4 mL or 1 tsp once/d; tinc (1:5) 3–6 mL or 1–2 tsp once/d; powdered ext (4:1) 250–500 mg once/d; Remifemin Menopause (standardized ext brand name) 20 mg bid **Notes/SE:** Hypotension, bradycardia, N/V, anorexia, HA, miscarriage, nervous system & visual disturbances **Interactions:** ↑ Effects of antihypertensives, estrogen HRT, oral contraceptives, hypnotics, sedatives; tinc may cause a reaction w/ disulfiram & metronidazole; ↑ antiproliferative effect w/ tamoxifen; ↓ effects of ferrous fumarate, ferrous gluconate, ferrous sulfate **Labs:** May ↓ LH levels & plt counts **NIPE:** Tinc contains large % of EtOH, ⊘ use in PRG or lactation or give to children

Chamomile (*Matricaria recutita*)
Uses: Antiinflammatory, antipyretic, antimicrobial, antispasmodic, astringent, sedative **Action:** Ingredients include α-bisabolol oil, which ↓ inflammation, antispasmodic activity, ↑ healing times for burns & ulcers, & inhibits ulcer formation; apigenin contributes to the anti-inflammatory effect, antispasmodic & sedative effect; azulene inhibits histamine release; chamazulene reduces inflammation & has antioxidant & antimicrobial effects **Available forms:** Teas 3–5 g (1 tbsp) flower heads steeped in water tid–qid, also use as a gargle or compress; fluid ext 1:1 -45% EtOH 1–3 mL tid **Notes/SE:** Allergic reactions if Pt allergic to Compositae family (ragweed, sunflowers, asters), eg, angioedema, eczema, contact dermatitis & anaphylaxis **Interactions:** ↑ Effects of CNS depressants, EtOH, anticoagulants, antiplts; ↑ risk of miscarriage; ↓ effects of drugs metabolized by CY 450 3A4, eg, alprazolam, atorvastatin, diazepam, ketoconazole, verapamil **Labs:** Monitor anticoagulant levels **NIPE:** ⊘ in PRG, lactation, children < age 2 y, patients w/ asthma or hay fever

Chondroitin Sulfate
Uses: Combine w/ glucosamine to Rx arthritis; use as an anticoagulant **Action:** Attracts fluid & nutrients into the joints; inhibits thrombi **Available forms:** 1200 mg once/d, PO, & usually given w/ glucosamine 1500 mg once/d, PO for normal weight adults; **Notes/SE:** Diarrhea, dyspepsia, HA, N/V, restlessness **Interactions:** ↑ Effects of anticoagulants, aspirin, NSAIDs **Labs:** None **NIPE:** ⊘ in PRG & lactation

Dong Quai (*Angelica polymorpha, sinensis*)
Uses: Dysmenorrhea, PMS, menorrhagia, chronic pelvic infection, irregular menstruation. Other reported uses include anemia, HTN, HA, rhinitis, neuralgia, & hepatitis **Action:** Root exts contain at least six coumarin derivatives that have anticoagulant, vasodilating, antispasmodic, & CNS-stimulating activity. Studies demonstrate weak estrogen-agonist actions of the ext **Available forms:** Caps 500 mg, 1–2 caps PO, tid; liq ext 1–2 gtt, tid; tea 1–2 g, tid **Notes/SE:** Diarrhea, bleeding, photosensitivity, fever **Interactions:** ↑ Effects of anticoagulants, antiplts, estrogens, warfarin; ↑ anticoagulant activity w/ chamomile, dandelion, horse chestnut, red clover; ↑ risk of disulfiram-like reaction w/ disulfiram, metronidazole; **Labs:** ↑ PT, PTT, INR

NIPE: Photosensitivity—use sunscreen, ⊘ if breast-feeding or PRG; tincs & exts contain EtOH up to 60%; stop herb 14 d prior to dental or surgical procedures

Echinacea (*Echinacea purpurea*)
Uses: Immune system stimulant; prevention/Rx of colds, flu; as supportive therapy for colds & chronic infections of the resp tract & lower urinary tract **Action:** Stimulates phagocytosis & cytokine production & ↑ resp cellular activity; topically exerts anesthetic, antimicrobial, & antiinflammatory effects **Available forms:** Caps w/ powdered herb equivalent to 300–500 mg, PO, tid; pressed juice 6–9 mL, PO, once/d; tinc 2–4 mL, PO, tid (1:5 dilution); tea 2 tsp (4 g) of powdered herb in 1 cup of boiling water **Notes/SE:** Fever, taste perversion, urticaria, angioedema; **Contra:** ⊘ in Pts w/ autoimmune Dz, collagen Dz, HIV, leukemia, MS, TB **Interactions:** ↑ Risk of disulfiram-like reaction w/ disulfiram, metronidazole; ↑risk of exacerbation of HIV or AIDS w/ echinacea & amprenavir, other protease inhibitors; ↓ effects of azathioprine, basiliximab, corticosteroids, cyclosporine, daclizumab, econazole vaginal cream, muromonab-CD3, mycophenolate, prednisone, tacrolimus **Labs:** ↑ ALT, AST, lymphocytes, ESR **NIPE:** Large doses of herb interferes w/ sperm activity; ⊘ w/ breast-feeding or PRG; ⊘ continuously for longer than 8 wk w/o a 3-wk break in Rx

Ephedra/Ma Huang
Uses: CNS stimulant, appetite suppressant, weight-loss herb, asthma, headaches, nasal congestion, arthralgia **Action:** Active ingredient of ext is ephedrine that stimulates CNS, ↑ HR, BP, & peripheral vasoconstriction; acts on β-receptors & α-receptors **Available forms:** Ext 1–3 mL, PO, tid; tea 1–5 g herb in 1 pt boiling water; caps max daily dose of 300 mg **Notes/SE:** Anxiety, confusion, dizziness, HA, insomnia, irritability, restlessness, nervousness, arrhythmias, HTN, palpitations, constipation, urinary retention, uterine contractions, dermatitis **Contra:** ⊘ Narrow-angle glaucoma, seizures, CAD, PRG, lactation **Interactions:** ↑ Sympathomimetic effects w/ BBs, guanethidine, yohimbe; ↑ cardiac rhythm disturbance w/ anesthetics, cardiac glycosides, halothane; ↑ psychotic episodes w/ caffeine, EtOH; ↑ effects of CNS stimulants, pseudoephedrine, theophylline ; ↑ risk of HTN crisis w/ MAOIs, oxytocics, phenelzine, TCAs; ↓ effects of oral hypoglycemics **Labs:** ↑ ALT, AST, total bilirubin, urine bilirubin, serum glucose **NIPE:** Tincs & exts contain EtOH; linked to several deaths; monitor for behavioral mood changes

Feverfew (*Tanacetum parthenium*)
Uses: Antiinflammatory for arthritis, asthma, digestion problems, fever, migraines, menstrual complaints, threatened abortion **Action:** Active ingredient, parthenolide, inhibits serotonin release, prostaglandin synthesis, plt aggregation, & histamine release from mast cells; several ingredients inhibit activation of polymorphonuclear leukocytes & leukotriene synthesis **Available forms:** Freeze-dried leaf ext 25 mg once/d; caps 300 mg–400 mg tid PO; tinc 15–ñ30 gtt once/d to 0.2–0.7 mg of parthenolide **Notes/SE:** Mouth ulcers, muscle stiffness, joint pain, GI upset, rash **Contra:** ⊘ in PRG & lactation or w/ ragweed allergy **Interactions:** ↑ Effects of anticoagulants,

antiplts, ↓ effects of Fe absorption **Labs:** ↑ PT, INR, PTT **NIPE:** ⊘ DC herb abruptly or may experience joint stiffness & pain, headaches, insomnia

Garlic (*Allium sativum*) **Uses:** Antithrombotic, antilipidemic, antitumor, antimicrobial, antiasthmatic, antiinflammatory **Action:** Inhibits gram(+) & gram(−) organisms, exerts cholesterol-lowering by preventing gastric lipase fat digestion & fecal excretion of sterols & bile acids & it inhibits free radicals **Available forms:** Tea, tabs, caps, ext, oil, dried powder, syrup, fresh bulb **Notes/SE:** Dizziness, diaphoresis, HA, N/V, hypothyroidism, contact dermatitis, allergic reactions, oral mucosa irritation, systemic garlic odor, ↓ Hgb production, lysis of RBCs **Interactions:** ↑ Effects of anticoagulants, antiplts, insulin, oral hypoglycemics; ↓ effects w/ acidophilus **Labs:** ↓ Total cholesterol, LDL, triglycerides, plt aggregation, iodine uptake; ↑ PT, serum IgE **NIPE:** ⊘ in PRG, lactation, prior to surgery, GI disorders; report bleeding, bruising, petechiae, tarry stools, monitor CBC, PT

Ginger (*Zingiber officinale*) **Uses:** Antiemetic ↓ N/V; antiinflammatory relieves pain & swelling of muscle injury, osteoarthritis & rheumatoid arthritis; antispasmodic action relieves colic, flatulence & indigestion; antiplt; antipyretic; antioxidant; antiinfective against gram(+) & gram(−) bacteria **Action:** Antiinflammatory effect inhibits prostaglandin, thromboxane, & leukotriene biosynthesis; antiemetic effects due to action on the GI tract; antiplt effect due to the inhibition of thromboxane formation; + inotropic effect on CV system **Available forms:** Dosage form & strength depends on Dz process *General use:* Dried ginger caps 1 g once/d, PO; fluid ext 0.7–2 mL once/d, PO, (2:1 ratio); tabs 500 mg bid–qid, PO; tinc 1.7–5 mL once/d, PO, (1:5 ratio) **Interactions:** ↑ Risk of bleeding w/ anticoagulants, antiplts; ↑ risk of disulfiram-like reaction w/ disulfiram, metronidazole **Labs:** ↑ PT **NIPE:** Store herb in cool, dry area; ⊘ in PRG, lactation; lack of standardization for herb dosing

Ginkgo Biloba **Uses:** Effective w/ circulatory disorders, cerebrovascular Dz, & dementia; used to improve alertness & attention span **Action:** Ext flavonoids release neurotransmitters & inhibit monoamine oxidase, which enhances cognitive function; vascular protective action results from relaxation of blood vessels, ↑ tissue perfusion, inhibition of plt aggregation; eradicates free radicals & ↓ polymorphonuclear neutrophils **Available forms:** Dosage depends on diagnosis *General uses:* Tabs & caps 40–ñ80 mg tid, PO; tinc 0.5 mL tid, PO; ext 40–80 mg tid, PO **Notes/SE:** Anxiety, diarrhea, flatulence, HA, heart palpitations, N/V, restlessness **Interactions:** ↑ Effect of MAOIs; ↑ risk of bleeding w/ anisindione, dalteparin, dicumerol, garlic, heparin, salicylates, warfarin; ↑ risk of coma w/ trazodone; ↓ effect of carbamazepine, gabapentin, insulin, oral hypoglycemics, phenobarbital, phenytoin; ↓ seizure threshold w/ bupropion, TCAs **Labs:** ↑ PT **NIPE:** ⊘ in PRG & lactation; tincs contain up to 60% EtOH; ⊘ 2 wk prior to surgery

Ginseng (*Panax quinquefolius*) **Uses:** ↑ Physical endurance, concentration, appetite, sleep & stress resistance; ↓ fatigue; antioxidant; aids in glucose control **Action:** Dried root contains ginsenosides, which ↑ natural killer cell activity, & nuclear RNA synthesis, & motor activity **Available forms:** No standard dosage *General use:* Caps 200 mg–500 mg once/d, PO; tea 3 g steeped in boiling water tid PO, tinc 1–2 mg once/d, PO (1:1 dilution) **Notes/SE:** Anxiety, anorexia, chest pain, diarrhea, HTN, N/V, palpitations **Interactions:** ↑ Effects of estrogen, hypoglycemics, CNS stimulants, caffeine, ephedra; ↑ risk of bleeding w/ ibuprofen; ↑ risk of HA, irritability & visual hallucinations w/ MAOIs; ↓ effects of anisindione, dicumarol, furosemide, heparin, warfarin **Labs:** ↑ Digoxin level falsely; ↓ glucose, PT, INR **NIPE:** ⊘ Use continuously for > 3 mo; ⊘ during PRG or lactation; eval for ginseng abuse syndrome w/ symptoms of diarrhea, depression, edema, HTN, insomnia, rash & restlessness

Glucosamine Sulfate (chitosamine) **Uses:** Used w/ chondroitin for the Rx of arthritis **Action:** Stimulate the production of cartilage components **Available forms:** Caps/tabs 1500 mg once/d, PO & chondroitin sulfate 1200 mg once/d, PO for adults of normal weight **Notes/SE:** Abdominal pain, anorexia, constipation or diarrhea, drowsiness, HA, heartburn, N/V, rash **Interactions:** ↑ Effects of hypoglycemics; **Labs:** Monitor serum glucose levels in diabetics **NIPE:** Take w/ food to reduce GI effects; no uniform standardization of herb

Hawthorn (*Crataegus laevigata*) **Uses:** Rx of HTN, arrhythmias, heart failure, stable angina pectoris, insomnia **Action:** ↑ myocardial contraction by ↓ oxygen consumption, ↓ peripheral resistance, dilating coronary blood vessels, ACE inhibition **Available forms:** Tinc 1–2 mL (1:5 ratio) tid, PO; liq ext 0.5–1 mL, (1:1 ration) tid, PO **Notes/SE:** Arrhythmias, fatigue, hypotension, N/V, sedation **Interactions:** ↑ Effects of antihypertensives, cardiac glycosides, CNS depressants,& herbs such as adonis, lily of the valley, squill ↓; effects of Fe **Labs:** False ↑ of digoxin **NIPE:** ⊘ in PRG & lactation; many tincs contain EtOH

Kava Kava (*Piper methysticum*) **Uses:** ↓ Anxiety, stress, & restlessness; sedative effect **Action:** Appears to act directly on the limbic system **Available forms:** Standardized ext (70% kavalactones) 100 mg bid–tid, PO **Notes/SE:** ↓ Reflexes, HA, dizziness, visual changes, hematuria, SOB **Interactions:** ↑ Effects of antiplts, benzodiazepines, CNS depressants, MAOIs, phenobarbital; ↑ absorption when taken w/ food; ↑ in parkinsonian symptoms w/ kava & antiparkinsonian drugs **Labs:** ↑ ALT, AST, urinary RBCs; ↓ albumin, total protein, bilirubin, urea, plts, lymphocytes **NIPE:** ⊘ Take for > 3 mo; ⊘ during PRG & lactation

Licorice (*Glycyrrhiza glabra*) **Uses:** Expectorant, shampoo, GI complaints **Action:** ↑ Mucous secretions, ↓ peptic activity, ↓ scalp sebum secretion **Available forms:** Liq ext, bulk dried root, tea; 15 g once/d PO of licorice root; intake > 50 g once/d may cause toxicity **Notes/SE:** HTN, arrhythmias, edema, hypokalemia, HA, lethargy, rhabdomyolysis **Interactions:** ↑ Drug effects of diuretics, corticosteroids, may prolong QT interval w/ loratadine, procainamide, quinidine, terfenadine; **Labs:** None **NIPE:** Monitor for electrolyte & ECG changes, HTN, mineralocorticord-like effects; toxicity more likely w/ prolonged intake of small doses than one large dose

Melatonin (MEL) **Uses:** Insomnia, jet lag, antioxidant, immunostimulant **Action:** Hormone produce by the pineal gland in response to darkness; declines w/ age **Available forms:** ER caps 1–3 mg once/d 2 h before hs, PO **Notes/SE:** HA, confusion, sedation, HTN, tachycardia, hyperglycemia **Interactions:** ↑ anxiolytic effects of benzodiazepines; ↑ risk of insomnia w/ cerebral stimulants, methamphetamine, succinylcholine **Labs:** None **NIPE:** ⊘ during PRG & lactation

Milk thistle (*Silybum marianum*) **Uses:** Rx of hepatotoxicity, dyspepsia, liver protectorant **Action:** stimulates protein synthesis, which leads to liver cell regeneration **Available forms:** Tinc 70–120 mg (70% silymarin) tid, PO **Notes/SE:** Diarrhea, menstrual stimulation, N/V **Interactions:** ↑ Effects of drugs metabolized by the cytochrome P-450, CYP3A4, CYP2C9 enzymes **Labs:** ↑ PT; ↓ LFTs, serum glucose **NIPE:** ⊘ in PRG & lactation; ⊘ in Pts allergic to ragweed, chrysanthemums, marigolds, daisies

Saw Palmetto (*Serenoa repens*) **Uses:** Rx of benign prostatic hypertrophy (BPH) stages 1 & 2 (inhibits testosterone-5-α-reductase), ↑ sperm production, ↑ breast size (estrogenic), ↑ sexual vigor, mild diuretic, treat chronic cystitis **Action:** Theorized that sitosterols inhibit conversion of testosterone to dihydrotestosterone (DHT), which reduces the prostate gland, also competes w/ DHT on receptor sites resulting in antiestrogenic effects **Available forms:** Caps/tabs 160 mg bid, PO; tinc 20–30 gtt qid (1:2 ration); fluid ext, standardized 160 mg bid PO or 320 mg once/d PO **Notes/SE:** Abdominal pain, back pain, diarrhea, dysuria, HA, HTN, N/V, impotence **Contra:** ⊘ PRG, lactation **Interactions:** ↑ Effects of adrenergics, anticoagulants, antiplts, hormones, Fe **Labs:** May affect semen analysis, may cause false – PSA **NIPE:** Take w/ meals to ↓ GI upset, do baseline PSA prior to taking herb, no standardization of herb content

Spirulina (*Spirulina spp*) **Uses:** Rx of obesity & as a nutritional supplement **Action:** Contains 65% protein, all amino acids, carotenoids, B-complex vitamins, essential fatty acids & Fe; has been shown to inhibit replicating viral cells **Available forms:** Caps/tabs or powder admin 3–5 g ac, PO **Notes/SE:** Anorexia, N/V **Interactions:** ↑ Effects of anticoagulants; ↓ effects of thyroid hormones due to high iodine content; ↓ absorption of vitamin B_{12} **Labs:** ↑ Serum Ca, serum alkaline phosphatase; monitor PT, INR **NIPE:** May contain ↑ levels of Hg & radioactive ion content

St. John's Wort (*Hypericum perforatum*) **Uses:** Depression, anxiety, antiinflammatory, antiviral **Action:** MAOI in vitro, not in vivo; bacteriostatic & bactericidal, ↑ capillary blood flow, uterotonic activity in animals **Available forms:** Teas, tabs, caps, tinc, oil ext for topical use **Notes/SE:** Photosensitivity (use sunscreen)rash, dizziness, dry mouth, GI distress **Interactions:** Enhance MAOI activity, EtOH, narcotics, MAOIs, sympathomimetics **Labs:** ↑ GH; ↓ digoxin, serum iron, serum prolactin, theophylline; **NIPE:** ⊘ in PRG, breast-feeding, or in children; ⊘ w/ SSRIs, MAOIs, EtOH, ⊘ sun exposure

Tea Tree (*Melaleuca alternifolia*) Uses: Rx of superficial wounds (bacterial, viral,& fungal), insect bites, minor burns, cold sores, acne **Action:** Broad-spectrum antibiotic activity against *E. coli, S. aureus, C. albicans* **Available forms:** Topical creams, lotions, oint, oil apply topically PRN **Notes/SE:** Ataxia, contact dermatitis, diarrhea, drowsiness, GI mucosal irritation **Interactions:** ↓ Effects of drugs that affect histamine release **Labs:** ↑ Neutrophil count **NIPE:** Caution Pt to use externally only; ⊘ apply to broken skin

Valerian (*Valeriana officinalis*) Uses: Antianxiety, antispasmodic, dysmenorrheal, restlessness, sedative **Action:** Inhibits uptake & stimulates release of GABA, which ↑ GABA concentration extracellularly & causes sedation **Available forms:** Ext 400–900 mg PO 30 min < HS, tea 2–3 g (1 tsp of crude herb) qid, PRN, tinc 3–5 mL (½–1 tsp) (1:5 ratio) PO qid, PRN **Notes/SE:** GI upset, HA, insomnia, N/V, palpitations, restlessness, vision changes **Interactions:** ↑ Effects of barbiturates, benzodiazepines, opiates, EtOH, catnip, hops, kava, passion flower, skullcap; ↓ effects of MAOIs, phenytoin, warfarin **Labs:** ↑ ALT, AST, total bilirubin, urine bilirubin **NIPE:** Periodic check of LFTs, unknown effects in PRG & lactation, full effect may take 2–4 wk, taper herb to avoid withdrawal symptoms after long-term use

Yohimbine (*Pausinystalia yohimbe*) Uses: Rx for impotence, aphrodisiac **Action:** Peripherally affects autonomic nervous system by ↓ adrenergic activity & ↑ cholinergic activity; ↑ blood flow **Available forms:** Tabs 5.4 mg tid, PO; doses at 20–30 mg/d may ↑ BP & heart rate **Notes/SE:** Anxiety, dizziness, dysuria, genital pain, HTN, tachycardia, tremors **Interactions:** ↑ Effects of CNS stimulants, MAOIs, SSRIs, caffeine, ETOH; ↑ risk of toxicity w/ α-adrenergic blockers, phenothiazines; ↑ yohimbe toxicity w/ sympathomimetics; ↑ BP w/ foods containing tyramine **Labs:** ↑ BUN, creatinine **NIPE:** ⊘ w/ caffeine-containing foods w/ herb, may exacerbate mania in patients w/ psychiatric disorders

TABLE 1
Quick Guide to Dosing of Acetaminophen Based on the Tylenol Product Line

	Suspension[a] Drops and Original Drops 80 mg/0.8 mL Dropperful	Chewable[a] Tablets 80-mg tabs	Suspension[a] Liquid and Original Elixir 160 mg/5 mL	Junior[a] Strength 160-mg Caplets/Chewables	Regular[b] Strength 325-mg Caplets/Tablets	Extra Strength[b] 500-mg Caplets/Gelcaps
Birth–3 mo/ 6–11 lb/ 2.5–5.4 kg	$\frac{1}{2}$ dppr[c] (0.4 mL)					
4–11 mo/ 12–17 lb/ 5.5–7.9 kg	1 dppr[c] (0.8 mL)		$\frac{1}{2}$ tsp			
12–23 mo/ 18–23 lb/ 8.0–10.9 kg	$1\frac{1}{2}$ dppr[c] (1.2 mL)		$\frac{3}{4}$ tsp			
2–3 y/24–35 lb/ 11.0–15.9 kg	2 dppr[c] (1.6 mL)	2 tab	1 tsp			
4–5 y/36–47 lb/ 16.0–21.9 kg		3 tab	$1\frac{1}{2}$ tsp			

263

TABLE 1
(Continued)

	Suspension[a] Drops and Original Drops 80 mg/0.8 mL Dropperful	Chewable Tablets 80-mg tabs[a]	Suspension[a] Liquid and Original Elixir 160 mg/5 mL	Junior[a] Strength 160-mg Caplets/ Chewables	Regular[b] Strength 325-mg Caplets/ Tablets	Extra Strength[b] 500-mg Caplets/ Gelcaps
6–8 y/48–59 lb/ 22.0–26.9 kg		4 tab	2 tsp	2 cap/tab		
9–10 y/60–71 lb/ 27.0–31.9 kg		5 tab	2½ tsp	2½ cap/ tab		
11 y/72–95 lb/ 32.0–43.9 kg		6 tab	4 tsp	3 cap/tab		
Adults & children ≥ 12 y ≥ 96 lb ≥ 44.0 kg				4 cap/tab	1 or 2 caps/ tabs	2 caps/ gel

[a]Doses should be administered 4 or 5 times daily. Do not exceed 5 doses in 24 h.

[b]No more than 8 dosage units in any 24-h period. Not to be taken for pain for more than 10 days or for fever for more than 3 days unless directed by a physician.

[c]Dropperful.

264

TABLE 2
Common Drug Levels[a]

Drug	When to Sample	Therapeutic Levels	Usual Half-Life	Potentially Toxic Levels
Antibiotics				
Gentamicin	Peak: 30 min after 30-min infusion (peak level not necessary if extended-interval dosing: 6 mg/kg/dose) Trough: <0.5 h before next dose	Peak: 5–8 µg/mL Trough: <2 µg/mL <1.0 µg/mL for extended intervals (6 mg/kg/dose) (peak levels not needed with extended-interval dosing)	2 h	Peak: >12 µg/mL
Tobramycin Amikacin Vancomycin	Same as above Same as above Peak: 1 h after 1-h infusion Trough: <0.5 h before next dose	Same as above Peak: 20–30 µg/mL Peak: 30–40 µg/mL	Same as above 2 h 6–8 h	Same as above Peak: >35 µg/mL Peak: >50 µg/mL Trough: >15 µg/mL

265

**TABLE 2
(Continued)**

Drug	When to Sample	Therapeutic Levels	Usual Half-Life	Potentially Toxic Levels
Anticonvulsants				
Carbamazepine	Trough: just before next oral dose	8–12 µg/mL (monotherapy) 4–8 µg/mL (polytherapy)	15–20 h	Trough: >12 µg/mL
Ethosuximide	Trough: just before next oral dose	40–100 µg/mL	30–60 h	Trough: >100 µg/mL
Phenobarbital	Trough: just before next dose	15–40 µg/mL	40–120 h	Trough: >40 µg/mL
Phenytoin	May use free phenytoin to monitor[b] Trough: just before next dose	10–20 µg/mL	Concentration-dependent	>20 µg/mL
Primidone	Trough: just before next dose (primidone is metabolized to phenobarb; order levels separately)	5–12 µg/mL	10–12 h	>12 µg/mL
Valproic acid	Trough: just before next dose	50–100 µg/mL	5–20 h	>100 µg/mL

266

Bronchodilators

Drug	Timing	Therapeutic level	Half-life	Toxic level
Caffeine	Trough: just before next dose	Adults 5–15 µg/mL Neonates 6–11 µg/mL	Adults 3–4 h Neonates 30–140 h	20 µg/mL
Theophylline (IV)	IV: 12–24 h after infusion started	5–15 µg/mL	Nonsmoking adults 8 h Children and smoking adults 4 h	>20 µg/mL
Theophylline (PO)	Peak levels: not recommended Trough level: just before next dose	5–15 µg/mL		

Cardiovascular Agents

Drug	Timing	Therapeutic level	Half-life	Toxic level
Amiodarone	Trough: just before next dose	1–2.5 µg/mL	30–100 days	>2.5 µg/mL
Digoxin	Trough: just before next dose (levels drawn earlier than 6 h after a dose will be artificially elevated)	0.8–2.0 ng/mL	36 h	>2 ng/mL

TABLE 2
(Continued)

Drug	When to Sample	Therapeutic Levels	Usual Half-Life	Potentially Toxic Levels
Disopyramide	Trough: just before next dose	2–5 μg/mL	4–10 h	>5 μg/mL
Flecainide	Trough: just before next dose	0.2–1.0 μg/mL	11–14 h	>1.0 μg/mL
Lidocaine	Steady-state levels are usually achieved after 6–12 h	1.2–5.0 μg/mL	1.5 h	>6.0 μg/mL
Procainamide	Trough: just before next oral dose	4–10 μg/mL NAPA + Procaine: 5–30 μg/mL	Procaine: 3–5 h NAPA: 6–10 h	>10 μg/mL >30 μg/mL NAPA + Procaine: 0.5 μg/mL
Quinidine	Trough: just before next oral dose	2–5 μg/mL	6 h	
Other Agents				
Amitriptyline plus nortriptyline	Trough: just before next dose	120–250 ng/mL		
Nortriptyline	Trough: just before next dose	50–140 ng/mL		
Lithium	Trough: just before next dose	0.5–1.5 mEq/mL	18–20 h	>1.5 mEq/mL

Imipramine plus desipramine	Trough: just before next dose	150–300 ng/mL
Desipramine	Trough: just before next dose	50–300 ng/mL
Methotrexate	By protocol	<0.5 μmol/L after 48 h
Cyclosporine	Trough: just before next dose	Highly variable Renal: 150–300 ng/mL (RIA) Hepatic: 150–300 ng/mL	Highly variable
Doxepin	Trough: just before next dose	100–300 ng/mL
Trazodone	Trough: just before next dose	900–2100 ng/mL

aResults of therapeutic drug monitoring must be interpreted in light of the complete clinical situation. For information on dosing or interpretation of drug levels contact the pharmacist or an order for a pharmacokinetic consult may be written in the patient's chart. Modified and reproduced with permission from the Pharmacy and Therapeutics Committee Formulary, 41st ed., Thomas Jefferson University Hospital. Philadelphia, PA.

bMore reliable in cases of uremia and hypoalbuminemia.

TABLE 3
Local Anesthetic Comparison Chart for Commonly Used Injectable Agents

Agent	Proprietary Names	Onset	Duration	Maximum Dose mg/kg	Maximum Dose Volume in 70-kg Adult[a]
Bupivacaine	Marcaine, Sensoricaine	7–30 min	5–7 h	3	70 mL of 0.25% solution
Lidocaine	Xylocaine, Anestacon	5–30 min	2 h	4	28 mL of 1% solution
Lidocaine with epinephrine (1:200,000)		5–30 min	2–3 h	7	50 mL of 1% solution
Mepivacaine	Carbocaine	5–30 min	2–3 h	7	50 mL of 1% solution
Procaine	Novocaine	Rapid	30 min–1 h	10–15	70–105 mL of 1% solution

[a]To calculate the maximum dose if not a 70-kg adult, use the fact that a 1% solution has 10 mg of drug per milliliter.

270

TABLE 4
Comparison of Systemic Steroids

Drug	Relative Equivalent Dose (mg)	Mineralo-corticoid Activity	Duration (h)	Route
Betamethasone	0.75	0	36–72	PO, IM
Cortisone (Cortone)	25.00	2	8–12	PO, IM
Dexamethasone (Decadron)	0.75	0	36–72	PO, IV
Hydrocortisone (Solu-Cortef, Hydrocortone)	20.00	2	8–12	PO, IM, IV
Methylprednisolone acetate (Depo-Medrol)	4.00	0	36–72	PO, IM, IV
Methylprednisolone succinate (Solu-Medrol)	4.00	0	8–12	PO, IM, IV
Prednisone (Deltasone)	5.00	1	12–36	PO
Prednisolone (Delta-Cortef)	5.00	1	12–36	PO, IM, IV

TABLE 5
Topical Steroid Preparations

Agent	Common Trade Names	Potency	Apply
Alclometasone dipropionate	Aclovate, cream, oint 0.05%	Low	bid/tid
Amcinonide	Cyclocort, cream, lotion, oint 0.1%	High	bid/tid
Betamethasone			
Betamethasone valerate	Valisone cream, lotion 0.01%	Low	qd/bid
Betamethasone valerate	Valisone cream 0.01, 0.1%, oint, lotion 0.1%	Intermediate	qd/bid
Betamethasone dipropionate	Diprosone cream 0.05%	High	qd/bid
Betamethasone dipropionate	Diprosone aerosol 0.1%		qd/bid
Betamethasone dipropionate, augmented	Diprolene oint, gel 0.05%	Ultrahigh	bid (2 wk max)
Clobetasol propionate	Temovate cream, gel, oint, scalp, soln 0.05%	Ultrahigh	qd–qid
Clocortolone pivalate	Cloderm cream 0.1%	Intermediate	bid–qid
Desonide	DesOwen, cream, oint, lotion 0.05%	Low	
Desoximetasone			
Desoximetasone 0.05%	Topicort LP cream, gel 0.05%	Intermediate	
Desoximetasone 0.25%	Topicort cream, oint	High	
Dexamethasone base	Aeroseb-Dex aerosol 0.01%	Low	bid–qid
	Decadron oint 0.1%		
Diflorasone diacetate	Psorcon cream, oint 0.05%	Ultrahigh	bid/qid
Fluocinolone			
Fluocinolone acetonide 0.01%	Synalar cream, soln 0.01%	Low	bid/tid
Fluocinolone acetonide 0.025%	Synalar oint, cream 0.025%	Intermediate	bid/tid

272

Fluocinolone acetonide 0.2%	Synalar-HP cream 0.2%	High	bid/tid
Fluocinonide 0.05%	Lidex, anhydrous cream, gel, soln 0.05%	High	bid/tid oint
	Lidex-E aqueous cream 0.05%		
Flurandrenolide	Cordran cream, oint 0.025%	Intermediate	bid/tid
	cream, lotion, oint 0.05%	Intermediate	bid/tid
	tape, 4 μg/cm²	Intermediate	qd
Fluticasone propionate	Cutivate cream 0.05%, oint 0.005%	Intermediate	bid
Halobetasol	Ultravate cream, oint 0.05%	Very High	bid
Halcinonide	Halog cream 0.025%, emollient base 0.1% cream, oint, solution 0.1%	High	qd/tid
Hydrocortisone			
Hydrocortisone	Cortizone, Caldecort, Hycort, Hytone, etc. aerosol 1%, cream: 0.5, 1, 2.5%, gel 0.5%, oint 0.5, 1, 2.5%, lotion 0.5, 1, 2.5%, paste 0.5%, soln 1%	Low	tid/qid
	Corticaine cream, oint 0.5, 1%	Low	tid/qid
Hydrocortisone acetate	Locoid oint, soln 0.1%	Intermediate	bid/tid
Hydrocortisone butyrate	Westcort cream, oint 0.2%	Intermediate	bid/tid
Hydrocortisone valerate			

273

TABLE 5
(Continued)

Agent	Common Trade Names	Potency	Apply
Mometasone furoate	Elocon 0.1% cream, oint, lotion	Intermediate	qd
Prednicarbate	Dermatop 0.1% cream	Intermediate	bid
Triamcinolone			
Triamcinolone acetonide 0.025%	Aristocort, Kenalog cream, oint, lotion 0.025%	Low	tid/qid
Triamcinolone acetonide 0.1%	Aristocort, Kenalog cream, oint, lotion 0.1%	Intermediate	tid/qid
	Aerosol 0.2 mg/2-sec spray		
Triamcinolone acetonide 0.5%	Aristocort, Kenalog cream, oint 0.5%	High	tid/qid

TABLE 6
Comparison of Insulins

Type of Insulin	Onset (h)	Peak (h)	Duration (h)
Ultra Rapid			
Humalog (lispro)	Immediate	0.5–1.5	3–5
NovoLog (insulin aspart)	Immediate	0.5–1.5	3–5
Rapid			
Regular Iletin II	0.25–0.5	2.0–4.0	5–7
Humulin R	0.5	2.0–4.0	6–8
Novolin R	0.5	2.5–5.0	5–8
Velosulin	0.5	2.0–5.0	6–8
Intermediate			
NPH Iletin II	1.0–2.0	6–12	18–24
Lente Iletin II	1.0–2.0	6–12	18–24
Humulin N	1.0–2.0	6–12	14–24
Novulin L	2.5–5.0	7–15	18–24
Novulin 70/30	0.5	7–12	24
Prolonged			
Ultralente	4.0–6.0	14–24	28–36
Humulin U	4.0–6.0	8–20	24–28
Lantus (insulin glargine)	4.0–6.0	No peak	24
Combination Insulins			
Humalog Mix (lispro protamine/ lispro)	0.25–0.5	1–4	24

TABLE 7
Commonly Used Oral Contraceptives[a]

Monophasics

Drug (Manufacturer)	Estrogen (µg)	Progestin (mg)
Alesse 21, 28 (Wyeth-Ayerst)	Ethinyl estradiol (20)	Desogestrel (0.15)
Apri 28 (Barr)	Ethinyl estradiol (30)	Desogestrel (0.15)
Aviane 28 (Barr)	Ethinyl estradiol (20)	Levonorgestrel (0.1)
Brevicon 28 (Watson)	Ethinyl estradiol (35)	Norethindrone (0.5)
Cryselle 28 (Barr)	Ethinyl estradiol (30)	Norgestrel (0.3)
Demulen 1/35 21, 28 (Pfizer)	Ethinyl estradiol (35)	Ethynodiol diacetate (1)
Demulen 1/50 21, 28 (Pfizer)	Ethinyl estradiol (50)	Ethynodiol diacetate (1)
Desogen 28 (Organon)	Ethinyl estradiol (30)	Desogestrel (0.15)
Estrostep 28 (Warner-Chilcott)[b]	Ethinyl estradiol (20, 30, 35)	Norethindrone acetate (1)
Junel Fe 1/20 21, 28 (Barr)	Ethinyl estradiol (20)	Norethindrone acetate (1)
Junel Fe 1.5/30 21, 28 (Barr)	Ethinyl estradiol (30)	Norethindrone acetate (1.5)
Kariva 28 (Barr)	Ethinyl estradiol (20, 0, 10)	Desogestrel (0.15)
Lessina 28 (Barr)	Ethinyl estradiol (20)	Levonorgestrel (0.1)
Levlen 28 (Berlex)	Ethinyl estradiol (30)	Levonorgestrel (0.15)
Levlite 28 (Berlex)	Ethinyl estradiol (20)	Levonorgestrel (0.1)
Levora 28 (Watson)	Ethinyl estradiol (30)	Levonorgestrel (0.15)
Loestrin Fe 1.5/30 21, 28 (Warner-Chilcott)	Ethinyl estradiol (30)	Norethindrone acetate (1.5)
Loestrin Fe 1/20 21, 28 (Warner-Chilcott)	Ethinyl estradiol (20)	Norethindrone acetate (1)
Lo/Ovral 21, 28 (Wyeth-Ayerst)	Ethinyl estradiol (30)	Norgestrel (0.3)
Low-Ogestrel 28 (Watson)	Ethinyl estradiol (30)	Norgestrel (0.3)
Microgestin Fe 1/20 21, 28 (Watson)	Ethinyl estradiol (20)	Norethindrone acetate (1)
Microgestin Fe 1.5/30 21, 28 (Watson)	Ethinyl estradiol (30)	Norethindrone acetate (1.5)

Brand	Estrogen (mcg)	Progestin (mg)
Mircette 28 (Organon)	Ethinyl estradiol (20, 0, 10)	Desogestrel (0.15)
Modicon 28 (Ortho-McNeil)	Ethinyl estradiol (35)	Norethindrone (0.5)
MonoNessa 28 (Watson)	Ethinyl estradiol (35)	Norgestimate (0.25)
Necon 1/50 28 (Watson)	Mestranol (50)	Norethindrone (1)
Necon 0.5/35, 28 (Watson)	Ethinyl estradiol (35)	Norethindrone (0.5)
Necon 1/35 28 (Watson)	Ethinyl estradiol (35)	Norethindrone (1)
Nordette 21, 28 (King)	Ethinyl estradiol (30)	Levonorgestrel (0.15)
Nortrel 0.5/35 28 (Barr)	Ethinyl estradiol (35)	Norethindrone (0.5)
Nortrel 1/35 21, 28 (Barr)	Ethinyl estradiol (35)	Norethindrone (1)
Noriyl 1/35 28 (Watson)	Ethinyl estradiol (35)	Norethindrone (1)
Noriyl 1/50 28 (Watson)	Mestranol (50)	Norethindrone (1)
Ogestrel 28 (Watson)	Ethinyl estradiol (50)	Norgestrel (0.5)
Ortho-Cept 28 (Ortho-McNeil)	Ethinyl estradiol (30)	Desogestrel (0.15)
Ortho-Cyclen 28 (Ortho-McNeil)	Ethinyl estradiol (35)	Norgestimate (0.25)
Ortho-Novum 1/35 28 (Ortho-McNeil)	Ethinyl estradiol (35)	Norethindrone (1)
Ortho-Novum 1/50 28 (Ortho-McNeil)	Mestranol (50)	Norethindrone (1)
Ovcon 35 21, 28 (Warner Chilcott)	Ethinyl estradiol (35)	Norethindrone (0.4)
Ovcon 50 28 (Warner Chilcott)	Ethinyl estradiol (50)	Norethindrone (1)
Ovral 21, 28 (Wyeth-Ayerst)	Ethinyl estradiol (50)	Norgestrel (0.5)
Portia 28 (Barr)	Ethinyl estradiol (30)	Levonorgestrel (0.15)
Sprintec 28 (Barr)	Ethinyl estradiol (35)	Norgestimate (0.25)
Yasmin 28 (Berlex)	Ethinyl estradiol (30)	Drospirenone (3)
Zovia 1/50 28 (Watson)	Ethinyl estradiol (50)	Ethynodiol diacetate (1)
Zovia 1/35E 28 (Watson)	Ethinyl estradiol (35)	Ethynodiol diacetate (1)

TABLE 7
(Continued)

Drug (Manufacturer)	Estrogen (µg)	Progestin (mg)
Multiphasics		
Cyclessa 28 (Organon)	Ethinyl estradiol (25)	Desogestrel (0.1, 0.125, 0.15)
Enpresse 28 (Barr)	Ethinyl estradiol (30, 40, 30)	Levonorgestrel (0.05, 0.075, 0.125)
Necon 10/11 21, 28 (Watson)	Ethinyl estradiol (35)	Norethindrone (0.5, 1)
Necon 7/7/7 (Watson)	Ethinyl estradiol (35)	Norethindrone (0.5, 0.75, 1)
Nortel 7/7/7 28 (Barr)	Ethinyl estradiol (35)	Norethindrone (0.5, 0.75, 1)
Ortho Tri-Cyclen 21, 28 (Ortho-McNeil)[b]	Ethinyl estradiol (25)	Norgestimate (0.18, 0.215, 0.25)
Ortho Tri-Cyclen lo 21, 28 (Ortho-McNeil)	Ethinyl estradiol (35, 35, 35)	Norgestimate (0.18, 0.215, 0.25)
Ortho-Novum 10/11 21 (Ortho-McNeil)	Ethinyl estradiol (35, 35)	Norethindrone (0.5, 1.0)
Ortho-Novum 7/7/7 21 (Ortho-McNeil)	Ethinyl estradiol (35, 35, 35)	Norethindrone (0.5, 0.75, 1.0)
Tri-Levlen 28 (Berlex)	Ethinyl estradiol (30, 40, 30)	Levonorgestrel (0.05, 0.075, 0.125)
Tri-Nessa 28 (Watson)	Ethinyl estradiol (35)	Norgestimate (0.18, 0.215, 0.25)
Tri-Norinyl 21, 28 (Watson)	Ethinyl estradiol (35, 35, 35)	Norethindrone (0.5, 1.0, 0.5)
Triphasil 21, 28 (Wyeth-Ayerst)	Ethinyl estradiol (30, 40, 30)	Levonorgestrel (0.05, 0.075, 0.125)
Tri-Sprintec (Barr)	Ethinyl estradiol (35)	Norgestimate (0.18, 0.215, 0.25)
Trivora-28 (Watson)	Ethinyl estradiol (30, 40, 30)	Levonorgestrel (0.05, 0.075, 0.125)
Velivet (Barr)	Ethinyl estradiol (25)	Desogestrel (0.1, 0.125, 0.15)

Progestin Only

Camila (Barr)	None	Norethindrone (0.35)
Errin (Barr)	None	Norethindrone (0.35)
Jolivette 28 (Watson)	None	Norethindrone (0.35)
Micronor (Ortho-McNeil)	None	Norethindrone (0.35)
Nor-QD (Watson)	None	Norethindrone (0.35)
Nora-BE 28 (Ortho-McNeil)	None	Norethindrone (0.35)
Ovrette (Wyeth-Ayerst)	None	Norgestrel (0.075)

Extended-Cycle Combination

Seasonale (Duramed)	Ethinyl estradiol (30)	Levonorgestrel (0.15)

Based on data published in the *Medical Letter* Volume 2 (Issue 24) August 2004.

[a]The designations 21 and 28 refer to number of days in regimen available.

[b]Also approved for acne.

TABLE 8
Some Common Oral Potassium Supplements

Brand Name	Salt	Form	mEq Potassium/ Dosing Unit
Glu-K	Gluconate	Tablet	2 mEq/tablet
Kaochlor 10%	KCl	Liquid	20 mEq/15 mL
Kaochlor S-F 10% (sugar-free)	KCl	Liquid	20 mEq/15 mL
Kaochlor Eff	Bicarbonate/ KCl/citrate	Effervescent tablet	20 mEq/tablet
Kaon elixir	Gluconate	Liquid	20 mEq/15 mL
Kaon	Gluconate	Tablets	5 mEq/tablet
Kaon-Cl	KCl	Tablet, SR	6.67 mEq/tablet
Kaon-Cl 20%	KCl	Liquid	40 mEq/15 mL
KayCiel	KCl	Liquid	20 mEq/15 mL
K-Lor	KCl	Powder	15 or 20 mEq/packet
Klorvess	Bicarbonate/ KCl	Liquid	20 mEq/15 mL
Klotrix	KCl	Tablet, SR	10 mEq/tablet
K-Lyte	Bicarbonate/ citrate	Effervescent tablet	25 mEq/tablet
K-Tab	KCl	Tablet, SR	10 mEq/tablet
Micro-K	KCl	Capsules, SR	8 mEq/capsule
Slow-K	KCl	Tablet, SR	8 mEq/tablet
Tri-K	Acetate/bicarbonate and citrate	Liquid	45 mEq/15 mL
Twin-K	Citrate/gluconate	Liquid	20 mEq/5 mL

SR = sustained release.

TABLE 9
Tetanus Prophylaxis

History of Absorbed Tetanus Toxoid Immunization	Clean, Minor Wounds		All Other Wounds[a]	
	Td[b]	TIG[c]	Td[d]	TIG[c]
Unknown or <3 doses	Yes	No	Yes	Yes
<3 doses	No[e]	No	No[f]	No

[a]Such as, but not limited to, wounds contaminated with dirt, feces, soil, saliva, etc; puncture wounds; avulsions; and wounds resulting from missiles, crushing, burns, and frostbite.

[b]Td = tetanus-diphtheria toxoid (adult type), 0.5 mL IM.
  - For children <7 y, DPT (DT, if pertussis vaccine is contraindicated) is preferred to tetanus toxoid alone.
  - For persons >7 y, Td is preferred to tetanus toxoid alone.
  - DT = diphtherio-tetanus toxoid (pediatric), used for those who cannot receive pertussis.

[c]TIG = tetanus immune globulin, 250 U IM.

[d]If only 3 doses of fluid toxoid have been received, then a fourth dose of toxoid, preferably an adsorbed toxoid, should be given.

[e]Yes, if >10 y since last dose.

[f]Yes, if >5 y since last dose.

Source: Based on guidelines from the Centers for Disease Control and Prevention and reported in MMWR.

TABLE 10
Oral Anticoagulant Standards of Practice

Thromboembolic Disorder	INR	Duration
Deep Venous Thrombosis		
High-risk surgery (prophylaxis)	10 mg night before surgery 5 mg night of surgery	Short term only
Treatment: single episode	2–3	3–6 mo
Recurrent systemic embolism	2–3	Indefinite
Prevention of Systemic Embolism		
Atrial fibrillation (AF)[a]	2–3	Indefinite
AF: cardioversion	2–3	3 wk prior; 4 wk post sinus rhythm
Valvular heart disease	2–3	Indefinite
Cardiomyopathy	2–3	Indefinite
Acute Myocardial Infarction		
Prevention of systemic embolization	2–3	<3 mo
Prevention of recurrence	2.5–3.5	Indefinite
Prosthetic Valves		
Tissue heart valves	2–3	3 mo
Bileaflet mechanical valves in aortic position	2–3	2–3 mo Indefinite
Other mechanical prosthetic valves[b]	2.5–3.5	Indefinite

[a]With high-risk factors or multiple moderate risk factors.

[b]May add aspirin 81 mg to warfarin in patients with ball–cage valves or with additional risk factors.

INR = international normalized ratio.

Source: Based on data published in *Chest* 2001;119 Supplement 1S–307S.

TABLE 11
Serotonin 5-HT₁ Receptor Agonists

Drug	Initial Dose	Repeat Dose	Max. Dose/24h	Supplied
Almotriptan (Axert)	6.25 or 12.5 mg PO	× 1 in 2 h	25 mg	Tabs 6.25, 12.5 mg
Frovatriptan (Frova)	2.5 mg PO	in 2 h	7.5 mg	Tabs 2.5 mg
Naratriptan (Amerge)	1 or 2.5 mg PO[a]	in 4 h	5 mg	Tabs 1, 2.5 mg
Rizatriptan (Maxalt)	5 or 10 mg PO[b]	in 2 h	30 mg	Tabs 5, 10 mg Disintegrating tabs 5, 10 mg
Sumatriptan (Imitrex)	25, 50, or 100 mg PO 5–20 mg intranasally 6 mg SC	in 2 h in 2 h in 1 h	200 mg 40 mg 12 mg	Tabs 25,50 mg Nasal spray 5, 20 mg Inj 12 mg/mL
Zolmitriptan (Zomig)	2.5 or 5 mg PO	in 2 h	10 mg	Tabs 2.5,5 mg

Precautions/contraindications: [C, M]; ischemic heart disease, coronary artery vasospasm, Prinzmetal's angina, uncontrolled HTN, hemiplegic or basilar migraine, ergots, use of another serotonin agonist within 24 h, use with MAOI. Side effects: dizziness, somnolence, paresthesias, nausea, flushing, dry mouth, coronary vasospasm, chest tightness, HTN, GI upset.

[a]Reduce dose in mild renal and hepatic insufficiency (2.5 mg/d MAX); contraindicated with severe renal (CrCl <15 mL/min) or hepatic impairment.

[b]Initiate therapy at 5 mg PO (15 mg/d max) in patients receiving propranolol.

INDEX

A

A-K Beta (levobunolol), 12, 154

V/T/S (erythromycin [topical]), 10, 108–109

Abacavir (Ziagen), 3, 23

Abarelix (Plenaxis), 5, 23

Abbokinase (urokinase), 15, 246–247

Abciximab (ReoPro), 15, 23–24

Abelcet (amphotericin B lipid complex), 3, 39

Abilify (aripiprazole), 9, 43

Acarbose (Precose), 11, 24

Accolate (zafirlukast), 20, 252

Accupril (quinapril), 6, 209

Accutane (isotretinoin [13-*cis* retinoic acid]), 10, 148

Acebutolol (Sectral), 6, 24

Aceon (perindopril erbumine), 6, 196

Acetaminophen
[APAP] (Tylenol), 19, 24–25
dosing guide, 263t–264t
with butalbital w/wo caffeine (Fioricet, Medigesic, Repan, Sedapap-10, Two-Dyne, Triapin, Axocet, Prenilin Forte), 18, 25
and chlorpheniramine, phenylephrine, hy-

drocodone, caffeine (Hycomine), 20, 137–138
with codeine (Tylenol No. 1, 2, 3, 4), 18, 25
and hydrocodone (Lorcet, Vicodin), 19, 136–137
and oxycodone (Percocet, Tylox), 19, 189–190
and propoxyphene (Darvocet), 19, 206

Acetaminophen/tramadol (Ultracet), 19, 241

Acetazolamide (Diamox), 7, 12, 25–26

Acetic acid and aluminum acetate (Otic Domeboro), 11, 26

Acetylcysteine (Mucomyst), 1, 20, 26

Achromycin V (tetracycline), 3, 233

Aciphex (Rabeprazole), 14, 210

Acitretin (Soriatane), 9, 26

Acova (argatroban), 15, 43

ActHIB (haemophilus B conjugate vaccine), 16, 133

Actidose (charcoal), 1, 70–71

Actimmune (interferon gamma-1b), 16, 145

Actiq (fentanyl [transmucosal system]), 19, 117

Activase (alteplase [recombinant tPA]), 15, 32

Actonel (risedronate), 12, 213

Actos (piogliazone), 11, 199–200

Acular (ketorolac [ophthalmic]), 13, 150

Acyclovir (Zovirax), 4, 9, 27

Adalat CC (nifedipine), 7, 180–181

Adalat (nifedipine), 7, 180–181

Adalimumab (Humira), 16, 27

Adapin (doxepin), 8, 100

Adefovir (Hepsera), 4, 27

Adenocard (adenosine), 6, 27–28

Adenosine (Adenocard), 6, 27–28

Adrenalin (epinephrine), 7, 20, 105

Adriamycin (doxorubicin), 5, 100–101

Adrucil, (fluorouracil [5-FU]), 5, 121

Advair Diskus (fluticasone proprionate and salmeterol xinafoate), 20, 123

Advil (ibuprofen), 19, 140

AeroBid (flunisolide), 20, 120

Afrinol (pseudoephedrine), 20, 207–208

Agenerase (amprenavir), 3, 40

Aggrastat (tirofiban), 15, 237–238

Aggrenox (dipyridamole and aspirin), 15, 97

AK-

Dex Ophthalmic (dexamethasone [ophthalmic]), 13, 89

Neo-Dex Ophthalmic (dexamethasone and neomycin), 12, 178

Poly Bac Ophthalmic (bacitracin and polymyxin B), 12, 49

Spore HC Ophthalmic (bacitracin, neomycin, polymyxin B, and hydrocortisone [ophthalmic]), 12, 49

Spore Ophthalmic (bacitracin, neomycin, and polymyxin B [ophthalmic]), 12, 49

Tracin Ophthalmic (bacitracin) 12, 49

AKTob (tobramycin [ophthalmic]), 13, 238

Alamast (pemirolast), 13, 193

Alavert (loratadine), 1, 159

Albalon-A Ophthalmic (naphazoline and antazoline), 13, 176

Albumin (Albuminar, Buminate, Albutein), 15, 28

Albuminar (albumin), 15, 28

Albutein (albumin), 15, 28

Albuterol and ipratropium (Combivent), 20, 28

Albuterol (Proventil, Ventolin, Volmax), 20, 28

Alclometasone dipropionate, 272t

Aldactazide (hydrochlorothiazide and spironolactone), 7, 136

Aldactone (spironolactone), 7, 222–223

Aldara (imiquimod cream), 5, 10, 142

Aldesleukin [Interleukin-2, IL-2] (Proleukin), 5, 28–29
Aldomet (methyldopa), 7, 167
Aldosterone antagonist, classification of, 6
Alefacept (Amevive), 9, 29
Alendronate (Fosamax), 12, 29
Aleve (naproxen), 19, 176
Alfenta (alfentanil), 18, 29–30
Alfentanil (Alfenta), 18, 29–30
Alfuzosin (Uroxatral), 21, 30
Alginic acid, aluminum hydroxide, and magnesium trisilicate (Gaviscon), 30
Alginic acid (Gaviscon), 13, 30
Alimta (pemetrexed), 5, 193
Alinia (nitazoxanide), 3, 181
Alka-Mints (calcium carbonate), 13, 58–59
Alkeran (Melphalan [L-Pam]), 4, 162–163
Alkylating agents, classification of, 4
Allegra (fexofenadine), 1, 118
Alloprim (allopurinol), 16, 30
Allopurinol (Zyloprim, Lopurin, Alloprim), 16, 30
Almotriptan (Axert), 18, 30, 283t
Alomide (lodoxamide), 12, 13, 158
Alosetron (Lotronex), 14, 30–31
Aloxi (palonosetron), 14, 191
Alpha$_1$-adrenergic blockers, classification of, 7
Alpha$_1$-protease inhibitor (Prolastin), 20, 31
Alphagan (brimonidine), 12, 55
Alprazolam (Xanax), 8, 31

Alprostadil
[intracavernosal] (Caverject, Edex), 21, 31–32
[Prostaglandin E$_1$] (Prostin VR), 8, 31
[urethral suppository] (Muse), 21, 32
Altace (ramipril), 6, 210
Alteplase [recombinant tPA] (Activase), 15, 32
AlternaGEL (aluminum hydroxide), 13, 33
Altocor (lovastatin), 7, 160
Altretamine (Hexalen), 4, 32–33
Alum (ammonium aluminum sulfate), 21, 37
Aluminum acetate and acetic acid (Otic Domeboro), 11, 26
Aluminum hydroxide (Amphojel, AlternaGEL), 13, 33
with magnesium carbonate (Gaviscon), 13, 33
with magnesium hydroxide (Maalox), 13, 33
with magnesium hydroxide and simethicone (Mylanta, Mylanta II, Maalox Plus), 13, 33–34
with magnesium trisilicate and alginic acid (Gaviscon), 30
with magnesium trisilicate (Gaviscon, Gaviscon-2), 13, 34
Alupent (metaproterenol), 20, 165
Amantadine (Symmetrel), 4, 9, 34

Amaryl (glimepiride), 11, 130

Ambien (zolpidem), 9, 254

AmBisome (amphotericin B liposomal), 3, 39

Amcill (ampicillin), 2, 39–40

Amcinonide, 272t

Amerge (naratriptan), 18, 176–177

Amevive (alefacept), 9, 29

Amicar (aminocaproic acid), 15, 35

Amifostine (Ethyol), 1, 34

Amikacin (Amikin), 1, 34–35, 265t

Amikin (amikacin), 1, 34–35

Amiloride and hydrochlorothiazide (Moduretic), 7, 136

Amiloride (Midamor), 7, 35

Amino-Cerv pH 5.5 Cream, 18, 35

Aminocaproic acid (Amicar), 15, 35

Aminoglutethimide (Cytadren), 5, 35

Aminoglycosides, classification of, 1

Aminophylline, 20, 36

Amiodarone (Cordarone, Pacerone), 6, 36, 267t

Amitriptyline (Elavil), 8, 19, 37

Amitriptyline plus nortriptyline, 268t

Amlodipine (Norvasc), 7, 37

Amlodipine/atorvastatin (Caduet), 8, 37

Ammonium aluminum sulfate (Alum), 21, 37

Amnesteem (isotretinoin [13-*cis* retinoic acid]), 10, 148

Amoxicillin (Amoxil, Polymox), 2, 37–38

and clavulanic acid (Augmentin), 2, 38

Amoxil (amoxicillin), 2, 37–38

Amphojel (aluminum hydroxide), 13, 33

Amphotec (amphotericin B cholesteryl), 3, 39

Amphotericin B

cholesteryl (Amphotec), 3, 39

(Fungizone), 3, 9, 38–39

lipid complex (Abelcet), 3, 39

liposomal (AmBisome), 3, 39

Ampicillin (Amcill, Omnipen), 2, 39–40

Ampicillin–sulbactam (Unasyn), 2, 40

Amprenavir (Agenerase), 3, 40

Anakinra (Kineret), 16, 40–41

Anaprox (naproxen), 19, 176

Anaspaz (hyoscyamine), 14, 21, 139

Anastrozole (Arimidex), 5, 41

Ancef, cefazolin, 2, 63–64

Androderm (testosterone), 11, 232

Androgel (testosterone), 11, 232

Anectine (succinylcholine), 17, 225

Anestacon Topical (lidocaine), 6, 18, 156

Anesthetics [local]

classification of, 18

comparison chart (commonly used injectables), 270t

Angiomax (bivalirudin), 15, 54

Angiotensin-converting enzyme inhibitors, classification of, 6

angiotensin II receptor antago-
    nists, classification of, 6
anistreplase (Eminase), 15, 41
nsaid (flurbiprofen), 19, 122
antacids, classification of, 13
antazoline and naphazoline (Al-
    balon-A Ophthalmic), 13,
    176
anthra-Derm (anthralin), 9, 41
anthralin (Anthra-Derm), 9, 41
antiallergenic agents, classifica-
    tion of, 1
antianxiety agents, 8
antiarrhythmic agents, classifica-
    tion of, 6
antibacterial agents (miscella-
    neous), classification of,
    3–4
antibiotics/antimicrobial agents,
    classification of, 1–3
antibiotics/antineoplastic agents,
    classification of, 4–5
anticoagulants
    classification of, 15
    [oral] standards of practice,
    282t
anticonvulsants, classification
    of, 8
antidepressants, classification
    of, 8
antidiabetic agents, classifica-
    tion of, 11
antidiarrheals, classification of, 13
antidotes, classification of, 1
antiemetics, classification of,
    13–14
antifungals, classification of, 3
antigout agents, classification of,
    16

Antihemophilic factor VIII (Mono-
    clate), 15, 41
Antihistamines, classification of, 1
Antihypertensive agents (cen-
    trally acting), classifica-
    tion of, 7
Antilirium (physostigmine), 1,
    199
Antimetabolites, classification of,
    5
Antimicrobial agents
    classification of, 1–3
    (miscellaneous), classification
    of, 4
Antimycobacterials, classifica-
    tion of, 3
Antineoplastic agents, classifica-
    tion of, 4–5
Antiparkinson agents, classifica-
    tion of, 9
Antiplatelet agents, classification
    of, 15
Antiprotozoals, classification of,
    3
Antipsychotics, classification of,
    9
Antipyrine and benzocaine (Au-
    ralgan), 11, 18, 51
Antiretrovirals, classification of,
    3–4
Antithrobotic agents, classifica-
    tion of, 15
Antithymocyte globulin [ATG]
    (ATGAM), 42
Antitussives, decongestants, and
    expectorants, classifica-
    tion of, 19–20
Antiulcer agents, classification
    of, 14

Antivert (meclizine), 14, 162

Antivirals, classification of, 4

Anturane (sulfinpyrazone), 16, 227

Anusol-HC Suppository (hydrocortisone [rectal]), 14, 138

Anusol Ointment (pramoxine), 10, 14, 18, 203

Anzemet (dolasetron), 13, 99

Apokyn (apormorphine), 9, 42

Apomorphine (Apokyn), 9, 42

Apraclonidine (Iopidine), 12, 42

Aprepitant (Emend), 13, 42–43

Apresoline (hydralzine), 8, 135

Aprotinin (Trasylol), 15, 43

Aquachloral (chloral hydrate), 9, 71

AquaMEPHYTON (Phytonadione [vitamin K]), 10, 199

Aranesp (darbepoetin alfa), 15, 87

Arava (leflunomide), 17, 152

Ardeparin (Normiflo), 15, 43

Aredia (pamidronate), 11, 191

Argatroban (Acova), 15, 43

Arimidex (anastrozole), 5, 41

Aripiprazole (Abilify), 9, 43

Arixtra (fondaparinux), 15, 124

Arnica (*Arnica montana*), 21, 255

Aromasin (exemestane), 5, 115

Artane (trihexyphenidyl), 9, 244

Artificial tears (Tears Naturale), 13, 43

Asacol (mesalamine), 14, 164

Aspirin

(Bayer, Ecotrin, St. Joseph's), 15, 19, 44

with butalbital, caffeine, and codeine (Fiorinal with codeine), 18, 45

and butalbital compound (Fio inal), 18, 44–45

with codeine (Empirin No. 2, 3 4), 18, 45

and hydrocodone (Lortab ASA), 1, 19, 137

and oxycodone (Percodan, Percodan-Demi), 19, 190

and propoxyphene (Darvon Compound-65, Darvon-N with Aspirin), 19, 206

Astelin (azelastine), 1, 48

Astragalus (*Astragalus membranaceus*), 255

Atacand (candesartan), 6, 59–60

Atarax (hydroxyzine), 1, 8, 9, 139

Atazanavir (Reyataz), 4, 45

Atenolol

(Tenormin), 6, 46

and chlorthalidone (Tenoretic) 6, 46

ATGAM (antithymocyte globulin [ATG]/lymphocyte immune globulin), 16, 42, 160

Ativan (lorazepam), 8, 159

Atomoxetine (Strattera), 9, 46

Atorvastatin (Lipitor), 7, 46–47

Atorvastatin/amlodipine (Caduet), 8, 37

Atovaquone (Mepron), 4, 47

Atovaquone/proguanil (Malarone), 4, 47

Atracurium (Tracrium), 17, 47

atropine, 6, 47, 139–140
  and scopolamine,
    hyoscyamine, phenobar-
    bital (Donnatal), 14,
    139–140
Atrovent (ipratropium), 20, 146
Augmentin (amoxicillin and
  clavulanic acid), 2, 38
Auralgan (benzocaine and an-
  tipyrine), 11, 18, 51
Avandia (rosiglitazone), 11, 215
Avapro (irbesartan), 6, 146
Avastin (bevacizumab), 5, 53
Avelox (moxifloxacin), 2, 174
Aventyl (nortriptyline), 8, 184
Avinza XR (morphine), 19,
  173–174
Avita (tretinoin/topical [retinoic
  acid]), 5, 10, 242
Avlosulfon (dapsone), 3, 87
Avodart (dutasteride), 21, 102
Axert (almotriptan), 18, 30,
  283t
Axid (Nizatidine), 14, 183
Axocet (acetaminophen with bu-
  talbital w/wo caffeine), 18,
  25
Azactam (aztreonam), 3, 48–49
Azathioprine (Imuran), 16,
  47–48
Azelastine (Astelin, Optivar), 1,
  48
Azithromycin (Zithromax), 2, 48
Azmacort (triamcinolone), 20,
  242
Azopt (brinzolamide), 12, 55
Aztreonam (Azactam), 3, 48–49
Azulfidine (sulfasalazine), 15,
  226–227

B
B & O Supprettes (belladonna
  and opium suppositories),
  21, 51
Baciduent (bacitracin [topical]),
  9, 49
Bacitracin
  and neomycin, polymyxin B,
    hydrocortisone [oph-
    thalmic] (AK spore HC
    Ophthalmic, Cortisporin
    Ophthalmic), 12, 49
  and neomycin, polymyxin B,
    hydrocortisone [topical]
    (Cortisporin), 9, 49
  and neomycin, polymyxin B, li-
    docaine [topical]
    (Clomycin), 10, 49
  and neomycin, polymyxin B
    [ophthalmic] (AK Spore
    Ophthalmic, Neosporin
    Ophthalmic), 12, 49
  and neomycin, polymyxin B
    [topical] (Neosporin Oint-
    ment), 9, 49
  [ophthalmic] (AK-Tracin Oph-
    thalmic), 12, 49
  and polymyxin B [ophthalmic]
    (AK Poly Bac Ophthalmic,
    Polysporin Ophthalmic),
    12, 49
  and polymyxin B [topical]
    (Polysporin), 9, 49
  [topical] (Baciguent), 9, 49
Baclofen (Lioresal), 17, 49–50
Bactocill (oxacillin), 2, 188
Bactrim, trimethoprim–sulfamethoxazole [co-trimox-
  azole], 3, 245

Bactroban (muprirocin), 10, 174

Balsalazide (Colazal), 14, 50

Basiliximab (Simulect), 16, 50

Bayer (aspirin), 15, 19, 44

BCG [Bacillus Calmette-Guérin] (TheraCys, Tice BCG), 5, 50

Becaplermin (Regranex Gel), 21, 50–51

Beclomethasone (Beconase, Vancenase, Nasal Inhaler), 20, 51 (QVAR), 20, 51

Beconase (beclomethasone), 20, 51

Belladonna and opium suppositories (B & O Supprettes), 21, 51

Benadryl (diphenhydramine), 1, 9, 96

Benazepril (Lotensin), 6, 51

Benemid (probenecid), 16, 204

Benign prostatic hyperplasia medications, classification of, 21

Bentyl (Dicyclomine), 14, 92–93

Benylin DM (dextromethorphan), 20, 90–91

Benzamycin (erythromycin and benzoyl peroxide), 108

Benzocaine and antipyrine (Auralgan), 11, 18, 51

Benzonatate (Tessalon Perles), 19, 51–52

Benzoyl peroxide and erythromycin (Benzamycin), 108

Benztropine (Cogentin), 9, 52

Bepridil (Vascor), 7, 52

Beractant (Survanta), 20, 52

Beta-adrenergic blockers, classification of, 6

Betagan (levobunolol), 12, 154

Betamethasone, 271t, 272t and clotrimazole (Lotrisone), 3, 10

Betapace AF (sotalol), 6, 222

Betapace (sotalol), 6, 221–222

Betaseron (interferon beta1b), 16, 145

Betaxolol (Kerlone), 6, 52 [ophthalmic] (Betoptic), 52

Bethanechol (Urecholine, Duvoid), 21, 53

Betopic (betaxolol [ophthalmic]), 52

Bevacizumab (Avastin), 5, 53

Bextra (valdecoxib), 19, 247

Biaxin (clarithromycin), 2, 77–78

Bicalutamide (Casodex), 5, 53

Bicarbonate. See Sodium bicarbonate

Bicillin (penicillin g benzathine), 3, 194

Bicitra (sodium citrate), 21, 220

BiCNU (Carmustine [BCNU]), 4, 61–62

Bisacodyl (Dulcolax), 14, 54

Bismuth subsalicylate (Pepto-Bismol), 13, 53–54

Bisoprolol (Zebeta), 6, 54

Bitolterol (Tornalate), 20, 54

Bivalirudin (Angiomax), 15, 54

Black Cohosh (Cimicifuga racemosa), 21, 255–256

Blenoxane (bleomycin sulfate), 4, 54–55

Bleomycin sulfate (Benoxane), 4, 54–55

Bleph-10 (sulfacetamide), 13, 226

Blephamide (sulfacetamide and prednisolone), 11, 13, 226

Blocadren (timolol), 6, 236–237

Bortezomib (Velcade), 5, 55

Brethine (terbutaline), 18, 20, 231–232

Brevibloc (esmolol), 6, 109

Bricanyl (terbutaline), 18, 20, 231–232

Brimonidine (Alphagan), 12, 55

Brinzolamide (Azopt), 12, 55

Bromocriptine (Parlodel), 9, 55

Bronchodilators, classification of, 20

Brontex (guaifenesin and codeine), 20, 132–133

Budesonide (Rhinocort, Pulmicort), 1, 20, 56

Bumetanide (Bumex), 7, 56

Bumex (Bumetanide), 7, 56

Buminate (albumin), 15, 28

Bupivacaine (Marcaine), 18, 56, 270t

Buprenex (buprenorphine), 18, 56

Buprenorphine (Buprenex), 18, 56

Bupropion (Wellbutrin, Zyban), 8, 56

BuSpar (buspirone), 8, 57

Buspirone (BuSpar), 8, 57

Busuflan (Myleran, Buslfex), 4, 57

Busulfex (busulfan), 4, 57

Butcher's Broom (Ruscus aculeatus), 21, 255

Butorphanol (Stadol), 18, 57

C

Caduet (amlodipine/atorvastatin), 8, 37

Caffeine, 267t

Calan (verapamil), 7, 250

Calcipotriene (Dovonex), 10, 58

Calcitonin (Cibacalcin, Miacalcin), 11, 58

Calcitriol (Rocaltrol), 11, 58

Calcium acetate (Calphron, Phos-Ex, PhosLo), 10, 58

Calcium carbonate (Tums, Alka-Mints), 13, 58–59

Calcium channel antagonists, classification of, 7

Calcium glubionate (Neo-Calglucon), 10, 59

Calcium salts [Chloride, Gluconate, Gluceptate], 10, 59

Calfactant (Infasurf), 20, 59

Calphron (calcium acetate), 10

Camptosar (irinotecan), 5, 146

Cancidas (caspofungin), 3, 62–63

Candesartan (Atacand), 6, 59–60

Capoten (captopril), 6, 60

Capsaicin (Capsin, Zostrix), 10, 18, 60

Capsin (capsaicin), 10, 18, 60

Captopril (Capoten), 6, 60

Carafate (sucralfate), 14, 226

Carbamazepine (Tegretol), 8, 60, 266t

Carbapenems, classification of, 1

Carbidopa/Levodopa (Sinemet), 9, 61

Carbocaine (mepivacaine), 270t

Carboplatin (Paraplatin), 4, 61

Cardene (nicardipine), 7, 179–180

Cardiovascular agents, classification of, 6

Cardizem (diltiazem), 7, 94–95

Cardura (doxazosin), 6, 21, 100

Carisoprodol (Soma), 17, 61

Carmustine [BCNU] (BiCNU, Gliadel), 4, 61

Carteolol (Cartrol, Ocupress Ophthalmic), 6, 12, 62

Cartia XT (diltiazem), 7, 94–95

Cartrol (carteolol), 6, 12, 62

Carvedilol (Coreg), 6, 62

Casodex (bicalutamide), 5, 53

Caspofungin (Cancidas), 3, 62–63

Cataflam (diclofenac), 19, 92

Catapres (clonidine), 7, 79–80

Cathartics/laxatives, classification of, 14

Caverject (alprostadil [intracavernosal]), 21, 31–32

Ceclor (cefaclor), 2, 63

Cedax (ceftibuten), 2, 68

Cefaclor (Ceclor), 2, 63

Cefadroxil (Duricef, Ultracef), 2, 63

Cefazolin (Ancef, Kefzol), 2, 63–64

Cefdinir (Omnicef), 2, 64

Cefditoren (Spectracef), 2, 64

Cefepime (Maxipime), 2, 64–65

Cefixime (Suprax), 2, 65

Cefizox (ceftizoxime), 2, 68

Cefmetazone (Zefazone), 2, 65

Cefobid (cefoperazone), 2, 66

Cefonicid (Monocid), 2, 65–66

Cefoperazone (Cefobid), 2, 66

Cefotan (cefotetan), 2, 66–67

Cefotaxime (Claforan), 2, 66

Cefotetan (Cefotan), 2, 66

Cefoxitin (Mefoxin), 2, 67

Cefpodoxime (Vantin), 2, 67

Cefprozil (Cefzil), 2, 67–68

Ceftazidime (Fortaz, Ceptaz, Tazidime, Tazicef), 2, 68

Ceftibuten (Cedax), 2, 68

Ceftin [oral] (cefuroxime), 2, 69

Ceftizoxime (Cefizox), 2, 68

Ceftriaxone (Rocephin), 2, 68–69

Cefuroxime (Ceftin [oral], Zinacef [parenteral]), 2, 69

Cefzil (cefprozil), 2, 67–68

Celebrex (celecoxib), 19, 69

Celecoxib (Celebrex), 19, 69–70

Celexa (citalopram), 8, 77

CellCept (mycophenolate mofetil), 16, 174–175

Cenestin (estrogen [conjugated-synthetic]), 17, 112

Central nervous sytem agents, classification of, 8–9

Cephalexin (Keflex, Keftab), 2, 69–70

Cephalosporins, classification of, 2

Cephradine (Velosef), 2, 70

Cephulac (lactulose), 14, 151

Ceptaz, ceftazidime, 2, 68

Cerebyx (fosphenytoin), 8, 126

Cerubidine (daunorubicin), 4, 87–88

Cerumenex (Triethanolamine), 11, 243

Cervidil Vaginal Insert (dinoprostone), 18, 95–96

Cetamide (sulfacetamide), 13, 226

Cetirizine (Zyrtec), 1, 70

Chamomile (Matricaria recutita), 22, 256

Charcoal (Superchar, Actidose, Liqui-Char Activated), 1, 70–71

Chemet (succimer), 1, 225

Chitosamine (glucosamine sulfate), 22, 259

Chlor-Trimeton (chlorpheniramine), 1, 72

Chloral hydrate (Aquachloral, Supprettes), 9, 71

Chlorambucil (Leukeran), 4, 71

Chlordiazepoxide (Librium, Mitran, Libritabs), 8, 71–72

Chloride (calcium salts), 10, 59

Chlorothiazide (Diuril), 7, 72

Chlorpheniramine (Chlor-Trimeton), 1, 72
and phenylephrine, acetaminophen, hydrocodone, caffeine (Hycomine), 20, 137–138

Chlorpromazine (Thorazine), 9, 73, 72–73

Chlorpropamide (Diabinese), 11, 73

Chlorthalidone (Hygroton), 7, 73
and atenolol (Tenoretic), 6, 46

Chlorzoxazone (Paraflex, Parafon Forte DSC), 17, 73–74

Cholecalciferol [Vitamin D_3] (Delta D), 10, 74

Cholestyramine (Questran, LoCHOLEST), 7, 74

Chondroitin sulfate, 22, 256

Chronulac (lactulose), 14, 151

Cialis (tadalafil), 21, 228

Cibacalcin (calcitonin), 11, 58

Ciclopirox (Loprox), 10, 74

Cidofovir (Vistide), 4, 74–75

Cilostazol (Pletal), 21, 75

Ciloxan (ciprofloxacin [ophthalmic]), 12, 76

Cimetidine (Tagamet), 14, 75

Cinacalcet (Sensipar), 12, 75

Cipro (ciprofloxacin), 2, 10, 75–76

Cipro HC Otic (ciprofloxacin [otic]), 11, 76

Ciprofloxacin
Cipro, 2, 10, 75–76
[ophthalmic] (Ciloxan), 12, 76
[otic] (Cipro HC Otic), 11, 76

Cisplatin (Platinol), 4, 76

Citalopram (Celexa), 8, 77

Cladribine (Leustatin), 5, 77

Claforan (cefotaxime), 2, 66

Claravis (isotretinoin [13-cis retinoic acid]), 10, 148

Clarinex (desloratadine), 1, 89

Clarithromycin (Biaxin), 2, 77–78

Claritin (loratadine), 1, 159

Clavulanic acid and amoxicillin (Augmentin), 2, 38

Clemastine fumarate (Tavist), 1, 78

Cleocin (clindamycin), 10, 78

Climara (estradiol [transdermal]), 17, 111

Clindamycin (Cleocin), 10, 78

Clinoril (sulindac), 19, 227

Clobetasol propionate, 272t

Clofazime (Lamprene), 3, 78

Clomycin, (bacitracin, neomycin, polymyxin B, and lidocaine [topical]), 10, 49

Clonazepam (Klonopin), 8, 78–79

Clonidine (Catapres), 7, 79–80

Clopidogrel (Plavix), 15

Clopra (metoclopramide), 14, 168

Clorazepate (Tranxene), 8, 80

Clotrimazole
(Lotrimin, Mycelex), 3, 80
and betamethasone (Lotrisone), 3, 10, 80

Clozapine (Clozaril), 9, 80–81

Clozaril (clozapine), 9, 80–81

Cocaine, 18, 81

Codeine, 19
and guaifenesin (Robitussin AC, Brontex), 20, 132–133

Cogentin (benztropine), 9, 52

Cognex (tacrine), 9, 227–228

Colace (docusate sodium), 14, 98

Colazal (balsalazide), 14, 50

Colchicine, 16, 81–82

Colesevelam (Welchol), 7, 82

Colestid (colestipol), 7, 82

Colestipol (Colestid), 7, 82

Colfosceril palmitate (Exosurf Neonatal), 20, 82

Colistin
and neomycin, hydrocortisone (Cortisporin-TC Otic Drops), 11, 178
and neomycin, hydrocortisone, and thonzonium (Cortisporin-TC Otic Suspension), 11, 178

CoLyte (polyethylene glycol-electrolyte solution), 14, 201

Combivent (albuterol and ipratropium), 20, 28

Combivir (zidovudine and lamivudine), 4, 253

Compazine (prochlorperazine), 9, 14, 205

Comtan (entacapone), 9, 104–105

Condylox Gel (podophyllin), 10, 201

Condylox (podophyllin), 10, 201

Contraceptives
classification of, 17–18
(emergency) classification of, 17–18
See also Oral contraceptives

Cordarone (amiodarone), 6, 36

Coreg (carvedilol), 6, 62

Corgard (nadolol), 6, 175

Corlopam (fenoldopam), 8, 116

Cortef (hydrocortisone [topical and systemic]), 11, 138

Cortifoam Rectal (hydrocortisone [rectal]), 14, 138

Cortisone, 271t–274t

Cortisone systemic, topical, 11

Cortisporin
(bacitracin, neomycin, polymyxin B, and hydrocortisone [topical]), 9, 49

Ophthalmic (bacitracin, neomycin, polymyxin B, and hydrocortisone [ophthalmic]), 12, 49

Ophthalmic and Otic (neomycin, polymyxin, and hydrocortisone), 11, 178

-TC Otic Drops (neomycin, colistin, and hydrocortisone), 11, 178

-TC Otic Suspension (neomycin, colistin, hydrocortisone, and thonzonium), 11, 178

Cortone (cortisone), 271t

Corvert (ibutilide), 6, 140

Cosmegen (dactinomycin), 4, 86

Cosopt (dorzolamide and timolol), 12, 100

Cotazym (pancrelipase), 191

Coumadin (warfarin), 15, 251–252

Cozaar (losartan), 6, 159–160

Creon (pancrelipase), 191

Crestor (rosuvastatin), 7, 215

Crixivan (indinavir), 4, 142–143

Cromolyn sodium (Intal, NasalCrom, Opticrom), 1, 20, 82–83

Cromolyn sodium (Opticrom), 13

Cyanocobalamin [vitamin B_{12}], 10, 83

Cyclobenzaprine (Flexeril), 17, 83

Cyclogyl (cyclopentolate), 13, 83

Cyclopentolate (Cyclogyl), 13, 83

Cyclophosphamide (Cytoxan, Neosar), 4, 83–84

Cyclosporine (Sandimmune, Neoral), 16, 84, 269t

Cyproheptadine (Periactin), 1, 84

Cystospaz (hyoscyamine), 14, 21, 139

Cytadren (aminoglutethimide), 5, 35–36

Cytarabine [ARA-C] (Cytosar-U), 5, 84–85

Cytarabine liposome (DepoCyt), 5, 85

Cytogan (cytomegalovirus immune globulin [CMV-IG IV]), 16, 85

Cytomegalovirus immune globulin [CMV-IG IV] (CytoGam), 16, 85

Cytomel (liothyronine), 12, 157

Cytosar-U (cytarabine [ARA-C]), 5, 84–85

Cytotec (misoprostol), 14, 171

Cytovene (ganciclovir), 4, 127–128

Cytoxan (cyclophosphamide), 4, 83–84

D

Dacarbazine (DTIC), 5, 85

Daclizumab (Zenapax), 16, 85–86

Dactinomycin (Cosmegen), 4, 86

Dalfopristin–quinupristin (Synercid), 3, 209–210

Dalgan (dezocine), 19, 91

Dalmane (flurazepam), 9, 122

Dalteparin (Fragmin), 15, 86

Danaparoid (Orgaron), 15, 86–87

Dantrium (dantrolene), 17

Dantrolene (Dantrium), 17

Dapsone (Avlosulfon), 3, 87

Darbepoetin Alfa (Aranesp), 15, 87

Darvocet (propoxyphene and acetaminophen), 19, 206

Darvon
(propoxyphene), 19, 206
Compound-65 (propoxyphene and aspirin), 19, 206
-N with Aspirin (propoxyphene and aspirin), 19, 206

Daunomycin (daunorubicin), 4, 87–88

Daunorubicin (Daunomycin, Cerubidine), 4, 87–88

Daypro (oxaprozin), 19, 188

DDAVP (desmopressin), 11, 15, 89

Decadron
(dexamethasone), 11, 89–90, 271t, 272t
Ophthalmic (dexamethasone [ophthalmic]), 13, 89

Declomycin (demeclocycline), 12, 88

Delavidine (Rescriptor), 3, 88

Delta D (cholecalciferol [Vitamin D_3]), 10, 74

Demadex (torsemide), 7, 240

Demeclocycline (Declomycin), 12, 88

Demerol (meperidine), 19, 163

Denavir (penciclovir), 4, 10, 193–194

Depakene (valproic acid), 8, 247–248

Depakote (valproic acid), 8, 247–248

Depo-Provera (medroxyprogesterone), 17, 18, 162

DepoCyt (cytarabine liposome), 5, 85

Dermatologic agents, classification of, 9–10

Desipramine (Norpramin), 8, 88–89, 269t

Desloratadine (Clarinex), 1, 89

Desmopressin (DDAVP, Stimate), 11, 15, 89

Desonide, 272t

Desoximetasone, 272t

Desyrel (trazodone), 8, 241–242

Detrol LA (tolterodine), 21, 239–240

Detrol (tolterodine), 21, 239–240

Detussin (hydrocodone and pseudoephedrine), 20, 137

Dexacort Phosphate Turbinaire (dexamethasone), 20

Dexamethasone
base, 272t
(Decadron), 11, 89–90, 271t, 272t
[nasal] (Dexacort Phosphate Turbinaire), 20, 89
and neomycin (AK-Neo-Dex Ophthalmic, NeoDecadron Ophthalmic), 12, 178
and neomycin, polymyxin B, (Maxitrol), 12, 178
[ophthalmic] (AK-Dex Ophthalmic, Decadron Ophthalmic), 13, 89

DexFerrum (iron dextran), 10, 146–147

Dexmethasone and tobramycin (TobraDex), 13, 238

Dexpanthenol (Ilopan-Choline Oral, Ilopan), 14, 90

Dextran 40 (Rheomacrodex), 15, 90

Dextrazoxane (Zinecard), 1, 90

Dextromethorphan (Mediquell, Benylin DM, Pedia-Care 1), 20, 90–91 and guaifenesin, 20, 133

Dey-Drop (silver nitrate), 13, 21, 218

Dezocine (Dalgan), 19, 91

DiaBeta (glyburide), 11, 131

Diabinese (chlorpropamide), 11, 73

Dialose (docusate potassium), 14, 98

Diamox (acetazolamide), 7, 12, 25–26

Diazepam (Valium), 8, 17, 91

Diazoxide (Hyperstat, Pro-glycem), 12, 91–92

Dibucaine (Nupercainal), 10, 14, 18, 92

Diclofenac (Cataflam, Voltaren), 19, 92

Dicloxacillin (Dynapen, Dycill), 2, 92

Dicyclomine (Bentyl), 14, 92–93

Didanosine [ddI] (Videx), 3, 93

Didronel (etidronate disodium), 11, 114

Dietary supplements, classification of, 10

Diflucan (fluconazole), 3, 119–120

Diflunisal (Dolobid), 19, 93

Digibind, digoxin immune fab, 1, 94

Digoxin Immune Fab (Digibind), 1, 94

Digoxin (Lanoxin, Lanoxicaps), 6, 7, 93–94, 267t

Dilacor (diltiazem), 7, 94–95

Dilantin (phenytoin), 8, 198–199

Dilatrate-SR (isosorbide dinitrate), 8, 147–148

Dilaudid (hydromorphone), 19, 138

Diltia XT (diltiazem), 7, 94–95

Diltiazem (Cardizem, Cartia XT, Dilacor, Diltia XT, Tiamate, Tiazac), 7, 94–95

Dimenhydrinate (Dramamine), 13, 95

Dimethyl sulfoxide [DMSO] (Rimso 50), 21, 95

Dinoprostone (Cervidil Vaginal Insert, Prepidil Vaginal Gel), 18, 95–96

Diovan (valsartan), 6, 248

Dipentum (olsalazine), 14, 185

Diphenhydramine (Benadryl), 1, 9, 96

Diphenoxylate with atropine (Lomotil), 13, 96

Diphtheria, tetanus toxoids, and acellular pertussis adsorbed, hepatitis B (recombinant), and inactivated poliovirus vaccine (IPV) combined (Pediarix), 16, 96

Dipivefrin (Propine), 12, 96–97

Diprivan (propofol), 9, 206

Dipyridamole and aspirin (Aggrenox), 15, 97

Dipyridamole (Persantine), 15, 97

Dirithromycin (Dynabac), 2, 97

Disopyramide (Norpace, NA-Pamide), 6, 97–98, 268t

Ditropan (oxybutynin), 21, 189

Ditropan XL (oxybutynin), 21, 189

Diuretics, classification of, 7

Diuril (chlorothiazide), 7, 72

Dobutamine (Dobutrex), 7, 98

Dobutrex (dobutamine), 7, 98

Docetaxel (Taxotere), 5, 98

Docusate calcium (Surfak), 14, 98

Docusate potassium (Dialose), 14, 98

Docusate sodium (DOS, Colace), 14, 98

Dofetilide (Tikosyn), 6, 98–99

Dolasetron (Anzemet), 13, 99

Dolobid (diflunisal), 19, 93

Dolophine (methadone), 19, 166

Dong Quai (*Angelic polymorpha, sinensis*), 22, 256–257

Donnatal (hyoscyamine, atropine, scopolamine, and phenobarbital), 14, 139–140

Dopamine (Intropin), 7, 99

Doral (quazepam), 9, 208

Dornase alfa (Pulmozyme), 20, 99

Dorzolamide and timolol (Cosopt), 12, 100

Dorzolamide (Trusopt), 12, 99

DOS (docusate sodium), 14, 98

Dovonex (calcipotriene), 10, 58

Doxazosin (Cardura), 6, 21

Doxepin
  (Sinequan, Adapin), 8, 100, 269t
  [topical] (Zonalon), 10, 100

Doxorubicin (Adriamycin, Rubex), 5, 100–101

Doxycycline (Vivramycin), 3, 101

Dramamine (dimenhydrinate), 13, 95

Dronabinol (Marinol), 13, 101

Droperidol (Inapsine), 13, 101

Drotrecogin alfa (Xigris), 21, 101–102

Droxia (hydroxyurea), 5, 138–139

Drug levels (common drugs), 265t–269t

Dryvax (smallpox vaccine), 219

DTIC (dacarbazine), 5, 85

Dulcolax (bisacodyl), 14, 53

Duragesic (fentanyl [transdermal]), 19, 117

Duramorph (morphine), 19, 173–174

Duricef, cefadroxil, 2, 63

Dutasteride (Avodart), 21, 102

Duvoid (bethanechol), 21, 53

Dyazide (hydrochlorothiazide and triamterene), 7, 136

Dycill (dicloxacillin), 2, 92

Dynabac (dirithromycin), 2, 97

DynaCirc (isradipine), 7, 148

Dynapen (dicloxacillin), 2, 92

Dyrenium (triamterene), 7, 243

E

E-Mycin (erythromycin), 2, 107–108

Ear (otic) agents, classification of, 11

Echothiophate idoine (Phospholine Ophthalmic), 12, 102

Ecinacea (*Ecinacea purpurea*), 22, 257

Econazole (Spectazole), 3, 10, 102

Ecotrin (aspirin), 15, 19, 44

Edex (alprostadil [intracavernosal]), 21, 31–32

Edrophonium (Tensilon), 17, 102

E.E.S. (erythromycin), 2, 107–108

Efalizumab (Raptiva), 10, 103

Efavirenz (Sustiva), 3, 103

Effer-syllium (psyllium), 14, 208

Effexor (venlafaxine), 8, 249

Efudex (fluorouracil [topical, 5-FU]), 121

Elavil (amitriptyline), 8, 19, 37

Eldepryl (selegiline), 9, 216–217

Elidel (pimecrolimus), 10, 199

Eligard (leuprolide), 5, 18, 153

Elimite (permethrin), 10, 196

Elitek (rasburicase), 5, 214

Ellence (epirubicin), 5, 105–106

Elmiron (pentosan polysulfate), 21, 196

Elspar (L-Asparaginase), 5, 43–44

Emadine (emadastine), 13, 103

Emcyt (estramustine phosphate), 5, 111

Emedastine (Emadine), 13, 103

Emend (aprepitant), 13, 42–43

Eminase (anistreplase), 15, 41

EMLA (lidocaine and prilocaine), 18, 156

Empirin No. 2, 3, 4 (aspirin with codeine), 18, 45

Emtricitabine (Emtriva), 4, 103

Emtriva (emtricitabine), 4, 103

Enalapril (Vasotec), 6, 103–104

Enbrel (etanercept), 16, 113

Endocrine system agents, classification of, 11–12

Enfuvirtide (Fuzeon), 4, 104

Engerix-B (hepatitis B vaccine), 16, 135

Enoxaparin (Lovenox), 15, 104

Entacapone (Comtan), 9, 104–105

Enulose (lactulose), 14, 151

Enzone (pramoxine with hydrocortisone), 10, 14, 203

Enzymes, classification of, 14

Ephedra/Ma Huang, 22, 257

Ephedrine, 20, 105

Epinephrine (Adrenalin, SusPhrine, EpiPen), 7, 20, 105

EpiPen (epinephrine), 7, 20, 105

Epirubicin (Ellence), 5, 105–106

Epivir
-HBV (lamivudine), 4, 151–152
(lamivudine), 4, 151–152

Eplerenone (Inspra), 6, 106

Epoetin alfa [erythropeoietin/EPO] (Epogen, Procrit), 15, 106

Epogen (epoetin alfa [erythropeoietin/EPO]), 15, 106

Epoprostenol (Flolan), 8, 106–107
Eprosartan (Teveten), 6, 107
Eptifibatide (Integrilin), 15, 107
Equinil (meprobamate), 8, 163–164
Ergamisol (levamisole), 5, 154
Ertaczo (sertaconazole), 3, 217
Ertapenem (Invanz), 1, 107
Ery-Tab (erythromycin), 2, 107–108
Erycette (erythromycin [topical]), 10, 108–109
Eryderm (erythromycin [topical]), 10, 108–109
Erythromycin
  (E-Mycin, E.E.S., Ery-Tab), 2, 107–108
  and benzoyl peroxide (Benzamycin), 108
  [ophthalmic] (Ilotycin Ophthalmic), 12, 108
  and sulfisoxazole (Eryzole, Pediazole), 2, 108
  [topical] (A/T/S, Eryderm, Erycette, T-Stat), 10, 108–109
Eryzole, erythromycin and sulfisoxazole, 2, 108
Escitalopram (Lexapro), 8, 109
Esidrix (Hydrochlorothiazide), 7, 136
Eskalith (lithium carbonate), 9, 157–158
Esmolol (Brevibloc), 6, 109
Esomeprazole (Nexium), 14, 109
Estazolam (ProSom), 9, 109–110

Esterified estrogens (Estratab, Menest), 17, 110
Esterified estrogens with methyltestosterone (Estratest), 17, 110
Estinyl (ethinyl estradiol), 18, 113
Estrace (Estradiol), 17, 110
Estracyt (estramustine phosphate), 5, 111
Estraderm (estradiol [transdermal]), 17, 111
Estradiol
  (Estrace), 17, 110
  cypionate and medroxyprogesterone acetate (Lunelle), 17, 111
  [transdermal] (Estraderm, Climara, Vivelle), 17, 111
Estramustine phosphate (Estracyt, Emcyt), 5, 111
Estratab (esterified estrogens), 17, 110
Estratest (esterified estrogens with methyltestosterone), 17, 110
Estrogen
  [conjugated with medroxyprogesterone] (Prempro, Premphase), 17, 112
  [conjugated with methylprogesterone] (Premarin with methylprogesterone), 18, 112
  [conjugated with methyltestosterone] (Premarin with methyltestosterone), 18, 112–113
  [conjugated] (Premarin), 17, 111–112

[conjugated-synthetic] (Cen-estin), 17, 112
supplementation agents, clas-sification of, 17–18
Etanercept (Enbrel), 16, 113
Ethambutol (Myambutol), 3, 113
Ethinyl estradiol
    (Estinyl, Feminone), 18, 113
    and levonorgestrel (Preven), 17, 113
    and norelgestromin (Ortho Evra), 113–114
Ethosuximide (Zarontin), 8, 114, 266t
Ethyol (amifostine), 1, 34
Etidronate disodium (Didronel), 11, 114
Etodolac (Lodine), 19, 114
Etonogestrel/ethinyl estradiol (NuvaRing), 17, 114–115
Etoposide [VP-16] (VePesid, Toposar), 5, 115
Eulexin (flutamide), 5, 122–123
Evista (raloxifene), 12, 210
Exelon (rivastigmine), 9, 214
Exemestane (Aromasin), 5, 115
Exosurf Neonatal (colfosceril palmitate), 20, 82
Exsel Shampoo (selenium sul-fide), 10, 217
Eye (ophthalmic) agents, classi-fication of, 12–13
Ezetimibe (Zetia), 7, 115

F

Famciclovir (Famvir), 4, 115
Famotidine (Pepcid), 14, 116
Famvir (famciclovir), 4, 115

Faslodex (fulvestrant), 5, 126
Feldene (piroxicam), 19, 200
Felodipine (Plendil), 7, 116
Femara (letrozole), 5, 153
FemHRT (norethindrone ac-etate/ethinyl estradiol), 18, 183
Feminone (ethinyl estradiol), 18, 113
Fenofibrate (Tricor), 7, 116
Fenoldopam (Corlopam), 8, 116
Fenoprofen (Nalfon), 19, 116–117
Fentanyl
    (Sublimaze), 19, 117
    [transdermal] (Duragesic), 19, 117
    [transmucosal system] (Actiq), 19, 117
Fergon (ferrous gluconate), 10, 117
Ferrlecit (ferrous gluconate com-plex), 10, 118
Ferrous gluconate complex (Ferrlecit), 10, 118
Ferrous gluconate (Fergon), 10, 117
Ferrous sulfate, 118
Feverfew (*Tanacetum parthe-nium*), 22, 257–258
Fexofenadine (Allegra), 1, 118
Filgrastim [G-CSF] (Neupogen), 15, 118
Finasteride (Proscar, Propecia), 10, 21, 118
Fioricet (acetaminophen with bu-talbital w/wo caffeine), 18, 25
Fiorinal (aspirin and butalbital compound), 18, 44–45

Fiorinal with codeine (aspirin with butalbital, caffeine, and codeine), 18, 45

Flagyl (metronidazole), 3, 10, 169

Flamp (fludarbine phosphate), 5, 120

Flavoxate (Urispas), 21, 119

Flecainide (Tambocor), 6, 119, 268t

Flexeril (cyclobenzaprine), 17, 83

Flolan (epoprostenol), 8, 106–107

Flomax (tamsulosin), 21, 229

Flonase (fluticasone) [nasal], 20, 123 [oral, nasal], 20

Florinef (fludrocortisone acetate), 11, 120

Flovent (fluticasone [oral]), 20, 123

Floxin (ofloxacin), 2, 12, 185

Floxuridine (FUDR), 5, 119

Fluconazole (Diflucan), 3, 119–120

Fludara (fludarbine phosphate), 5, 120

Fludarabine phosphate (Flamp, Fludara), 5, 120

Fludrocortisone acetate (Florinef), 11, 120

Flumadine (rimantadine), 4, 212–213

Flumazenil (Romazicon), 1, 120

FluMist (influenza virus vaccine live [intranasal]), 16, 144

Flunisolide (AeroBid, Nasalide), 20, 120

Fluocinolone, 272t–273t

Fluoroqinolones, classification of, 2

Fluorouracil [5-FU] (Adrucil), 5, 121 [topical, 5-FU] (Efudex), 121

Fluoxetine (Prozac, Sarafem), 8, 121

Fluoxymesterone (Halotestin), 5, 121–122

Fluphenazine (Prolixin, Permitil), 9, 122

Flurandrenolide, 273t

Flurazepam (Dalmane), 9, 122

Flurbiprofen (Ansaid), 19, 122

FluShield (influenza vaccine), 16, 143–144

Flutamide (Eulexin), 5, 122–123

Fluticasone [oral, nasal] (Flonase, Flovent), 20, 123

Fluticasone proprionate, 273t and sameterol xinafoate (Advair Diskus), 20, 123

Fluvastatin (Lescol), 7, 123

Fluvirin (influenza vaccine), 16, 143–144

Fluvoxamine (Luvox), 8, 123–124

Fluzone (influenza vaccine), 16, 143–144

Folex (methotrexate), 5, 17, 167

Folic acid, 10, 124

Fondaparinux (Arixtra), 15, 124

Foradil Aerolizer (Formoterol), 20, 124–125

Formoterol (Foradil Aerolizer), 20, 124–125

Fortaz, ceftazidime, 2, 68

Forteo (teriparatide), 12, 232

Fortovase (saquinavir), 4, 215–216

Fosamax (alendronate), 12, 29

Fosamprenavir (Lexiva), 3, 125

Foscarnet (Foscavir), 4, 125

Foscavir (foscarnet), 4, 125

Fosfomycin (Monurol), 3, 125

Fosinopril (Monopril), 6, 126

Fosphenytoin (Cerebyx), 8, 126

Fragmin (dalteparin), 15, 86

Frova (frovatriptan), 18, 283t

Frovatriptan (Frova), 18, 283t

FUDR (floxuridine), 5, 119

Fulvestrant (Faslodex), 5, 126

Fungizone (amphotericin B), 3, 9, 38–39

Furadantin (nitrofurantoin), 21, 182

Furosemide (Lasix), 7, 126–127

Fuzeon (enfuvirtide), 4, 104

G

G-Mycitin (gentamicin), 1
[topical], 10

Gabapentin (Neurontin), 8, 127

Gabitril (tiagabine), 8, 235–236

Galantamine (Reminyl), 9, 127

Gallium nitrate (Ganite), 11, 127

Gamimune (immune globulin [IV]), 16, 142

Gammar IV (immune globulin [IV]), 16, 142

Ganciclovir (Cytovene, Vitrasert), 4, 127–128

Ganite (gallium nitrate), 11, 127

Garamycin (gentamicin), 1
[ophthalmic], 12, 130
[topical], 10, 130

Garlic (*Allium sativum*), 22, 258

Gastrointestinal agents, classification of, 13–15

Gatifloxacin (Tequin), 2, 128

Gaviscon
(alginic acid), 13
(alginic acid, aluminum hydroxide, and magnesium trisilicate), 30
(aluminum hydroxide with magnesium carbonate), 13, 33
(aluminum hydroxide with magnesium trisilicate), 13, 34

Gaviscon II (aluminum hydroxide with magnesium trisilicate), 13, 34

Gefitinib (Iressa), 5, 128

Gemcitabine (Gemzar), 5, 128–129

Gemfibrozil (Lopid), 7, 129

Gemtuzumab Ozogamicin (Mylotarg), 5, 129

Gemzar (Gemcitabine), 5, 128–129

Genoptic (gentamicin [ophthalmic]), 12, 130

Gentacidin (gentamicin [ophthalmic]), 12, 130

Gentak (gentamicin [ophthalmic]), 12, 130

Gentamicin (Garamycin G-Mycitin), 1, 129, 265t
[topical], 10

Gentamicin [ophthalmic] (Garamycin, Genoptic, Gentacidin, Gentak), 12, 130

Gentamicin and prednisolone [ophthalmic] (Pred-G Ophthalmic), 130

Ginger (*Zingiber officinale*), 22, 258

Ginko biloba, 22, 258

Ginseng (*Panax quinquefolius*), 22, 258–259

Glaucoma agents, classification of, 12

Gleevec (imatinib), 5, 141

Gliadel (Carmustine [BCNU]), 4, 61–62

Glimepiride (Amaryl), 11, 130

Glipizide (Glucotrol), 11, 130–131

Glucagon, 11, 131

Gluceptate (calcium salts), 10, 59

Gluconate (calcium salts), 10, 59

Glucophage (metformin), 11, 165–166

Glucosamine sulfate (chitosamine), 22, 259

Glucotrol (glipizide), 11, 130–131

Glucovance (glyburide/metformin), 11, 131

Glyburide (DiaBeta, Micronase, Glynase), 11, 131

Glyburide/metformin (Glucovance), 11, 131

Glylcerine suppository, 14, 131–132

Glynase (glyburide), 11, 131

Glyset (miglitol), 11, 171

Goedon (ziprasidone), 9, 253–254

GoLYTELY (polyethylene glycol-electrolyte solution), 14, 201

Gonadorelin (Lutrepulse), 18, 132

Goserelin (Zoladex), 5, 132

Granisetron (Kytril), 13, 132

Guaifenesin and
codeine (Robitussin AC, Brontex), 20, 132–133
dextromethorphan, 20, 133
hydrocodone (Hycotuss Expectorant), 20, 137

Guaifenesin (Robitussin), 20

H

H-BIG (hepatitis B immune globulin), 16, 135

Habitrol (nicotine transdermal), 21, 180

Haemophilus B conjugate vaccine (ActHIB, HibTITER, Pedvax-HIB, Prohibit), 16, 133

Halcion (triazolam), 9, 243

Haldol (haloperidol), 9, 133–134

Halobetasol, 273t

Haloperidol (Haldol), 9, 133–134

Haloprogin (Halotex), 10, 134

Halotestin (fluoxymesterone), 5, 121–122

Halotex (haloprogin), 10, 134

Havrix (hepatitis A vaccine), 16, 134

Hawthorn (*Crataegus laevigata*), 22, 259

Hematologic agents, classification of, 15

Hematopoietic stimulants, classification of, 15

Heparin, 15, 134

Hepatitis A (inactivated) and hepatitis B recombinant vaccine (Twinrix), 16, 124–135

Hepatitis A vaccine (Havrix, Vaqta), 16, 134

Hepatitis B immune globulin (HyperHep, H-BIG), 16, 135

Hepatitis B vaccine (Engerix-B, Recombivax HB), 16, 135

Hepsera (adefovir), 4, 27

Herceptin (trastuzumab), 5, 241

Hespan (hetastarch), 15, 135

Hetastarch (Hespan), 15, 135

Hexalen (altretamine), 4, 32–33

HibTITER (haemophilus B conjugate vaccine), 16, 133

Hiprex (methanamine), 21, 166

Histussin-D (hydrocodone and pseudoephedrine), 20, 137

Hivid (zalcitabine), 4, 252

Holoxan (ifosfamide), 4, 140–141

Homatropine and hydrocodone (Hycodan, Hydromet), 20, 137

Hormone/synthetic substitutes, classification of, 11

Hormones, classification of, 5

Humira (adalimumab), 16, 27

Hycamtin (topotecan), 5, 240

Hycodan (hydrocodone and homatropine), 20, 137

Hycomine (hydrocodone, chlorpheniramine, phenylephrine, acetaminophen, and caffeine), 20, 137

Hycotuss Expectorant (hydrocodone and guaifenesin), 20, 137

Hydralazine (Apresoline), 8, 135

Hydrea (hydroxyurea), 5, 138–139

Hydrochlorothiazide (HydroDIURIL, Esidrix), 7, 136

and amiloride (Moduretic), 7, 136

and spironolactone (Aldactazide), 7, 136

and triamterene (Dyazide, Maxzide), 7, 136

Hydrocodone and

acetaminophen, chlorpheniramine, phenylephrine, and caffeine (Hycomine), 20, 137

acetaminophen (Lorcet, Vicodin), 19, 136–137

aspirin (Lortab ASA), 19, 137

guaifenesin (Hycotuss Expectorant), 20, 137

homatropine (Hycodan, Hydromet), 20, 137

ibuporfen (Vicoprofen), 19, 137

pseudoephedrine (Detussin, Histussin-D), 20, 137

Hydrocortisone

bacitracin, neomycin, and polymyxin B [ophthalmic] (AK Spore HC Ophthalmic, Cortisporin Ophthalmic), 12, 49

bacitracin, neomycin, and polymyxin B [topical] (Cortisporin), 9, 49

Hydrocortisone (*cont.*)
colistin, and neomycin (Cortisporin-TC Otic Drops), 11, 178
colistin, neomycin, and thonzonium (Cortisporin-TC Otic Suspension), 11, 178
neomycin, and polymyxin (Cortisporin Opthalmic and Otic), 11, 178
and polymyxin B (Otobiotic Otic), 11, 201–202
and pramoxine (Enzone, Proctofoam-HC), 10, 203
[rectal] (Anusol-HC Suppository, Cortifoam Rectal, Proctocort), 14, 138
[topical and systemic] (Cortef, Solu-Cortef), 11, 138, 271t, 273t
Hydrocortone (hydrocortisone), 271t
HydroDIURIL (Hydrochlorothiazide), 7, 136
Hydromet (hydrocodone and homatropine), 20, 137
Hydromorphone (Dilaudid), 19, 138
Hydroxyurea (Hydrea, Droxia), 5, 138–139
Hydroxyzine (Atarax, Vistaril), 1, 8, 9, 139
Hygroton (chlorthalidone), 7, 73
Hyoscyamine (Anaspaz, Cystospaz, Levsin), 14, 21, 139
Hyoscyamine, atropine, scopolamine, and phenobarbital (Donnatal), 14, 139–140

Hypercalcemia agents, classification of, 11
HyperHep (hepatitis B immune globulin), 16, 135
Hyperstat (diazoxide), 12, 91–92
Hytrin (terazosin), 6, 21, 231

I
Ibuprofen
(Motrin, Rufen, Advil), 19, 140
and hydrocodone (Vicoprofen), 19, 137
Ibutilide (Corvert), 6, 140
Idamycin (idarubicin), 5, 140
Idarubicin (Idamycin), 5, 140
Ifex (ifosfamide), 4, 140–141
Ifosfamide (Ifex, Holoxan), 4, 140–141
Ilopan-Choline Oral (dexpanthenol), 14, 90
Ilopan (dexpanthenol), 14, 90
Ilotycin Ophtahlmic (erythromycin [ophthalmic]), 12, 108
Imatinib (Gleevec), 5, 141
Imdur (isosorbide mononitrate), 8, 148
Imipnem–cilastatin (Primaxin), 1, 141
Imipramine plus desipramine, 269t
Imipramine (Tofranil), 8, 19, 141
Imiquimod Cream 5(Aldara), 10, 142
Imitrex (sumatriptan), 18, 227
Immune globulin [IV] (Gamimune N, Sandoglobulin, Gammar IV), 16, 142

Immune system agents, classification of, 16

Immunomodulators, classification of, 16

Immunosuppressive agents, classification of, 16

Imodium (loperamide), 13, 158

Imuran (azathioprine), 16, 47–48

Inamrinone [Amrinone] (Inocor), 7, 142

Inapsine (droperidol), 13, 101

Indapamide (Lozol), 7, 142

Inderal (propranolol), 6, 206–207

Indinavir (Crixivan), 4, 142–143

Indocin (indomethacin), 19, 143

Indomethacin (Indocin), 19, 143

Infasurf (calfactant), 20, 59

INFeD (iron dextran), 10, 146

Infergen (interferon alfacon-1), 16, 145

Infliximab (Remicade), 14, 143

Influenza vaccine (Fluzone, FluShield, Fluvirin), 16, 143–144

Influenza virus vaccine live [intranasal] (FluMist), 16, 144

INH (isoniazid), 3, 147

Innohep (tinzaparin), 15, 237

Inocor (inamrinone [amrinone]), 7, 142

Inotropic/pressor agents, classification of, 7

Inspra (eplerenone), 6, 106

Insulin/s, 144, 275t

Intal (cromolyn sodium), 1, 20, 82–83

Integrilin (eptifibatide), 15, 107

Interferon alfa-2b and ribavirin combinationation (Rebetron), 4, 145

Interferon alfa (Roferon-A, Intron A), 16, 144–145

Interferon alfacon-1 (Infergen), 16, 145

Interferon beta-1b (Betaseron), 16, 145

Interferon gamma-1b (Actimmune), 16, 145–146

Intron A (interferon alfa), 16, 144–145

Intropin (dopamine), 7, 99

Invanz (ertapenem), 1, 107

Iopidine (apraclonidine), 12, 42

Ipecac syrup (OTC Syrup), 1, 146

Ipratropium and albuterol (Combivent), 20, 28

Ipratropium (Atrovent), 20, 146

Irbesartan (Avapro), 6, 146

Iressa (gefitinib), 5, 128

Irinotecan (Camptosar), 5, 146

Iron dextran (DexFerrum, INFeD), 10, 146–147

Iron sucrose (Venofer), 10, 147

Ismo (isosorbide mononitrate), 8, 148

Isoniazid (INH), 3, 147

Isoproterenol (Isuprel), 7, 20, 147

Isoptin (verapamil), 7, 250

Isordil (isosorbide dinitrate), 8, 147

Isosorbide dinitrate (Isordil, Sorbitrate, Dilatrate-SR), 8, 147–148

Isosorbide mononitrate (Ismo, Imdur), 8, 148

Isotretinoin [13-*cis* retinoic acid] (Accutane, Amnesteem, Claravis, Sotret), 10, 148

Isradipine (DynaCirc), 7, 148

Isuprel (isoproterenol), 7, 20, 147

Itraconazole (Sporanox), 3, 149

K

K-Lor (potassium supplements), 10, 202

Kabikinase (streptokinase), 15, 224

Kadian SR (morphine), 19, 173–174

Kaletra (lopinavir/ritonavir), 4, 158–159

Kao-Spen (kaolin-pectin), 13, 149

Kaochlor (potassium supplements), 10, 202

Kaodene (kaolin-pectin), 13, 149

Kaolin-pectin (Kaodene, Kao-Spen, Kapectolin, Parepectolin), 13, 149

Kaon (potassium supplements), 10, 202

Kapectolin (kaolin-pectin), 13, 149

Kava Kava (*Piper methysticum*), 22, 259

Kayexalate (sodium polystyrene sulfonate), 21, 221

Keflex, cephalexin, 2, 69–70

Keftab, cephalexin, 2, 69–70

Kefzol, cefazolin, 2, 63–64

Keppra (levetiracetam), 8, 154

Kerlone (betaxolol), 6, 52

Ketek (telithromycin), 2, 229–230

Ketoconazole (Nizoral), 3, 10, 149–150

Ketolide, classification of, 2

Ketoprofen (Orudis, Oruvail), 19, 150

Ketorolac (Toradol), 19, 150 [ophthalmic] (Acular), 13, 150

Ketotifen (Zaditor), 13, 151

Kineret (anakinra), 16, 40–41

Klonopin (clonazepam), 8, 78–79

Klorvess (potassium supplements), 10, 202

Kwell (lindane), 10, 156

Kytril (granisetron), 13, 132

L

L-Asparaginase (Elspar, Oncaspar), 5, 43–44

Labetalol (Trandate, Normodyne), 6, 151

Lac-Hydrin (lactic acid and ammonium hydroxide [ammonium lactate]), 10, 151

Lactic acid and ammonium hydroxide [ammonium lactate] (Lac-Hydrin), 10, 151

Lactinex Granules (lactobacillus), 13, 151

Lactobacillus (Lactinex Granules), 13, 151

Lactulose (Chronulac, Cephulac, Enulose), 14, 151

Lamictal (lamotrigine), 8, 152

Lamisil (terbinafine), 3, 10, 231
Lamivudine
(Epivir, Epivir-HBV), 4, 151–152
and zidovudine (Combivir), 4, 253
Lamotrigine (Lamictal), 8, 152
Lamprene (clofazimine), 3, 78
Lanoxicaps (digoxin), 6, 7, 93–94
Lanoxin (digoxin), 6, 7, 93–94
Lansoprazole (Prevacid), 14, 152
Lasix (furosemide), 7, 126–127
Latanoprost (Xalatan), 12, 152
Leflunomide (Arava), 17, 152
Lepirudin (Refludan), 15, 152–153
Lescol (fluvastatin), 7, 123
Letrozole (Femara), 5, 153
Leucovorin (Wellcovorin), 5, 153
Leukeran (chlorambucil), 4, 71
Leukine (sargramostim [GM-CSF]), 15, 216
Leuprolide (Lupron, Viadur, Eligard), 5, 18, 153
Leustatin (cladribine), 5, 77
Levalbuterol (Xopenex), 20, 153–154
Levamisole (Ergamisol), 5, 154
Levaquin (levofloxacin), 2, 154
Levatol (penbutolol), 6, 193
Levetiracetam (Keppra), 8, 154
Levitra (vardenafil), 21, 248
Levo-Dromoran (levorphanol), 19, 155
Levobunolol (A-K Beta, Betagan), 12, 154
Levocabastine (Livostin), 12, 154

Levofloxacin (Levaquin, Quixin Ophthalmic), 2, 154
Levonorgestrel
(Plan B), 17, 155
and ethinyl estradiol (Preven), 17
implant (Norplant), 17, 155
Levophed (norepinephrine), 7, 183
Levorphanol (Levo-Dromoran), 19, 155
Levothyroxine (Synthroid, Levoxyl), 12, 155–156
Levoxyl (levothyroxine), 12, 155–156
Levsin (hyoscyamine), 14, 21, 139
Lexapro (escitalopram), 8, 109
Lexiva (fosamprenavir), 3, 125
Libritabs (chlordiazepoxide), 8, 71–72
Librium (chlordiazepoxide), 8, 71–72
Licorice (*Glycyrrhiza glabra*), 22, 259
Lidocaine
(Anestacon Topical, Xylocaine), 6, 18, 156, 268t, 270t
polymyxin B, neomycin, and bacitracin [topical] (Clomycin), 10, 49
and prilocaine (EMLA, LMX), 18, 156
Lindane (Kwell), 10, 156
Linezolid (Zyvox), 3, 157
Lioresal (baclofen), 17, 49–50
Liothyronine (Cytomel), 12, 157

Lipid-lowering agents
  classification of, 7
    antihypertensive combina-
      tions, 8
Lipitor (atorvastatin), 7, 46–47
Liqui-Char Activated (charcoal),
  1, 70–71
Lisinopril (Prinivil, Zestril), 6, 157
Lithium, 268t
Lithium carbonate (Eskalith,
  Lithobid), 9, 157–158
Lithobid (lithium carbonate), 9,
  157–158
Livostin (levocabastine), 12, 154
LMX (lidocaine and prilocaine),
  18, 156
LoCHOLEST (cholestyramine),
  7, 74
Lodine (etodolac), 19, 114
Lodoxamide (Alomide), 12, 13,
  158
Lomefloxacin (Maxaquin), 2, 158
Lomotil (diphenoxylate with at-
  ropine), 13, 96
Loniten (minoxidil), 8, 10, 171
Loperamide (Imodium), 13, 158
Lopid (gemfibrozil), 7, 129
Lopinavir/ritonavir (Kaletra), 4,
  158–159
Lopressor (metoprolol), 6, 169
Loprox (ciclopirox), 10, 74
Lopurin (allopurinol), 16, 30
Lorabid (loracarbef), 2, 159
Loracarbef (Lorabid), 2, 159
Loratadine (Claritin, Alavert), 1,
  159
Lorazepam (Ativan), 8, 159
Lorcet (hydrocodone and aceta-
  minophen), 19, 136–137

Lortab ASA (hydrocodone and
  aspirin), 19, 137
Losartan (Cozaar), 6, 159–160
Lotensin (benazepril), 6, 51
Lotrimin (clotrimazole), 3, 80
Lotrisone (clotrimazole and be-
  tamethasone), 3, 10, 80
Lotronex (alosetron), 14, 30–31
Lovastatin (Mevacor, Altocor), 7,
  160
Lovenox (enoxaparin), 15, 104
Lowsium (magaldrate), 13, 160
Lozol (indapamide), 7, 142
Lugol's solution [potassium io-
  dide] (SSKI, Thyro-Block),
  12
Lunelle (estradiol cypionate and
  medroxyprogesterone ac-
  etate), 17, 111
Lupron (leuprolide), 5, 18, 153
Lutrepulse (gonadorelin), 18,
  132
Luvox (fluvoxamine), 8, 123–124
Lymphocyte immune globulin
  [antithymocyte
  globulin/ATG] (Atgam),
  16, 42, 160
Lysodren (mitotane), 5, 172

M
Ma Huang/Ephedra, 22, 257
Maalox (aluminum hydroxide
  with magnesium hydrox-
  ide), 13, 33
Maalox Plus (aluminum hydroxide with magnesium hy-
  droxide and simethicone),
  13, 33–34

Macrobid (nitrofurantoin), 21, 182

Macrodantin (nitrofurantoin), 21, 182

Macrolides, classification of, 2

Mag-Ox, 400, 10, 161

Magaldrate (Riopan, Lowsium), 13, 160

Magnesium carbonate with aluminum hydroxide (Gaviscon), 13, 33

Magnesium citrate, 14, 160

Magnesium hydroxide with aluminum hydroxide (Maalox), 13, 33

Magnesium hydroxide with aluminum hydroxide and simethicone (Mylanta, Mylanta II, Maalox Plus), 13, 33–34

Magnesium hydroxide (Milk of Magnesia), 14, 160

Magnesium oxide (Mag-Ox 400), 10, 161

Magnesium sulfate, 10, 18, 161

Magnesium trisilicate, aluminum hydroxide, and alginic acid (Gaviscon), 30

Magnesium trisilicate with aluminum hydroxide (Gaviscon, Gaviscon-2), 13, 34

Malarone (atovaquone/proguanil), 4, 47

Mannitol, 7, 161

Marcaine (bupivacaine), 18, 56

Marinol (dronabinol), 13, 101

Matulane (procarbazine), 4, 204–205

Mavik (trandolapril), 6, 241

Maxair (pirbuterol), 20, 200

Maxalt (rizatriptan), 283t

Maxaquin (lomefloxacin), 2, 158

Maxipime (cefepime), 2, 64–65

Maxitrol (neomycin, polymyxin B, and dexamethasone), 12, 178

Maxzide (hydrochlorothiazide and triamterene), 7, 136

Mechlorethamine (Mustargen), 4, 161–162

Meclizine (Antivert), 14, 162

Medicinal herbs (commonly used), classification of, 21–22

Medigesic (acetaminophen with butalbital w/wo caffeine), 18, 25

Mediquell (dextromethorphan), 20, 90–91

Medroxyprogesterone acetate and estradiol cypionate (Lunelle), 17, 111

Medroxyprogesterone (Provera, Depo-Provera), 17, 18, 162

Mefoxin (cefoxitin), 2, 67

Megace (megestrol acetate), 5, 21, 162

Megestrol acetate (Megace), 5, 21, 162

MEL (melatonin), 22, 260

Melatonin (MEL), 22, 260

Mellaril (thioridazine), 9, 235

Meloxicam (Mobic), 19, 162

Melphalan [L-Pam] (Alkeran), 4, 162–163

Memantine (Namenda), 9, 163

Menest (esterified estrogens), 17, 110

Meningococcal polysaccharide vaccine (Menomune), 16, 163

Menomune (meningococcal polysaccharide vaccine), 16, 163

Meperidine (Demerol), 19, 163

Mepivacaine, 270t

Mepivacaine (Carbocaine), 270t

Meprobamate (Equanil, Miltown), 8, 163–164

Mepron (atovaquone), 4, 47

Mercaptopurine [6-MP] (Purinethol), 5, 164

Meridia (sibutramine), 11, 218

Meropenem (Merrem), 1, 164

Merrem (meropenem), 1, 164

Mesalamine (Rowasa, Asacol, Pentasa), 14, 164

Mesna (Mesnex), 1, 164

Mesnex (mesna), 1, 164

Mesoridazine (Serentil), 9, 165

Metamucil (psyllium), 14, 208

Metaprel (metaproterenol), 20, 165

Metaproterenol (Alupent, Metaprel), 20, 165

Metaxalone (Skelaxin), 17, 165

Metformin (Glucophage), 11, 165–166

Metformin/glyburide (Glucovance), 11

Methadone (Dolophine), 19, 166

Methanimine (Hiprex, Urex), 21, 166

Methergine (methylergonovine), 18, 167–168

Methimazole (Tapazole), 12, 166

Methocarbamol (Robaxin), 17, 166–167

Methotrexate (Folex, Rheumatrex), 17, 167, 269t

Methotrexate (MRX, Folex, Rheumatrex), 5

Methyldopa (Aldomet), 7, 167

Methylergonovine (Methergine), 18, 167–168

Methylprednisolone (Solu-Medrol), 11, 168, 271t

Methyltestosterone with esterified estrogens (Estratest), 17

Metoclopramide (Reglan, Clopra, Octamide), 14, 168

Metolazone (Mykrox, Zaroxolyn), 7, 168

Metoprolol (Lopressor, Toprol XL), 6, 169

MetroGel (metronidazole), 3, 10, 169

Metronidazole (Flagyl, Metro-Gel), 3, 10, 169

Mevacor (lovastatin), 7, 160

Mexiletine (Mexitil), 6, 169–170

Mexitil (mexiletine), 6, 169–170

Mezlin (mezlocillin), 2, 170

Mezlocillin (Mezlin), 2, 170

Miacalcin (calcitonin), 11, 58

Micardis (telmisartan), 6, 230

Miconazole (Monistat), 3, 10, 18, 170

Micro-K (potassium supplements), 10, 202

Micronase (glyburide), 11, 131

Midamor (amiloride), 7, 35

Midazolam (Versed), 9, 170

Mifeprex (mifepristone [RU486]), 18, 170

Mifepristone [RU486] (Mifeprex), 18, 170

Miglitol (Glyset), 11, 171

Migraine headache medications, classification of, 18

Milk of Magnesia (magnesium hydroxide), 14, 160

Milk thistle (*Silybum marianum*), 22, 260

Milrinone (Primacor), 7, 171

Miltown (meprobamate), 8, 163–164

Mineral oil, 14, 171

Minipress (prazosin), 6, 203

Minoxidil (Loniten, Rogaine), 8, 10, 171

MiraLax (polyethylene glycol [PEG] 3350), 201

Mirapex (pramipexole), 9, 202–203

Mirtazapien (Remeron), 8, 171

Miscellaneous therapeutic agents, classification of, 21–22

Misoprostol (Cytotec), 14, 171–172

Mitomycin (Mutamycin), 5, 172

Mitotane (Lysodren), 5, 172

Mitotic inhibitors, classification of, 5

Mitoxantrone (Novantrone), 5, 172

Mitran (chlordiazepoxide), 8, 71–72

Moban (molindone), 9, 173

Mobic (meloxicam), 19, 162

Modafinil (Provigil), 172–173

Moduretic (hydrochlorothiazide and amiloride), 7, 136

Moexipril (Univasc), 6, 173

Molindone (Moban), 9, 173

Mometasone furoate, 274t

Monistat (miconazole), 3, 10, 18, 170

Monocid (cefonicid), 2, 65–66

Monoclate (antihemophilic factor VIII), 15, 41

Monopril (Fosinopril), 6, 126

Montelukast (Singulair), 1, 20, 173

Monurol (fosfomycin), 3, 125

Morphine (Avinza XR, Du- amorph, MS Contin, Ka- dian SR, Roxanol), 19, 173–174

Motrin (ibuprofen), 19, 140

Moxifloxacin (Avelox), 2, 174

MRX (methotrexate), 5

MS Contin (morphine), 19, 173–174

Mucomyst (acetylcysteine), 1, 19, 20, 26

Mupirocin (Bactroban), 10, 174

Muromonab-CD3 (Orthoclone OKT3), 16, 174

Muscle relaxants, classification of, 17

Musculoskeletal agents, classi- fication of, 16–17

Muse (alprostadil [urethral sup- pository]), 21, 32

Mustargen (mechlorethamine), 4, 161–162

Mutamycin (mitomycin), 5, 172

Myambutol (ethambutol), 3, 113

Mycelex (clotrimazole), 3, 80

Myciguent (neomycin sulfate), 10, 179

Mycobutin (rifabutin), 3, 211–212

Mycolog-II (triamcinolone and nystatin), 3, 243

Mycophenolate mofetil (Cell-Cept), 16, 174–175

Mycostatin (nystatin), 3, 10, 18, 184

Mykrox (metolazone), 7, 168

Mylanta (aluminum hydroxide with magnesium hydroxide and simethicone), 13, 33–34

Mylanta II (aluminum hydroxide with magnesium hydroxide and simethicone), 13, 33–34

Myleran (busulfan), 4, 57

Mylicon (simethicone), 13, 218

Mylotarg (gemtuzumab ozogamicin), 5, 129

N

Nabumetone (Relafen), 19, 175

Nadolol (Corgard), 6, 175

Nafcillin (Nallpen), 2, 175

Naftifine (Naftin), 10, 175

Naftin (naftifine), 10, 175

NaHCO₃ (sodium bicarbonate), 10

Nalbuphine (Nubain), 19, 175

Nalfon (fenoprofen), 19, 116–117

Nallpen (nafcillin), 2, 175

Naloxone (Narcan), 1, 176

Naltrexone (ReVia), 21, 176

Namenda (memantine), 9, 163

NAPamide (disopyramide), 6, 97–98

Naphazoline and antazoline (Albalon-A Ophthalmic), 13, 176

Naphazoline and pheniramine acetate (Naphcon A), 13, 176

Naphcon A (naphazoline and pheniramine acetate), 13, 176

Naprosyn (naproxen), 19, 176

Naproxen (Aleve, Naprosyn, Anaprox), 19, 176

Naratriptan (Amerge), 18, 176–177

Narcan (naloxone), 1, 176

Narcotics, classification of, 18–19

Nardil (phenelzine), 8, 197

Nasal Inhaler (beclomethasone), 20

NasalCrom (cromolyn sodium), 1, 20, 82–83

Nasalide (flunisolide), 20, 120

Nateglinide (Starlix), 11, 177

Natrecor (nesiritide), 7, 179

Navane (thiothixene), 9, 235

Navelbine (vinorelbine), 5, 251

Nebcin (tobramycin), 1, 238

NebuPent (pentamidine), 4, 195

Nedocromil (Tilade), 20, 177

Nefazodone (Serzone), 8, 177

Nelfinavir (Viracept), 4, 177

Nembutal (pentobarbital), 8, 9, 195–196

Neo-Calglucon (calcium glubionate), 10, 59

Neo-Synephrine (phenyle-
phrine), 7, 198
NeoDecadron Ophthalmic (dexamethasone and
neomycin), 12, 178
Neomycin, 1
bacitracin, polymyxin B, and lidocaine [topical]
(Clomycin), 10, 49
bacitracin, and polymyxin B
[ophthalmic] (AK Spore
Ophthalmic, Neosporin
Ophthalmic), 12, 49
bacitracin, and polymyxin B
[topical] (Neosporin Ointment), 9, 49
colistin, hydrocortisone, and
thonzonium (Cortisporin-
TC Otic Suspension), 11,
178
colistin, and hydrocortisone
(Cortisporin-TC Otic
Drops), 11, 178
and dexamethasone (AK-Neo-
Dex Ophthalmic,
NeoDecadron Oph-
thalmic), 12, 178
polymyxin B, and dexamethasone (Maxitrol), 12, 178
polymyxin B, hydrocortisone,
and bacitracin [oph-
thalmic] (AK Spore HC
Ophthalmic, Cortisporin
Ophthalmic), 12, 49
polymyxin B, hydrocortisone,
and bacitracin [topical]
(Cortisporin), 9, 49
and polymyxin B (Neosporin
Cream), 178

polymyxin B, and pred-
nisolone (Poly-Pred Oph-
thalmic), 12, 178–179
polymyxin, and hydrocortisone
(Cortisporin Ophthalmic
and Otic), 11, 178
Neomycin-polymyxin bladder irri-
gant (Neosporin GU Irrig-
ant), 21, 178
Neomycin sulfate (Myciguent),
10, 179
Neoral (cyclosporine), 16, 84,
269t
Neosar (cyclophosphamide), 4,
83–84
Neosporin
Cream (neomycin and
polymyxin B), 178
GU Irrigant (neomycin-
polymyxin bladder irrig-
ant), 21, 178
Ointment (bacitracin,
neomycin, and polymyxin
B [topical]), 9, 49
Ophthalmic (bacitracin,
neomycin, and polymyxin
B [ophthalmic]), 12, 49
Nesiritide (Natrecor), 7, 179
Neulasta (pegfilgrastim), 15,
192–193
Neumega (oprelvekin), 15, 186
Neupogen (filgrastim [G-CSF]),
15, 118
Neuromuscular blockers, classi-
fication of, 17
Neurontin (gabapentin), 8, 127
Neutrexin (trimetrexate), 4, 245
Nevirapine (Viramune), 4, 179
Nexium (esomeprazole), 14, 109

Niacin (Niaspan), 7, 179

Niaspan (niacin), 7, 179

Nicardipine (Cardene), 7, 179–180

Nicoderm CQ (nicotine transdermal), 21, 180

Nicorette (nicotine gum), 21, 180

Nicotine gum (Nicorette), 21, 180

Nicotine nasal spray (Nicotrol NS), 21, 180

Nicotine transdermal (Habitrol, Nicoderm CQ, Nicotrol), 21, 180

Nicotrol (nicotine transdermal), 21, 180

Nicotrol NS (nicotine nasal spray), 21, 180

Nifedipine (Procardia, Procardia XL, Adalat, Adalat CC), 7, 180–181

Nilandron (nilutamide), 5, 181

Nilutamide (Nilandron), 5, 181

Nimodipine (Nimotop), 7, 9, 181

Nimotop (nimodipine), 7, 9, 181

Nipride (nitroprusside), 8, 182–183

Nisoldipine (Sular), 7, 181

Nitazoxanide (Alinia), 3, 181

Nitro-Bid IV (nitrogylcerin), 8, 182

Nitro-Bid Ointment (nitrogylcerin), 8, 182

Nitrodisc (nitrogylcerin), 8, 182

Nitrofurantoin (Macrodantin, Furadantin, Macrobid), 21, 182

Nitrogen mustards, classification of, 4

Nitroglycerin (Nitrostat, Nitrolingual, Nitro-Bid Ointment, Nitro-Bid IV, Nitrodisc, Transderm-Nitro), 8, 182

Nitrolingual (nitrogylcerin), 8, 182

Nitropress (nitroprusside), 8, 182–183

Nitroprusside (Nipride, Nitropress), 8, 182–183

Nitrosoureas, classification of, 4

Nitrostat (nitrogylcerin), 8, 182

Nix (permethrin), 10, 196

Nizatidine (Axid), 14, 183

Nizoral (ketoconazole), 3, 10, 149–150

Nolvadex (tamoxifen), 5, 228–229

Nonnarcotic agents, classification of, 19

Nonsteroidal antiinflammatory agents, classification of, 19

Norcuron (vecuronium), 17, 249

Norelgestromin and ethinyl estradiol (Ortho Evra), 113–114

Norepinephrine (Levophed), 7, 183

Norethindrone acetate/ethinyl estradiol (FemHRT), 18, 183

Norflex (orphenadrine), 17, 187

Norfloxacin (Noroxin), 2, 183–184

Norgestrel (Ovrette), 17, 184

Normiflow (ardeparin), 15, 43

Normodyne (labetalol), 6, 151

Noroxin (norfloxacin), 2, 183–184

Norpace (disopyramide), 6, 97–98

Norplant (levonorgestrel implant), 17, 155

Norpramin (desipramine), 8, 88–89

Nortriptyline (Aventyl, Pamelor), 8, 184, 268t

Norvasc (amlodipine), 7, 37

Norvir (ritonavir), 213–214

Novafed (pseudoephedrine), 20, 207–208

Novantrone (mitoxantrone), 5, 172

Novocaine (procaine), 270t

Nubain (nalbuphine), 19, 176

Numorphan (oxymorphone), 19, 190

Nupercainal (dibucaine), 10, 14, 18, 92

NuvaRing (etonogestrel/ethinyl estradiol), 17, 114–115

Nystatin (Mycostatin), 3, 10, 18, 184

Nystatin and triamcinolone (Mycolog-II), 3, 243

Ocuflox Ophthalmic (ofloxacin), 2, 12, 185

Ocupress Ophthalmic (carteolol), 6, 62

Ofloxacin (Floxin, Ocuflox Ophthalmic), 2, 12, 185

Olanzapine (Zyprexa, Zyprexa Zydis), 9, 185

Olopatadine (Patanol), 13, 185

Olsalazine (Dipentum), 14, 185

Omalizumab (Xolair), 20, 185–186

Omeprazole (Prilosec), 14, 186

Omnicef (cefdinir), 2, 64

Omnipen (ampicillin), 2, 39–40

Oncaspar (L-Asparaginase), 5, 43–44

Oncovin (vincristine), 5, 250–251

Ondansetron (Zofran), 14, 186

Ophthalmic antibiotics, classification of, 12–13

Oprelvekin (Neumega), 15, 186

Opticrom (cromolyn sodium), 1, 13, 20, 82–83

Optivar (azelastine), 1, 48

Oral contraceptives
  monophasic, 186–187, 276t–277t
  multiphasic, 186–187, 277t–278t
  progestin only, 186–187, 279t

Oramorph SR (morphine), 19, 173–174

Orgaron (danaparoid), 15, 86–87

Orinase (tolbutamide), 11, 239

Orlistat (Xenical), 21, 187

Orphenadrine (Norflex), 17, 187

O

Ob/Gyn agents, classification of, 17–18

Obesity, classification of, 11

Occupress Ophthalmic (carteolol), 6, 12

Octamide (metoclopramide), 14, 168

Octreotide (Sandostatin, Sandostatin LAR), 13, 184–185

Ortho Evra (ethinyl estradiol and norelgestromin), 113–114
Orthoclone OKT3 (muromonab-CD3), 16, 174
Orudis (ketoprofen), 19, 150
Oruvail (ketoprofen), 19, 150
Oseltamivir (Tamiflu), 4, 187
Osteoporosis agents, classification of, 12
OTC Syrup (ipecac syrup), 1, 146
Otic Domeboro (acetic acid and aluminum acetate), 11, 26
Otobiotic Otic (Polymyxin B and hydrocortisone), 11, 201–202
Ovrette (norgestrel), 17, 184
Oxacillin (Bactocill, Prostaphlin), 3, 188
Oxaprozin (Daypro), 19, 188
Oxazepam (Serax), 8, 188
Oxcarbazepine (Trileptal), 8, 188
Oxiconazole (Oxistat), 3, 10, 188–189
Oxistat (oxiconazole), 3, 10, 188–189
Oxybutynin (Ditropan, Ditropan XL), 21, 189
Oxybutynin transdermal system (Oxytrol), 21, 189
Oxycodone [dihydrohydroxycodeinone] (OxyContin, OxyIR, Roxicodone), 19, 189
  and acetaminophen (Percocet, Tylox), 19, 189–190
  and aspirin (Percodan, Percodan-Demi), 19, 190
OxyContin (oxycodone), 19, 189

OxyIR (oxycodone), 19, 189
Oxymorphone (Numorphan), 19, 190
Oxytocin (Pitocin), 18, 190
Oxytrol (oxybutynin transdermal system), 21, 189

P

Pacerone (amiodarone), 6, 36
Paclitaxel (Taxol), 5, 190–191
Pain medications, classification of, 18–19
Palivizumab (Synagis), 4, 191
Palonosetron (Aloxi), 14, 191
Pamelor (nortriptyline), 8, 184
Pamidronate (Aredia), 11, 191
Pancrease (pancrelipase), 191
Pancrelipase (Pancrease, Cotazym, Creon, Ultrase), 191
Pancuronium (Pavulon), 17, 191–192
Pantoprazole (Protonix), 14, 192
Paraflex (chlorzoxazone), 17, 73–74
Parafon Forte DSC (chlorzoxazone), 17, 73–74
Paraplatin (carboplatin), 4, 61
Paregoric [camphorated tincture of opium], 13, 192
Parepectolin (kaolin-pectin), 13, 149
Parlodel (bromocriptine), 9, 55
Paroxetine (Paxil), 8, 192
Patanol (olopatadine), 13, 185
Pavulon (pancuronium), 17, 191–192
Paxil (paroxetine), 8, 192

PediaCare 1 (dextromethorphan), 20, 90–91

Pediarix (diphtheria, tetanus toxoids, and acellular pertussis adsorbed, hepatitis B [recombinant], and inactivated poliovirus vaccine [IPV] combined), 16, 96

Pediazole, erythromycin and sulfisoxazole, 2, 108

Pedvax-HIB (haemophilus B conjugate vaccine), 16, 133

Peg interferon alfa-2a (Pegasys), 4, 193

Peg interferon alfa-2b (PEG-Intron), 16, 193

PEG-Intron (peg interferon alfa-2b), 16, 193

Pegasys (peg interferon alfa 2a), 4, 193

Pegfilgrastim (Neulasta), 15, 192–193

Pemetrexed (Alimta), 5, 193

Pemirolast (Alamast), 13, 193

Pen-Vee K (pennicillin v), 3, 194–195

Penbutolol (Levatol), 6, 193

Penciclovir (Denavir), 4, 10, 193–194

Penicillin g. aqueous (potassium or sodium) (Pfizerpen, Pentids), 2, 194

Penicillins, classification of, 2–3

Pennicillin G Benzathine (Bicillin), 3, 194

Pennicillin G Procaine (Wycillin), 3, 194

Pennicillin V (Pen-Vee K, Veetids), 3, 194–195

Pentam 300 (pentamidine), 4, 195

Pentamidine (Pentam 300, Nebu-Pent), 4, 195

Pentasa (mesalamine), 14, 164

Pentazocine (Talwin), 19, 195

Pentids (penicillin g. aqueous [potassium or sodium]), 2

Pentobarbital (Nembutal), 8, 9, 195–196

Pentosan polysulfate (Elmiron), 21, 196

Pentoxifylline (Trental), 15, 196

Pepcid (fomotidine), 14, 116

Pepto-Bismol (bismuth subsalicylate), 13, 53–54

Percocet (oxycodone and acetaminophen), 19, 189–190

Percodan-Demi (oxycodone and aspirirn), 19, 190

Percodan (oxycodone and aspirin), 19, 190

Pergolide (Permax), 9, 196

Periactin (cyproheptadine), 1, 84

Perindopril erbumine (Aceon), 6, 196

Permax (pergolide), 9, 196

Permethrin (Nix, Elimite), 10, 196

Permitil (fluphenazine), 9, 122

Perphenazine (Trilafon), 9, 197

Persantine (dipyridamole), 15, 97

Pfizerpen (penicillin g. aqueous [potassium or sodium]), 2, 194

Phenazopyridine (Pyridium), 21, 197

Phenelzine (Nardil), 8, 197

Phenergan (promethazine), 14, 205

Pheniramine acetate and naphazoline (Naphcon A), 13

Phenobarbital, 8, 9, 197–198, 266t

and scopolamine, hyoscyamine, and atropine (Donnatal), 14, 139–140

Phenylephrine, acetaminophen, hydrocodone, chlorpheniramine, and caffeine (Hycomine), 20, 137

Phenylephrine (Neo-Synephrine), 7, 198

Phenytoin (Dilantin), 8, 198–199, 266t

Phos-Ex (calcium acetate), 10

PhosLo (calcium acetate), 10

Phospholine Ophthalmic (echothiophate iodine), 12, 102

Phrenilin Forte (acetaminophen with butalbital w/wo caffeine), 18, 25

Physostigmine (Antilirium), 1, 199

Phytonadione [vitamin K] (AquaMEPHYTON), 10, 199

Pimecrolimus (Elidel), 10, 199

Pindolol (Visken), 6, 199

Pioglitazone (Actos), 11, 199–200

Piperacillin (Pipracil), 3, 200

Piperacillin–Tazobactam (Zosyn), 3, 200

Pipracil (piperacillin), 3, 200

Pirbuterol (Maxair), 20, 200

Piroxicam (Feldene), 19, 200

Pitocin (oxytocin), 18, 190

Pitressin (vasopressin), 15, 249

Pitressin (vasopressin [antidiuretic hormone, ADH]), 11

Plan B (levonorgestrel), 17, 155

Plasma protein fraction (Plasmanate), 15, 200–201

Plasmanate (plasma protein fraction), 15, 200–201

Platinol (cisplatin), 4, 76–77

Plavix (clopidogrel), 15

Plenaxis (abarelix), 5, 23

Plendil (felodipine), 7, 116

Pletal (cilostazol), 21, 75

Pneumococcal vaccine [polyvalent] (Pneumovax-23), 16, 201

Pneumococcal 7-valent conjugate vaccine (Prevnar), 16, 201

Pneumovax-23 (pneumococcal vaccine [polyvalent]), 16, 201

Podocon-25 (podophyllin), 10, 210

Podophyllin (Podocon-25, Condylox Gel 0.5 Condylox), 10, 201

Poly-Pred Ophthalmic (neomycin, polymyxin B, and prednisolone), 12, 178–179

Polycitra-K (potassium citrate and citric acid), 21, 202

Polyethylene glycol-electrolyte solution (goLYTELY, CoLyte), 14, 201

Polyethylene glycol [PEG] 3350 (MiraLax), 201

Polymox (amoxicillin), 2, 37–38

Polymyxin B and

bacitracin [ophthalmic] (AK Poly Bac Ophthalmic, Polysporin Ophthalmic), 12, 49

bacitracin [topical] (Polysporin), 9, 49

hydrocortisone, bacitracin, neomycin [ophthalmic] (AK Spore HC Ophthalmic, Cortisporin Ophthalmic), 12, 49

hydrocortisone, bacitracin, neomycin [topical] (Cortisporin), 9, 49

hydrocortisone (Otobiotic Otic), 11, 201–202

neomycin, bacitracin, lidocaine [topical] (Clomycin), 10, 49

neomycin, bacitracin [ophthalmic] (AK Spore Ophthalmic, Neosporin Ophthalmic), 12, 49

neomycin, dexamethasone (Maxitrol), 12, 178

neomycin (Neosporin Cream), 178

neomycin, prenisolone (Poly-Pred Ophthalmic), 12, 178–179

Polymyxin Band, neomycin, bacitracin [topical] (Neosporin Ointment), 9, 49

Polymyxin, neomycin, and hydrocortisone (Cortisporin Opthalmic and Otic), 11, 178

Polysporin (bacitracin and polymyxin B [topical]), 9, 49

Polysporin Ophthalmic (bacitracin and polymyxin B), 12, 49

Potassium citrate and citric acid (Polycitra-K), 21, 202

Potassium citrate (Urocit-K), 21, 202

Potassium clavulanate/ticarcillin (Timetin), 3, 236

Potassium iodide [Lugol's solution] (SSKI, Thyro-Block), 12, 21, 202

Potassium iodide (SSKI, Thyro-Block), 20

Potassium supplements (Kaon, Kaochlor, K-Lor, Slow-K, Micro-K, Klorvess), 10, 202, 280t

Pramipexole (Mirapex), 9, 202–203

Pramoxine (Anusol Ointment, Proctofoam-NS), 14, 18, 203

Pramoxine and hydrocortisone (Enzone, Proctofoam-HC), 10, 14, 203

Prandin (repaglinide), 11, 211

Pravachol (pravastatin), 7, 203

Pravastatin (Pravachol), 7, 203

Prazosin (Minipress), 6, 203

Precose (Acarbose), 11, 24

Pred-G Ophthalmic (gentamicin and prednisolone [ophthalmic]), 130

Prednicarbate, 274t
Prednisolone, 11, 203–204, 271t
   and gentamicin [ophthalmic]
      (Pred-G Ophthalmic), 130
   and polymyxin B, neomycin
      (Poly-Pred Ophthalmic),
      12, 178–179
   and sulfacetamide (Ble-
      phamide), 11, 13, 226
Prednisone, 11, 204, 271t
Premarin (estrogen [conju-
      gated]), 17, 111–112
Premarin with methylproges-
      terone (estrogen
      [conjugated with
      methylprogesterone]), 18,
      112
Premarin with methyltestos-
      terone (estrogen
      [conjugated with
      methyltestosterone]), 18,
      112–113
Premphase (estrogen [conju-
      gated with medroxyprog-
      esterone]), 17, 112
Prempro (estrogen [conjugated
      with medroxyproges-
      terone]), 17, 112
Prepidil Vaginal Gel (dinopros-
      tone), 18, 95–96
Prevacid (lansoprazole), 14, 152
Preven (ethinyl estradiol and lev-
      onorgestrel), 17, 113
Prevnar (pneumococcal 7-valent
      conjugate vaccine), 16,
      201
Priftin (rifapentine), 3, 212
Prilocaine and lidocaine (EMLA,
      LMX), 18

Prilosec (omeparazole), 14, 186
Primacor (milrinone), 7, 171
Primaxin (imipnem–cilastatin), 1,
      141
Primidone, 266t
Prinivil (lisinopril), 6, 157
Priscoline (tolazoline), 8, 238–239
Pro-Banthine (propantheline),
      15, 206
Probenecid (Benemid), 16, 204
Procainamide (Pronestyl, Pro-
      can), 6, 204, 268t
Procaine (Novocaine), 270t
Procan (procainamide), 6, 204
Procarbazine (Matulane), 4,
      204–205
Procardia (nifedipine), 7,
      180–181
Procardia XL (nifedipine), 7,
      180–181
Prochlorperazine (Compazine),
      9, 14, 205
Procotfoam-NS (pramoxine), 14,
      203
Procrit (epoetin alfa [erythro-
      peoietin/EPO]), 15,
      106
Proctocort (hydrocortisone [rec-
      tal]), 14, 138
Proctofoam-HC (pramoxine with
      hydrocortisone), 10, 14,
      203
Proctofoam-NS (pramoxine), 10,
      18
Proglycem (diazoxide), 12,
      91–92
Prograf (tacrolimus), 10, 16, 228
Proguanil/atovaquone
      (Malarone), 4, 47

Prohibit (haemophilus B conjugate vaccine), 16, 133

Prokine (sargramostim [GM-CSF]), 15, 216

Prolastin (alpha$_1$-protease inhibitor), 20, 31

Proleukin (aldesleukin [Interleukin-2, IL-2]), 5, 28–29

Prolixin (fluphenazine), 9, 122

Proloprim (trimethoprim), 21, 244–245

Promethazine (Phenergan), 14, 205

Pronestyl (procainamide), 6, 204

Propafenone (Rythmol), 6, 205–206

Propantheline (Pro-Banthine), 15, 206

Propecia (finasteride), 10, 21, 118

Propine (dipivefrin), 12, 96–97

Propofol (Diprivan), 9, 206

Propoxyphene (Darvon), 19, 206
    and acetaminophen (Darvocet), 19, 206
    and aspirin (Darvon Compound-65, Darvon-N with Aspirin), 19, 206

Propranolol (Inderal), 6, 206–207

Propylthiouracil [PTU], 12, 207

Proscar (finasteride), 10, 21, 118

ProSom (estazolam), 9, 109–110

Prostaphlin (oxacillin), 2, 188

Prostin Vr (alprostadil [Prostaglandin E$_1$]), 8, 31

Protamine, 15, 207

Protonix (pantoprazole), 14, 192

Protopic (tacrolimus), 10, 16, 228

Proventil (albuterol), 20, 28

Provera (medroxyprogesterone), 17, 18, 162

Provigil (modafinil), 172–173

Prozac (fluoxetine), 8, 121

Pseudoephedrine and hydrocodone (Detussin, Histussin-D), 20, 137

Pseudoephedrine (Sudafed, Novafed, Afrinol), 20, 207–208

Psyllium (Metamucil, Serutan, Effer-Syllium), 14, 208

Pulmicort (budesonide), 1, 20, 56

Pulmozyme (dornase alfa), 20, 99

Purinethol (Mercaptopurine [6-MP]), 5, 164

Pyrazinamide, 3, 207

Pyridium (phenazopyridine), 21, 197

Pyridoxine (vitamin B$_6$), 10, 208

Q

Quazepam (Doral), 9, 208

Quelicin (succinylcholine), 17, 225

Questran (cholestyramine), 7, 74

Quetiapine (Seroquel), 9, 209

Quinaglute (quinidine), 6, 209

Quinapril (Accupril), 6, 209

Quinidex (quinidine), 6, 209

Quinidine (Quinidex, Quinaglute), 6, 209, 268t

Quinupristin–Dalfopristin (Synercid), 3, 209–210
Quixin Ophthalmic (levofloxacin), 2, 154
QVAR (beclomethasone), 20, 51

R

Rabeprazole (Aciphex), 14, 210
Raloxifene (Evista), 12, 210
Ramipril (Altace), 6, 210
Ranitidine hydrochloride (Zantac), 14, 210–211
Rapamune (sirolimus), 16, 219
Raptiva (efalizumab), 10, 103
Rasburicase (Elitek), 5, 211
Rebetron (interferon alfa-2b and ribavirin combinationation), 4, 145
Recombinivax HB (hepatitis B vaccine), 16, 135
Refludan (lepirudin), 15, 152–153
Reglan (metoclopramide), 14, 168
Regranex Gel (becaplermin), 21, 50–51
Relafen (nabumetone), 19, 175
Relenza (zanamivir), 4, 252–253
Remeron (mirtazapine), 8, 171
Remicade (infliximab), 14, 143
Reminyl (galantamine), 9, 127
Remodulin (treprostinil sodium), 8, 242
Renagel (sevelamer), 21, 217
Renova (tretinoin/topical [retinoic acid]), 5, 10, 242
ReoPro (abciximab), 15, 23–24
Repaglinide (Prandin), 11, 211

Repan (acetaminophen with butalbital w/wo caffeine), 18, 25
Requip (ropinirole), 9, 214–215
Rescriptor (delavirdine), 3, 88
Respiratory agents, classification of, 19–20
Respiratory inhalants, classification of, 20
Restoril (temazepam), 9, 230
Retavase (reteplase), 15, 211
Reteplase (Retavase), 14, 15, 211
Retin-A (tretinoin/topical [retinoic acid]), 5, 10, 242
Retinoic acid (tretinoin) [topical] (Retin-A, Avita, Renova), 5, 10
Retrovir (zidovudine), 4, 253
ReVia (naltrexone), 21, 176
Reyataz (atazanavir), 4, 45
Rheomacrodex (dextran 40), 15, 90
Rheumatrex (methotrexate), 5, 17, 167
Rhinocort (budesonide), 1, 20, 56
Ribavirin and interferon alfa-2b combination (Rebetron), 4, 145
Ribavirin (Virazole), 4, 211
Rifabutin (Mycobutin), 3, 211–212
Rifadin (rifampin), 3, 212
Rifampin (Rifadin), 3, 212
Rifapentine (Priftin), 3, 212
Rimantadine (Flumadine), 4, 212–213
Rimexolone (Vexol Ophthalmic), 12, 13, 213

Rimso 50 (dimethyl sulfoxide [DMSO]), 21, 95
Riopan (magaldrate), 13, 160
Risedronate (Actonel), 12, 213
Risperdal (risperidone), 9, 213
Risperidone (Risperdal), 9, 213
Ritonavir (Norvir), 213–214
Ritonavir/lopinavir (Kaletra), 4, 158–159
Rivastigmine (Exelon), 9, 214
Rizatriptan (Maxalt), 283t
Robaxin (methocarbamol), 17, 166–167
Robitussin AC (guaifenesin and codeine), 20, 132–133
Robitussin (guaifenesin), 20
Rocaltrol (calcitriol), 11, 58
Rocephin (ceftriaxone), 2, 68–69
Rocuronium (Zemuron), 17, 214
Rofecoxib (Vioxx), 19, 214
Roferon-A (interferon alfa), 16, 144–145
Rogaine (minoxidil), 8, 10, 171
Romazicon (flumazenil), 1, 120
Ropinirole (Requip), 9, 214–215
Rosiglitazone (Avandia), 11, 215
Rosuvastatin (Crestor), 7, 215
Rowasa (mesalamine), 14, 164
Roxanol (morphine), 19, 173–174
Roxicodone (oxycodone), 19, 189
Rubex (doxorubicin), 5, 100–101
Rufen (ibuprofen), 19, 140
Rythmol (propafenone), 6, 205–206

S

St. John's Wort (*Hypericum perforatum*), 22, 260

St. Joseph's (aspirin), 15, 19, 44
Salmeterol (Serevent), 20, 215
Salmeterol xinafoate and fluticasone propionate (Advair Diskus), 20, 123
Sanctura (trospium chloride), 21, 246
Sandimmune (cyclosporine), 16, 84, 269t
Sandoglobulin (immune globulin [IV]), 16, 142
Sandostatin LAR (octreotide), 13, 184–185
Sandostatin (octreotide), 13, 184–185
Saquinavir (Fortovase), 4, 215–216
Sarafem (fluoxetine), 8, 121
Sargramostim [GM-CSF] (Prokine, Leukine), 15, 216
Saw Palmetto (*Serenoa repens*), 22, 260
Scopace (scopolamine), 14, 216
Scopolamine, hyoscyamine, atropine, and phenobarbital (Donnatal), 14, 139–140
Scopolamine (Scopace, Trans-Derm-Scop), 14, 216
Secobarbital (Seconal), 9, 216
Seconal (secobarbital), 9, 216
Sectral (acebutolol), 6, 24
Sedapap-10 (acetaminophen with butalbital w/wo caffeine), 18, 25
Sedative hypnotics, classification of, 9
Selegiline (Eldepryl), 9, 216–217

Selenium sulfide (Exsel Shampoo, Selsun Blue Shampoo, Selsun Shampoo), 10, 217

Selsun Blue Shampoo (selenium sulfide), 10, 217

Selsun Shampoo (selenium sulfide), 10, 217

Sensipar (cinacalcet), 12, 75

Septra, trimethoprim–sulfamethoxazole [co-trimoxazole], 3, 245

Serax (oxazepam), 8, 188

Serentil (mesoridazine), 9, 165

Serevent (salmeterol), 20, 215

Seroquel (quetiapine), 9, 209

Serotonin receptor agonists, 283, 283t

Sertaconazole (Ertaczo), 3, 217

Sertraline (Zoloft), 8, 217

Serutan (psyllium), 14, 208

Serzone (nefazodone), 8, 177

Sevelamer (Renagel), 21, 217

Sibutramine (Meridia), 11, 218

Sildenafil (Viagra), 21, 218

Silvadene (silver sulfadiazine), 10, 218

Silver nitrate (Dey-Drop), 13, 21, 218

Silver sulfadiazine (Silvadene), 10, 218

Simethicone and magnesium hydroxide with aluminum hydroxide (Mylanta, Mylanta II, Maalox Plus), 13, 33–34

Simethicone (Mylicon), 13, 218

Simulect (basiliximab), 16, 50

Simvastatin (Zocor), 7, 219

Sinemet (carbidopa/levodopa), 9, 61

Sinequan (doxepin), 8, 100

Singulair (montelukast), 1, 20, 173

Sirolimus (Rapamune), 16, 219

Skelaxin (metaxalone), 17, 165

Slow-K (potassium supplements), 10, 202

Smallpox vaccine (Dryvax), 219

Sodium bicarbonate ($NaHCO_3$), 10, 219–220

Sodium citrate (Bicitra), 21, 220

Sodium oxybate (Xyrem), 9, 220

Sodium phosphate (Visicol), 14, 221

Sodium polystyrene sulfonate (Kayexalate), 21, 221

Sodium Sulamyd (sulfacetamide), 13, 226

Solu-Cortef (hydrocortisone [topical and systemic]), 11, 138

Solu-Medrol (Methylprednisolone), 11, 168, 271t

Soma (carisoprodol), 17, 61

Somophyllin (theophylline), 20, 234

Sonata (zaleplon), 9, 252

Sorbitol, 14, 221

Sorbitrate (isosorbide dinitrate), 8, 147–148

Soriatane (acitretin), 9, 26

Sotalol (Betapace, Betapace AF), 6, 221–222

Sotret (isotretinoin [13-*cis* retinoic acid]), 10, 148

Sparfloxacin (Zagam), 2, 222

Spectazole (econazole), 3, 10, 102

Spectracef (cefditoren), 2, 64

Spiriva (tiotropium), 20, 237

Spironolactone (Aldactone), 7, 222–223

Spironolactone and hydro-chlorothiazide (Aldac-tazide), 7, 136

Spirulina (*Spirulina* spp), 22, 260

Sporanox (itraconazole), 3, 149

SSKI (potassium iodide), 20

SSKI (potassium iodide [Lugol's solution]), 12, 21, 202

Stadol (butorphanol), 18, 57

Starlix (nateglinide), 11, 177

Stavudine (Zerit), 4, 223

Stelazine (trifluoperazine), 9, 244

Sterile Talc Powder (talc), 21, 228

Steroids, 272t–274t

Steroids (systemic), 223–224, 271t

Stimate (desmopressin), 11, 15, 89

Strattera (atomoxetine), 9, 46

Streptase (streptokinase), 15, 224

Streptomycin, 1, 3, 224–225

Streptozocin (Zanosar), 4, 225

Stretokinase (Streptase, Kabiki-nase), 15, 224

Striant (testosterone), 11, 232

Sublimaze (fentanyl), 19, 117

Succimer (Chemet), 1, 225

Succinylcholine (Anectine, Quelicin, Sucostrin), 17, 225

Sucostrin (succinylcholine), 17, 225

Sucralfate (Carafate), 14, 226

Sudafed (pseudoephedrine), 20, 207–208

Sular (nisoldipine), 7, 181

Sulfacetamide (Bleph-10, Cetamide, Sodium Su-lamyd), 13, 226

Sulfacetamide and prednisolone (Blephamide), 11, 13, 226

Sulfamethoxazole [co-trimoxa-zole]–trimethoprim (Bactrim, Septra), 3201

Sulfasalazine (Azulfidine), 15, 226–227

Sulfinpyrazone (Anturane), 16, 227

Sulfisoxazole and erythromycin (Eryzole, Pediazole), 2, 108

Sulindac (Clinoril), 19, 227

Sumatriptan (Imitrex), 18, 227

Sumycin (tetracycline), 3, 233

Superchar (charcoal), 1, 70–71

Supprettes (chloral hydrate), 9, 71

Suprax (cefixime), 2, 65

Surfak (docusate calcium), 14, 98

Survanta (beractant), 20, 52

Sus-Phrine (epinephrine), 7, 20, 105

Sustiva (efavirenz), 3, 103

Symmetrel (amantadine), 4, 9, 34

Synagis (palivizumab), 4, 191

Synercid (quinupristin–dalfo-pristin), 3, 209–210

Synthroid (levothyroxine), 12, 155–156

T

T-Stat (erythromycin [topical]), 10, 108–109

Tabloid (6-Thioguanine [6-TG]), 5, 234–235

Tacrine (Cognex), 9, 227–228

Tacrolimus (Prograf, Protopic), 10, 16, 228

Tadalafil (Cialis), 21, 228

Tagamet (cimetidien), 14, 75

Talc (Sterile Talc Powder), 21, 228

Talwin (pentazocine), 19, 195

Tambocor (flecainide), 6, 119

Tamiflu (oseltamivir), 4, 187

Tamoxifen (Nolvadex), 5, 228–229

Tamsulosin (Flomax), 21, 229

Tapazole (methimazole), 12, 166

Tasmar (tolcapone), 9, 239

Tavist (clemastine fumarate), 1, 78

Taxol (paclitaxel), 5, 190–191

Taxotere (docetaxel), 5, 98

Tazarotene (Tazorac), 10, 229

Tazicef, ceftazidime, 2, 68

Tazidime, ceftazidime, 2, 68

Tazobactam–piperacillin (Zosyn), 3, 200

Tazorac (tazarotene), 10, 229

Tea Tree (*Melaleuca alternifolia*), 22, 261

Tears Naturale (artificial tears), 13, 43

Tegaserod maleate (Zelnorm), 15, 229

Tegretol (carbamazepine), 8, 60

Telithromycin (Ketek), 2, 229–230

Telmisartan (Micardis), 6, 230

Temazepam (Restoril), 9, 230

Tenecteplase (TNKase), 15, 230–231

Tenofovir (Viread), 4, 231

Tenoretic (atenolol and chlorthalidone), 6, 46

Tenormin (atenolol), 6, 46

Tensilon (edophonium), 17, 102

Tequin (gatifloxacin), 2, 128

Terazole 7 (terconazole), 18, 232

Terazosin (Hytrin), 6, 21, 231

Terbinafine (Lamisil), 3, 10, 231

Terbutaline (Brethine, Bricanyl), 18, 20, 231–232

Terconazole (Terazol 7), 18, 232

Teriparatide (Forteo), 12, 232

Tespa (triethylenetriphos-phamide), 4, 243–244

Tessalon Perles (benzonatate), 19, 51–52

Testim (testoterone), 11, 232

Testoderm (testoterone), 11, 232

Testoterone (AndroGel, Andro-derm, Striant, Testim, Testoderm), 11, 232

Tetanus immune globulin, 16, 232–233

Tetanus prophylaxis, 281t

Tetanus toxoid, 16, 233

Tetracycline (Achromycin V, Sumycin), 3, 233

Tetracyclines, classification of, 3

Teveten (eprosartan), 6, 107

Thalidomide (Thalomid), 5, 233–234

Thalomid (thalidomide), 5, 233–234

Theolair (theophylline), 20, 234

Theophylline (Theolair, Somophyllin), 20, 234, 267

TheraCys (BCG [Bacillus Calmette-Guérin]), 5, 50

Thiamine (vitamin B₁), 10, 234

Thiethylperazine (Torecan), 14, 234

Thio-Tepa (triethylenetriphosphamide), 4, 243–244

6-Thioguanine [6-TG] (Tabloid), 5, 234–235

Thioridazine (Mellaril), 9, 235

Thiothixene (Navane), 9, 235

Thonzonium, hydrocortisone, colistin, and neomycin (Cortisporin-TC Otic Suspension), 11, 178

Thorazine (chlorpromazine), 9, 13, 72–73

Thyro-Block (potassium iodide), 20

Thyro-Block (potassium iodide [Lugol's solution]), 12, 21, 202

Thyroid/antithyroid, classification of, 12

Tiagabine (Gabitril), 8, 235–236

Tiamate (diltiazem), 7, 94–95

Tiazac (diltiazem), 7, 94–95

Ticar (ticarcillin), 3, 236

Ticarcillin (Ticar), 3, 236

Tice BCG (BCG [Bacillus Calmette-Guérin]), 5, 50

Ticlid (ticlopidine), 15, 236

Ticlopidine (Ticlid), 15, 236

Tigan (trimethobenzamide), 14, 244

Tikosyn (dofetilide), 6, 98–99

Tilade (nedocromil), 20, 177

Timentin (ticarcillin/potassium clavulanate), 3, 236

Timolol (Blocadren), 6, 236–237

Timolol and dorzolamide (Cosopt), 12, 100

Timolol [opthalmic] (Timoptic), 12, 237

Timoptic (timolol [opthalmic]), 12, 237

Tinactin (tolnaftate), 10, 239

Tinzaprin (Innohep), 15, 237

Tioconazole (Vagistat), 18, 237

Tiotropium (Spiriva), 20, 237

Tirofiban (Aggrastat), 15, 237–238

TNKase (tenecteplase), 15, 230–231

Tobradex (tobramycin and dexmethasone), 13, 238

Tobramycin and dexamethasone (TobraDex), 13, 238

Tobramycin (Nebcin), 1, 238, 265t

Tobramycin [ophthalmic] (AKTob, Tobrex), 13, 238

Tobrex (tobramycin [ophthalmic]), 13, 238

Tofranil (imipramine), 8, 19, 141

Tolazamide (Tolinase), 11, 238

Tolazoline (Priscoline), 8, 238–239

Tolbutamide (Orinase), 11, 239

Tolcapone (Tasmar), 9, 239

Tolectin (tolmetin), 19, 239

Tolinase (tolazamide), 11, 238

Tolmetin (Tolectin), 19, 239

Tolnaftate (Tinactin), 10, 239

Tolterodine (Detrol, Detrol LA), 21, 239–240

Topamax (topiramate), 8, 240

Topiramate (Topamax), 8, 240

Toposar (etoposide [VP-16]), 115

Topotecan (Hycamtin), 5, 240

Toprol XL (metoprolol), 6, 169

Toradol (ketorolac), 19, 150

Torecan (thiethylperazine), 14, 234

Tornalate (bitotolterol), 20, 54

Torsemide (Demadex), 7, 240

Tracrium (atracurium), 17, 47

Tramadol (Ultram), 19, 241

Tramadol/acetaminophen (Ultracet), 19, 241

Trandate (labetalol), 6, 151

Trandolapril (Mavik), 6, 241

Trans-Derm-Scop (scopolamine), 216

Transderm-Nitro (nitrogylcerin), 8, 182

Tranxene (clorazepate), 8, 80

Trastuzumab (Herceptin), 5, 241

Trasylol (aprotinin), 15, 43

Trazodone (Desyrel), 8, 241–242, 269t

Trelstar Depot (triptorelin), 5, 245–246

Trelstar LA (triptorelin), 5, 245–246

Trental (pentoxifylline), 15, 196

Treprostinil sodium (Remodulin), 8, 242

Tretinoin (retinoic acid) [topical] (Retin-A, Avita, Renova), 5, 10, 242

Triamcinolone, 274t (Azmacort), 20, 242

and nystatin (Mycolog-II), 3, 243

Triamterene (Dyrenium), 7, 243

Triamterene and hydrochlorothiazide (Dyazide, Maxzide), 7, 136

Triapin (acetaminophen with butalbital w/wo caffeine), 18, 25

Triazolam (Halcion), 9, 243

Tricor (fenofibrate), 7, 116

Triethanolamine (Cerumenex), 11, 243

Triethylenetriphosphamide (Thio-Tepa, Tespa, TSPA), 4, 243

Trifluoperazine (Stelazine), 9, 244

Trifluridine (Viroptic), 13, 244

Trihexyphenidyl (Artane), 9, 244

Trilafon (perphenazine), 9, 197

Trileptal (oxcarbazepine), 8, 188

Trimethobenzamide (Tigan), 14, 244

Trimethoprim (Trimpex, Proloprim), 21, 244–245

Trimethoprim–sulfamethoxazole [co-trimoxazole] (Bactrim, Septra), 3, 245

Trimetrexate (Neutrexin), 4, 245

Trimpex (trimethoprim), 21, 244–245

Triptorelin (Trelstar Depot, Trelstar LA), 5, 245–246

Trospium chloride (Sanctura), 21, 246

Trovafloxacin (Trovan), 2, 246

Trovan (Trovafloxacin), 2, 246

Trusopt (dorzolamide), 12, 99

TSPA (triethylenetriphosphamide), 4, 243–244

Tums (calcium carbonate), 13, 58–59

Twinrix (hepatitis A [inactivated] and hepatitis B recombinant vaccine), 16, 134–135

Two-Dyne (acetaminophen with butalbital w/wo caffeine), 18, 25

Tylenol
(acetaminophen [APAP]), 19, 24–25
No. 1, 2, 3, 4 (acetaminophen with codeine), 18, 25

Tylox (oxycodone and acetaminophen), 19, 189–190

U

Ultracef, cefadroxil, 2, 63

Ultracet (tramadol/acetaminophen), 19, 241

Ultram (tramadol), 19, 241

Ultrase (pancrelipase), 191

Unasyn (ampicillin–sulbactam), 2, 40

Univasc (moexipril), 6, 173

Urecholine (bethanechol), 21, 53

Urex (methanimine), 21, 166

Urinary/genitourinary agents, classification of, 21

Urispas (flavoxate), 21, 119

Urocit-K (potassium citrate), 21, 202

Urokinase (Abbokinase), 15, 246–247

Uroxatral (alfuzosin), 21, 30

V

Vaccines/serums/toxoids, classification of, 16

Vaginal preparations, classification of, 18

Vagistat (tioconazole), 18, 237

Valacyclovir (Valtrex), 4, 247

Valcyte (valganciclovir), 4, 247

Valdecoxib (Bextra), 8, 17, 91

Valerian (*Valeriana officinalis*), 22, 261

Valganciclovir (Valcyte), 4, 247

Valium (diazepam), 8, 17, 91

Valproic acid (Depakene, Depakote), 8, 247–248, 266t

Valsartan (Diovan), 6, 248

Valtrex (valacyclovir), 4, 247

Vancenase (beclomethasone), 20, 51

Vancocin (vancomycin), 3, 248

Vancoled (vancomycin), 3, 248

Vancomycin (Vancocin, Vancoled), 3, 248, 265t

Vantin (cefpodoxime), 2, 67

Vaqta (hepatitis A vaccine), 16, 134

Vardenafil (Levitra), 21, 248

Varicella virus vaccine (Varivax), 16, 248–249

Varivax (varicella virus vaccine), 16, 248–249

Vascor (bepridil), 7, 52

Vasodilators, classification of, 8
Vasopressin [antidiuretic hormone, ADH] (Pitressin), 11, 15, 249
Vasotec (enalapril), 6, 103–104
Vecuronium (Norcuron), 17, 249
Veetids (penicillin v), 3, 194–195
Velban (vinblastine), 5, 250
Velbe (vinblastine), 5, 250
Velcade (bortezomib), 5, 55
Velosef, cephradine, 2, 70
Venlafaxine (Effexor), 8, 249
Venofer (iron sucrose), 10, 147
Ventolin (albuterol), 20, 28
VePesid (etoposide [VP-16]), 5, 115
Verapamil (Calan, Isoptin), 7, 250
Versed (midazolam), 9, 170
Vexol Opthalmic (rimexolone), 12, 213
VFEND (voriconazole), 3, 251
Viadur (leuprolide), 5, 18, 153
Viagra (sildenafil), 21, 218
Vibramycin (doxycycline), 3, 101
Vicodin (hydrocodone and acetaminophen), 19, 136–137
Vicoprofen (hydrocodone and ibuprofen), 19, 137
Videx (didanosine [ddI]), 3, 93
Vinblastine (Velban, Velbe), 5, 250
Vincasar PFS (vincristine), 5, 250–251
Vincristine (Oncovin, Vincasar PFS), 5, 250–251

Vinorelbine (Navelbine), 5, 251
Vioxx (rofecoxib), 19, 214
Viracept (nelfinavir), 4, 177
Viramune (nevirapine), 4, 179
Virazole (ribavirin), 4, 211
Viread (tenofovir), 4, 231
Viroptic (trifluridine), 13, 244
Visicol (sodium phosphate), 14, 221
Visken (pindolol), 6, 199–200
Vistaril (hydroxyzine), 1, 8, 9, 139
Vistide (cidofovir), 4, 74–75
Vitamin B_1 (thiamine), 10, 234
Vitamin B_6 (pyridoxine), 10, 208
Vitamin B_{12} (cyanocobalamin), 10, 83
Vitamin D_3 (cholecalciferol), 10, 74
Vitamin K [phytonadione] (AquaMEPHYTON), 10, 199
Vitrasert (ganciclovir), 4, 127–128
Vivelle (estradiol [transdermal]), 17, 111
Volmax (albuterol), 20, 28
Voltaren (diclofenac), 19, 92
Volume expanders, classification of, 15
Voriconazole (VFEND), 3, 251

W
Warfarin (Coumadin), 15, 251–252
Welchol (cholesevelam), 7, 82
Wellbutrin (bupropion), 8, 56–57